William Wales, J. Robertson

The Elements of Navigation

Vol. I

William Wales, J. Robertson

The Elements of Navigation
Vol. I

ISBN/EAN: 9783337078201

Printed in Europe, USA, Canada, Australia, Japan

Cover: Foto ©Andreas Hilbeck / pixelio.de

More available books at **www.hansebooks.com**

THE

ELEMENTS

OF

NAVIGATION.

VOLUME THE FIRST.

THE

ELEMENTS OF NAVIGATION;

CONTAINING THE

THEORY and PRACTICE.

With the neceſſary TABLES,

And COMPENDIUMS for finding

The LATITUDE and LONGITUDE at SEA.

To which is added,

A TREATISE OF MARINE FORTIFICATION.

Compoſed for the Uſe of

The ROYAL MATHEMATICAL School at CHRIST'S HOSPITAL,

The ROYAL ACADEMY at PORTSMOUTH,

And the GENTLEMEN of the NAVY.

IN TWO VOLUMES.

By J. ROBERTSON,

Late Librarian to the Royal Society, and formerly Head-Maſter of the Royal Academy, at Portſmouth.

The FIFTH EDITION, with ADDITIONS.

Carefully reviſed and corrected by

WILLIAM WALES,

Maſter of the Royal Mathematical School, Chriſt's Hoſpital, London.

LONDON,

Printed for C. NOURSE, in the STRAND,

MDCCLXXXVI.

TO

JOHN EARL OF

SANDWICH,

&c. &c. &c.

FIRST COMMISSIONER

OF THE

Boards of Admiralty and Longitude.

MY LORD,

WHILE the public voice is unanimous in applauding your humanity towards the Artificers, in general, of His Majesty's Dock-yards, and your attention to restore the Royal Navy of Britain to the respectable state from which it had been suffered to decline since the last War, Philosophers not only admire these noble acts, but likewise, your generous encouragement to improve Geographical, Nautical, and Natural Knowledge.

Such exertions of your Lordſhip's extraordinary Mental and Official Abilities, will undoubtedly be tranſmitted with honour to the lateſt poſterity: And your laudable example muſt inſpire a regard for Works intended to promote public utility.

The Author of *The Elements of Navigation*, notwithſtanding the favourable reception which the former impreſſions have met with from Britiſh Mariners, thinks himſelf extremely happy that this improved Edition is permitted to appear under your Lordſhip's Patronage.

That you may long enjoy the Opportunity as well as Inclination of promoting uſeful Arts and Learning, is a hope ſincerely entertained by,

My LORD,

Your LORDSHIP'S

moſt obedient

and humble Servant,

Nov. 1. 1772.

John Robertſon.

TO THE

RIGHT WORSHIPFUL

Sir ROBERT LADBROKE, Knt. Alderman,

PRESIDENT;

THE

Worſhipful THOMAS BURFOOT, Eſq.

TREASURER;

And the reſt of the

WORSHIPFUL GOVERNORS

OF

Chriſt's Hoſpital, London:

This Book, containing the Elements of Navigation, and a Treatiſe on Marine Fortification, firſt publiſhed for the Uſe of the Children in the Royal Mathematical School, when they were under my Care, is, as a grateful acknowledgement for paſt favours, addreſſed by

Your WORSHIPS' moſt humble Servant,

Nov. 1. 1772. John Robertſon.

ADVERTISEMENT.

IN this Edition, the Editor has carefully corrected the errors which had crept into the former; he has recomputed the Tables in Book V. Art. 308, 309, and 310, of the Sun's Longitude, Right Afcenfion, and Declination, and has alfo revifed, as far as his materials extended, the Geographical Table, and added the names of fuch places as his own obfervations, or thofe of other perfons, have furnifhed him with; fo that he flatters himfelf it is the moft extenfive and correct of any extant. On the whole, he prefumes, this Edition will be found as worthy of the approbation of the public in general, and of feamen in particular, as thofe which were printed under the Author's infpection.

THE

PREFACE.

IT having been part of my employment for many years past, to instruct youth in the theoretical and practical parts of Navigation; I was naturally led to draw up rules and examples fitted to the years and capacity of the scholar: some of the precepts, from time to time were altered, according as I had observed how they were comprehended by the majority of my pupils; until at length I had put together a set of materials, which I found sufficient for teaching this Art.

Upon my being intrusted by the governors of Christ's Hospital (in the beginning of the year 1748) with the care of the Royal Mathematical school there, founded by King Charles the second, I had a great opportunity of experiencing the method I had before used; and finding it fully answered my expectation, I determined to print it for the use of that school: but as those children are to be instructed in the mathematical sciences, on which the art of Navigation is founded, I judged it proper, on their account, to introduce the subjects of Arithmetic, Geometry, Trigonometry, &c. for which reason, this treatise is distinguished by the title of Elements of Navigation.

After my appointment (in the year 1755) to be head master of the Royal Marine Academy at Portsmouth, founded by King George the second, I also found that this book was sufficiently intelligible to beginners of middling capacities; and therefore, in the second edition, in the year 1764, the manner in which it was first composed was continued, except the removing of the book of Astronomy, from being the 8th. into the place of the 5th.; whereby the books of Plane Sailing, Globular Sailing, and Days Works, which together nearly comprehend the art of Navigation, follow in succession. There were indeed some variations in the modes of expression in a few places; but the additions in every [illegible] were [illegible] rather to extend the notions of learners, than to supply any deficiency existing in the former edition; except some of the additions in the 9th. book, which were not yet well known at the time of the first impression.

The work is divided into ten parts or books, each being a distinct treatise; the preceding ones contain the necessary elements which are wanted in those that follow. The demonstration of the several propositions are given as concisely as I could contrive, to carry with them a sufficient degree of evidence: Throughout the whole of the elementary parts, brevity and perspicuity were considered; but the practical parts are more fully treated on, and intended to include every useful particular, worthy of the mariner's notice.

In the elementary parts, where it is not easy to introduce new matter, there will be found the common principles treated in a manner, which, it is apprehended, is better adapted to beginners; and such new lights thrown on several particulars, as will render them more obvious than in the view wherein they have been commonly seen.

The treatise of Fortification annexed, is the result of many years application; and is delivered in a very different mode from what other writers have taken; for among the multitude which I have seen, they generally begin with the fortifying of a town, the most difficult part of the art, and end with works the most easy to contrive and execute: Herein the works of the simplest construction are begun with, and the learner gradually advanced to the fortifying of a town: Indeed the limits chosen for this tract have caused some articles to be briefly mentioned, and others to be totally omitted; nevertheless, it is conceived that, in its present state, it may be of considerable use to Marine Officers, and even furnish some hints not altogether unworthy the notice of the Gentlemen of the Army.

The Maritime parts of these Elements, contained in the vii[th], viii[th], *and* ix[th] *books, are also delivered in a manner somewhat different from what is seen in other writers; who, for the most part copying from one another, have not much contributed towards perfecting the art of Navigation; the writers indeed have been many, but the improvers have been very few;* Wright, Norwood, *and* Halley, *having done the most of what has been discovered since a little before the beginning of the 17th century: However, in the method here taken, it is apprehended that the proper judges will find some few improvements, as well in the art itself as in the manner of communicating it to learners.*

The common treatises of Navigation, which, on account of their small bulk and easy price, are vended among the British Mariners, seem not to be written with an intention to excite in their readers a desire

desire to pursue the Sciences, farther than they are handled *in those books; so that it is no wonder our seamen in general had so little mathematical knowledge; for the person who could keep a* trite *journal, formed on the most easy occurrences, has been reckoned a good artist; but whenever those occurrences have not happened, the journalist has been at a loss, and unable to find the ship's place with any tolerable degree of precision; and such accidents have probably contributed to the distress which many ships crews have experienced, and which a little more knowledge among them might have prevented, or at least have lessened.*

*About the middle of the 16th century, Navigation began to be considered as an art, in a great measure dependent on the Mathematical sciences; and on such a plan has it been cultivated by the labours of the most judicious, who have applied themselves towards its perfection; and although the art has been enriched by the observations of some learned men in different nations, yet it has so happened, that the chief of the improvements, and particularly the mathematical ones *, were first published in Britain.*

Into this work are collected most, if not all, of the useful and curious particulars relating to the art of Navigation; there are also interspersed historical remarks of inventions, with the names of many eminent men, and their works; these were intended as incentives to inspire learners and our seamen with a desire not only of knowing the things herein treated of from their foundations, but of pushing their inquiries into such other parts of the sciences as may procure to themselves pleasure, profit, and respect, and render them more useful to their country by the skill resulting from such acquisitions.

I have always thought that the chief motives which ought to induce a person to appear as a writer should be, either that he has something new to publish, or that he has arranged the parts of a known subject, in a method more regular and useful than had been done before; in either of these cases he cannot be a proper judge, unless he has seen the pieces extant on that subject, or at least, those of the most eminent authors already published: On these principles I was led to examine what had been done by the different writers on Navigation; and having perused most of their books, of which I

* See the following dissertation.

could get information, I had an opportunity of discovering the steps by which this art has risen to its present perfection, and consequently of knowing the most material parts of the history of its progress: Among other things, I could not avoid remarking a mistake which has crept into many of the modern books of Navigation; which is, that Wright's *invention of making a true sea-chart was stolen by* Mercator, *and published as his own. I suspect this story had its rise in a book printed in the year* 1675 *by* Edward Sherburne, *intitled* "*The Sphere of Marcus Manilius made an* English Poem, with Annotations and an Astronomical Appendix."

My enquiries into these matters induced the late learned Dr. James Wilson *to review and complete his observations on the same subject, and produced his Dissertation on the History of the Art of Navigation; which he was pleased to give me leave to publish with the second edition of this work.*

There are few persons, however knowing and careful, who may not commit, and overlook, inadvertencies in their own compositions, which may be discovered by others: therefore at my request the greatest part of the manuscript for the first edition was read and examined by two of my friends *, *well acquainted with the theory and practice of Navigation; who, by their judicious observations, enabled me to improve several articles: Some part of the additions to the 2d Edition, received much elegance and perspicuity through the friendly advice and communications of the late learned Dr.* Henry Pemberton, F. R. S.

The second Edition of these Elements having also been well received by the Public; Dr. Wilson *took the pains to revise his Dissertation, which he improved in many particulars: And I have also endeavoured to retain their favourable opinions of my labours, by giving Compendiums for performing the operations of the new methods of finding the latitude and longitude of a ship at sea; and some other alterations and additions which I conceived would render this third Edition more generally useful.*

Nov. 1, 1772.

---

* William Mountaine, Esq. F. R. S. and Mr. William Payne.

C O N T E N T S.

THIS treatiſe in two volumes contains ten books; each is divided into ſeveral ſections, and numbered with the Roman numerals.

The particular articles are numbered by the common figures, each book beginning with the number 1.

The references made from one article of the treatiſe to another is of two kinds.

Firſt. When in the ſame book. Then the number of the article referred to, is put in a parentheſis. Thus (27), refers to the article numbered 27 in the ſame book.

Second. When in another book. Then the number of the book in Roman figures, and of the article in common figures, is put in a parentheſis. Thus (II. 160) refers to the 160th article of the ſecond book.

In the following contents, the ſections refer to the number of the page: the particulars to the number of the article.

Vol. I. BOOK I. ARITHMETIC.

From Page 1 to Page 42.

Diviſion

BOOK II. GEOMETRY.

From Page 43 to Page 88.

BOOK III. PLANE TRIGONOMETRY.

From Page 89 to Page 124.

BOOK

CONTENTS.

BOOK IV. OF SPHERICS.

From Page 125 to Page 193.

BOOK V. ASTRONOMY.

From Page 195 to Page 328.

Fourteen

BOOK VI. GEOGRAPHY, &c.

From Page 329 to Page 400.

VOL. II. BOOK VII. OF PLANE SAILING.

From Page 1 to Page 130.

Propositions

CONTENTS.

BOOK VIII. OF GLOBULAR SAILING.

From Page 131 to Page 224.

BOOK IX.

BOOK IX. OF DAYS WORKS.

From Page 225 to Page 341.

Journal

CONTENTS.

FORTIFICATION.

PART I. OF LAND FORTIFICATIONS.

From Page 1 to Page 52.

PART II. OF MARINE FORTIFICATIONS.

From Page 52 to Page 76.

CONTENTS.

In this Treatise are XVI. Plates.

ERRATA.

VOLUME I.

P. 34, l. 7 and 8, from the bottom, and p. 98, l. 9, *for* Nepier, *read* Napier. ——P. 63, l. 28, 29, and 30, *for* BC, *r.* AC.——P. 71, l. 4, *for* $\frac{D}{C}$, *r.* $\frac{C}{D}$.——P. 77, l. 22, *for* (art.) 145, *r.* 146.——P. 129, l. 22, *for* (art.) 213, *r.* 212. ——P. 132, l. 9, *for* ABS, *r.* ABL; l. 28, *for* AF, *r.* FR, and *for* AR, *r.* FR; l. 29, *for* AR, *r.* FR; and l. 31, *for* ABE, *r.* BAE.——P. 138, l. 19, *for* Ap, *r.* AC.——P. 223, l. 4, *for* VIII *q* IX, *r.* VIII *q* IV.——P. 225, l. 40, *for* ♎ ☉, *r.* ♈ ☉.——P. 337, l. 30, p. 388, l. 37, and p. 389, l. 27, *for* Manilla, *r.* Manila.——P. 35[illegible], in the title, *for* Geograpay, *r.* Geography.——P. 395, catch-word, *for* Siera, *r.* Siara.

VOLUME II.

P. 144, l. 2, 10, 26, 41, 42, and 44, *for* Napeir, *r.* Napier.——P. 301, l. 4 and 5, *for* Regulus, *r.* Spica Virginis.——P. 307, l. 6, *for* enlightened limb, *r.* center.——P. 351, l. 9 and 16, *for* IV., *r.* VI.

A

DISSERTATION

ON THE

RISE AND PROGRESS

OF THE

Modern ART OF NAVIGATION.

IT has been much diſputed to whom the world was obliged for the mariner's compaſs. A late *Italian* writer indeed contends, after many *, that the honour of the invention is due to *Flavio Gioja* of *Amalfi* in *Campania*, who lived about the beginning of the 14th century †, though others ſay it came from the Eaſt, and was earlier known in *Europe* ‡. However that may be, it is certain, this wonderful diſcovery gave riſe to the preſent art of navigation; which ſeems to have made ſome progreſs during the voyages, that were begun in the year 1420, by *Henry* Duke of *Viſeo* ‖. This learned Prince, brother to *Edward* King of *Portugal*, was particularly knowing in coſmography, and ſent for one maſter *James* from the iſland of *Majorca*, to teach navigation, and make inſtruments and charts for the ſea §.

Theſe voyages being greatly extended, the art was improved under the ſucceeding monarchs of that nation. For *Roderic* and *Joſeph*, phyſicians to King *John* the Second, together with one *Martin de Bohemia*, a *Portugueſe* native of the iſland of *Fayal*, ſcholar to *Regiomontanus*, about the year 1485, calculated tables of the Sun's declination, for the uſe of the ſailors, and recommended the aſtrolabe for taking obſervations at ſea ¶.

The famous *Chriſtopher Columbus* is ſaid, before he attempted the diſcovery of *America*, to have conſulted *Martin de Bohemia*, with others, and during the courſe of his voyage to have inſtructed the *Spaniards* in

---

* Suitable to that verſe of *Pannormitana*,

Prima dedit nautis uſum magneti Amalphis.

† See Signor *Gregorio Grimaldi*'s Diſſertation on this ſubject in the *Memoirs* of the *Etruſcan* Academy of *Cortona*, tom. iii. p. 193, printed at *Rome* in 1742.

‡ *Hiſtoire des Mathematiques, par M. Montucla, à Paris*, 1758.

‖ *Marianæ* Hiſt. *Hiſpan.* lib. xx. cap. 11. and lib. xxvi. cap. 17. *Moguntiæ*, 1605.

§ Decados d'Aſia par J. di Burnos, lib. xvi. 1552.

¶ *Maffeii* Hiſtor. *Indic.* lib. i. p. 6. printed at *Florence* in 1588.

navigation *; for the improvement of which art, the Emperor *Charles* the Fifth afterwards founded a lecture at *Seville* †.

The variation of the sea-compass could not be long a secret. *Columbus*, on the 14th of September 1492, observed it, as his son *Ferdinand* asserts ‡, though others seem to attribute that discovery to *Sebastian Cabot* ||. And as this variation differs in different places, *Gonzales d' Oviedi* found there was none at the *Azores* §; where some geographers have thought fit in their maps to make their first meridian to pass through one of those islands; it not being then known, that the variation altered in time.

The use of the *Cross-Staff* now began to be introduced amongst the Sailors. This very ancient instrument being described by *John Werner* of *Nuremberg*, in his *Annotations* on the first book of *Ptolemy's Geography*, printed in 1514; he recommends it for observing the distance between the Moon and some star, in order thence to determine the longitude. *Werner* seems to have been the greatest geometer, as well as astronomer, of the time. In 1522, he published a tract ¶, containing a specimen of the conics, with some solid problems, and also he there determined the precession of the equinox more exactly than it had been done.

But the art of navigation still remained very imperfect, from the constant use of the plane-chart, the gross errors of which must have often misled the mariner, especially in voyages far distant from the equator. Its precepts were probably at first only set down on the earliest sea-charts, as that custom is continued to this day; and larger directions have been usually premised by the *Dutch*, to collections of their charts called *Wagoner*'s, from the name of the publisher: The *Dutch* call these collections also by many other affected titles, such as *Fiery-Columns*, *Sea-Beacons*, *Mirrors*, *Atlasses*, &c.

At length there were published in *Spanish* two treatises, containing a system of the art, which were in great vogue; the first by *Pedro de Medina* at *Valladolid*, 1545, called *Arte de Nauegar*; the other at *Seville*, in 1556, by *Martin Cortes*, with this title, *Breve Compendio de la Sphera, y de la Arte de Nauegar con nueuos Instrumentos y Reglas.* The author of this last tract says, he composed it at *Cadiz* in 1545.

These seem to have been the oldest writers, who had fully handled this subject; for *Medina*, in his dedication to *Philip* Prince of *Spain*,

* La Historia general y natural de las Indias par Gonzalles de Miedo, en Sevilla, 1535. And Descriptione de las Indias Occidentale, de Antonio de Herrera, en Madrid, 1601.

† *Hackluyt*, in the dedication of his first volume of Voyages, printed in 1599.

‡ In *Columbus*'s life written in *Spanish*, which is very scarce, but it was printed in *Italian* at *Venice* in 1571.

|| See *Livio Sanuto*'s *Geographia*, at the same place in 1585. Dr. *William Gilbert*, *de Magnete*. *London*, 1600; and *Purchas*'s *Pilgrim*, in 1625, vol. I.

§ *Cabot*, a *Venetian* by birth, first served our King *Henry* the seventh, then the King of *Spain*, and lastly, returning to *England*, he was constituted grand pilot by King *Edward* the sixth, with an annual salary of above 160 pounds. Of this famous navigator and his expeditions, many writers have made mention, both foreigners and *English*, as *Peter Martyr*, *Ramuseo*, *Herrera*, *Holinshed*. Lord *Bacon*, and particularly *Hackluyt* and *Purchas*, in their Collections of Voyages.

¶ *Opera Mathematica* at *Nuremberg*, in quarto.

laments,

laments, that multitudes of ſhips daily periſhed at ſea, becauſe there were neither teachers of the art, nor books by which it might be learnt; and *Cortes*, in his dedication, boaſts to the Emperor, that he was the firſt who had reduced navigation into a *compendium*, enlarging much on what he had performed *.

Medina gave ridiculous directions, how to gueſs at the place of the horizon, when it could not be ſeen; as alſo he defended the errors of the plane-chart, and advanced againſt the variation of the magnetic needle ſuch abſurd arguments, as *Ariſtotle* and his followers had done to prove the impoſſibility of the Earth's motion. But *Cortes* briefly and clearly made out the errors of the plane-chart, and ſeemed to reflect on what had been ſaid againſt the variation of the compaſs, when he adviſed the mariner rather to be guided by experience, than to mind ſubtle reaſonings. Beſides he endeavoured to account for this variation, in imagining the needle to be influenced by a magnetic pole (which he called the point attractive) different from that of the world, and this notion has been farther proſecuted by others.

However, *Medina*'s book, being perhaps the firſt of its kind, was ſoon tranſlated into *Italian*, *French*, and *Flemiſh* †, ſerving for a long time as a guide to navigators of foreign countries.

But *Cortes* was our favourite author, a tranſlation of whoſe work by Mr. *Richard Eden* was, on the recommendation of that great navigator Mr. *Stephen Borrough*, and the encouragement of the Society for making diſcoveries at ſea, publiſhed at *London* in 1561: which underwent various impreſſions ‡, whilſt that of *Medina*, though tranſlated within twenty years after the other, ſeems to have been neglected, notwithſtanding the encomiums beſtowed on it by Mr. *John Frampton*, the tranſlator.

A ſyſtem of navigation at that time conſiſted of ſome ſuch particulars as theſe: An account of the *Ptolemaic* hypotheſis, and the circles of the ſphere; of the roundneſs of the Earth, its longitudes, latitudes, climates, and eclipſes of the luminaries; a kalendar; how to find the prime, epact, &c. and by the laſt the Moon's age, and thence the tides; a deſcription of the ſea-compaſs, not forgetting the loadſtone, with ſomething about the variation, called its north-eaſting and north-weſting, for the diſcovering of which, by night as well as by day, *Cortes* ſaid, an inſtrument might be eaſily contrived; tables of the Sun's declination for four years §,

---

* The learned Don *Nicolo Antonio*, in his *Bibliotheca Hiſpanica*, printed at *Rome* in 16[illegible]2, tom. i. p. 323. puts down a book, intitled, *Tradado de la Sphera y del marear con el regimento de las alturas*, written by *Franciſco Falero*, a *Portugueze*, and printed at *Seville* in 1535; but perhaps there is a miſtake in the date. He alſo mentions an edition of *Cortes* in 1551.

† The *Italian* and *French* tranſlations were printed in 1554, the firſt at *Venice*, the other at *Lions*; the *Flemiſh* edition, I have ſeen, was at *Antwerp* in 1580; perhaps it had been printed before.

‡ In the latter editions ſome miſtakes in the tranſlation are corrected.

§ *Cortes* ſets down the places of the Sun for a twelvemonth, with an equation-table to correct thoſe places, ſerving for many years to come; and alſo another table to find the Sun's declination from his longitude being given.

in order to find the latitude, from his meridian altitude; to do the same thing by those called the guard-stars in the north, and the crosiers in the south; of the course of the Sun and Moon; the length of the days; of time and its divisions; to find the hour of the day, and by the nocturnal that of the night; and lastly, a description of the sea-chart, on which to discover where the ship is, they made use of a small table, that shewed, upon an alteration of one degree in the latitude, how many leagues were run on each rhumb, together with the departure from the meridian. Besides some instruments were described, especially by *Cortes*; as one to find the place and declination of the sun, with the days and place of the Moon; certain dials, the astrolabe and cross-staff, with a complex machine to discover the hour and latitude at once.

And after this manner the art continued to be treated, though from time to time improvements were made by the following authors.

As *Werner* had proposed to find the longitude by observations on the Moon; so *Gemma Frisius*, in a tract intitled *De Principiis Astronomiæ et Cosmographiæ*, printed at *Antwerp* in 1530, advised the keeping of the time by means of small clocks or watches for the same purpose, then, as he says, lately invented. He also contrived a new sort of cross-staff, which he describes in his treatise *De Radio Astronomico et Geometrico*, printed at the same place 1545, and in his additions to *Peter Apian*'s Cosmography, gives the figure of an instrument, he calls a *Nautical Quadrant*, as very useful in navigation, promising to write largely on the subject; accordingly, in an edition he made *anno* 1553, of his above-mentioned book *De Principiis Astronomiæ*, &c. he delivers several *nautical axioms*, as he calls them, which with some alterations were repeated by his son *Cornelius Gemma*, in a posthumous piece of his father on the *Universal Astrolabe*, published in 1556. *Gemma Frisus* died in 1555, aged 45 years.

With us Dr. *William Cunningham*, in his *Cosmographical Glass*, printed in 1559, amongst other things briefly treats of navigation, especially shewing the use of the *Nautical Quadrant*, much praising that instrument.

But a greater genius than these undertook this subject; for the famous mathematician *Pedro Nunez*, or *Nonius*, having so early as 1537 published a book, written in the *Portuguese* language, to explain a difficulty in navigation proposed to him by the commander Don *Martin Alphonso de Susa*; which was thirty years after printed at *Basil*, in *Latin*, with the addition of a second book, the whole intitled *de Arte et Ratione Navigandi*; where he exposes, both truly and learnedly, the errors of the plane-chart; and besides gives the solution of several curious Astronomical Problems, amongst which is that of determining the latitude from two observations of the Sun's altitude and the intermediate azimuth being given. He also delivers many useful advices about the art of navigation, particularly how to perform its operations on the globe. He observed, that though the oblique rhumbs are spiral lines, yet the direct course of a ship will always be the arch of some great circle, whereby the angle with the meridians will continually change; all that the steersman can here do for the preserving of the original rhumb is to correct these deviations, as soon as they appear sensible. But thus the ship will in reality describe a course without the rhumb-line intended; and therefore his calculations for assigning the latitude, where any rhumb-line crosses the several meridians,

ridians, will be in ſome meaſure erroneous. He alſo again ſets down his method of diviſion of a quadrant by concentric circles *, which he had deſcribed in his ingenious treatiſe *de Crepuſculis*, printed in 1542, imagining it had been practiſed by *Ptolemy*. There were alſo added other tracts of his, but the completeſt edition of his *Latin* works was made by himſelf at *Coimbra* in 1573. His treatiſe of *Algebra*, written in *Spaniſh*, was printed at *Antwerp* ſix years before.

In 1577 Mr. *William Bourne* publiſhed his treatiſe †, intitled, *A Regiment for the Sea*, which he deſigned as a ſupplement to *Cortes*, whom he frequently quotes. Beſides many things common with others, *Bourne* gives a table of the places and declinations of thirty-two principal ſtars, in order to find the latitude and hour; as alſo a larger tide-table than that publiſhed by Mr. *Leonard Digges*, in 1556 ‡. He ſhews, by conſidering the irregularities in the Moon's motion, the errors of the ſailors in finding her age by the epact; and alſo in their determining the hour from obſerving upon what point of the compaſs the Sun and Moon appeared. He adviſes in ſailing towards high latitudes to keep the reckoning by the globe, as there the plane-chart errs moſt. He deſpairs of our ever being able to find the longitude by any inſtrument, unleſs the variation of the compaſs ſhould be cauſed by ſome ſuch attractive point, as *Cortes* had imagined. Though of this he doubts, and as he had ſhewn how to find the variation of the compaſs at all times, he adviſes to keep an account of the obſervations, as uſeful to diſcover thereby the place of a ſhip; which advice the famous *Simon Stevin* proſecuted at large in a treatiſe publiſhed at *Leyden* in 1599, intitled *Portuum inveſtigandorum Ratio Metaphraſto Hugone Grotio*; the ſubſtance of which was the ſame year printed at *London* in *Engliſh*, by Mr. *Edward Wright*, intitled *The Haven-finding Art*.

But the moſt remarkable thing in this ancient tract is, the deſcribing of the way by which our ſailors eſtimated the rate a ſhip made in her courſe, by an inſtrument called the *log*. This was ſo named from the piece of wood, or log, that floats in the water, while the time is reckoned during which the line that is faſtened to it is veering out. The author of this device is not known, and I find no farther mention of it till 1607, in an *Eaſt-India* voyage, publiſhed by *Purchas*; but from that time its name occurs in other voyages, that are amongſt his collections. And henceforward it became famous, being taken notice of, both by our own authors, and by foreigners; as by *Gunter* in 1623, *Snellius* in 1624, *Metius* in 1631, *Oughtred* in 1633, *Herigone* in 1634, *Saltonſtall* in 1636, *Norwood* in 1637, *Fournier* in 1643; and indeed by almoſt all the ſucceeding writers on navigation, of every country. And it continues to be ſtill in uſe as at firſt, though attempts have been often made to im-

* The admirable diviſion, now ſo much in uſe, is a very great improvement of this; ſo that when the famous Dr. *Edmund Halley*, the Royal Aſtronomer, received that by adapting it to his *Mural Arch*, ſome body here named it *A Nonius*, in which he has been followed by many.

† He had ten years before publiſhed what he calls *Rules of Navigation*, as appears from his *Almanac*, printed in 1571.

‡ In his treatiſe, intitled, *A Prognoſtication everlaſting*, fol. 23.

prove it, and other contrivances proposed to supply its place. Many of these have succeeded in quiet water, but proved useless in a troubled sea.

A following edition of this book was revised by the author, where, in the preface, he sets forth the gross ignorance of the old ship-masters, repeating some of the insipid jests they made use of to justify their want of knowledge in their art. Amongst the additions, he enlarges on the account of the log-line. And at the end subjoins an *Hydrographical Discourse touching the five several Passages into Cathay.*

Bourne published other tracts, as one called *Inventions* or *Devises*, where he describes a method by *wheel-work* of measuring the velocity of a ship at Sea, which artifice he attributes to one Mr. *Humfrey Cole.*

At *Antwerp*, in 1581, *Michael Coignet*, a native of the place, published a small treatise, intitled, *Instruction nouvelle des Points plus excellents & necessaires touchant l'Art de Naviger* *. This served as a supplement to *Medina*, whose mistakes *Coignet* well exposed. He there shewed, that as the rhumbs are spirals, making endless revolutions about the poles, numerous errors must arise from their being represented by straight lines on the sea-charts; and expressed his hopes of discovering a rule to remedy those errors; saying, that most of the speculations, delivered by the great mathematician, *Peter Nonius*, for that purpose, were scarce practicable; and therefore in a manner useless to sailors. In treating of the Sun's declination, he took notice of the gradual decrease in the obliquity of the ecliptic, a point long disputed, but now settled from the theory of attraction. He also described the cross-staff with three transverse pieces, as it is at present made, which he acknowledged to be then in common use amongst the mariners; but he preferred that of *Gemma Frisius.* He likewise gave some instruments of his own invention, which are now quite laid aside, except perhaps his nocturnal. As the old sea-table, mentioned above, erred more and more in advancing towards the poles; he set down another to be used by such as sailed beyond the 60th degree of latitude. At the end of the book is delivered a method of sailing on a parallel of latitude by means of a ring dial, and a 24 hour glass; on which the author very much values himself.

The same year Mr. *Robert Norman* † published a discovery, he had long before made, of the dipping of the magnetic needle, in a small pamphlet called *The Newe Attractive*, where he shews how to determine its quantity; and in speaking of the loadstone, he disputes against *Cortes*'s notion, that the variation of the compass was caused by a point fixed in the heavens, contending that it should be sought for in the earth, and proposes how to discover its place. He also treats of the various sorts of compasses, setting forth at large the dangers that must arise from the then prevailing practice of not fixing, on account of the variation, the wire directly under the *flower-de-luce*; as compasses made in different

---

* It had been published in *Flemish*, but the *French* edition is the fullest. *Coignet* died in 1623, leaving many mathematical manuscripts, see *Valerii Andreæ Bibliotheca Belgica*, printed at *Louvain* in 1643.

† He is commended for an excellent Artist by our authors, as *Bourne*, *Burrough*, Sir *Humfrey Gilbert*, *Hues*, *Potter*, *Blundeville*, *Wright*, and Dr. *Gilbert.*

countries have it placed differently. *Bourne* indeed had warned againſt this abuſe, and there are many things common to both authors.

To *Norman*'s piece is always ſubjoined, Mr. *William Burrough's Diſcourſe of the Variation of the Cumpaſs or Magneticall Needle.* The author had been a famous navigator, having uſed the ſea from fifteen years of age, and for his merit promoted to be Controller of the navy by Queen *Elizabeth* *. He ſhews how to determine the variation ſeveral ways, ſetting down many obſervations of it made by an azimuth-compaſs of *Norman*'s invention, but improved by himſelf. He demonſtrates the falſhood of the rules commonly uſed, to find the latitude by the guard-ſtars. He particularizes many errors in the then ſea-charts, occaſioned by the neglect of the variation; adding, *But of theſe coaſtes* (towards the north), *and of the inwarde partes of the countries of* Ruſſia, Muſcovia, &c. *I have made a perfect plat and deſcription, by myne owne experience in ſundrie voiages and travailes, bothe by ſea and lande to and fro in theſe partes, which I gave to her Majeſtie in* anno 1578. And laſtly, he juſtly finds fault with *Coignet*'s inſtrument, called a *nautical hemiſphere*; but ſpeaks too ſeverely againſt the writers of navigation, concluding thus,

But as I haue alreadie ſufficientlie declared, the cumpas ſheweth not alwaies the pole of the worlde, but varieth from the ſame diverſly, and in ſayling deſcribeth circles accordyngly. Whiche thing, if Petrus Nonius, *and the reſt that haue written of Navigation, had jointlie conſidered in the tranſlation of their rules and Inſtruments, then might they haue been more auaileable to the uſe of Navigation; but they perceivyng the difficultie of the thyng, and that if they had dealt therewith, it would have utterly overwhelmed their former plauſible conceits, with* Pedro de Medina *(who, as it appeareth, hauyng ſome ſmall ſuſpicion of the matter, reaſoneth very clerkly, that it is not neceſſary that ſuch an abſurdity as the Variation, ſhould be admitted in ſuch an excellent art as Navigation is) they haue all thought beſt to paſſe it over with ſilence.*

The *Spaniards* too continued to publiſh treatiſes of the art; particularly at *Seville* was printed in 1585 an excellent *Compendium* by *Roderico Zamorano*; which is written clearly and with brevity, not being incumbered with ſuch idle ſpeculations as abound in *Medina* and *Cortes*. The author was Royal Lecturer at *Seville*, and contributed much to the reforming the ſea charts; as we are told by his ſucceſſor, *Andres Garcia de Ceſpedes*, who alſo publiſhed a treatiſe of navigation at *Madrid*, in 1606.

As globes may be very ſerviceable for the mariner, Mr. *Edward Mullineux* ſet forth in 1592, at the charges of Mr. *William Sanderſon* merchant †, a pair much larger than thoſe the famous geographer *Gerard Mercator* publiſhed in 1541. On the terreſtrial one were deſcribed many new diſcovered countries, and traced out the reſpective voyages round the world by Sir *Francis Drake* in 1577, and Mr. *Thomas Candiſh* in 1586, with the progreſs Sir *Martin Frobiſher* had made towards the north in 1576, to a place called his *Straits*.

---

* *Hackluyt*'s Voyages, vol. i. p. 417, printed in 1599.

† Mr. *Sanderſon* was commended for his knowledge as well as generoſity to ingenious men.

These globes were accompanied with a tract containing their uſes written in *Engliſh*; but in 1594 Mr. *Robert Hues* publiſhed a more elaborate one in *Latin*; wherein, amongſt others, he ſolves by the globe the problem of determining the latitude from two heights of the Sun obſerved with the intermediate time being given *; and in the laſt part of his book, he performs the uſual queſtions in navigation, premiſing a diſcourſe on the rhumb-lines, where he attempts to refute what *Gemma Friſius* had aſſerted, who ſays, that they meet in the poles. At the concluſion he highly praiſes a treatiſe of Mr. *Thomas Hariot*, hoping it would be ſoon publiſhed, in which that author had treated of this ſubject upon geometrical principles, with great ſagacity and judgment. But all the manuſcripts of that great mathematician were loſt, except his *Artis Analyticæ Praxis*, which was publiſhed long after his death in 1631; wherein is firſt advanced that idea of algebraic equations, which has been ever ſince followed.

Hues † was a perſon of letters, and beſides had been far at ſea. Amongſt other curious particulars, he gives a good account of the attempts that had been made at various times to meaſure the Earth. In the *Epiſtle* to Sir *Walter Rawley* he takes an occaſion to enumerate the many diſcoveries of our mariners in very different parts of the world. His book was received with great applauſe, and has been indeed a pattern for ſuch as afterwards handled the ſame ſubject. It has been often printed abroad, particularly in 1617 with the notes of *John Iſaac Pontanus*, who omitted the *Epiſtle* and the mentioning of *Hariot*. However from this mutilated edition it was tranſlated into *Engliſh* by one Mr. *John Chilmead*, and publiſhed in 1639.

Amongſt our ſailors none were more famous than Captain *John Davis* ‡, who gave name to the ſtraits which he diſcovered; and great matters were expected from his long experience and ſkill. In 1594 he publiſhed a ſmall treatiſe, intitled, *The Seaman's Secrets*. This is written with brevity, though ſomewhat pedantically, and was eſteemed in its time, an eighth edition being printed in 1657; ſo that it ſeems to have ſupplanted *Cortes*. *Davis* treats of plane ſailing, calling it *horizontal*, and ſets down the form of keeping a reckoning at Sea. He likewiſe ſhews how to ſail by the globe, and boaſts of what he intended to do; much commending great circle ſailing, without deſcribing it, as alſo

---

* This problem has been diſcuſſed by Dr. *Henry Pemberton*, in the Philoſophical Tranſactions, vol. li. part. 2d. 1760, p. 910, where he has alſo given ſome improvements in trigonometry.

† There is an account of *Hues* and *Hariot* in *Anthony Wood's Athen. Oxon.* vol. i. printed in 1721, as being both members of that Univerſity.

‡ Several of his voyages are in *Hackluyt's* and *Purchas's* collections. He and Captain *Abraham Kendal* are greatly praiſed by Sir *Robert Dudley*, in his *Arcano del Mare*, as keeping a perfect reckoning by the way of longitude and latitude, where are given two of their *Journals*. This *Dudley* was a natural ſon of the great Earl of *Leiceſter*, and had commanded, in 159[illegible], a fleet againſt the *Spaniards*; but retiring to *Florence*, he aſſumed the titles of Duke of *Northumberland* and Earl of *Warwick*. His *Arcano* was printed at that place in two volumes in 1646 and 1647.

what

what he calls *paradoxal*; that is, by a projection on the plane of the equator with spiral rhumbs, saying, he will publish a chart for that purpose. But above all, he extols the use of calculations in the cases of navigation, and promises to handle that subject.

At the end of the book is given the figure of a staff of his contrivance, to make a back observation. Of this the author is so vain as to say, *Than which instrument (in my opinion) the seaman shall not finde any so good, and in all clymates of so great certaintie, the invention and demonstration whereof, I may boldly challenge to appertain unto my selfe (as a portion of the talent which God hath bestowed upon me) I hope without abuse or offence to any.*

This instrument seems to have for some time been in use; for *Adrian Metius*, in his treatise, intitled *Astronomiæ Institutio*, printed in 1605, gives a figure of it from an original, in the possession of M. *Frederic Hautman*, governor of *Amboyna*. But it soon yielded to one of a more commodious form, which is now commonly called *Davis's Quadrant* *; as if it was also of his invention, and that perhaps only because a back observation is made by both instruments, so the quadrant itself was at first styled a *Staff* and *Back-Staff*.

The famous traveller Signor *Pietro della Valle* passing, in 1623, from *Ormus* to *Surat* aboard an *English* vessel, where observing this quadrant much practised by the seamen, as it was quite new to him, takes an occasion to shew its use very distinctly, and says, they told him, that it had been lately invented and called *David's Staff* † from its author. Also Captain *Charles Saltonstall*, in his *Navigation*, describes it under the name of a *Back-Staff*; and in Captain *Thomas James's* famous voyage for discovering a north-west passage, begun in 1631, amongst the many instruments, he carried along with him, are mentioned two of Mr. *Davis's Back-staves*, which were doubtless these quadrants.

Contemporary with *Davis* was Mr. *Richard Polter*, who, it is said, had been a principal master aboard the *Royal Navy*. He wrote a very small book intitled *The Pathway to Perfect Sailing*, where, from an observation he made in 1586, he would infer ‡, that different loadstones communicated different degrees of variation to the magnetic needle, and therefore despises the publishing observations of that kind, as needless. His book was not printed till 1644, nor did it deserve to be published at all, as it abounds with mistakes, and is written fantastically, obscurely and arrogantly.

But all this while the plane-chart, notwithstanding its errors were frequently complained of, continued to be followed; as its use is easy, and serves tolerably well in short voyages, especially near the equator.

---

* It is called by the *French Quartier Anglois*.

† *David Staff, che in lingua Inglese vale à dir legno di David Viaggi*; *Part* 3. *Letter* 1. *à Roma*. This author not only praises the Captain *Nicholas Woodcock*, and other officers, but also the common sailors, for their care and skill; and says, the *Portuguese* lose great number of ships for not being so exact in their observations as the *English*.

‡ Whereas he should have thence concluded the variation altered, as was discovered afterwards.

However,

However, a way to remedy these errors had, for some time, been inquired after. And *Gerrard Mercator* seems to be the first, who conceived the means of effecting this, in a manner convenient for seamen, by continuing to represent both the meridians and parallels of latitude by parallel straight lines, as in the plane-chart, but gradually augmenting the distances between the degrees of latitude in advancing from the equator towards either pole, that the rhumbs also might be extended into straight lines, so that a straight line drawn between any two places, laid down in this chart by their longitudes and latitudes, should make an angle with the meridians, expressing the rhumb leading from one to the other. But though *Mercator*, in 1569, set forth an universal map thus constructed *, it does not appear upon what principles he proceeded; probably, by observing in a globe furnished with rhumbs, what meridians the rhumbs passed at each degree of latitude. That he knew not the genuine principles, I shall make evident; our countryman, Mr. *Edward Wright*, was certainly the first who discovered them.

Wright insinuates, but without sufficient grounds, that this enlargement of the intervals between the parallels had been suggested before by *Cortes* †, and even by *Ptolemy* himself.

As to *Cortes*, he speaks of the number of the degrees of latitude, and not the extent of them; for his expression amounts to no more than this, that the degrees of latitude are to be numbered from the equator, and consequently both northwards and southwards from that line the numbers affixed to them must continually increase; and from any place having latitude (suppose Cape *St. Vincent* in *Spain*, which is his instance) the degrees of latitude will be denoted by numbers increasing towards the pole, and decreasing towards the equator. He had before expressly directed, that they should be all equal by measurement on a scale of leagues adapted to the map ‡.

The passage in *Ptolemy* ||, referred to by *Wright* §, does indeed relate to the proportion between the distances of the parallels and meridians, but contains no shadow of *Mercator*'s scheme: for instead of proposing any gradual enlargement of the distances of the parallels in a general chart; that passage relates only to particular maps, and is more distinctly explained in the first chapter of his last book; where he advises explicitly not to confine a system of such maps to one and the same scale, but to plan them out by a different measure, as occasion shall require, with this only caution; that the degrees of longitude should in each bear in some measure that proportion to the degrees of latitude, which the magnitude of the respective parallels bear to a great circle of the sphere; and subjoins, that in particular maps, if this proportion be observed in regard to the

---

* See his life, written by his intimate friend, *Gaulterus Ghymmius*, which was prefixed to an enlarged edition of his *Atlas*, published at *Duisbourg*, in 1595, by *Rameldus* his son, a year after his father's death. *Gerrard Mercator* was born in 1512.

† See the 2d chapter of *Wright*'s book.

‡ *Part* 3d. cap. 2d. fol. 58.

|| *Geograph.* lib. ii. cap. 1.

§ In an advertisement set down on his universal map, at the end of his second edition of his book; and in this mistake he has been followed by others.

middle

middle parallel, the inconvenience will not be great, though the meridians ſhould be ſtraight parallels to each other; wherein his deſign is plainly no other, than that the maps ſhould in ſome ſort repreſent the figures of the countries they are drawn for. *Mercator*, who drew maps for *Ptolemy*'s tables *, underſtood him in no other ſenſe, thinking it an improvement not to regulate the meridians by one parallel, but by two; one diſtant from the northern, and the other from the ſouthern extremity of the map by a fourth part of the whole depth; whereby in his maps, though the meridians are ſtraight lines, they are generally drawn inclining to each other towards the pole.

But *Mercator*'s univerſal map, mentioned above, though the author deſigned it for the benefit of ſailors, was ſo far from being readily adopted, that ſome of the moſt ſkilful amongſt them objected to its uſefulneſs. Thus Mr. *Burrough* ſays of it — *By augmenting his degrees of latitude towards the poles, the ſame is more fitte for ſuche to beholde, as ſtudie in coſmographie, by readyng authours upon the lande, then to bee uſed in Navigation at the ſea.*

And Mr. *Thomas Blundeville*, in his *Briefe Deſcription of Univerſal Mappes and Cardes*, firſt printed in 1589, gives an account of this map, obſerving that *Barnardus Puteanus* of *Bruges* had publiſhed, in 1579, one altogether like it. And though *Blundeville* is ſo particular, as to ſet down numbers expreſſing the diſtances between each parallel of latitude in thoſe maps, yet he ſeems to ſlight them, by ſaying, that no better rules than thoſe given by *Ptolemy* can be deviſed. But what is delivered by this *geographer* about the conſtruction of a general map, is a very indifferent performance, altogether unworthy the author of the *Almageſt*, and not in the leaſt correſponding with the ſagacity ſhewn in two treatiſes on the *Planiſphere* and *Analemma*, which the *Arabians* have handed down to us as *Ptolemy*'s †.

Maginus alſo, at the end of his *Geographia Univerſa*, (the former part of which is a tranſlation of *Ptolemy*'s) firſt printed at *Venice*, in 1596, mentions this map of *Mercator*, and gives even a ſketch of it; but ſeems to have no diſtinct conception of the author's deſign.

That *Mercator*'s map was not rightly deſcribed, is manifeſt from the numbers given by *Blundeville*; and that he was ignorant of a genuine method of dividing the meridian, appears from a paſſage in his life, where the writer ſays *Mercator* often aſſured him, that this extending a ſphere into a plane anſwered to the quadrature of the circle, as that nothing ſeemed to be wanting but the demonſtration.

However, our authors now began to entertain favourable thoughts of it, perhaps from the report that Mr. *Wright* was about to treat on that ſubject. Dr. *Thomas Hood*, to the firſt edition which he gave of *Bourne*'s *Regiment* in 1592, added a *Dialogue* of his own, called *The Mariner's Guide*, written only to ſhew the uſe of the plane chart, where he acknowledges and ſets forth its errors, and highly praiſes *Mercator*'s, ſaying, he

---

* In an edition he made of *Ptolemy*'s *Geography*, in 1584.

† Theſe were publiſhed by *Fed. Commandinus*, one at *Venice*, in 1518, the other at *Rome*, in 1562.

had

had composed a treatise concerning it; but the indistinct account he gives of it, shews it would not be this author's lot to render it fit for the use of navigation. And Mr. *Blundeville*, in the following editions of his above-mentioned tract, omitted the commendation he had given of *Ptolemy*'s method of delineating an *universal map*.

Mercator's scheme was not indeed contrived for representing the parts of a country in a just proportion to each other; but is appropriated to the use of mariners, who sail upon rhumbs by the guidance of the compass; which our countryman, Mr. *Edward Wright*, perfected *, by discovering a true way of dividing the meridian. An account of this he sent from *Caius* college, in *Cambridge*, where he was then a fellow, to his friend the above-mentioned Mr. *Blundeville*, containing a short table for that purpose, with a specimen of a chart so divided, together with the manner of dividing it. All which *Blundeville* published, in 1594, amongst his *Exercises*, in that part which treats of navigation †; where he has well delivered what had been before written on that art; insomuch that his book was long in great repute, a seventh edition having been printed in 1636. To the second edition, *Anno* 1606, and following ones, was added his former discourse of universal maps.

In 1597, the Reverend Mr. *William Barlowe*, in his *Navigator's Supply*, gave a demonstration of this division as communicated by a friend; saying, *This manner of carde has been publiquely extant in print these thirtie yeares at least* ‡, *but a cloude (as it were) and thicke miste of ignorance doth keepe it hitherto concealed: And so much the more, because some who were reckoned for men of good knowledge, have by glauncing speeches (but never by any one reason of moment) gone about what they could to disgrace it.*

This book of *Barlowe*'s contains descriptions of several instruments for the use of navigation, the principal of which is an *azimuth compass*, with two upright sights §; and as the author was very curious in making experiments on the loadstone, he discourses well and largely on the sea-compass; and still farther handles that subject in a tract he published some years after, intitled, *Magnetical Advertisements*.

At length, in 1599, Mr. *Wright* himself printed his famous treatise, intitled, *The Correction of certain Errors in Navigation*, which had been written many years before; where he shews the reason of this division ‖,

---

* Some of our modern writers have said, *Mercator* took the hint from *Wright*, but that is a mistake; for *Mercator*'s map was published thirty years before *Wright*'s book, who frequently refers to it. See *Edward Sherburn*'s translation of the first book of *Manilius*, in 1675, p. 86.

† Chap. 29.

‡ He should have said 28 only.

§ Many of these instruments are in the *Arcano del Mare*, together with the demonstration above mentioned.

‖ Maps with their meridians thus divided had been published at *Amsterdam* by *Jodocus Hondius*, who, when in *London*, working as an engraver, learnt the manner of doing it from Mr. *Wright*'s *Manuscript*; the fourth chapter of which he had transcribed into one of his maps. *Hondius* afterwards in his letters, both to Mr. *Briggs*, and also to Mr. *Wright*, begged pardon for not having acknow-

the manner of constructing his table, and its uses in navigation, with other improvements: A book, as Dr. *Halley* says, *well deserving the perusal of all such as design to use the sea**.

In the preface, *Wright* complains of the obstinacy of our mariners, for not liking an improvement in their art, saying, that they were like those whose ignorance Master *Bourne* had exposed, repeating *Bourne*'s very words.

"Though this great improvement in navigation by *Wright* has been embraced and followed by all proper judges; yet some undiscerning persons have of late, even amongst us, found fault with it, particularly *Henry Wilson*, author of a Treatise on Navigation, by a proposal for a *curvilinear sea-chart*, in 1720; and the Rev. Mr. *West*, of *Exeter*, in a posthumous piece, printed in 1762. But their *cavils* were sufficiently obviated; those of the first by Mr. *Haselden*, in his *Mercator*'s *Chart*, and in his *Reply*, both printed in 1722; and of the second, by Mr. *William Mountaine*, in the Philosophical Transactions, vol. LIII. p. 69. *Anno* 1763."

In 1610 a second edition of Mr. *Wright*'s book was published, and dedicated to Prince *Henry*, his royal pupil †, where the author inserted farther improvements; particularly, he proposed an excellent way of determining the magnitude of the Earth; at the same time recommending, very judiciously, the making our common measures in some settled proportion to that of a degree on its surface, that they might not depend on the uncertain length of a barley-corn.

Some of his other improvements were; The Table of Latitudes for dividing the meridian, computed to minutes; whereas before it was but to every tenth minute, and the short table sent by him to *Blundeville* to degrees only: An instrument, he calls the Sea-rings, by which the variation of the compass, altitude of the Sun, and time of the day, may be determined readily at once in any place, provided the latitude be known: The correcting of the errors arising from the excentricity of the eye in observing by the cross-staff: A total amendment in the Tables of the declinations and places of the Sun and stars, from his own observations, made with a six-foot quadrant, in the years 1594, 95, 96, and 97: A sea-quadrant, to take altitudes by a forward or backward observation, and likewise with a contrivance for the ready finding the latitude by the height of the pole-star, when not upon the meridian. And that his book might be the better understood by beginners, in this edition is subjoined a translation of the above-mentioned *Zamorano*'s *Compendium*; he correct-

---

acknowledged the obligation. See *Wright*'s preface, where he complains of *Hondius*'s piratical edition, and farther relates, how his book, a copy of which having been presented to the Earl of *Cumberland*, had liked to have come out under the name of a famous navigator, whom, from some circumstances there mentioned, I imagine to have been *Abraham Kendal*.

* *Philosophical Transactions*, for 1696, N° 219.

† In 1657 a 3d edition was published by Mr. *Joseph Moxon*, where the dedication is unadvisedly left out, and at the end is added by the editor the above-mentioned *Haven-finding Art*, as also *Wright*'s universal map, improved by the discoveries made since his time.

ing fome miftakes in the original, and adding a large table of the variation of the compafs obferved in very different parts of the world, to fhew it is not occafioned by any magnetical pole.

This excellent perfon was allowed fifty pounds a year (no inconfiderable fum at that time) by the *Eaft India* Company, for reading a lecture of navigation; he alfo projected the conveying water to *London*, but was prevented from executing his fcheme by defigning men, which is frequently the cafe. Whilft he led a ftudious and retired life, his reputation was fo far known, that Queen *Elizabeth* granted, in 1589, a *difpenfation* for his abfence from the univerfity, in order to accompany the Earl of *Cumberland* in the expedition to the *Azores*; as I am informed by Sir *James Burrough*, Mafter of *Caius* College, whofe fine tafte in architecture, part of the new buildings in *Cambridge* fhew, they rendering the reft of thofe buildings a difgrace to that famous feat of learning, which has produced many great men, as, (to mention here only mathematicians) *Wright*, *Briggs*, *Oughtred*, Dr. *Pell*, *Fofter*, *Horrox*, *Bainbridge*, Bifhop *Ward*, Dr. *Wallis*, Dr. *Barrow*, *Rooke*, Sir *Ifaac Newton*, *Cotes*, and Dr. *Brook Taylor*.

Wright's improvements on *Mercator*'s chart became foon known abroad.

In 1608 were publifhed the *Hypomnemata Mathematica* of the abovementioned *Simon Stevin*, compofed for the ufe of Prince *Maurice*. In the part concerning navigation, the author, having treated of failing on a great circle, and fhewn how to draw mechanically the rhumbs on a globe, fets down *Wright*'s two tables of latitude and of rhumbs, in order to defcribe thofe lines more accurately; and in an appendix he commends *Hues*, fhews a miftake committed by *Nonius* in relation to the rhumbs, and pretends to have difcovered an error in *Wright*'s latter table; but *Wright* himfelf, in the fecond edition of his book, has fully anfwered all *Stevin*'s objections, demonftrating that they arofe from his grofs way of calculating.

And in 1624 the learned *Willebrordus Snellius*, Profeffor of the Mathematics at *Leyden*, publifhed his *Typhis Batavus**, a treatife of navigation on *Wright*'s plan, written fomewhat obfcurely. In the introduction are praifed *Nonius*, *Mercator*, *Stevin*, *Hues*, and *Wright*. But fince what had been performed by our artifts on this fubject, is not there particularly declared, as are the improvements made by the others; it has happened that fome have attributed *Wright*'s principal difcovery to this author. Thus *Albert Girard*, who in 1634 publifhed a *French* tranflation of *Stevin*'s Works with notes, in one of them obferves, that *Snellius* had calculated, what he calls, *Tabulæ Canonicæ Parallelorum*, to minutes as far as 70 degrees, whereas *Wright* had fet forth in 1610 fuch a table fo calculated to 89 degrees 59 minutes; notwithftanding which M. *de Lagni*, in the Memoirs of the Royal Academy of Sciences at *Paris* for 1703, treating of the *Corrected Chart*, fays, *c'eft Willebrord Snellius qui*

* In 1617 had been publifhed his *Eratofthenes Batavus*, where is given an account of his meafuring the earth.

en eſt l'inventeur. But the *French* writers now acknowledge our countryman to have been its author*.

Snellius was followed in *Holland* by *Adrian Metius*, in a treatiſe, intitled, *Primum Mobile*, printed at *Amſterdam*, in 1631; and in *France* by the learned *Peter Herigone*, in his *Curſus Mathematicus*, where, in the dedication of the fourth tome to the Marſhal *Baſſompire*, the author ſays, *Artem navigandi in cenſu Mathematices non repoſuere plerique noſtrum, neque ſanè in hunc ordinem aſcribi meruit, quandiu cœcâ tantùm nautarum praxi celebrata eſt; nunc verò cùm inventis tabulis loxodromicis (quas nos primùm Gallis exhibemus) formam certam firmaſque leges acceperit ſine injuriâ omitti non poteſt.* But to return to our countrymen.

Mr. *Wright*, in the 12th chapter, having ſhewn how to find the place of a ſhip on his chart, obſerved, the ſame might be performed more accurately by calculation; but conſidering, as he ſays, that the latitudes, and eſpecially the courſes at ſea, could not be determined ſo preciſely, he forbore ſetting down particular examples; as the mariner may be allowed to ſave himſelf this trouble, and only mark out upon his chart, when truly conſtructed, the ſhip's way after the manner then uſually practiſed.

However, in 1614†, Mr. *Raphe Handſon*, among his nautical queſtions ſubjoined to a tranſlation of *Pitiſcus's Trigonometry*, ſolved very diſtinctly every caſe of navigation, by applying arithmetical calculations to *Wright*'s table of latitudes, or of meridional parts, as it has ſince been called.

And beſides, though the method *Wright* diſcovered for determining the change of longitude by a ſhip ſailing on a rhumb, is the adequate means of performing it; *Handſon* propoſed two ways of approximation for that purpoſe, without the aſſiſtance of *Wright*'s diviſion of the meridian line. The firſt was computed by the arithmetical mean between the co-ſines of both latitudes; the other by the ſame mean between their ſecants, as an alternative, when *Wright*'s book was not at hand, though this latter is wider from the truth than the firſt; and farther he ſhewed by the aforeſaid calculations, how much each of theſe *compendiums* deviates from the truth, and alſo how erroneouſly the computations on the principles of the plain-chart differ from them all.

There is another method of approximation, by what is called The Middle Latitude‡, which, though it errs more than that by the arithmetical mean between the co-ſines; yet being leſs operoſe, is that generally uſed by our ſailors; notwithſtanding the arithmetical mean between the logarithmic co-ſines, equivalent to the geometrical mean between the co-ſines themſelves, hath been ſince propoſed by Mr. *John Baſſat*‖, which in high latitudes is ſomewhat preferable.

---

* ——— *c'eſt qu'on* [illegible] *de les cartes réduites, invention admirable, de laquelle* [illegible] *à* [illegible] Wright, *quoiqu'on l'ait ſouvent attribuée à* Mercator. Hiſt. de l'Acad. Royale des Sciences, An. 1753, p. 275.

† It was reprinted in 1635.

‡ [illegible] works, firſt printed in 1623.

‖ [illegible], in a dialogue which was publiſhed after the author's death, in an appendix to the *Pathway to perfect Sailing*. [illegible] had been a teacher of

The computation by the middle latitude, will always fall short of the true change of longitude; that, by the geometrical mean, will always exceed; but that, by the arithmetical mean, fall short in latitudes above 45 degrees, and exceed in lesser latitudes. However, none of these methods, when the change in latitude is sufficiently small, will deviate greatly from the real change in longitude.

About this time logarithms * began to be introduced into the practice of the mathematics; and as they are of excellent use in the art of navigation, we shall here say something about their original.

These were invented by *John Napier*, Baron of *Marchistoun* in *Scotland*, as appears from his treatise, intitled, *Mirifici Logarithmorum Canonis Descriptio*, first printed in 1614 †. Soon after, the author communicated to Mr. *Henry Briggs*, Professor of geometry at *Gresham* college in *London* ‡, another form of logarithms; with which Mr. *Briggs* was so well pleased, that he immediately set about computing a very large table of them, which he published in 1624, with his *Arithmetica Logarithmica* ‖. But in the mean time, as a specimen, he printed in 1617 a few copies for his own use and that of his friends, of a very small one, not exceeding a thousand natural numbers.

From this table Mr. *Edmund Gunter*, Mr. *Briggs*'s colleague in Astronomy, computed one of artificial sines and tangents to every minute of the quadrant, which he published in 1620, being the first of its kind §. And when he made an edition of his works three years after, both these tables were subjoined to his book.

---

of navigation at *Chatham*, and well made out what he undertook, that a ship would return to the place it departed from, by sailing on the same rhumb, contrary to what *Fuller* and others had maintained. At the end of this discourse, he applies his compendium to the three principal problems in sailing.

* The foundation of logarithms is a property of two series of numbers, one in arithmetical, the other in geometrical proportion; which property is declared by *Archimedes* in his *Arenarius*.

† In 1619 was made, after the author's death, a second edition, with his farther improvements in Spherical Trigonometry.

‡ He was in 1619 appointed by Sir *Henry Saville*, his professor of geometry at *Oxford*.

‖ *Adrian Vlacq* made an edition of this book at *Tergou*, in 1628, where the table of logarithms was continued by him to one hundred thousand numbers, though the logarithms themselves are but to ten places, whereas in *Briggs*'s book they were to fourteen. Some copies of *Vlacq*'s tables were purchased by our booksellers, and published at *London*, with an *English* explanation premised, dated 1631.

§ *Vlacq* also published, at the same place, in 1633, his *Trigonometria Artificialis*, with tables of logarithmic sines and tangents to every tenth second of the quadrant. *Vlacq*'s tables have a great reputation for their exactness, as *Sherwin*'s first edition in 1706, and *Gardiner*'s in 1742, have amongst us. M. *de Fontenelle*, in the History of the Academy of Sciences for 1717, commends an edition of *Vlacq*'s smaller tables, made at *Lyons*, in 1670, as does M. *de la Lande*, in his Astronomy, printed at *Paris*, in 1761, tables published there in 1760.

There

There he applied to navigation, according to *Wright*'s table of meridional parts; as well as to other branches of the mathematics, his admirable Ruler *, on which were inscribed the logarithmic lines for numbers and for sines and tangents of arches. He also greatly improved the Sector † for the same purposes. And he shewed how to take a back observation by the cross-staff, whereby the error, arising from the excentricity of the eye, is avoided; describing likewise an instrument of his invention, named by him a Cross-Bow, for taking altitudes of the Sun or stars, with some contrivances for the more ready collecting the latitude from the observation ‡.

The discoveries relating to the logarithms were carried to *France* by Mr. *Edmund Wingate*, who, going to *Paris* in 1624, published in that city two small tracts in *French* ‖, and dedicated them both to *Gaston*, the King's only brother. In the first he teaches the use of *Gunter*'s ruler, and in the other, of the tables of logarithms and artificial sines and tangents, as modelled according to *Napier*'s last form, attributed by *Wingate* to *Briggs*, which is a mistake; as appears from the dedication of *Napier*'s *Rabdologia*, printed in 1616, and from what Mr. *Briggs* himself said in the preface of his *Arithmetica Logarithmica*.

The Reverend Mr. *William Oughtred* projected this ruler into a circular arch, shewing fully its uses in a treatise first printed in 1633, intitled, *The Circles of Proportion*; where, in an appendix, are well handled several important points in navigation. It has been made in the form of a Sliding *Ruler*. See *Seth Partridge*'s use of the double scale in 1662.

As by the logarithmic tables all trigonometrical calculations are greatly facilitated; so the first author, who, I find, has applied them to the cases of sailing, was Mr. *Thomas Addison*, in his treatise, intitled, *Arithmetical Navigation*, printed in 1625. He also gives two traverse tables with their uses, the one to quarter points of the compass, the other to degrees.

Mr. *Henry Gellibrand*, Mr. *Gunter*'s successor at *Gresham* College, published his discovery of the changes in the variation of the compass in a small quarto pamphlet, intitled, *A Discourse Mathematical on the Variation of the Magnetical Needle*, printed in 1635. This extraordinary *phenomenon* he found out by comparing the observations made at different times near the same place by Mr. *Burrough*, Mr. *Gunter*, and himself,

---

* This Ruler is so constantly in the practice of our artists, that it has got the name of *The Gunter*.

† The uses of a Sector had been shewn by Dr. *Robert Hood*, in a tract he published in 1598.

‡ This ingenious person died 1626, aged 45 years. His works have been several times reprinted with successive additions; the second edition was made in 1636 from his own manuscript; then from those of Mr. *Samuel Foster* Professor of Astronomy at *Gresham* College, again by Mr. *Henry Bond*, and Mr. *William Leybourn*. The fullest and last, being the fifth, was in 1673.

‖ These were afterwards printed at *London* in *English* with improvements.

all perſons of great ſkill and experience in theſe matters. And this diſcovery was ſoon known abroad *, for father *Athanaſius Kircher*, in his treatiſe intitled *Magnes*, firſt printed at *Rome* in 1641, ſays our countryman Mr. *John Greaves* had informed him of it, and then gives a letter of the famous *Marinus Merſennus*, containing a very diſtinct account thereof. *Gellibrand* had been famous, for the part he bore in the *Trigonometria Britannica* of his deceaſed friend Mr. *Briggs*, which was printed in 1633, at *Tergou*, under the care of *Adrian Vlacq*. *Gellibrand* alſo, in 1635, publiſhed in *Engliſh* an *Inſtitution Trigonometricall*.

In 1631 Mr. *Richard Norwood* had publiſhed an excellent treatiſe of *Trigonometry*, adapted to the invention of logarithms, particularly in applying *Napier*'s general canons †. The author having, as he ſays, acquired his knowledge in the mathematics at ſea ‡, eſpecially ſhewed the uſe of trigonometry in the three principal kinds of navigation. And towards the farther improvement of that art, he undertook a laborious work for examining the diviſion of the log-line.

As altitudes of the Sun are taken on ſhip-board, by obſerving his elevation above the viſible horizon; to collect from thence the Sun's true altitude with correctneſs, *Wright* obſerves it to be neceſſary, that the dip of the horizon below the obſerver's eye ſhould be brought into the account, which cannot be calculated without knowing the magnitude of the earth. Hence he was led to propoſe different methods for finding this; but complains, that the moſt effectual was out of his power to execute; and therefore contented himſelf with a rude attempt, in ſome meaſure ſufficient for his purpoſe: and the dimenſions of the Earth deduced by him correſponded ſo well with the uſual diviſions of the log-line, that as he wrote not an expreſs treatiſe on navigation, but only for the correcting ſuch errors, as prevailed in general practice, the log-line did not fall under his notice. But Mr. *Norwood*, for regulating this inſtrument upon genuine principles, put in execution the method Mr. *Wright* recommends, as the moſt perfect for meaſuring the dimenſion of the Earth, with the true length of the degrees of a great circle upon it; and, in 1635, actually meaſured the diſtance between *London* and *York*; from whence, and the ſummer-ſolſtitial altitudes of the Sun obſerved on the meridian at both places, he found a degree on a great circle of the Earth to contain 367196 *Engliſh* feet, equal to 57300 *French* fathoms or toiſes, which is very exact; as appears from many meaſures, that have been made ſince that time.

---

* In the Hiſtory of the Royal Academy of Sciences at *Paris* for 1712, p. 19. it is ſaid by M. *de Fontenelle*, that the learned *Peter Gaſſendi* was the principal diſcoverer of this property; but *Gaſſendi* himſelf acknowledged that he had before received information of *Gellibrand*'s diſcoveries. *Gaſſend.* Oper. vol. ii. p. 152, *Lugd.* 1658.

† A very advantageous report of it was made by M. *Mariotte* at a meeting, in 1668, of the Academy. *Du Hamel*, Hiſt. Acad. Scient. p. 51. 1701.

‡ From a ſailor he became a teacher, ſtyling himſelf before his books, A Reader of the Mathematics in *London*.

Of

Of this affair Mr. *Norwood* gives a full and clear account in his treatiſe, called *The Seaman's Practice*, firſt publiſhed in 1637. There, with unaffected modeſty, he apologizes for the hardineſs of a private perſon's undertaking ſo difficult a taſk; and very cautiouſly points out the true reaſon, how ſo great a mathematician as *Snellius* had failed in his attempt. He alſo ſhews various uſes of his diſcovery, particularly for correcting the groſs errors hitherto committed in the diviſions of the log-line. But ſuch neceſſary amendments have been little attended to by the ſailors, whoſe obſtinacy in adhering to inveterate miſtakes has been always complained of by the beſt writers on navigation. This improvement has at length, however, made its way into practice: few navigators of reputation uſing now the old meaſure of 42 feet to a knot.

Farther, Mr. *Norwood* likewiſe there deſcribes his own excellent method of *ſetting down and perfecting a Sea-Reckoning*, uſing a traverſe-table, which method he had followed and taught for many years; and beſides, ſhews how to rectify the courſe, by the variation of the compaſs being conſidered; as alſo how to diſcover currents, and to make proper allowance on their account.

This treatiſe, and that of *Trigonometry*, were continually reprinted, as the principal books for learning ſcientifically the art of Navigation. What he had delivered, eſpecially in the latter of them, concerning this ſubject, was contracted as a manual for ſailors, in a very ſmall piece, called his *Epitome*, which uſeful performance has gone through numberleſs editions.

No alterations were ever made in *The Seaman's Practice*, till in the 12th edition, printed in 1676, after the author's deceaſe, there began to be inſerted, at page 59, the following paragraph in a ſmaller character [*About the year* 1672, *Monſieur* Picart *has publiſhed an account in* French, *concerning the meaſure of the Earth, a breviate whereof may be ſeen in the* Philoſophical Tranſactions, N° 112, *wherein he concludes one* degree *to contain* 365184 Engliſh *feet, nearly agreeing to Mr.* Norwood's *experiment.*] And this advertiſement is continued in the ſubſequent editions, as I find it in one printed ſo lately as 1732.

Norwood's meaſure therefore, though it was not known to the great Sir *Iſaac Newton* in his youth, was not buried in oblivion, on account of the confuſions occaſioned by our civil wars, as M. *de Voltaire* has been pleaſed to ſay *; on the contrary, it has been conſtantly commended by our writers on navigation: as by Mr. *Henry Bond*, ſoon after its publication, in a note at page 107 of the *Seaman's Kalendar*, which ancient book he reprinted and improved, whoſe uſe, through numberleſs editions, is continued amongſt our ſailors to this day; by Mr. *Henry Phillips* in his *Geometrical Seaman* in 1652, and in his *Advancement of Navigation* in 1657; by Mr. *John Collins* in his *Navigation by the Plane Scale*, in 1659; by the reverend Dr. *John Newton* in his *Mathematical Elements*, in 1660; Mr. *John Seller* in his *Practical Navigation*, in 1669; Mr. *John Brown* in his *Triangular Quadrant* in 1671.

---

* *Elemens de la Philoſophie de* Newton, chap. xviii. printed at *Paris* in 17.8.

And in the *Philosophical Transactions* for 1676, N° 126, there is given a very particular account of it. Nor had it escaped the royal notice; for when King *James*, in 1690, honoured the observatory at *Paris* with a visit, he informed the gentlemen, then present, of this measure of the Earth; and upon their acquainting his Majesty how that had been determined by Mr. *Picard*, the King wished the two measures might be compared together *.

But that it was not commonly known in *France* is no wonder, seeing our books were not then so much inquired after as at present by that polite and learned people.

In the *Journal des Sçavans* for *December* 1666, it was observed of Dr. *Hooke's Micrographia, qu'il est écrit en une langue que peu de personnes entendent*; but long after, in the same *Journal* for *February* 1750, it is said of the *English* tongue, that it was *une langue que tous les vrais savans devroient savoir*. And now, as *Norwood* is taken notice of in the latter editions of Sir *Isaac Newton's Principia*, his name and merit indeed are become universally known. Insomuch that a particular account of his measure is given by M. *de Maupertuis*, in the preface to his Treatise of the figure of the Earth, printed at *Paris* in 1738; wherein he describes his method of determining the length of a degree on the Earth in *Lapland*; and *Norwood* is mentioned by two learned *Spanish* sea officers, D. *Jorge Juan*, and D. *Antonio d'Ulloa*, i. their voyage printed at *Madrid* in 1748, which was undertaken, as they were appointed to accompany the *French* mathematicians, sent to measure a degree near the equator.

About the year 1645 Mr. *Bond* published in *Norwood's Epitome* a very great improvement in *Wright*'s method, by a property in his meridian line, whereby its divisions are more scientifically assigned, than the author himself was able to effect; which was from this theorem, That these divisions are analogous to the excesses of the logarithmic tangents of half the respective latitudes augmented by 45 degrees above the logarithm of the radius.

This he afterwards explained somewhat more fully in the third edition of *Gunter*'s works, printed in 1653, where, after observing that the logarithmic tangents from 45° upwards increase in the same manner (as he expresses it) that the secants added together do, if every half degree be accounted as one whole degree of *Mercator*'s meridional line; his rule for computing the meridional parts appertaining to any two latitudes (supposed on the same side of the equator) is laid down to this effect; To take the logarithmic tangent, rejecting the radius, of half each latitude augmented by 45 degrees, and dividing the difference of those numbers by the logarithmic tangent of 45° 30′, the radius being likewise rejected, and the quotient will be the meridional parts required, expressed in degrees. And this rule is the immediate consequence from the general theorem, That the degrees of latitude bear to 1 degree (or 60 minutes, which in *Wright*'s table stands as the meridional parts for 1 degree) the same proportion as the logarithmic tangent of half any latitude augmented by 45 degrees, and the radius neglected, to the like tangent

* *Du Hamel*, Hist. Academ. Regal. Scient. p. 285.

of

of half a degree augmented by 45 degrees, with the radius likewise rejected.

But here was farther wanting the demonstration of this general theorem, which was at length supplied by that great mathematician, Mr. *James Gregory* of *Aberdeen*, in his *Exercitationes Geometricæ*, printed at *London* in 1668; and since more concisely demonstrated, together with a scientific determination of the divisor, by Dr. *Halley*, in the *Philosophical Transactions* for 1695, N° 219, from the consideration of the spirals into which the rhumbs are transformed in the stereographic projection of the sphere upon the plane of the equinoctial; which the excellent Mr. *Roger Cotes* has rendered still more simple, in his *Logometria*, first published in the *Philosophical Transactions* for 1714, N° 388.

It is moreover added in *Gunter*'s book, that if $\frac{1}{20}$ of this divisor (which does not sensibly differ from the logarithmic tangent of 45° 1′ 30″ curtailed of the radius) be used, the quotient will exhibit the meridional parts expressed in leagues: and this is the divisor set down in *Norwood*'s *Epitome*.

After the same manner the meridional parts will be found in minutes, if the like logarithmic tangent of 45° 0′ 30″ diminished by the radius be taken, that is, the number used by others * being 12633, when the logarithmic tables consist of eight places besides the index.

This Mr. *Bond*, who introduced so useful a discovery into the art, was a teacher of the mathematics in *London*, and employed to take care of and improve the impressions of the current treatises of navigation. In an edition of the *Seaman's Kalendar*, p. 103, he declared, he had discovered the longitude, by having found out the true theory of the magnetic variation; and to gain credit to his assertion, he foretold, that at *London* in 1657 there would be no variation of the compass, and from that time it would gradually increase the other way, which happened accordingly. Again, in the *Philosophical Transactions* for 1668, N° 40, he published a table of the variations for 49 years to come.

This joyful news to all sailors acquired Mr. *Bond* a great reputation; insomuch that the treatise he had composed, called *The Longitude found*, was in 1676 published by the special command of King *Charles* the Second, and ushered into the world with the approbation of several of the most eminent mathematicians of that time †.

But it was soon opposed, there being published at *London* a book in 1678, called *The Longitude not found*, written by one Mr. *Beckborrow*. And indeed as *Bond*'s hypothesis did not in any wise answer its author's sanguine expectations, the famous Dr. *Halley* again undertook this affair; and from a multitude of observations he would conclude, that the mag-

* See Mr. *Perkins*'s *Treatise of Navigation* in Vol. I. of Sir *Jonas Moore*'s *New System of the Mathematicks*, p. 203, printed at *London* in 1681. *Perkins*'s book was published by itself the year following, under the title of the *Seaman's Tutor*.

† In the *Philosophical Transactions* for the same year, N° 130, it is said, the Lord *Brounker*'s name was inserted by mistake.

netic needle was influenced by four poles. His speculations on this subject are delivered in the *Philosophical Transactions* for 1683, N° 148, and for 1692, N° 195. But this wonderful *phenomenon* seems to have hitherto eluded all our researches.

However, that excellent person in 1700 published a general map, on which were delineated curve lines expressing the paths, where the magnetic needle had the same variation. This was received with universal applause *, as it may lead to some discovery in so abstruse an affair, and at present be useful on many occasions in determining the longitude. The positions of these curves will indeed continually suffer alterations; but then they should be corrected from time to time; as they have been for the year 1744, and 1756, by two ingenious persons, Mr. *William Mountaine* and Mr. *James Dodson*, Fellows of the Royal Society. The latter died not long after he had been chosen, for his merit, mathematical master, at *Christ's Hospital*, in *London*.

Dr. *Halley* also gave, in the *Philosophical Transactions* for 1690, N° 183, a dissertation on the monsoons, containing many observations very useful for all such as sail to places that are subject to those winds.

The true principles of navigation having been settled by *Wright*, *Norwood*, and *Bond*, many authors amongst us trod in their steps, making some little improvements. It would be impossible to enumerate each particular. Of the writers already mentioned, *Phillips* and *Collins*, in the title pages of their books, declare what they aimed at; *Phillips* also, in his tract called the *Advancement of Navigation*, recommends a pendulum instead of a half minute glass, to estimate the time the log-line is running out. He also proposes to do the same thing by wheel-work. Besides, in the *Philosophical Transactions* for 1668, N° 34, he delivers a better method to determine the tides than what was commonly practised; for which purpose Mr. *John Flamsteed*, the Royal Astronomer, still gave more perfect directions in the same *Transactions* for 1683, N° 143; as likewise he first ordered a glass lens to be fixed on the shade vane, in what is called *Davis*'s quadrant †, which contrivance Dr. *Robert Hook*, Professor of Geometry at *Gresham* College, had before thought of ‡.

Seller's Practical Navigation, though without demonstrations, has the rules of sailing in the different kinds, as performed by calculation, by the plane scale, by the *Gunter*, and by the sinical quadrant, with various other matters relative to the art; as also the use of the azimuth-compass as now modelled, the ring-dial, the sea-ring, cross-staff, *Davis*'s quadrant,

* It is particularly commended in the History and Memoirs of the Royal Academy of Sciences at *Paris*, for the year 1701, 1705, 1706, 1708, and 1710. See also Mr. *Robins*'s Collections in his Introduction to Lord *Anson*'s Voyage round the World, made in 1743, &c. as also in the ninth chapter of the first book, and eighth of the third.

† See the above-mentioned *Perkins*'s Navigation, page 250.

‡ See Bishop *Thomas Sprat*'s excellent History of the Royal Society in 1667, page 246; and *Hook*'s Posthumous Works, published by *Richard Waller*, Esq. in 1705, p. 557.

plough,

plough, nocturnal, inclinatory needle and globe, together with all the necessary tables; the whole being delivered in a manner so well adapted to the general humour of mariners, that it has undergone numberless editions: the last, I have seen, was in 1739; but some late writers seem to have abated the run of this book.

As in sailing especial regard ought to be had to the lee-way a ship makes, so many authors have touched upon this point; but the allowances usually made on that account are very particularly set down by Mr. *John Buckler*, and published in a small tract first printed in 1702, intitled, *A New Compendium of the whole Art of Navigation*, written by Mr. *William Jones*.

We ought not here to pass over in silence the very useful invention of Dr. *Gowin Knight*, which is the making *artificial magnets*, that are of greater efficacy than the natural ones. Though the Doctor has not thought fit to reveal his secret; yet others have found it out, who have made it public, particularly the Rev. *John Mitchel*, and Mr. *John Canton*; the first in a treatise of *Artificial Magnets*, printed in 1750; the other in the *Philosophical Transactions*, vol. XLVII. *Ann.* 1751.

The Earth being now universally agreed to be not a perfect globe, but a spheroid, whose diameter at the poles is shorter than any other; the Rev. Dr. *Patrick Murdoch* published a tract in 1741, where he accommodated *Wright*'s sailing to such a figure; and Mr. *Colin Maclaurin*, the same year, in the *Philosophical Transactions*, N° 461, gave a rule to determine the meridional parts of a spheroid, which speculation he farther treats of in his book of *Fluxions*, printed at *Edinburgh*, in 1742.

Though Sir *Isaac Newton* in his *Principia*, first printed in 1686, had demonstrated from the theory of gravity, that this must be the real form of the Earth, as it revolved about an axis; yet in the year 1718 M. *Cassini* again * undertook from observations to shew the contrary, and that the earth was a spheroid, having its longest diameter passing through its poles †; and in 1720 M. *de Mairan* advanced arguments, supposed to be strengthened by geometrical demonstrations, to confirm farther M. *Cassini*'s assertion. But in the *Philosophical Transactions* for 1725, N° 386, 387, 388, Dr. *Desaguliers* published a dissertation, wherein he made appear the weakness of the reasoning, and the insufficiency of the observations, as they were managed, to settle so nice an affair. He there also proposed a proper method for adjusting this point, when he says, *If any consequence of this kind could be drawn from actual measuring, a degree of latitude should be measured at the equator, and a degree of longitude likewise measured there; and a degree very northerly, as for example, a whole degree might be actually measured upon the* Baltic *sea, when frozen, in the latitude*

* In the Memoirs of the Royal Academy of Sciences at *Paris*, his father in 1701, and he in 1713, attempted to prove the Earth was an oblong spheroid.

† M. *John Bernouilli* in his *Essai d'une Nouvelle Physique Celeste*, printed at *Paris* in 1735, triumphs over Sir *Isaac Newton*; vainly imagining these precarious observations could invalidate what Sir *Isaac* had demonstrated.

of sixty degrees. There, according to M. *Cassini's last supposition, a degree would be* 56653 *toises; whereas at the equator it would be of* 58019 *toises, the difference being* 1366 *toises, about the two and fortieth part of a degree, which must be sensible; and likewise the degree of longitude would according to him be of* 56817 *toises, less by* 1202, or the *forty-eighth part, than a degree of* latitude at the same place.

On this admonition, in 1735, there were sent from *France* two sets of mathematicians, members of the Royal Academy of Sciences; one towards the pole, the other to the equator, in order to measure, at each place, the length of a degree on the meridian. The report they brought home, quite overset what had been urged in favour of the oblong figure; a degree towards the north, in the latitude of 66° 20′, being found to contain about 57438 toises, and near the equator but 56750.

This unwelcome news caused a degree to be again measured in *France*, which at length came out to be consonant with those which had been brought from very distant parts of the world. Thus these mathematicians confirmed by painful observations, what Sir *Isaac Newton* had, as M. *de Maupertuis* used to say, determined in his elbow-chair; Sir *Isaac* making the length of a degree under the pole to be 57382, and at the equator 56637 toises. And perhaps no observations can be exact enough to determine this matter more precisely.

But let us mention some of the foreign writers on navigation.

At *Rome*, in 1607, came forth a treatise, intitled, *Nautica Mediterranea*, written in *Italian* by *Bartolomew Crescenti*, the Pope's engineer. The author misses no opportunity of exposing the errors of *Medina*; but scarce gives any thing of his own, except a machine for measuring the way a ship made.

As the Jesuits have treated of most branches of learning, so this art has not been beneath their consideration; the three following authors having been of their society.

At *Paris*, in 1633, Father *George Fournier*, published an *Hydrography*, principally relating to navigation. The author would persuade us, that one of *Dieppe* had corrected the plane chart; and that the *Hollanders* learnt of the *French* the making charts so corrected; whereas this had been engraved long before at *Amsterdam*, by *Iodocus Hondius*, and others.

John Baptist Riccioli, in his *Geographia & Hydrographia Reformata*, printed at *Bologna* in 1661, inserts a treatise of navigation, collecting his materials from almost every writer, as he does in his *Almagest* and *Chronology*, which is indeed the chief merit of his works.

Father *Millet Dechalles* wrote on this subject after a more masterly manner, both in his *Cursus Mathematicus*, first printed at *Lyons* in 1674, and in a *French* treatise, published in 1677, intitled *L'Art de Naviger demontré par Principes*.

These three authors, besides treating of the different kinds of sailing, abound in methods for taking of altitudes, finding the variation, and estimating the way a ship makes, &c. They also describe a machine resembling that of *Crescenti*. *Riccioli* gives a very faulty measure of the Earth, made by himself; and *Dechalles* advises the use of a pendulum in reckoning by the log-line, as also of wheel-work for the same purpose, as *Phillips* and *Cole* had done.

But

But there were writers in *France* between *Fournier* and *Dechalles*. For in 1666, and the following years, there were printed at *Dieppe* several tracts handling different parts of navigation, composed by M. *G. Denys*, which have been often reprinted.

And in 1671 the Sieur *Blondel S. Aubin* published a book called, *L'Art de Naviger par le Quartier de Reduction*, describing an instrument * much in use amongst the *French* sailors, by which may be performed, as by the sinical quadrant, the operations of navigation, though not much more speedily than by the traverse table, and not at all so accurately. He also published in 1673 his *Tresor de la Navigation*, where the art is well treated of, particularly by calculations.

M. *Saverien*, in his *Marine Dictionary*, printed at *Paris* in 1758, says, that M. *Dassier* seems to have been the first of the *French* writers that shewed the use of *Gunter*'s scales [*échelles Angloises*] in his *Pilote expert*, printed in 1683.

At *Paris*, ten years after, was published the first part of a pompous work, intitled, *Le Neptune François*, by order of the *French* king, consisting of sea-charts, according to *Wright*'s scheme, made from the latest observations, and reviewed by Mess. *Pene*, *Cassini*, and others. As this contained the charts of *Europe* only, there were added others of different parts of the world, printed the same year at *Amsterdam*. The whole was preceded by a discourse of M. *Sauveur*, who had formed some of the charts, where he shews how to perform the problems of astronomy and navigation by scales; which discourse had been published by itself at *Paris*, in 1692.

M. *John Bouguer* composed, by authority, his *Traité Complet de la Navigation*, first printed in 1698, which was well received, as containing most of the practices then known; and Father *Pézenas*, Jesuit and Royal Professor of Hydrography at *Marseilles*, published there, in 1733, a tract, called, *Elemens de Pilotage*; and at *Avignon*, in 1741, a larger work, intitled, *Practique du Pilotage*. This author shews how to find the meridional parts by the *Artificial Tangents*, an old discovery amongst us, declared so long ago as 1645, in *Norwood's Epitome*; he also has been industrious in translating several of our mathematical books into *French*.

But in 1753 M. *Peter Bouguer*, son of the former, published a very elaborate treatise on this subject, intitled, *Nouveau Traité de Navigation*, which is written sensibly, the author being an excellent mathematician, and famous for other productions. He there gives a variation-compass † of his own invention, and attempts to reform the log, as he had done in the Memoirs of the Academy of Sciences for 1747. He is also very

* It is only a kind of skeleton of *Wright*'s universal map.

† Many of these sorts of compasses have been proposed at different times, as by M. *Buache*, in the Memoirs of the *French* Academy of Sciences for 1752, page 377; Captain *Christopher Middleton*, in the Philosophical Transactions, N° 450, *Ann.* 1738; and Dr. *Knight*, as improved by the ingenious Mr *John Smeaton*, *ibid.* N° 495, *Ann.* 1750.

particular

particular in determining the lunations more accurately than by the common methods, and in describing the corrections of the dead reckonings.

The excellent astronomer, M. *de la Caille*, in 1760, made an edition of M. *Bouguer*'s book, which he somewhat abridged and improved.

In 1766, came out at *Paris*, a treatise, with this title, *Abregé du Pilotage divisé en deux parties, ou on traite principalement des Amplitudes, des Loxodromies, dans l'hypothese de la Sphere et de Spheroide, des marées, des variations de l'aiman.*

The former part of this book was first published in 1693. Here the whole is improved by M. *le Monnier*.

Though the *Spaniards* were the earliest writers on navigation, yet they were very backward to adopt its improvements. Indeed *Antonio de Naiera* published at *Lisbon*, in 1628, a treatise, intitled, *Navegacion especulativa y practica*; where, though the author rectifies the tables of the Sun and fixed stars, from *Tycho Brahe*'s observations, he proceeds no farther in the theory of navigation than what had been advanced by *Nonius*, as followed by *Cespedes*. But of late, in 1712, was printed at the same place, *Arte de Navegar por Manuel Pimental*; where is shewn the use of *Wright*'s chart, which, in imitation of the *French*, the author calls *Charta Reduzida*. He likewise describes *Davis*'s quadrant, and mentions *Norwood* and *Picard*'s measures of the Earth. In 1757 a treatise was printed at *Cadiz*, intitled, *Compendio de Navigacion para el uso de los Cavelleros Guardias Marinas*, written by the ingenious gentleman mentioned above, Don *Jorge Juan*. This is a good performance, delivering very distinctly the several parts of the art, as now improved. Some things are here omitted, that usually occur in books on this subject; but for the knowledge of such particulars, references are made to tracts composed expressly for the use of the society of gentlemen, destined for the sea-service.

Bouguer and *Jorge Juan*, describe and commend the method of dividing instruments for taking of angles, published by *Peter Vernier*, in a treatise, intitled, *La Construction, &c. du quadrant nouveau*, printed at *Brussels*, in 1631. This division is an improvement of that of *Curtius*, as that of *Fererius* is of the division by diagonals *, and readily follows from the first *Lemma* of *Clavius*'s treatise on the *Astrolabe* †, as has been observed by *Pézenas*, in a book he published at *Avignon* in 1765, intitled, *Astronomie des Marins*.

As to their treating of *Wright*'s chart, I mentioned above *Snellius* and *Metius*. To an edition, in 1665, of *Vlacq*'s small tables of logarithms, &c. is added, by *Abraham de Gruel*, one of meridional parts, whose use he shews, with other parts of navigation, in his *Course of Mathematics*, written in *Dutch*, and printed at *Amsterdam* in 1676, as had been done by *John V*[illegible], in his *Flambeau reluissant où Thresor de la Navigation*, at the same place, in 1677.

---

* See Mr. *Robins*'s Mathematical Tracts, where these divisions are largely treated of.

† First printed at *Rome*, in 1693.

The *Dutch* are great navigators, and have been famous for their *Atlasses*, before which are premised treatises of navigation, as has been already observed. The oldest I have seen of these, was published at *Leyden* in 1584, intitled, *Spiegel der Zee-Vaert* (or *Mirror of Navigation*,) by *Lucas Jansz Waghenaer*. In their later *Atlasses* there is described an instrument to be used after the manner of *Davis*'s quadrant, but where instead of circular arches are substituted straight lines.

Notwithstanding all the improvements hitherto mentioned, the *sea-reckonings*, though kept by such as were deemed very skilful mariners, are often found widely different from the truth. But this often happens through negligence, as I have heard Dr. *Halley*, who had used the sea, say.

These errors would be avoided, if from time to time the latitude and longitude could be determined. The first is generally obtained by the meridian altitude and declination of the Sun being given. The declination is got by the help of tables of the Sun, with an easy trigonometrical operation.

But even the latitude could not be very exact, before the famous *Kepler* had determined the true form of the Earth's orbit *. Hence were fabricated his *Tabulæ Rudolphinæ*. Next, those of Mr. *Thomas Street* were in great request †. But they, in their turn, yielded to Dr. *Halley*'s, and his again to those of the accurate and elaborate *Mayer*; which, however, will want to be corrected hereafter: For, as Sir *Isaac Newton* has shewn, that all bodies mutually attract one another, the Earth will be disturbed in its motion by the actions of some of the other planets.

To find the longitude is a much more difficult affair. For this end, at present, the societies of learned men in *Europe* offer from time to time rewards to such as shall best treat of particular subjects in mathematicks or physicks. Some of these have been relating to navigation, when *Polleni*, *Bernouilli*, *Bouguer*, and others have obtained the prizes. And it is hoped, this institution may contribute to the advancement of the art.

Eclipses of the moon were used of old; and *Kepler* recommended those of the Sun as preferable ‖.

The satellites of *Jupiter* were no sooner discovered by the great *Galileo* §, than the frequency of their eclipses recommended them for this purpose; and amongst those who attempted this subject, none were more successful than Signor *Dominic Cassini*.

This great astronomer in 1688 published at *Bologna* tables for calculating the appearances of their eclipses, with directions for finding thence the longitudes of places; and being invited to *France* by *Lewis* the Fourteenth, he there published correcter tables in 1693. But the mutual attractions of the satellites on one another rendering their motions excessively irregular, the tables soon run out; insomuch that they require to be renewed from time to time, which has been performed by ingenious

* In his treatise *de Motu Martis*, in 1609.

† In his *Astronomia Carolina*, in 1661.

‖ *Tabulæ Rudolph.* printed at *Ulm* in 1627, cap. xvi. & xxxi.

§ In his *Sydereus Nuncius*, first printed at *Venice* in 1610.

persons.

perſons, as Dr. *James Pound*, Dr. *James Bradley* *, M. *Caſſini* the ſon, and M. *Peter Wargentin* †; ſo that now many of the common *Almanacs* ſet down, when theſe eclipſes happen throughout the year.

The Rev. *Nevil Maſkelyne*, D. D. our preſent Royal Aſtronomer, has publiſhed annually, ſince the year 1767, by order of the Commiſſioners of Longitude, a work entitled, *The Nautical Almanac and Aſtronomical Ephemeris*, containing not only the eclipſes of the ſatellites, but alſo many other tables, to enable the mariner to determine the longitude at ſea; particularly tables of the diſtances which the moon's center will have from that of the Sun, and from fixed ſtars, at every three hours, under the meridian of the Royal Obſervatory at *Greenwich*, and which have ſince beeen copied into the *Connoiſance des Temps* for theſe latter years by the editor of that work.

The large reward granted by the *Parliament* for a practical way of diſcovering the longitude at ſea, has put many upon the ſearch: inſomuch that ſeveral idle and abſurd ſchemes have been offered by ignorant and wrong-headed men. But the perfecting the methods propoſed long ago by *John Werner* and *Gemma Friſius*, ſeems at preſent to engage the attention of the public.

The theory of the moon, though much amended by the noble *Tycho Brahe* and Mr. *Jeremy Horrox* ‡, was found to be inſufficient to anſwer this end. But the cauſes of her various irregularities having been diſcovered by Sir *Iſaac Newton*, and her theory thence improved beyond expectation, gave great hopes of ſucceſs; which have ſince been happily fulfilled by means of the improvements which have ſince been made in the methods of computing the ſeveral quantities of theſe inequalities by M. *Euler*, and *Tobias Mayer* of *Gottingen* §: The former of theſe gentlemen having been happy in reducing Sir *Iſaac Newton*'s theory into neat analytical expreſſions, of which the latter availing himſelf, was, by a very ſingular addreſs of his own, enabled to bring out the greateſt quantities of the equations with eaſe and exactneſs, and thence to conſtruct tables

---

* He ſucceeded Dr. *Halley* at *Greenwich*, where he made a great number of Aſtronomical Obſervations, which, as they are moſt accurate, it is hoped will not be loſt. He became famous on obſerving and accounting for an apparent motion in the fixed ſtars, and called their aberration, which was immediately exhibited by the great mathematician Dr. *Brook Taylor* according to the exact theory of the Earth's motion. See Mr. *Robins*'s Mathematical Tracts, vol. II. page 276.

† *Wargentin*'s tables are much eſteemed; they were firſt publiſhed at *Stockholm* in the *Acta Societatis Regii Scientiarum Upſalenſis* for the year 1741, but ſince more correct from a new copy of the author's at *Paris* in 1759, by M. *de la Lande*. The ingenious author has rendered them yet more correct, and his labours on this head may be ſeen in the *Connoiſance des Temps* for 1766, and the *Nautical Almanac* for 1771, and 1779.

‡ This great genius died in 1641, ſcarce 23 years old. See his *Opera Poſthuma*, publiſhed by the famous Dr. *John Wallis* at *London*, in 1673. *Horrox* firſt obſerved the Tranſit of *Venus* over the Sun in 1639. He wrote an account of this *Phenomenon*, which was publiſhed by the great aſtronomer *Hevelius*, at *Dantzic*, in 1661.

§ *Com. Societ. Reg. Gottingenſ.* tom. II. page 283.

agreeing

agreeing to the moon's motion in every part of her orbit, with very surprising exactneſs. And this ingenious perſon has left behind him tables ſtill more exact *, for which the *Britiſh* Parliament have rewarded his widow with £. 3000, as alſo Mr. *Euler* with £. 300. Theſe tables were publiſhed in 1770, by Dr. *Maſkelyne*.

As to the method of *Gemma Friſius*, M. *Huygens* was perſuaded it might be accompliſhed by his inventions of pendulum clocks and watches; a deſcription of the firſt he publiſhed in a ſmall tract, printed at the *Hague*, in 1658; and of the ſecond, as improved, in the *Journal des Sçavans* for the month of *February*, 1675. And great expectations of ſucceſs had been raiſed from ſome trials made in a voyage with theſe watches of the firſt conſtruction, by Major *Holmes*; an account whereof is given in the Philoſophical Tranſactions, *Ann*. 1669. But the various accidents thoſe movements are liable to, ſoon cauſed that way to be laid aſide.

Notwithſtanding which, the ingenious Mr. *John Harriſon* has for many years paſt employed himſelf in contriving a machine, that ſhall be free from all imaginable inconveniencies; and his endeavours were ſo well approved of by gentlemen of the greateſt knowledge in theſe ſubjects, that the commiſſioners for the longitude thought ſit to allow him ſome gratifications for his pains. He was afterwards farther conſidered, upon diſcloſing the internal ſtructure of his machine, and the whole reward has ſince been given him by Parliament.

The difficulty of making obſervations at ſea with ſufficient exactneſs for finding the longitude, was feared to be inſurmountable; but attempts have not been wanting to overcome it. In the Hiſtory of the Royal Society, at page 246, we meet with the firſt mention of an invention in theſe words: *A new inſtrument for taking angles by reflection, by which means the eye at the ſame time ſees the two objects both as touching the ſame point, though diſtant almoſt to a ſemicircle; which is of great uſe for making exact obſervations at ſea.* A figure of this inſtrument, drawn by Dr. *Hook*, the inventor, is given in the Doctor's poſthumous works, with a deſcription, at page 503. But here, as one reflection only was made uſe of, it would not anſwer the purpoſe. However, this was at laſt effected by Sir *Iſaac Newton*, who communicated to Dr. *Halley*, about the year 1700, a paper of his own writing, containing a deſcription of an inſtrument with two reflections, which ſoon after the Doctor's death was found among his papers by Mr. *Jones*, who communicated it to the Royal Society, and it was publiſhed in the Philoſophical Tranſactions, N° 465, *Ann*. 1742.

How it happened that Dr. *Halley* never mentioned this in his lifetime, is very extraordinary; ſeeing *John Hadley*, Eſq. † had deſcribed,

* See his *Elogium* in the *Nova Acta Eruditorum*, for *March* 1762.

† Mr. *Hadley* being well acquainted with Sir *Iſaac Newton*, might have heard him ſay, *Hook's* propoſal could be perfected by means of a double reflection. However, Mr. *Hadley*, being a very ingenious perſon, might have hit on the ſame thought; as well as Mr. *Godfrey* of *Penſylvania* to whom the invention of this admirable inſtrument has been aſcribed by ſome gentlemen of that colony: This is not the only caſe, wherein different perſons have produced ſimilar inventions.

in N° 430, *Ann.* 1731, an instrument grounded on the same principles, which is so well esteemed, that our shops abound with them, accommodated with *Vernier's* division, as they are made by our most skilful workmen; and are now in general use amongst the skilful seamen of most of the maritime nations.

Though *Medina's* method for finding the place of the horizon was absurd; yet, for this end, several plausible ones have been proposed by ingenious persons, as Mess. *Elton*, *Hadley*, *Godfrey*, and *Leigh*; and that chiefly by applying a level to *Davis's* quadrant. Their devices are described in the Philosophical Transactions for 1732, 33, 34, and 37. And, lastly, an *Horizontal Top*, invented by the late Mr. *Serson*, who was unfortunately lost at sea aboard the *Victory* man of war, has been approved of, and published by Mr. *Smeaton* in the Philosophical Transactions, vol. XLVII. for 1752, part ii. page 352.

Some methods used for obtaining the place of the horizon, and of observing with Mr. *Hadley's Reflecting Sector*, are described by Mr. *Robertson*, in his *Elements of Navigation*; which treatise has deservedly met with the approbation of the public.

Thus have I endeavoured to trace out the principal steps by which the art of navigation has advanced to its present height; nor without hopes that the attempt may not prove altogether unacceptable to those whose business or curiosity lead them to be acquainted with this very useful branch of the mathematics: on the successful practising of which depends, in an especial manner, the flourishing state of our country.

This Dissertation, written at first by desire, is now reprinted with alterations. Though I may be thought to have dwelt too long on some particulars not directly relating to the subject; yet I hope that what is so delivered, will not be altogether unentertaining to the candid reader. As to any apology for having handled a matter quite foreign to my way of life, I shall only plead, that very young, living in a sea-port town, I was eager to be acquainted with an art that could enable the Mariner to arrive across the wide and pathless ocean at his desired harbour.

London. JAMES WILSON.

ADVER-

ADVERTISEMENT.

As it may be expected that four kinds of readers will look into this book, it was thought convenient to point out to some of them, the places where they may meet with what they more particularly want.

First. Those who having made a proficiency in the mathematics, will, it is likely, examine in what manner the subjects are here treated, and whether any thing new is contained therein: it is conceived that such readers will find some things which may recompence them for their trouble, in almost every one of the books.

Secondly. Those learners, who are desirous of being instructed in the art of Navigation in a scientific manner, and would chuse to see the reason of the several steps they must take to acquire it: To such persons, it is recommended that they read the whole book in the order they find it; or, if the learner is very young, he may omit the IVth and Vth books till after he is master of the VIth and VIIth.

Thirdly. That class of readers, which, with too much truth may be said, comprehends most of our mariners, who want to learn both the elements and the art itself by rote, and never trouble themselves about the reason of the rules they work by: As it is probable there ever will be many readers of this kind, they may be well accommodated in this work; thus, if they are not already acquainted with Arithmetic and Geometry, let them read the five first rules of Arithmetic, to page 20; thence proceed to the definitions and problems in Geometry, from page 43 to 58. In the book of Trigonometry, read pages 89, 90, 91, 92, 98, 99, and from 104 to 114: the whole of book VI. In book the VIIth they may read to page 35, and as much more as they please. In book VIII, let them read the sections III, IV, V, VI, from page 146 to page 182. In book V, they may read section III, and as many problems in the Vth and VIth sections as they can; and let them read the whole of the ninth book.

Fourthly.

Fourthly. That set of readers who will not be at the pains of learning any thing more than how to perform a day's work; such may herein meet with the practice almost independent of other knowledge. Let such persons make themselves acquainted with section IV. of book VI, and the use of the table at page 374; then learn the use of the Traverse Table at the end of book VII, which they will find exemplified between pages 8 and 35, Vol. II; also they must learn the use of the Table of Meridional parts at the end of Book VIII. After which, they may proceed to book IX, where they will find ample instructions in all the particulars which enter into a day's work. But with this scanty knowledge of things, they will be obliged to omit some parts, which it is well worth their pains to be acquainted with.

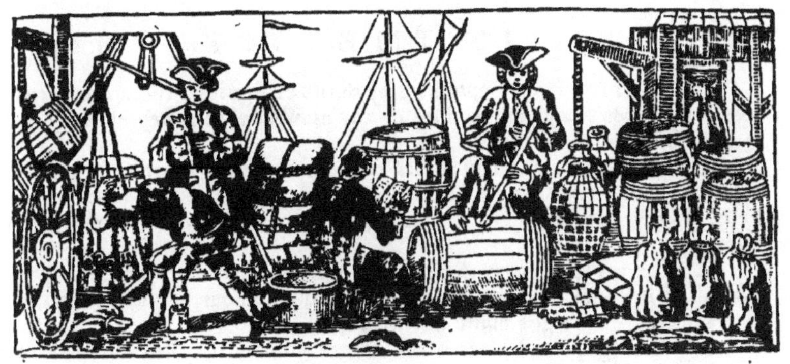

THE ELEMENTS OF NAVIGATION.

BOOK I.

OF ARITHMETICK.

SECTION I.

Definitions and *Principles*.

1. ARITHMETICK is a ſcience which teaches the properties of numbers; and how to compute or eſtimate the value of things.

2. An UNIT or UNITY, is any thing conſidered as one.

3. NUMBER, in general, is many units.

4. DIGITS or FIGURES are the marks by which numbers are denoted or expreſſed, and are the nine following.

Digits,	1.	2.	3.	4.	5.	6.	7.	8.	9.
Names,	One.	Two.	Three.	Four.	Five.	Six.	Seven.	Eight.	Nine.

And with theſe is uſed the mark 0, called cypher, which of itſelf ſtands for nothing; but being annexed to a digit, alters its value.

Thus 40 *ſignifies forty*; *and* 400 *ſtands for four hundred, &c.*

5. INTEGER, or WHOLE, NUMBERS, are ſuch as expreſs a number of things, each of which is conſidered as an unit.

Thus four pounds, twelve miles, thirty-four gallons, one hundred days, &c. are, in each caſe, called an integer number, or whole number.

6. FRACTIONAL NUMBERS, are thoſe which expreſs the value of ſome part or parts of an unit.

Thus one half, one quarter, three quarters, &c. are each the fractional parts of an unit.

7. NOTATION is the expressing by digits or figures any number proposed in words; and the reading of any number that is expressed by figures, is called NUMERATION.

8. DECIMAL NOTATION is that kind of numbering in which ten units of any inferior name are equal in value to an unit of the next superior.

9. Every number is said to consist of as many places as it contains figures.

10. The value of every digit in any number is changed according to the place it stands in; and the reading of any number consists in giving to each figure its right name and value.

11. The right hand place of an integer number is called the place of units; and from this place all numbers begin, whether *whole* or *fractional*; the integers increasing in order from the unit place towards the left; and the fractions decreasing in order from the unit place towards the right: and to distinguish decimal fractions from integers, there is always a point or comma (,) set on the left hand side of the fractional number; so that the integers stand on the left hand side of the mark, and the fractions on the right hand.

12. For the more convenient reading of numbers, they are divided into periods of six places each, beginning at the unit place; and each period into two degrees of three places each, the names and order of which are as follow: where X stands for the word tens, C for hundreds, and Th. for thousands.

13.

Integers															Decimal fractions												
		Second period						First period							First period						Second period						
		Degree			Degree			Degree			Degree				Degree			Degree			Degree			Degree			
&c.	Billions	C. Th. Millions	X. Th. Millions	Th. Millions	C. Millions	X. Millions	Millions	C. Thousands	X. Thousands	Thousands	Hundreds	Tens	Units		Tenths	Hundredths	Thousandths	X. Thousandths	C. Thousandths	Millionths.	X. Millionths	C. Millionths	Th. Millionths	X. Th. Millionths	C. Th. Millionths	Billionths	&c.
	5	4	3	2	1	2	3	4	5	6	7	8	9	,	8	7	6	5	4	3	2	1	2	3	4	5	

Decimal Fractions are also thus named,	Primes	Seconds	Thirds	Fourths	Fifths	Sixths	Sevenths	Eighths	Ninths	Tenths	Elevenths	Twelfths	&c.

The name of the first period is Units; of the second, Millions; of the third, Billions; of the fourth, Trillions; &c.

In the above order it may be observed, that each degree contains the names of Units, Tens, Hundreds; the first degree of a period contains the units of that period, and the second contains the thousandths thereof: so that from hence it will be easy to read a number consisting of ever so many places by the following directions.

14. RULE. 1st. Suppose the number parted into as many sets or degrees of three places each, beginning at the unit's place, as it will admit of; and if one or two places remain, they will be the units and tens of the next degree.

2d. Beginning at the left hand, read in each degree, as many hundreds, tens, and units, as the figures in those places of the degree express, adding the name thousands, if in the second degree of a period; and adding the name of the period, after reading the hundreds, tens, and units in its first degree.

Thus the integer number in the preceding table will be read.
Five billions, four hundred thirty two thousand, one hundred twenty three millions, four hundred fifty six thousand, seven hundred eighty nine.

15. All fractional numbers consist of two parts, which are usually written one above the other with a line drawn between them: the number below the line, called the *denominator*, shews into how many equal parts the unit is divided: the number above the line, called the *numerator*, shews by how many of these equal parts the value of that fraction is expressed.

Thus 9 pence, is 9 parts in twelve of a shilling; and may be written thus, $\frac{9}{12}$, *when a shilling is the unit.*

16. Those fractions, the denominators of which are 10, or 100, or 1000, or 10000, or 100000, &c. are called *decimal fractions*: but fractions with any other denominators are called *vulgar fractions.*

The vulgar fractions that most frequently occur, are these:

$\frac{1}{4}$, which is read one fourth, or one quarter.
$\frac{1}{3}$ - - - - - - - one third.
$\frac{1}{2}$ - - - - - - - one half.
$\frac{2}{3}$ - - - - - - - two thirds.
$\frac{3}{4}$ - - - - - - - three fourths, or three quarters.

17. As decimal fractions are parts of an unit divided into either 10, 100, 1000, 10000, &c. parts, according to the places in the fractional number; therefore they are read like whole numbers, only calling them so many parts of 10, or of 100, or of 1000, &c.

Thus a decimal fraction of	one two three four &c.	places, will be so many parts of	10, Ten. 100, Hundred. 1000, Thousand. 10000, Ten Thousand, &c.

18. Cyphers on the right hand of integers increase their value; on the left hand of a decimal fraction diminish its value: but on the left hand of integers, or on the right hand of fractions, do not alter their value.

 Thus

Thus	8 *is* 8 *units.*	*And*	,8 *is* 8 *parts in* 10		
	80 8 *tens.*		,08 8 *parts in* 100	*of an unit so divided.*	
	800 8 *hundreds.*		,008 8 *parts in* 1000		

When a fraction has no integer prefixed, it is convenient to put o in the place of units.

19. A Mixed Number, is when a fraction is annexed to a whole number.

Thus five and a half is called a mixed number, and is written $5\frac{1}{2}$, *or thus,* 5,5; *which is thus read, five and five tenths.*

20. Like names in different numbers are ſuch figures as ſtand equally diſtant from the place of units; or have the ſame denomination annexed to them.

Thus all numbers of pounds ſterling are like names, and ſo are all numbers of ſhillings; the like of any numbers of miles, &c.

21. Beſides the decimal notation explained in article 8, there are other kinds in common uſe; ſuch as the *duodecimal*, in which every ſuperior name contains 12 units of its next inferior name: the *Sexagenary*, or *Sexageſimal*, in which ſixty of an inferior name make one of its next ſuperior. The former is uſed by workmen in the meaſuring of artificers works in building; and the latter is uſed in the diviſion of a *Circle*, and of *Time*.

22. The following characters or marks are frequently uſed in Arithmetical computations, briefly to expreſs the manner of operation.

The mark + (more) belongs to addition; and ſhews that the numbers it ſtands between are to be added together.

Thus 12 + 3 *expreſſes the ſum of* 12 *and* 3; *or that* 3 *is to be added to* 12, *and is thus read,* 12 *more* 3.

The mark — (leſs) is for ſubtraction; and ſhews that the number following it, or on the right hand, is to be taken from the number preceding it, or on the left hand.

Thus 12 — 3, *expreſſes the difference between* 12 *and* 3; *or that* 3 *is to be ſubtracted from* 12, *and is thus read,* 12 *leſs* 3, *or* 12 *leſſened by* 3.

This mark × (into) for multiplication, ſhews that the numbers on each ſide of it are to be multiplied the one by the other.

Thus 12 × 3, *denotes the product of* 12 *into* 3; *or that* 12 *is to be multiplied by* 3.

Diviſion is expreſſed by ſetting the diviſor under the dividend with a line drawn between them, like a fraction.

Thus $\frac{12}{3}$, *expreſſes the quotient of* 12 *by* 3; *or that* 12 *is to be divided by* 3.

This ſign = (equal) ſhews that the reſult of the operation by the numbers or quantities on one ſide of it, is equal either to the numbers or quantities on the other ſide, or to the reſult of the operation by theſe numbers or quantities.

Thus 12+3=15; *and* 12—3=9; *and* 12×3=36; *and* $\frac{12}{3}$=4; *ſeverally ſhews the value of the preceding expreſſions.*

23. Tables

23. Tables of English Money, Weights, and Measures.

Money.

Farthings	Pence	Shill.	Pound
960 =	240 =	20 =	1 £.
48 =	12 =	1s.	
4 =	1d.		

Note, 1, 2, 3 farthings, are thus written, $\frac{1}{4}$, $\frac{1}{2}$, $\frac{3}{4}$.

Troy Weight.

Grains	Pennyw[ts]	Ounces	Pound
5760 =	240 =	12 =	1 lb.
480 =	20 =	1 oz.	
gr. 24 =	1 dwt.		

Note, Gold and Silver are weighed by Troy Weight.

Avoirdupoise Weight.

Drams	Ounces	Pounds	Hund.	Ton
573440 =	35840 =	2240 =	20 =	1
28672 =	1792 =	112 =	1 C.	
256 =	16 =	= 1lb.		
16 =	1 oz.			

Note, Provisions, Stores, &c. are weighed by the Avoirdupoise, or great weight.

Wine Measure.

Solid inch.	Pints.	Gall.	Hogsh.	Pipe	Tun
58212 =	2016 =	252 =	4 =	2 =	1
29106 =	1008 =	126 =	2 =	1 P.	
14553 =	504 =	63 =	1 Hhd.		
231 =	8 =	1			
		42 = 1 Tierce.			
		84 = 1 Puncheon.			

Dry Measure.

Pints	Gall.	Pecks	Bush.	Quarter
512 =	64 =	32 =	8 =	1
64 =	8 =	4 =	1	
16 =	2 =	1		
8 =	1			

Note, 4 bush. = 1 Comb: 10 qrs. = 1 Wey: 12 Weys = Last of Corn. 36 Bushels = 1 Chaldron of Coals.

Cloth Measure.

4 Nails	= 1	Quarter of a Yard.
4 Quarters	= 1	Yard.
5 Quarters	= 1	English ell.
3 Quarters	= 1	Flemish ell.
6 Quarters	= 1	French ell.
a Span	= 9	inches.
a Hand	= 4	inches.

Long Measure.

Barley corns	Inches	Feet	Yards	Poles	Furl.	Mile.
190080 =	63360 =	5280 =	1760 =	320 =	8 =	1
23760 =	7920 =	660 =	220 =	40 =	1	
594 =	198 =	$16\frac{1}{2}$ =	$5\frac{1}{2}$ =	1		
108 =	36 =	3 =	1			
36 =	12	1				
3 =	1					

Also 3 miles make 1 league.
And 20 leagues or 60 Sea miles make a degree.
But a degree contains about $69\frac{1}{2}$ miles of statute measure.
A fathom = 6 feet = 2 yards.

Time.

Seconds	Minutes	Hours	Days	Year
31556937 =	525948 =	8766 =	$365\frac{1}{4}$ =	1
86400 =	1440 =	24 =	1 day	
3600 =	60 =	1 hour.		
60 =	1			

Pence Table.

Pence	Sh. Pence	Pence	Sh. Pence
20 =	1 . 8	70 =	5 . 10
30 =	2 . 6	80 =	6 . 8
40 =	3 . 4	90 =	7 . 6
50 =	4 . 2	100 =	8 . 4
60 =	5 . 0	110 =	9 . 2

Even parts of a Pound Sterling.

s. d.	is	
10 . 0	$\frac{1}{2}$	of a Pound Sterling.
6 . 8	$\frac{1}{3}$	
5 . 0	$\frac{1}{4}$	
4 . 0	$\frac{1}{5}$	
3 . 4	$\frac{1}{6}$	
2 . 6	$\frac{1}{8}$	
2 . 0	$\frac{1}{10}$	

d.	is	of a Shilling, or	of a Pound.
6	$\frac{1}{2}$	[illegible]	
4	$\frac{1}{3}$	[illegible]	
3	$\frac{1}{4}$	[illegible]	
2	$\frac{1}{6}$	[illegible]	
$1\frac{1}{2}$	$\frac{1}{8}$		
$0\frac{3}{4}$	$\frac{1}{16}$		

24. SECTION II. ADDITION.

Addition *is the method of collecting ſeveral numbers into one ſum.*

Rule 1ſt. Write the given numbers under each other, ſo that like names ſtand under like names; that is units under units, tens under tens, &c. and under theſe draw a line.

2d. Add up the firſt or right hand upright row, under which write the overplus of the units of the ſecond row, contained in that ſum.

3. Add theſe units to the ſum of the ſecond row, under which write the overplus of the units of the third row, contained in that ſum.

And thus proceed until all the rows are added together.

Examples.

Ex. I. *Add* 28—76—47—18 *and* 12 *together.*

Theſe numbers being written under each other will ſtand thus. Say 2 and 8 is 10, and 7 is 17, and 6 is 23, and 8 is 31; then, becauſe 10 units in the right hand row make an unit in the next row; therefore in 31 there are 3 units of the ſecond row, and an overplus of 1; write down the 1, and add the 3 to the ſecond row, ſaying, 3 that is carried and 1 is 4, and 1 is 5, and 4 is 9, and 7 is 16, and 2 is 18, in which is one unit of the third row (had there been a 3d) and an overplus of 8; write down the 8, and add the 1 to the third row: but as there is no third row, the 1 carried muſt be written on the left hand of the 8; and 181 will be the ſum of the five given numbers.

28
76
47
18
12
181

Ex. II. *Add* 476—3784—18329—290—75—7638—*and* 46 *together.*

	476
	3784
The given numbers ſet in order will ſtand thus	18329
	290
	75
	7638
	46
The Sum	30638

Ex. III. *Add the numbers,* 10768—3489—28764—289—6438—19 *and* 438 *together.*

	10768
	3489
The given numbers placed as the rule directs, ſtand thus	28764
	289
	6438
	19
	438
The Sum	50205

Ex. IV. *Add theſe numbers together.*

	3720,45
	25,0036
	4179,802
	3,6284
Sum	7928,8840

Ex. V. *Add the following numbers together.*

	15836,071
	20,09
	34,7
	583,27008
Sum	16474,13108

In

In the two last examples, where there are both integer and fractional numbers, it may be obſerved, that like integer places, and like fractional places, ſtand under each other; and the manner of adding them together, is the ſame as explained in the firſt example.

25. It frequently happens, that numbers are to be added together, the names of which do not increaſe in a tenfold manner, as in the laſt Examples; ſuch as in adding different ſums of money, weights, or meaſures; in which, regard is to be had to the number of thoſe of a lower name, contained in one of its next greater name, as ſhewn in the preceding tables: Examples of which follow.

Ex. VI. *Add the following ſums of money together.*

£.	s.	d.
353	14	8½
276	10	4
89	17	5¼
34	12	10¾
754	15	4½

Ex. VII. *Add the following ſums of money together.*

£.	s.	d.
7683	08	2¼
954	19	9½
682	10	7¾
63	15	6¼
9384	14	2¼

In theſe two examples the carriage is by 4 in the farthings; by 12 in the pence; by 20 in the ſhillings; and by 10 in the pounds.

Ex. VIII. *Add the following Troy Weights together.*

lb.	oz.	dwt.	gr.
218	10	13	18
176	9	19	23
85	11	17	11
24	8	15	21
506	5	07	01

Carry for 24, 20, 12, 10.

Ex. IX. *Add the following Avoirdupoiſe Weights together.*

Tons.	Cwt.	qrs.	lb.	oz.
535	17	3	22	11
94	19	1	27	13
158	12	0	18	15
7	15	2	13	08
797	05	0	26	15

Carry for 16, 28, 4, 20, 10.

Ex. X. *Add the following parts of Time together.*

Weeks	Da.	Ho.	Min.	Sec.
21	4	18	37	59
11	6	13	25	47
19	3	23	59	28
38	4	08	22	39
91	5	16	25	53

Carry for 60, 60, 24, 7, 10.

Ex. XI. *Add the following parts of a Circle together.*

Deg.	′	″	‴	
176	32	59	43	25
85	59	27	31	59
114	28	45	59	14
67	12	38	24	47
444	13	51	39	25

Carry for 60, 60, 60, 60, 10

Explanation of Example VI.

Three farthings and 1 farthing is 4 farthings, and 2 farthings is 6 farthings; which is a penny halfpenny; ſet down ½ and carry 1.

Then 1 and 10 is 11, and 5 is 16, and 4 is 20, and 8 is 28 pence; which is 2 ſhillings and 4 pence: ſet down 4, and carry 2.

Again, 2 and 12 is 14, and 17 is 31, and 10 is 41, and 14 is 55 ſhillings; which is 2 pounds 15 ſhillings; ſet down 15 ſhillings, and carry 2 pounds. The reſt is eaſy.

26. SECTION III. SUBTRACTION.

Subtraction *is the method of taking one number from another, and ſhewing the remainder, or difference, or exceſs.*

The *ſubducend* is the number to be ſubtracted, or taken away.

The *minuend* is the number from which the ſubducend is to be taken.

Rule 1ſt. Under the minuend write the ſubducend, ſo that like names ſtand under like names; and under them draw a line.

2d. Beginning at the right-hand ſide, take each figure in the lower line from the figure ſtanding over it, and write the remainder, or what is left, beneath the line, under that figure.

3d. But if the figure below is greater than that above it, increaſe the upper figure by as many as are in an unit of the next greater name; from this ſum take the figure in the lower line, and write the remainder under it.

4th. To the next name in the lower line, carry the unit borrowed, and thus proceed to the higheſt denomination or name.

Examples.

Ex. I.	*From*	436565874	*the minuend,*
	Take	249853642	*the ſubducend,*
	Remains	186712232	*the difference.*

Here the five figures on the right of the ſubducend may be taken from thoſe over them: but the 6th figure, viz. 8, cannot be taken from the 5 above it. Now as an unit in the 7th place makes 10 in the 6th place, therefore borrowing this unit makes the 5, 15; then ſay, 8 from 15 leaves 7, which ſet down; and ſay 1 carried and 9 is 10, 10 from 6 cannot be had, but 10 from 16 leaves 6, ſet it down; then 1 carried and 4 is 5, 5 from 13 leaves 8; ſet it down: then 1 carried and 2 is 3, 3 from 4 leaves 1.

Ex. II.	*From*	7620908
	Take	3875092
	Remains	3745816

Ex. III.	*From*	327,9563
	Take	49,8697
	Remains	278,0866

Ex. IV.	*From*	30007,295
	Take	2536,876
	Leaves	27470,419

Ex. V.	*From*	5000,0000
	Take	479,6378
	Leaves	4520,3622

		£.	s.	d.
Ex. VI.	*Borrowed*	24	14	$6\frac{1}{2}$
	Paid	18	12	$4\frac{1}{4}$
	Remains	6	02	$2\frac{1}{4}$

		£.	s.	d.
Ex. VII.	*Lent*	294	15	$9\frac{1}{4}$
	Received	89	18	$10\frac{1}{4}$
	Remains	204	16	$10\frac{1}{2}$

Ex. VIII.

Ex. VIII. *In Sexagesimals.*

	°	′	″	‴	iv
From	76	28	37	49	32
Take	65	29	16	53	45
Leaves	10	59	20	55	47

Ex. IX. *In Sexagesimals.*

	°	′	″	‴	iv
From	218	46	32	50	18
Take	149	52	47	53	29
Leaves	68	53	44	56	49

27. QUESTIONS to exercise Addition and Subtraction.

QUEST. I. *The share of Jack's prize money was* 148£. 17*s.* 6*d*½; *and Tom received as much, beside* 7£. 18*s. smart money: How much money did Tom receive?*

	£.	s.	d.
Tom's prize money	148	17	6½
Smart money	7	18	0
Tom received	156	15	6½

QUEST. II. *The Spanish invasion was in the year* 1588, *and the French attempted an invasion in the year* 1744: *How many years were between these fruitless attempts?*

French	1744
Spanish	1588
Years between	156

QUEST. III. *What year was King George born in, he being* 67 *years old in the year* 1749?

Current year	1749
Age	67 subtr.
Year born in	1682

QUEST. IV. *Two ships depart from the same port, one having sailed* 835 *miles, is got* 48 *miles a-head of the other: Required the aftermost ship's distance?*

The first ship's distance	835
Their difference	48
Second ship's distance	787

QUEST. V. *A seaman who had received* 46£. 17*s.* 6*d. for wages, prize money, &c. meeting with bad company was tricked out of* 18 *guineas: Now John had reckoned to pay his wife's debts of* 13£. 16*s.* 6*d. and his landlady's bill of* 16£. 12*s.* *Required whether he can fulfil his intentions, and what the difference will be?*

	£.	s.	d.
Money lost	18	18	0
Wife's debt	13	16	6
Landlady's bill	16	12	0
Total	49	6	6
Money received	46	17	6
He will want	2	9	0

QUEST. VI. *Will and Frank talking of their ages in the year* 1749, *Will said he was born in the year of the Rebellion, in* 1715; *and Frank said he remembered he was ten years old the year King George the second was crowned in* 1727: *Required the age of each, and the difference of their ages?*

Current year	1749
Will was born	1715
Will's age	34
Current year	1749
King George crowned	1727
Years since	22
Frank's age then	10
Frank's age	32

So Will was oldest by two years.

28, SEC-

28. SECTION IV. MULTIPLICATION.

MULTIPLICATION *is the method of finding what a given number will amount to, when repeated as many times as is represented by another number.*

The number to be multiplied, is called the *Multiplicand.*

The number multiplied by, is called the *Multiplier.*

And the number which the multiplication amounts to, is called the *Product.*

Both multiplicand and multiplier are called *Factors.*

Before any operation can be performed in Multiplication, it is necessary that the learner should commit to memory the following table.

29. The MULTIPLICATION TABLE.

times	2	3	4	5	6	7	8	9	10	11	12
2	4	6	8	10	12	14	16	18	20	22	24
3		9	12	15	18	21	24	27	30	33	36
4			16	20	24	28	32	36	40	44	48
5				25	30	35	40	45	50	55	60
6					36	42	48	54	60	66	72
7						49	56	63	70	77	84
8							64	72	80	88	96
9								81	90	99	108
10									100	110	120
11										121	132
12											144

Observe, that in multiplying any figure in the upper line by any figure in the left-hand column, the product will stand right against the figure used in the left-hand column, and under that used in the upper line. Thus were 6 to be multiplied by 9, seek the greater figure 9 in the upper line, and right under it, against 6 in the left hand, stands 54 for the Product. And so of others.

The foregoing table being well known, the work of Multiplication will be performed as follows.

To multiply any number, as	37256
By any single figure, as by	7
Set them as in the margin, and proceed	260792

thus, 7 times 6 is 42, set down 2 and carry 4; 7 times 5 is 35 and 4 carried is 39, set down 9 and carry 3; 7 times 2 is 14 and 3 carried is 17, set down 7 and carry 1; 7 times 7 is 49 and 1 carried is 50, set down 0 and carry 5; 7 times 3 is 21 and 5 carried is 26, which set down, and the work is done. But for compound Multiplication take the following:

30. RULE 1st. Write the Factors so, that the right hand place of the Multiplier stands under the right hand place of the Multiplicand.

2d. Multiply the Multiplicand severally by every figure of the Multiplier, setting the first figure of each line under the figure then multiplying by.

3d. Add the several lines together; and their sum is the Product.

4th. From the right hand of the Product point off, for fractions, as many places as there are fractional places in both Factors; and those to the left of the mark of distinction are integers; those to the right are fractions.

5th. If

5th. If the number of places in the Product are not ſo many as the number of fractional places in both Factors, make up that number by writing cyphers on the left hand, and to theſe prefix the mark of diſtinction.

EXAMPLE I. *Multiply* 742 by 53.

Multiplicand	742	Factors.
Multiplier	53	
	2226	
	3710	
Product	39326	

The leſſer Factor being written under the greater Factor, as here ſhewn, and a line drawn under them; ſay 3 times 2 is 6, write 6 under the 3; then 3 times 4 is 12, write down 2 and carry 1; and 3 times 7 is 21, and 1 carried is 22, write the 22:- Again, 5 times 2 is 10, write 0 under the 5, and carry 1; and 5 times 4 is 20 and 1 carried is 21, write down 1 and carry 2; then 5 times 7 is 35, and 2 carried is 37, write down the 37: Now add the two lines together found by multiplying by 3 and by 5, and their ſum 39326 is the product required.

EXAMPLE II.

Multiply	28704
by	8631
	28704
	86112
	172224
	229632
	247744224 Product.

EXAMPLE III.

Multiply	3684,2795
by	7,594
	147371180
	331585155
	184213975
	257899565
	27978,4185230

Here, becauſe there are 4 fractional places in the Multiplicand, and 3 in the Multiplier, which together make 7, therefore 7 places are pointed off on the right of the product for fractions.

EXAMPLE IV.

Multiply	936,287
by	607,02
	1872574
	65540090
	56177220
	568344,93474

The cyphers in the Multiplier of this example are thus managed. Having multiplied by the 2 as before, ſay 0 times 7 is 0, write 0 under the 0, and proceed to the next figure 7, by which multiply as before, then coming to the ſecond 0, ſay, 0 times 7 is 0, write 0 under the place of the ſecond 0, and proceed to the next figure 6, by which multiply as before.

EXAMPLE V.

Multiply	0,34796
by	0,0258
	278368
	173980
	69592
	0,008977368

Here, becauſe there are 5 fractional places in one Factor, and 4 in the other, there ſhould be 9 fractional places in the Product; and there ariſing but 7, therefore two cyphers are ſet on the left hand to make 9 places.

31. SECTION V. DIVISION.

DIVISION *is the method of finding how often one number is contained in another; or may be taken from another.*

The number to be divided, is called the *Dividend.*

The number dividing by, is called the *Divisor.*

The *Quotient* is the number arising from the division, and shews how many times the Divisor is contained in the Dividend.

The operations in Division are performed as follow.

32. RULE 1st. On the right and left of the Dividend draw a crooked line; write the Divisor on the left side, and the Quotient, as it arises, on the right side of the Dividend.

2d. Seek how often the Divisor may be taken in as many figures on the left hand of the Dividend, as are just necessary; write the number of times it may be taken, in the Quotient; and there will be as many figures more in the Quotient, as there are figures remaining in the Dividend then not used.

3d. Multiply the Divisor by this Quotient-figure, set the Product under that part of the Dividend used; subtract, and to the right hand of the remainder bring down the next figure of the Dividend: Divide as before; and thus proceed until all the figures of the Dividend are used.

4th. If there is a remainder, to its right hand side annex a cypher or cyphers, as if brought down from the Dividend, and divide as before; and thus it is that fractions arise, viz. from the remainders in division.

5th. When any figure of the Dividend is taken down, or annexed, as before shewn, and the Divisor cannot be taken in the number thus increased; put o in the Quotient, and take down, or annex, another figure; and proceed in this manner, until the Divisor can be taken from the number.

6th. When fractions are concerned: From the number of fractional places used in the Dividend, take those in the Divisor; count the number of remaining places from the right of the Quotient, put the mark there; and those to the left are integers, those to the right fractions.

7th. If there arise not so many places in the Quotient as the 6th article requires, supply the places wanting with cyphers on the left, and to those prefix the fractional mark.

Ex. I. *Divide 3656 £. among 8 persons.*

```
8)3656(457
  32
  --
   45
   40
   --
    56
    56
    --
     0
```

Set the given numbers as in Art. 1st. Now the two left hand figures contain 8; then say 8 is contained in 36, 4 times; set 4 in the Quotient, and say 4 times 8 is 32, set 32 under 36, subtract, there remains 4, to which bring down the next figure of the Dividend 5, makes 45; then say 8 is contained in 45, 5 times; set 5 in the Quotient, and say 5 times 8 is 40; write 40 under 45, subtract, and to the remainder 5 take down 6, the next figure of the Dividend, makes 56; then say 8 is contained in 56, 7 times; write 7 in the Quotient, multiply 8 by 7 makes 56, which write under the other 56, and subtracting there remains o: So it may be concluded, that 3656 contains 8, 457 times: Or, if 3656 £. be divided among 8 persons, the share of each will be 457 £.

Ex. II.

Ex. II. *Divide* 3125 *by* 25.

```
25)3125(125
   25
   ---
    62
    50
   ---
    125
    125
   ---
     0
```

Ex. III. *Divide* 95269 *by* 47.

```
47)95269(2027
   94
   ---
See precept 5th. 126
                  94
                 ---
                 329
                 329
                 ---
                   0
```

Ex. IV. *Divide* 5859 *by* 124.

```
124)5859(47,25
    496
    ---
     899
     868
     ---
      310 for the Remaind.
      248 See precept 4th.
      ---
      620
      620
      ---
```

Ex. V. *Divide* 337,27368 *by* 6,28.

```
6,28)337,27368(53,706  for
     3140        the Quotient.
     ----        See precept 6th.
      2327
      1884
      ----
       4433
       4396
       ----
See precept 5th. 3768
                 3768
                 ----
```

Ex. VI. *Divide* 2,3569 *by* 673,4.

```
673,4)2,3569(35
      20202   Quot. 0,0035
      -----
       33670 See precepts
       33670 4th, 6th, 7th.
       -----
```

In Ex. VI. the 4 fractional places given in the Dividend, and the o used with the Remainder, make 5 fractional places; from which 1 place in the Divisor being taken, leaves 4 fractional places for the Quotient; but in the Quotient are only the two places 35, therefore 2 cyphers are prefixed, and makes ,0035, before which, for form sake, an o is set for the place of units.

33. When the Divisor does not exceed the number 12, the Division may be performed in one line; by making the Multiplication and Subtraction mentally, or in the mind, and carrying the Remainder, as so many tens, to the next figure.

34. In all operations of Division, it must be observed, that the Product of the Divisor by the Quotient figure must not exceed that part of the Dividend then using; and the Remainder, by subtracting the Product, must ever be less than the Divisor.

As the Quotient multiplied by the Divisor makes the Dividend;

So the Product of two numbers being divided by one of them, will give the other; that is, Division is proved by Multiplication, and Multiplication is proved by Division.

35. SECTION VI. REDUCTION.

Reduction *is the method of reducing numbers from one name, or denomination, to another; retaining the ſame value.*

Case I. *To reduce a number conſiſting of ſeveral names, to their leaſt name.*

Rule 1ſt. Multiply the firſt, or greater name, by the parts which an unit of that name contains of the next leſs name; adding to the Product the parts of the ſecond name in the given number.

2d. Multiply this ſum by the number of times that an unit of the next leſs name is contained in one of the ſecond name; adding to the Product the parts of the third name contained in the given number: And thus proceed, until the leaſt name in the given number is arrived at.

Ex. I. *In 23£. 14s. 6½d. how many farthings?*

```
        £.  s.  d.
        23  14  6½
        20
       ----
       474 Shillings.
        12
       ----
      5694 Pence.
         4
      -----
Anſwer 22778 Farthings.
```

Ex. II. *In 8lb. 10oz. of gold, how many grains?*

```
 lb. oz.
  8  10
 12
 ----
 106 Ounces.
  20
 ----
2120 Pennyweights.
  24
 ----
 8480
4240
 -----
50880 Grains.
```

Ex. III. *In a cannon weighing 2 Tons, 14C. 3qrs. 19lb. how many pounds?*

```
 T.  C. Qrs. lb.
 2  14   3   19
20
---
 54 C. weight.
  4
---
219 Qrs.
 28
---
1771
438
----
6151 Pounds.
```

Ex. IV. *In 36 deg. 48′. 27″. 56‴. how many thirds?*

```
   °    ′    ″    ‴
  36   48   27   56
  60
  ----
  2208 Minutes.
    60
  ------
132507 Seconds.
    60
  -------
7950476 Thirds.
```

An explanation of the firſt Ex. will make all the reſt plain. Since pounds is the greateſt name in the given number, and an unit thereof contains 20 of the next leſs name, or ſhillings; therefore multiply the pounds by 20, ſaying 0 times 3 is 0, to which adding the 4 in the 14s. makes 4; then 2 times 3 is 6, and the one, in the place of tens in the ſhillings, makes 7; then 2 times 2 is 4: Now multiply 474s. by 12, ſaying 12 times 4 is 48, and the 6 in the pence makes 54; write 4 and carry 5; then 12 times 7 is 84 and 5 is 89, &c. Laſtly, multiply the 5694 pence by 4, ſaying 4 times 4 is 16, and the two farthings in the given number is 18; write 8 and carry 1, &c.

36. Case

36. Case II. *A number of an inferior name being given; to find how many of each superior denomination are contained in it.*

Rule 1ſt. Divide the given number, by the number of times that one of its units is contained in an unit of the next ſuperior name.

2d. Divide this Quotient by the parts making one of the next name.

3d. Divide this Quotient by the parts making one of the next name: And proceed in this manner, until the higheſt name is obtained.

4th. Then the laſt Quotient, and the ſeveral remainders, will be the parts of the different names contained in the given number.

Ex. I. *In 22778 farthings, how many pounds, ſhillings, and pence?*

4)22778(2 Farthings.

12) 5694(6 Pence.

2,0) 47,4(14 Shillings.

23 Pounds.

Anſwer 23 £. 14*s.* 6½*d.*

Ex. II. *In 7950476 thirds of a degree, how many* ° ' '' '''?

6,0)795047,6(56 Thirds.

6,0)13250,7(27 Seconds.

6,0) 220,8(48 Minutes.

36 Degrees.

Anſwer 36°. 48'. 27''. 56'''.

Ex. III. *In 6151 pounds, how many Tons, Hundreds, Quarters, Pounds?*

28)6151(219
56
—
55
28
—
271
252
—
19 Pounds.

4)219(3 Qrs.

2,0)5,4(14 C.

2 Tons.

Anſwer 2 T. 14 C. 3 Qrs. 19 lb.

Ex. IV. *In 50880 grains, how many Pounds, Ounces, Pennyweights, Grs.*

24)50880(2120
48
—
28
24
—
48
48
—
0

2,0)212,0(0 dwt.

12) 106(10 oz.

8 lb.

Anſwer 8 lb. 10 oz.

Explanation of Ex. I. Since 4 of the given number make one of the next name, pence, then 22778 divided by 4, give 5694 pence, and a Remainder of 2 farthings; then 5694 pence divided by 12, the number of pence in one of the next name, ſhillings, the Quotient is 474 ſhillings, and a Remainder of 6 pence; then 474 ſhillings divided by 20, the number of ſhillings in one of the next name, pounds, the Quotient is 23 pounds, and a Remainder of 14 ſhillings. And by the 4th precept, the anſwer is collected.

A like operation will ſolve the other examples, having regard to the increaſe of the different names.

37. In any Diviſion, if the Diviſor has one or more cyphers on the right hand, thoſe cyphers may be pointed off; but then as many places muſt be pointed off from the Dividend, which places are not to be divided, but annexed to the right hand of the Remainder. See the above examples.

38. Case

38. Case III. *To reduce a vulgar fraction to its equivalent decimal fraction.*

Rule. To the Numerator annex one or more cyphers, divide this by the Denominator, and the Quotient will be the fraction sought.

If the Division does not end when six figures are found in the Quotient, the work need not be carried any farther.

Exam. I. *To reduce* $\frac{15}{423}$ *to its equivalent decimal fraction.*

```
423)15,00(0,03546
    1269
    ----
     2310
     2115
     ----
      1950
      1692
      ----
       2580
       2538
       ----
        420
```

Here 423 the Denominator is made the Divisor, and 15 the Numerator is set for the Dividend, to which annexing a cypher or two for fractional places, seek how often the Divisor can be had in 15, the integral part of the Dividend; and as it cannot be taken, put o in the Quotient for the place of units: Then taking in one fractional place, seek how oft the Divisor can be had in 150, say o times, and put another o in the Quotient for the place of primes: Now taking in two fractional places to the 15, the Divisor will be contained in it thrice, and thus proceed until the Division ends, or till 6 places arise in the Qotient: But in this example, as the 6th place would be o, it is omitted, because cyphers on the right hand of decimal fractions are of no signification, as will evidently appear, Notation of Fractions being well understood.

Ex. II. *Reduce* $\frac{1}{2}$ *to a decimal fraction.*

2)1,0(0,5 Answer.

Ex. III. *Reduce* $\frac{1}{4}$ *to a decimal fraction.*

4)1,00(0,25 Answer.

Ex. IV. *Reduce* $\frac{3}{4}$ *to a decimal fraction.*

4)3,00(0,75 Answer.

Ex. V. *Reduce* $\frac{5}{8}$ *to a decimal fraction.*

8)5,000(0,625 Answer.

Ex. VI. *Reduce* $\frac{1}{3}$ *to a decimal fraction.*

3)1,00(0,33, &c. Answer.

Ex. VII. *Reduce* $\frac{7}{12}$ *to a decimal fraction.*

12)7,0000(0,5833 &c. Answ.

39. In the two last Quotients, it may be observed, that 3 would continually arise; such decimal fractions are called circulating, or recurring fractions: These have a peculiar kind of operation belonging to them, which the inquisitive reader will find in a book intitled *A General Treatise of Mensuration**, the third edition, published in the year 1767; and also in other books.

* By the Author of these Elements.

40. Case IV. *To reduce a number consisting of different names, to a decimal fraction of its greatest name.*

Rule 1st. Write the given names orderly under one another, the least name being uppermost; and on their left side draw a line: Let these be reckoned as Dividends.

2d. Against each name, on the left hand, write the number making one of its next superior name: And let these be the Divisors to the former Dividends.

3d. Begin with the upper one, and write the Quotient of each division as fractions, on the right of the Dividend next below it; then let this mixed number be divided by its Divisor, &c.

And the last Quotient will be the decimal fraction sought.

Ex. I. *Reduce* 15*s.* $9\frac{3}{4}$*d. to the fractional part of a pound sterling.*

4	3
12	9,75
20	15,8125
	0,790625

First set the three farthings, the 9 pence, the 15 shillings and 0 pounds under one another; and against the farthings set 4, against the pence set 12, and against the shillings, 20; then the three with cyphers supposed to be annexed, being divided by 4, the Quotient ,75 is written on the right hand of the 9 pence; and the mixed number 9,75 with cyphers annexed as they are wanted, being divided by 12, the Quotient ,8125 is written on the right hand of the 15*s.* then this mixed number 15,8125 being divided by 20, the Quotient 0,790625£. is the answer.

Ex. II. *Reduce* 1*s.* $2\frac{1}{4}$*d. to the fractional part of a pound sterling.*

4	1
12	2,25
20	1,1875
	0,059375

Answer 1*s.* $2\frac{1}{4}$*d.*=0,059375£.

Ex. III. *Reduce* 48′. 17″. 53‴. *to the fractional part of a degree.*

60	53
60	17,883333
60	48,298055
	0,804967

Answ. 48′. 17″. 53‴.=0,804967 Deg

Ex. IV. *Reduce* 8*oz.* 15*dwt.* 18*gr. to the fractional part of a pound troy.*

24 {	4	18
	6	(4.5
20		15,75
12		8,7875
		0.732291

Ans. 8oz. 15dwt. 18 gr =0,732291lb.

Ex. V. *Reduce* 3*qrs.* 19*lb.* 14*oz. to the fractional part of a C. weight.*

16 {	4	14
	4	(3,5
28 {	4	19,875
	7	(4.96875
4		3,709821
		0,927455

Answ. 3qr. 19lb. 14oz=0,927455 C.

41. Here because 24 is a number too great to divide by in one line, therefore it is broken into the parts 4 and 6, which multiplied together make 24.

Here the 16 is broken into the numbers 4 and 4; and 28 into 4 and 7; and 14 is divided by 4; and the Quotient 3,5 by 4, &c.

42. Case V. *To reduce a decimal fraction of a superior name, to its value in inferior denominations.*

Rule 1st. Multiply the given fraction by the number that an unit of its name contains units of the next lesser name; from the right hand of the Product point off as many places as there are in the given fraction.

2d. Multiply the places, so pointed off, by as many as an unit of this name contains of the next less name; point off as before.

And thus proceed until the multiplication is made by the least name.

3d. Then the integers, or the numbers on the left of the distinguishing marks in each Product, will be the parts in each name, which together are equal to the given fraction.

Example I. *What number of shillings, pence, and farthings, are equal in value to 0,790625£. sterling.*

£.	0,790625
	20
s.	15,812500
	12
d.	9,750000
	4
far.	3,000000

Here an unit of the given name £. contains 20 of the next less name, shillings; then multiplying by 20, and pointing off 6 places on the right, because the given number 0,790625 contains 6 fractional places, the Product is 15,812500 shillings; then the fractions of this number, *viz.* 812500 multiplied by 12, the number that an unit of this name contains of the next less name, and the product pointed as before, there arises 9,750000 pence; the fractions of this number multiplied by 4, gives 3,000000 farthings; then the parts pointed off on the left, *viz.* 15s. 9¾d. are the value of the given fraction.

Example II. *What is the value of 0,056285£. sterling?*

£.	0,056285
	20
s.	1,1257|00
	12
d.	1,5084
	4
far.	2,0336

Example III. *What is the value of 0,58695 degrees?*

Deg.	0,58695
	60
Min.	35,217|00
	60
Sec.	13,02|0
	60
Thirds	0,120

Example IV. *What is the value of 0,732291lb. troy?*

This example worked as above, by multiplying by 12, 20, 24, the value will be found to be

8oz. 15dwts. 18gr. nearly.

Example V. *What is the value of 0,927455 part of a C. weight?*

By operating as above, multiplying by 4, 28, 16, the answer will be

3qrs. 19lb. 14oz. nearly.

43. Quest.

43. QUESTIONS to exerciſe the preceding rules.

QUEST. I. *A ſloop with the captain and 26 hands take a prize which ſold for 1578 £. of which each ſeaman had 45 £. and the captain the reſt: How much was his ſhare?*

26 Men
45 £. to each

130
104

ſubtract 1170 £. the crew's ſhare.
from 1578 £. the whole prize.

remains 408 £. the captain's ſhare.

QUEST. II. *A boat's crew of 15 men got by plunder 321 £. How much was the ſhare of each?*

15)321(21 £.
30

21
15

remains 6 £. which
mult. by 20 s. in 1 £.

15)120 s. (8 s.
120

Anſwer 21 £. 8 s. to each.

QUEST. III. *A ſeaman, whoſe wages are 35 s. 6 d. a month, returns home at the end of 29 months; he having taken up 12 £. 18 s.: How much has he to receive?*

s. d.
35 6
mult. by 12

426 pence a month,
mult. by 29 months,

3834
852

12)12354 pence

2,0) 102,9 6 d.

from 51 £. 9 s. 6 d. = wages,
take 12 £. 18 s. 0 d. received,

remains 38 £. 11 s. 6 d. to receive.

QUEST. IV. *Six meſs-mates, who propoſe to live well during an Eaſt-India voyage of 22 months, agree to expend among them 5 s. a day, beſides the ſhip's allowance: Now one of them having but 25 s. a month, how will matters ſtand with him at the end of the voyage?*

Now 28 days, at 5 s. a day, makes 140 s. or 7 £. a month; which for 22 months, is 154 £.

Then a ſixth part of 154 £. is 25 £. 13 s. 4 d. for each man.

Alſo 25 s. a month for 22 months makes 27 £. 10 s. for wages; which will overpay his expences, by 1 £. 16 s. 8 d.

QUEST. V. *In 306 crowns, how many half crowns and pence?*

Anſwer { 612 half crowns.
18360 pence.

QUEST. VI. *In 30 chalders of coals, each of 36 buſhels, how many pecks?*

Anſwer 4320 pecks.

QUEST. VII. *A ſeaman's ſhare of a prize was 14 guineas, 32 moidores, 12 thirty-ſix ſhillings pieces, and 52 piſtoles at 17 s. each: How much ſterling did the whole come to?*

Anſwer 123 £. 14 s.

QUEST. VIII. *Suppoſe a ſhip ſails $5\frac{1}{2}$ miles an hour for 14 days: How many degrees and minutes has ſhe ſailed in the whole; 60 ſea miles making one degree?*

Anſwer 30 deg. 48 min.

SECTION VII. Of PROPORTION:

Or, THE RULE OF THREE.

44. Four numbers are ſaid to be proportional, when by comparing them together by two and two, they either give equal Products or equal Quotients.

Suppoſe theſe four numbers 3 8 12 32

In comparing them together by multiplication,

The Product	of 3 and 8 is 24;	of 12 and 32 is 384,	unequal.
	of 3 and 12 is 36;	of 8 and 32 is 256,	unequal.
	of 3 and 32 is 96;	of 8 and 12 is 96,	equal.

Therefore 3 8 12 32, are called proportional numbers.

Now let them be compared together by diviſion.

The Quotient	of 8 by 3 is 2,6&c.	of 32 by 12 is 2,6 &c.	equal.
	of 12 by 3 is 4	of 32 by 8 is 4,	equal.
	of 32 by 3 is 10,6&c.	of 12 by 8 is 1,5,	unequal.

Therefore by this compariſon, the numbers are ſaid to be proportional.

In this kind of comparing four numbers together, there is no need to try for more equal Products, or Quotients, than one ſet of either ſort; for either caſe will determine the proportionality independent of the other.

But it muſt be obſerved, that among four proportional numbers, there will be but one ſet of equal Products, and two ſets of equal Quotients, the ſmaller numbers being Diviſors.

45. When four numbers are to be written as proportionals, they muſt be placed in ſuch order, that the Product of the firſt and fourth be equal to the Product of the ſecond and third.

A queſtion is ſaid to belong to the *Rule of Three*, when three numbers or terms are given to ſind a fourth proportional, which is the anſwer to the queſtion.

And in order to reſolve ſuch queſtions, the three given terms muſt be firſt placed in a proper order, which is called ſtating the terms of the queſtion.

46. Queſtions in the *Rule of Three* are ſtated, and reſolved by the following precepts.

1ſt. Conſider of what kind the fourth term, or number ſought, will be, whether money, weight, meaſure, time, &c. and among the three numbers given in the queſtion let that which is of the ſame kind with what is required be placed for the third term.

2d. From the nature of the queſtion, determine whether the number ſought will be greater or leſs than the number which is placed for the third term.

3d. If the fourth term will be greater than the third, ſet the greater of the remaining two terms for the ſecond, and the leſs for the firſt.

But if the fourth term is to be leſs than the third, ſet the greater of the remaining two terms for the firſt, and the leſs for the ſecond.

Then in either caſe, the given three terms are ſtated.

4th. Reduce thoſe terms which conſiſt of more names than one, to one name; and obſerve that the firſt and ſecond terms are always to be of the ſame name.

5th. Multiply the ſecond and third terms together, divide the product by the firſt term, and the Quotient will be the fourth term, of the ſame name the third term was reduced to.

47. QUEST. I. *If 4 yards of cloth coſt 18 s. what will 24 yards coſt?*

Here it is plain, that the term ſought, or the worth of 24 yards, will be money; therefore the given money 18 *s.* is ſet for the third term; and as the worth of 24 yards muſt be greater than the worth of 4 yards, therefore the 24 is ſet for the 2d term, and the 4 for the 1ſt. Then the 2d term 24 being multiplied by the 3d, 18, the Product is 432, which divided by the 1ſt term 4, the Quotient or 4th term is 108, which are ſhillings, the ſame name of the 3d term; then 108 ſhillings divided by 20, gives 5 £. 8 *s.*

```
yds.  yds.   s.
 4 — 24 — 18
      18
     ———
     192
      24
     ———
  4)432( 108 ſhillings.
  ———  ———
  2,0) 10,8 ſhillings.
       ———
        5 pounds.
```

Anſwer 5 £. 8 *s.*

QUEST. II. *If I lend 200 £. for 12 months, how long ought I to have the uſe of 150 £. to recompence me?*

Here the anſwer or 4th term is to be time; therefore let 12 months, the given time, be ſet for the 3d term: Now it is evident, that the 150 £. being leſs than the 200 £. muſt be kept a longer time, and ſo the 4th term will be greater than the 3d term: Therefore the 200 is put for the 2d term, and the 150 for the 1ſt. Then the 2d term multiplied by the 3d, the Product will be 2400; which being divided by the 1ſt term, the Quotient 16 is the 4th term; and becauſe the 3d term was months, the 4th term will be months.

```
 £.    £.    m.
150 — 200 — 12
             12
           ———
15,0)240,0(16 months.
      15
     ———
      90
      90
     ———
```

Anſwer 16 months.

QUEST. III. *What will 1836 lb. of raisins come to, at the rate of 6 s. 8 d. for 24 lb.?*

Here as money is the thing sought, money must be the 3d term: And as 6 s. 8 d. consists of two names, they must be reduced to one name, *viz.* pence.

```
lb.    lb.      s.  d.
24 —— 1836 ——— 6   8
                6   8
    1836       12
      80       —
    ———      80d.=3d term.
24)146880(6120d.=4th term.
   144     ———
   ———   | 12)6120
     28  |    ———
     24  | 2,0)51,0 ( 10s.
     ——  |     ———
     48       25 £.
     48
     ——
      0
```

Here the 2d term being multiplied by the 3d, and the Product divided by the first, the quotient is 6120 pence; which being valued, gives 25 £. 10 s.

QUEST. IV. *If 20 yards of cloth, 5 quarters wide, will serve to hang a room: How many yards of 4 quarters wide will serve to hang the same room?*

Here yards of length are required; then 20 yards must be the 3d term.

```
qrs.  qrs.   yds.
4 ——— 5 ——— 20
              5
             ——
        4)100(
          ———
Answer 25 yards.
```

QUEST. V. *What will 420 yards of cloth come to, at 14 s. 10¼ d. for 1 ell English?*

The term sought being money, the 14 s. 10¼ d. must be the 3d term, and be reduced to farthings; also the 1st and 2d terms are to be reduced to quarters of a yard.

```
Ell Eng. yds.      s.   d.
1 ——— 420 ——— 14  10¼
1      420      14  10¼
5        4      12
——     ———    | ———
5     1680    | 178
       715    |   4
      ————    | ———
      8400    | 715 far.=3d term.
     1680
    11760
    —————
  5)1201200(
    —————
  4)240240  farthings=4th term.
    ——————
 12)60060  pence.
    —————
 2,0)500,5  5 shillings.
    —————
     250  pounds.
   Answer 250 £. 5 s.
```

The Divisor 5 being a single digit, the Quot. is written under the Divid.

QUEST. VI. *A owes to B 463 £. but compounds for 7 s. 6 d. in the pound: How much must B receive for his debt?*

Here composition money is the thing sought; then the 3d term must be the composition money, *viz.* 7 s. 6 d.

```
£.     £.        s.  d.
1 ——— 463 ——— 7   6
       90    | 12
     ————    | ——
12)41670(6d. | 90 pence.
 2,0)347,2 (12s.
     ———
     173
Answer 173 £. 12 s. 6 d.
```

48. As it will be more convenient in most cases to reduce such numbers, or terms, which consist of several names, to the fractional parts of their greatest name, than to reduce them to their lowest name; therefore in the solution of some of the following questions, the inferior parts of the given terms are reduced by Case IV. of Reduction; and the answers are valued by Case V.

QUEST.

QUEST. VII. *If 8lb. of pepper cost 4s. 8d.: What will 7 C. 3qrs. 14lb. come to at that rate?*

```
lb.   C.  qrs. lb.      s.  d.
8 —— 7   3   14 —— 4   8
     4                12
     —                —
     31               56
     28      882lb.   —
     ——       56
     262     ——
     62     5292
     ——    4410
     882   ——
     ——   8)49392
          ——
         12)6174   6d.
          ——
        2,0)51,4   14s.
          ——
           25 £.
```

Anſwer 25 £. 14s. 6d.

QUEST. VIII. *One bought 4 Hhds. of ſugar, each containing 6 C. 2qrs. 14lb. at 2£. 8s. 6d. for each C. weight: What did the whole come to?*

```
C.     C. qrs. lb.      £. s. d.
1 —— 6   2   14 —— 2  8  6
```

Now 1 C. weight is 112lb.
And 4 Hh. at 6C. 2q. 14lb=2968lb.
Alſo 2£. 8s. 6d. is 582d.
Then the Product of the 2d and 3d terms is 1727376.
Which divided by the 1ſt term 112, the Quotient is 15423 pence, whoſe value is 64£. 5s. 3d.

QUEST. IX. *What is the intereſt of 584£. for a year, at 5 per cent. per annum: Or at the rate of 5£. for the uſe of 100£. for a year?*

Here intereſt is the term required; therefore 5£. the intereſt of 100£. is to be the 3d term: And as the 4th term, or the intereſt of 584£. is greater than the 3d term; then the 2d term is to be greater than the 1ſt.

```
£.         £.        £.
100 —— 584 —— 5
            5
1,00)29,20( See Caſe V. of
     —      Reduction.
      20
      ——
     4,00
      ——
```

Anſwer 29 £. 4s.

QUEST. X. *What is the intereſt of 387£. 12s. for three years and 4 months, at $3\frac{1}{2}$ per cent. per annum?*

Find the intereſt for 1 year; then thrice that, together with $\frac{1}{3}$ of one year, will be the intereſt ſought.

```
£.        £.          £.
100 —— 387,6 —— 3,5
           3,5
          ——
         19380
        11628
         ——
  100) 1356,60(
        13,566 for 1 year.
             3
         ——
        40,698 for 3 years.
1/3 of 1 year=4,522 for 4 months.
The ſum 45,220 is the intereſt.
         ——
```

Anſwer 45 £. 4s. 5d.

QUEST. XI. *What is the intereſt of 542£. 10s. for 219 days, at 5£. per cent. per annum?*

To ſolve this queſtion, find the intereſt for 1 year; multiply this intereſt by 219, and divide the Product by 365, the Quotient will be the anſwer; and is 16£. 5s. 6d.

QUEST. XII. *For how long muſt 487£. 10s. be at ſimple intereſt, at $4\frac{1}{2}$£. per cent. per annum. to gain 95£. 1s. 3d.?*

Find what will be the intereſt of 487£. 10s. for 1 year; divide 95£. 1s. 3d. by this intereſt, and the Quotient will be $4\frac{1}{3}$ years.

QUEST. XIII. *One bought 14 pipes of wine, and is allowed 6 months credit: But for ready money gets it 6d. in a gallon cheaper: How much did he save by paying ready money?*

Answer 44£. 2

QUEST. XIV. *A clothier sold 50 pieces of kersey, each piece containing 34 ells Flemish, at the rate of 8s. 4d. per ell English: What did the whole come to?*

Answer 425£.

QUEST. XV. *One bought 3 tons of oil for 153£. 9s. which having leaked 74 gallons, he would make the prime-cost of the remainder: How must it be sold per gallon?*

Now 1 T.=252 Gall. And 3 T.=756
Subtract the gallons leaked= 74

Remains 682

G. G. £.
Then 682 —— 1 —— 153,45
Answer 4s. 6d. a gallon.

QUEST. XVI. *A broker sold $\frac{2}{5}$ of $\frac{3}{4}$ of a ship for 147£. 11s. 3d.: How much was the whole ship valued at?*

Now $\frac{2}{5}$ of $\frac{3}{4}=\frac{2}{5}\times\frac{3}{4}=\frac{6}{20}=\frac{3}{10}$ by art. 38.
For 2×3=6, a new numerator.
And 5×4=20, a new denominator.
Also 147£. 11s. 3d.=147,5625. art. 40.

share share £.
Then 0,3 —— 1 —— 147,5625 art. 46.

Answer 491£. 17s. 6d.

QUEST. XVII. *At 13£. for 100lb. of goods: What will 895lb. come to, allowing 4lb. upon every 100lb. for tret, or waste?*

Since 4lb. is to be allowed on the 100lb. therefore 104lb. is given for 100.

lb. lb. £.
Then 104 —— 895 —— 13

Answer 111£. 17s. 6d.

QUEST. XVIII. *One has cloth which cost 2s. 8d. a yard: For how much must it be sold a yard on 3 months credit, to gain 25£. per cent. per annum?*

mon. mon. £. £.
First 12 — 3 — 25 — 6,25
£. £. £.
Secondly 100—6,25——0,133333
By multiplying and dividing, the 4th term will be found 2d.
Then 2s. 8d.+2d.=2s. 10d. a yard, the selling price.

QUEST. XIX. *If 100 pounds of sugar be worth 36s. 8d. What will be the worth of 875lb. rebating 4lb. upon every 100lb. for tare?*

Here the buyer has 100lb. on paying for 96lb.

lb. lb. lb.
Then 100 —— 96 —— 875
And the 4th term will be 840lb.
Also 100 —— 840 —— 1,833333

Then the 4th term will be 15£. 8s. and so much will the sugar come to.

QUEST. XX. *A chapman bought 81 kerseys for 135£.: How must he sell them per piece to gain 15£. per cent?*

Find how much 135£. will be advanced to, at 15£. per cent.

Then this sum divided by 81 will be the selling price of each piece.

£. £. £. £.
Now 100 — 115 — 135 — 155,25
Then 81) 155,25 (1,916666£.
Answer 1£. 18s. 4d. a-piece.

QUEST.

QUEST. XXI. *A merchant who is to receive a sum of money, is offered ducats at 6s. 4d. which are worth but 6s. 2½d. or chequins at 8s. 2d. each, that are worth but 8s: By which specie will he sustain the least loss?*

6s. 2½d.=74, 5d. } the real value.
8s. 0 d.=96 }
6s. 4 d.=76 } the advan. val.
8s. 2 d.=98 }

r. val. r. val. ad. val. ad. val.
Then 74,5 —— 96 —— 76 —— 97,93

But the chequins are valued at 98 d. Therefore the ducats are most advantageous.

QUEST. XXII. *One who had sold a parcel of cloths at 2s. 10d. a yard on 3 months credit, found he had gained 25£. per cent. per annum: What did the cloth cost per yard?*

mo. £. mo. £.
Now 12——25——3——6,25
And 100+6,25=106,25 £.
£. £. £.
Then 106,25—100—0,14166

The fourth term to which will be a fraction, the value of which will be 2s. 8d. which is the prime cost per yard of the cloth.

QUEST. XXIII. *A person wants 750 pieces of foreign coin, each worth 11s. 4d. How much will they come to, allowing the broker the worth of 2 pieces upon every 100?*

Now 100 —— 102 —— 750 —— 765. He must pay for 765 pieces, which will come to 433 £. 10s.

QUEST. XXIV. *A gentleman would exchange 729 pieces of 4s. 2d. each into sterling money: How much will he receive for them, allowing the broker 1¼£. per cent.?*

P. P. £. £.
Now 1—729—0,208333—151,875
the worth of the pieces.
Then 101,25—100—151,875—150£.
He will receive 150£. for them.

QUEST. XXV. *A grocer bought 4¼ C. of pepper for 15£. 17s. 4d. which proving to be damaged, he is willing to lose 12½£. per cent. For how much must he sell it a lb.?*

Since he is to lose 12½ per cent. he must take 87£. 10s. for 100£. Now diminish the 15£. 17s. 4d. in this proportion, and this sum divided by the pounds in 4¼ C. will give 7d. for what each pound is to be sold at.

QUEST. XXVI. *Suppose 42 gallons of honey be valued at 2£. and the duty is 15£. per cent. on this value, and a drawback of 5£. per cent. on the duty for prompt payment: What will the ready money duty of 672 gallons come to?*

Now 42G. : 672G. : : 2£. : 32£.
And 100£. : 15£. : : 32£. : 4,8£.
Also 100£. : 95£. : : 4,8£. : 4,56£.

Answer 4£. 11s. 2½d.

The Rule of Proportion is of almost universal use in all business where computation is required; as in buying and selling, values of stocks and their dividends; the interest and discount of money; the customs and duties on goods, &c. But the designed brevity of this book will not permit farther illustrations.

SEC-

SECTION VIII. OF THE POWERS OF NUMBERS, AND OF THEIR ROOTS.

49. *The* Power *of a number, is a product arising by multiplying that number by itself, the product by the same number, this product by the same number again, &c. to any number of multiplications.*

50. The given number is called the first power or root.
The Product of the 1st power by itself, is the second power, or square.
The Product of the 2d power by the 1st, is the 3d power, or cube.
The Product of the 3d power by the 1st, is the 4th power, &c.

51. Here follow the 1st, 2d, and 3d powers of the nine digits.

Roots, or 1st power	1	2	3	4	5	6	7	8	9
Squares, or 2d power	1	4	9	16	25	36	49	64	81
Cubes, or 3d power	1	8	27	64	125	216	343	512	729

Ex. I. *What is the 2d power, or square of the number 24?*

24×24=576 is the 2d power.

Ex. II. *What is the 3d power, or cube of 38?*
Now 38×38=1444 the 2d power.
Then 1444×38=54872 the 3d power.

The figure, or number, shewing the name of any power, is called the index of that power.

Thus 1 is the index of the first power: 2 is the index of the 2d power; 3 of the third power, *&c.* Also $\frac{1}{2}$ is the index of the square root; $\frac{1}{3}$, the index of the cube root, *&c.*

52. Any number may be considered as a power of some other number.

Thus 64 may be taken as the 2d power of 8, and the third power of 4, *&c.*

53. The root of a given number, considered as a power, is a number which being raised to the index of that power, will either be equal to the given number, or approach very near to it.

54. *To extract the Square Root of a given number.*

Rule 1st. Begin at the unit's place, put a point over it, and also over every next figure but one, reckoning to the left for integers, and to the right for fractions; and there will be as many integer places in the root, as there are points over the integers in the given number.

The figure under a point, with its left-hand place, is called a period.

2d. Under the left-hand period write the greatest square contained in it, and set the root thereof in the Quotient; subtract the square, and to the remainder bring down the next period, as in Division.

3d. On the left of this Remainder write the double of the Root or Quotient for a Divisor; seek how often this may be had in the Remainder, except the right-hand place; write what ariseth both in the Root, and on the right of the Divisor.

4th. Multiply this increased Divisor by the last Quotient-figure; subtract, and to the Remainder bring down the next period; double the Root for a Divisor, and proceed as before.

55. Fractional places will arise in the Root, by annexing to the Remainders, periods of two cyphers each, and renewing the operation.

Ex. I. *What is the Square Root of* 1444?

Put a point over the units place 4, and alſo over the place of 100s. Now the number conſiſts of 2 periods, and will have 2 integer places in the Root: Then the greateſt Square in 14, the left-hand period, is 9, and its Root is 3; write 9 under the period, and three in the Root; now 9 from 14 leaves 5, to which annex the next period 44; the Root 3 doubled makes 6, which in 54 is contained 8 times, annex 8 to the 3 in the Quotient, and to the Diviſor 6, makes the Root 38 and the Diviſor 68; then 8 times 68 is 544; and there remaining 0, on ſubtraction, it may be concluded, that 38 is the true Root.

```
      1444 (38 Root.
      9
68)   544
      544
```

Ex. II. *What is the Square Root of* 36372961?

```
        36372961 (6031 Root.
        36
1203)   3729
        3609
12061)  12061
        12061
```

Ex. III. *What is the Square Root of* 1,0609?

```
     1,0609 ( 1,03 Root.
     1
203) 0609
      609
```

Ex. IV. *What is the Square Root of* 24681024?

Anſwer 4968.

Ex. V. *What is the Square Root of* 911236798,794365?

Anſwer 30186,699, &c.

```
         911236798,794366 ( 30186,6
601 )    1123
6028 )   52267
60366 )  404398
603726 ) 4220279
           597923
              &c.
```

Here the products are omitted, the multiplication and ſubtraction being made in the mind.

Ex. VI. *What is the Square Root of* 76395820?

```
              76395820 (8740,4702
              64
167 )         1239
              1169
1744 )        7058
              6976
174804 )      822000
              699216
1748087 )     12278400
              12236609
174809402 )   4179100000
              3496188804
               682911196
```

In the VIth Example, after all the periods given were brought down, there remained 8220, to which a period of two cyphers was annexed, and the operation renewed, and continued until 4 decimal places were obtained in the Root; every period brought down giving one place.

56. To

56. *To extract the Cube Root of a given Number.*

Rule 1ſt. Over the unit place of the given number put a point, and alſo over every third figure from the unit place, to the left for integers, and to the right for fractions; and the root will have as many integer places, as there are points, or periods, in the integral part of the given number.

2d. Under the left hand period, write the greateſt Cube it contains, the root of which ſet in the Quotient: Subtract the Cube from the period, and to the Remainder annex the remaining periods; call this the Reſolvend.

3d. To the Quotient annex as many cyphers as there were periods remaining; call this the Root.

4th. Divide the Reſolvend by the Root, add the Quotient to thrice the Square of the Root, let the Sum be a Diviſor to the Reſolvend, and the Quotient-figures annexed to the right of the firſt Root, without the cyphers, will be the Cube Root ſought.

5th. If the ſecond figure of the Root be 1, or 0; then generally 3 or 4 figures of the Root will be obtained at the firſt operation: But if the ſecond figure exceeds 2, it will be beſt to find only two places at firſt.

6th. To renew the operation; ſubtract the Cube of the figures found in the Root from the given number; then form a Diviſor, and divide as directed in the fourth precept; and this will give the Root true to 5 or ſix places: For each operation commonly triples the figures found in the laſt Root.

Ex. I. *What is the Cube Root of* 9800344?

Put a point over the unit place 4, another over the place of thouſands, and another over that of millions; and becauſe there are 3 points, there will be 3 places in the Root. Under the left hand period 9, write 8, the greateſt Cube in it, and its Root 2 write in the Quotient, then ſubtracting, the Reſolvend is 1800344: Now becauſe there are two periods remaining, therefore two cyphers annexed to the Root 2, make it 200, by which dividing the Reſolvend, the Quotient is 9001; alſo the ſquare of 200 is 40000, the triple thereof 120000 being added to 9001, makes 129001 for a Diviſor, by which dividing 1800344, the Quotient is 14 nearly, and is taken as 14, becauſe it is much nearer to it than to 13; now 14 being annexed to the former Root 2, makes 214, the Root ſought. For 214×214×214=9800344.

```
        9800344(2
        8
        -------
2,00) 18003,44 Reſolvend.
        -------
        9001 = Quotient.
      120000=thrice the Sq. of the R.
      ------
      129001)1800344(14
              129001
              ------
               510344
               516004
               ------
          The Root is 214.
```

Ex. II.

Ex. II. *What is the Cube Root of* 518749442875?

```
        .  .  .  .
        518749442875(8
        512
8,000)  6749442,875
         843680
        192000000                  .
        192843680( 6749442875 (035
                    578531040
                    964132475
                    964218400
```

In this example, because 3 periods were remaining, and consequently 3 places more to be found; therefore in the last division a point is put over the 3d place from the right hand, and the Divisor is first to be tried in the Dividend as far as this point, in which as it cannot be taken, 0 is put in the Quotient, &c. here the last figure 5 is too much, but it is much nearer to 5 than to 4; then 035 annexed to the first Root 8, makes 8035 for the Root.

Ex. III. *What is the Cube Root of* 114604290,028?

```
      .  .  .  .
      114604290,028
       64
4,00) 50604290
      126510
      480000
      606510) 50604290 (8
```

```
   48
   48
  384
  192
 2304
   48
18432
 9216
110592
```

Here 480 is taken for the Root at the first operation.

```
Then 114604290,028(48
      110592

480)  4012290   The work of the Division is supposed to be done
                   on a waste paper.
        8358,9   the Quotient.
      691200  = triple the Square of 480, viz. 230400×3.

Divisor 699558,9) 4012290,028 (5736
          ...     34977945
                               To  480 the first Root
                   5144955     Add   5,736
                   4896912
                               Sum 485,736
                    248043
                    209807
                     38176
```

57. Here, instead of bringing down the figures of the Dividend to the Remainders, the Divisor is lessened each time, by pointing off a place on the right; but regard is to be had to the carriage which will arise from the places thus omitted.

SECTION IX. OF NUMERAL SERIES.

58. *A rank of three or more numbers that increaſe or decreaſe by an uniform progreſſion, is called a Numeral Series.*

59. If the Progreſſion is made by equal differences, that is by the conſtant addition or ſubtraction of the ſame number; the series is called an *Arithmetic Progreſſion.*

Thus

1	2	3	4	5	6	7	8	9	&c. increaſing by adding 1,
3	6	9	12	15	18	21	24	27	&c. increaſing by adding 3,
49	43	37	31	25	19	13	7	1	&c. decreaſing by ſubducting 6,

are ranks of numbers in Arithmetic Progreſſion: And of ſuch ranks there may be an infinite variety.

60. If the Progreſſion is made by a conſtant multiplication or diviſion with the ſame number, the ſeries is called a *Geometric Progreſſion.*

Thus

1	2	4	8	16	32	64		&c. increaſing by 2,
1	5	25	125	625	3125	15625		&c. increaſing by 5,
6561	2187	729	243	81	27	9	3	&c. decreaſing by 3,
16384	4096	1024	256	64	16	4	1	&c. decreaſing by 4,

are ranks of numbers in Geometric Progreſſion: And of ſuch ranks there may be an infinite variety.

61. The common Multiplier or Diviſor is called the *ratio.*

Thus 2 is the ratio in the 1ſt rank, 5 in the 2d rank, 3 is the ratio in the 3d rank, and 4 in the 4th rank.

62. In any ſeries of terms in Arithmetic Progreſſion, the ſum of any two terms, conſidered as extremes, is equal to the ſum of any two terms taken as means equally diſtant from the extremes.

Thus in 3 terms (where the 1ſt and 3d are extremes, and the other the mean) viz. 6 . 9 . 12, then $6+12=9+9=18$.
And in 4 terms, viz. 13 . 19 . 25 . 31.
Then $13+31=19+25=44$.
Alſo in the terms 49 . 43 . 37 . 31 . 25 . 19 . 13 . 7 . 1.
Then $49+1=43+7=37+13=31+19=25+25=50$.

63. In a ſeries of terms in Geometric Progreſſion, the Product of any two terms conſidered as extremes, is equal to the Product of any two intermediate equidiſtant terms conſidered as means.

Thus in 3 terms, viz. 5 . 25 . 125 . *Or* 3 . 9 . 27.
Then $5\times125=25\times25=625$. *Alſo* $3\times27=9\times9=81$.
And in 4 terms 4 . 8 . 16 . 32 .
Then $32\times4=16\times8=128$.
Alſo in the terms 1 . 4 . 16 . 64 . 256 . 1024 . 4096 . 16384 .
Then $16384\times1=4096\times4=1024\times16=256\times64=16384$.

64. In

64. In any Arithmetic Progression, the sum of any two terms lessened by the first term; or their difference increased by the first term, will be a term also in that progression.

Thus in the Progression 1 . 3 . 5 . 7 . 9 . 11 . 13 . 15 . 17 . 19 . 21 *&c.*
Then $7+11=18$, and $18-1=17$ is a term of the Progression.
Also $11-7=4$, and $4+1=5$ is a term of the Progression.

65. In any Geometric Progression, the product of any two terms divided by the first term; or the Quotient of any two terms multiplied by the first term, will give a term also in that series.

Thus in the Progression 3 . 6 . 12 . 24 . 48 . 96 . 192 . 384 . 768 *&c.*
Then $\frac{12\times 96}{3}=384$; and $\frac{192}{12}\times 3=48$, are terms in the Progression.

66. If over a series of terms in Geometric Progression, be written a series of terms in Arithmetic Progression, the first term of which is 0, and common difference is 1, term for term; then any term in the Arithmetic Series, will shew how far its corresponding term in the Geometric Series is distant from the first term.

Thus { 0 1 2 3 4 5 6 *&c.* Arithmetic Series.
{ 1 3 9 27 81 243 729 *&c.* Geometric Series.

Here 729 is distant from the 1st term, 6 terms; 243 is distant 5 terms, 81 is distant 4 terms.

67. The terms of the Arithmetical Series are called indices to the terms of the Geometric Series.

Thus 5 *is the index to* 243; 3 *is the index to* 27; 1 *is the index to* 3; *&c.*

68. Problem I. *In an Arithmetic Progression: Given the first term, the common difference, and the number of terms.*
Required the last term.

Rule. Subtract 1 from the number of terms, multiply the remainder by the common difference; to the product add the first term, and the sum will be the last term.

Ex. I. *Suppose* 1 *and* 9 *to be the first and second terms, of an Arithmetic Progression of* 1074 *terms: What is the last term?*

Here $9-1=8$ is the com. diff. Now $1074-1=1073$.
And $1073\times 8=8584$. Then $8584+1=8585=$ last term.

Ex. II. *A person agrees to discharge a certain debt in a year, by weekly payments, viz. the first week* 5s. *the* 2d *week* 8s. &c. *constantly increasing each week by* 3s.: *How much was the last payment?*

$5=$ 1st. term.	Now $52-1=51$.
$3=$ com. diff.	And $51\times 3=153$.
$52=$ N° of terms.	Then $153+5=158\,s.=7$ £. 18 s. $=$ last Payment.

69. Pro-

69. PROBLEM II. *In an Arithmetic Progression: Given the first term, last term, and the number of terms.*

Required the sum of all the terms.

RULE. Add the first and last terms together, the sum multiplied by half the number of terms, gives the sum of all the terms.

Ex. I. *Required the sum of the first* 1000 *numbers in their natural order.*

Here 1=1st term, 1=com. diff.
1000=N° of terms, its $\frac{1}{2}$ is 500.
Now 1000+1=1001.
Then 1001×500=500500 is the sum required.

Ex. II. *A debt is to be discharged in a year by weekly payments equally increasing; the 1st to be 5s. and the last 7£. 18s. How much was the debt?*

Here 7£. 18s =158s.=last term.
52=N° of terms, its $\frac{1}{2}$ is 26.
Now 158+5=163.
Then 163×26=4238s.=211£. 18s. is the sum of the terms, or debt.

Ex. III. *Suppose a basket and 500 stones were placed in a straight line, a yard distant from one another: Required in what time a man could bring them one by one to the basket, allowing him to walk at the rate of 3 miles an hour?*

Between the basket and stones are 500 spaces, which is the number of terms.
Now 500+1=501. Then 501×250=125250=sum of the terms.
But as he goes backwards and forwards, he walks 250500 yards.
Which divided by 1760 (the yards in 1 mile) gives 142,329 miles.
Which at 3 miles an hour, will take 47 h. 26 min. 35 seconds nearly.

70. PROBLEM III. *In a Geometric Progression: Given the first term, the ratio and the last term.*

Required the sum of all the terms.

RULE. Multiply the last term by the common ratio, from the Product subtract the first term for a Dividend.

Subtract 1 from the ratio for a Divisor; then divide, and the Quotient will be the sum of all the terms.

Ex. I. *Suppose the first term of a series to be* 3, *the ratio* 3, *and the last term* 6561: *Required the sum of all the terms.*

Now	6561=last term.	And	3=ratio.
Mult. by	3=ratio.	Sub.	1
	19683=Product.	Rem.	2=Divisor.
Subtr.	3=first term.		
	19680=Dividend.		

Then 2)19680(9840 is the sum of all the terms.

Ex. II. *Let the first term be* 2, *the second term* 10, *and the last term* 156250: *Required the sum of all the terms.*

Here 2) 10 (5 is the common ratio.
Now 156250×5=781250. And 781250—2=781248=Dividend.
Also 5—1=4 the Divisor.
Then 4) 781248 (195312 is the sum of all the terms.

71. PRO-

71. PROBLEM IV. *In a Geometric Progression: Given the first term, the ratio, and the number of terms.*

Required the last term.

RULE 1st. Write down 6 or 7 of the leading terms in the Geometric Series, and over them their Indices.

2d. Add together the most convenient indices to make an index less by unity than the number expressing the place of the term sought.

3d. Multiply together the terms of the Geometric Series, belonging to those indices which were added; make the product a dividend.

4th. Raise the first term to a power whose index is one less than the number of terms multiplied; make the result a Divisor to the former Dividend, and the Quotient will be the term sought.

Ex. I. *What is the 12th term of a Geometric Series, the first term of which is 3, and second term is 6?*

Now $\frac{6}{3} = 2$ is the common ratio.

And { 0 . 1 . 2 . 3 . 4 . 5 . 6 &c. Indices.
3 . 6 . 12 . 24 . 48 . 96 . 192 &c. Geometric terms.

Then $6+5=11$, is the index to the 12th term.

And $192 \times 96 = 18432$, is the Dividend.

The number of terms multiplied together is 2; and $2-1=1$, the power to which the first term 3 is to be raised; but the first power of 3 is 3.

Then $\frac{18432}{3} = 6144$ is the 12th term of the given series.

Ex. II. *A Person being asked to dispose of a fine horse, said he would sell him on condition of having one farthing for the 1st nail in his shoes, two farthings for the 2d nail; one penny for the 3d nail; two pence for the 4th; four pence for the 5th; 8 pence for the 6th, &c.; doubling the price of every nail to 32, the number of nails in the four shoes: How much would that horse be sold for at that rate?*

Here the first term is 1, the ratio 2, and the number of terms 32.

First. To find the last term.

Now { 0 . 1 . 2 . 3 . 4 . 5 . 6 . 7 . 8 &c. Indices.
1 . 2 . 4 . 8 . 16 . 32 . 64 . 128 . 256 &c. Geometric terms.

And 31 is the index to the 32d term.

Then $8+8=16$; $16+8=24$; $24+7=31$.

The 1st term being 1, any power thereof is 1; so the 4th article of the rule is useless in this question.

Now $256 \times 256 = 65536$ is the 17th term.
$65536 \times 256 = 16777216$ is the 25th term.
$16777216 \times 128 = 2147483648$ is the 32d term.

Then 2147483648
×2
= 4294967296
−1 the 1st term.

$2-1=1$) 4294967295 the sum of the terms: or the price, in farthings, of the horse.

4 | 4294967295
12 | 1073741823 ¾ f.
20 | 89478485 - 3 d.
4473924 - 5 s.

Answer 4473924 £. 5s. 3¾d.

SECTION X. OF LOGARITHMS.

72. LOGARITHMS *are a ſeries of numbers ſo contrived, that by them the work of multiplication may be performed by addition; and the operation of diviſion may be done by ſubtraction.*

73. Or, Logarithms are the Indices to a ſeries of numbers in Geometrical Progreſſion.

Thus		0	1	2	3	4	5	6	&c. Indices or Logarithms.
		1	2	4	8	16	32	64	&c. Geometric Progreſſion.
	or		0	1	2	3	4	5	&c. Indices or Logarithms.
			1	3	9	27	81	243	&c. Geometric Series.
	or		0	1	2	3	4	5	&c. Indices or Logarithms.
			1	10	100	1000	10000	100000	&c. Geometric Series.

Where the ſame Indices ſerve equally for any Geometric Series.

74. Hence it is evident, there may be as many kinds of Indices or Logarithms, as there can be taken kinds of Geometric Series.

But the Logarithms moſt convenient for common uſes, are thoſe adapted to a Geometric Series increaſing in a tenfold Progreſſion, as in the laſt of the examples above.

75. In the Geometric Series 1 . 10 . 100 . 1000 . &c. between the terms 1 and 10, if the numbers 2 . 3 . 4 . 5 . 6 . 7 . 8 . 9 were interpoſed, to them might Indices be alſo adapted in an Arithmetic Progreſſion, ſuited to the terms interpoſed between 1 and 10, conſidered as a Geometric Progreſſion: Alſo proper Indices may be found to all the numbers that can be interpoſed between any two terms of the Geometric Series.

But it is evident that all the Indices to the numbers under 10 muſt be leſs than 1; that is, are fractions: Thoſe to the numbers between 10 and 100 muſt fall between 1 and 2; that is, are mixed numbers conſiſting of 1 and ſome fraction: And ſo the Indices to the numbers between 100 and 1000 will fall between 2 and 3; that is, are mixed numbers conſiſting of two and ſome fraction: And ſo of the other Indices.

76. Hereafter, the integral part only of theſe Indices will be called the Index; and the fractional part will be called the Logarithm: And the computing of thoſe fractional parts is called the making of Logarithms; the moſt troubleſome part of this work is to make the Logarithms of the *prime numbers*; that is, of ſuch numbers which cannot be divided by any other number than by itſelf and unity.

77. *To find the Logarithms of prime numbers.*

RULE 1ſt. Let the ſum of the propoſed number and its next leſs number be called A.

2d. Divide 0,868588963 * by A, reſerve the Quotient.

* The number 0,868588963 is the Quotient of 2 divided by 2,302585093, which is the Logarithm of 10, according to the firſt form of the Lord *Nepier*, who was the inventor of Logarithms. The manner by which *Nepier*'s Log. of 10 is found, may be ſeen in many books of Algebra; but is here omitted, becauſe this treatiſe does not contain the elements of that ſcience: However, thoſe who have not opportunity to enter thoroughly into this ſubject, had better grant the truth of one number, and thereby be enabled to try the accuracy of any Logarithm in the tables, than to receive thoſe tables as truly computed, without any means of examining the certainty thereof.

3d. Divide the reserved Quotient by the Square of A, reserve this Quotient.

4th. Divide the last reserved Quotient by the Square of A, reserving the Quotient; and thus proceed as long as division can be made.

5th. Write the reserved Quotients orderly under one another, the first being uppermost.

6th. Divide these Quotients respectively by the odd numbers 1 . 3 . 5 . 7 . 9 . 11, &c. that is, divide the first reserved Quotient by 1, the 2d by 3, the 3d by 5, the 4th by 7, &c. let these Quotients be written orderly under one another, add them together, and their sum will be a Logarithm.

7th. To this Logarithm, add the Logarithm of the next less number, and the sum will be the Logarithm of the number proposed.

Ex. I. *Required the Logarithm of the number* 2.

Here the next less number is 1, and $2+1=3=A$.
And the Square of A is 9. Then;

$$\frac{0,868588963}{3}=,289529654. \quad \text{And} \quad \frac{,289529654}{1}=,289529654$$

$$\frac{0,289529654}{9}=,032169962. \quad \& \quad \frac{,032169962}{3}=,010723321$$

$$\frac{0,032169962}{9}=,003574440. \quad \& \quad \frac{,003574440}{5}=,000714888$$

$$\frac{0,003574440}{9}=,000397160. \quad \& \quad \frac{,000397160}{7}=,000056737$$

$$\frac{0,000397160}{9}=,000044129. \quad \& \quad \frac{,000044129}{9}=,000004903$$

$$\frac{0,000044129}{9}=,000004903. \quad \& \quad \frac{,000004903}{11}=,000000445$$

$$\frac{0,000004903}{9}=,000000545. \quad \& \quad \frac{,000000545}{13}=,000000042$$

$$\frac{0,000000545}{9}=,000000060. \quad \& \quad \frac{,000000060}{15}=,000000004$$

To this Log.	0,301029994
Add the Log. of	1=0,000000000
Their sum is the Log. of	2=0,301029994

This process needs no other explanation than comparing it with the rule.

That the manner of computing these Logarithms may be familiar to the Reader, the operations of making several of them are here subjoined.

 Ex. II.

Ex. II. *Required the Logarithm of the number* 3.

Here the next less number is 2; and $3+2=5=A$, whose Square is 25.

$\frac{0,868588963}{5}=,173717792$. And $\frac{,173717792}{1}=,173717792$

$\frac{0,173717792}{25}=6948712$. & $\frac{6948712}{3}=,002316327$

$\frac{0,006948712}{25}=277948$. & $\frac{277948}{5}=,000055590$

$\frac{0,000277948}{25}=11118$. & $\frac{11118}{7}=,000001588$

$\frac{0,000011118}{25}=445$. & $\frac{445}{9}=,000000049$

$\frac{0,000000445}{25}=18$. & $\frac{18}{11}=,000000002$

To this Logarithm	0,176091258
Add the Log. of 2	0,301029994
The sum is the Logarithm of 3	0,477121252

78. Since the Logarithms are the Indices of numbers considered in a Geometric Progression; therefore the sums, or differences of these Indices, will be Indices or Logarithms belonging to the Products, or Quotients, of such terms in the Geometric Progression as correspond to those Logarithms which were added or subtracted (71).

Ex. III. *Required the Log. of* 4.

Now $4=2\times2$.

Then to the Log. of 2	0,301029994
Add the Log. of 2	0,301029994
Sum is the Log. of 4	0,602059988

Ex. IV. *Required the Log. of* 6.

Now $3\times2=6$.

Then to the Log. of 3	0,477121252
Add the Log. of 2	0,301029994
Sum is the Log. of 6	0,778151246

Ex. V. *Required the Log. of* 10.

In the original Series, 1 is assumed for the Logarithm of 10.

Ex. VI. *Required the Log. of* 5.

Now 10 divided by 2 gives 5.

Then from Log. of 10	1,000000000
Take Log. of 2	0,301029994
Leaves the Log. of 5	0,698970006

Ex. VII. *Required the Log. of* 8.

Now $8=2\times2\times2$.

Therefore the Log. of 2 taken thrice gives the Log. of the number 8

The Log. of 2 is	0,301029994
Which multiplied by	3
Gives the Log. of 8	0,903089982

Ex. VIII. *Required the Log. of* 9.

Now $9=3\times3$.

Therefore the Log. of 3 doubled gives the Log. of 9.

The Log. of 3 is	0,477121252
Which multiplied by	2
Gives the Log. of 9	0,954242504

Ex. IX. *Required the Logarithm of 7.*

Here 6 is the next leſs. Then $7+6=13=A$; and $169=$Square of A.

$\frac{0,868588963}{13}=,066814536$. And $\frac{,066814536}{1}=,066814536$

$\frac{0,066814536}{169}=$ 395352. & $\frac{395352}{3}=$ 131784

$\frac{0,000395352}{169}=$ 2339. & $\frac{2339}{5}=$ 468

$\frac{0,000002339}{169}=$ 14. & $\frac{14}{7}=$ 2

To this Logarithm	0,066946790
Add the Logarithm of 6	0,778151246
The ſum is the Logarithm of 7	0,845098036

The Log. of 12 is equal to the ſum of the Logs. of 3 & 4, or of 2 & 6.
The Log. of 14 is equal to the ſum of the Logs. of 7 & 2.
of 15 — of 3 & 5.
of 16 — of 4 & 4, or of 8 & 2.
of 18 — of 3 & 6, or of 9 & 2.
of 20 — of 4 & 5, or of 10 & 2.

79. The Logs. of the prime numbers 11, 13, 17, 19, are to be found as in the examples I. II. IX. and in like manner is the Log. of any other prime number to be found; but it may be obſerved, that the operation is ſhorter in the larger prime numbers; for any number exceeding 400, the firſt Quotient added to the Logarithm of its next leſſer number, will give the Logarithm ſought, true to 8 or 9 places; and therefore it will be very eaſy to examine any ſuſpected Logarithm in the tables.

80. The manner of diſpoſing the Logarithms, when made, into tables, is various: But in this treatiſe they are ordered as follows.

Any number under 100, *or not exceeding two places, and its Logarithm, are found in the firſt page of the table*, where they are placed in adjoining columns; and diſtinguiſhed by the title *Num.* for the common numbers; and by *Log.* for the Logarithms.

Theſe tables are at the end of Book IX.

A number of three or four places being given, its Logarithm is thus found.

Seek for a page in which the given number ſhall be contained between the two numbers marked at the top, annexed to the letter N: Then right againſt the three firſt figures of the given number, found in the column ſigned *Num*, and in the column ſigned by the fourth, ſtands the Logarithm belonging to that number of four places.

If the number conſiſted of 3 places only; then theſe places found as before directed, the Logarithm ſtnads againſt them in the column ſigned 0.

Thus, *to find the Logarithm of* 5738. Seek for a page in which ſtands at top N° 5200 to 5800; then in the column ſigned N° find 573, right againſt which in the column ſigned 8 at top or bottom ſtands, 75876, which is the Logarithm to 5738, excluſive of its Index.

81. *A Logarithm being given, its number is thus found.*

Seek for a page in which the three firſt figures of the given Logarithm are found at top annexed to the letter *L*; then in one of the columns ſigned with the figures 0, 1, 2, 3, 4, 5, 6, 7, 8, 9, find a number the neareſt to the given Logarithm; againſt this number in the column ſigned N°, ſtand three figures; to the right of theſe annex the figure with which the column was ſigned at top or bottom, and this will be the number correſponding to the given Logarithm, not regarding the Index.

82. All numbers conſiſting of the ſame figures, whether they be integral, fractional, or mixed, have the fractional parts of their Logarithms the ſame.

If the following examples be well attended to, there will be no difficulty in finding the Logarithm to a propoſed number, or the number to a propoſed Logarithm, within the limits of the table of Logarithms here uſed.

Num.	Logarithms.	Logarithms.	Numbers.
5874	3,76893	0,37295	2,360
587,4	2,76893	1,28631	19,33
58,74	1,76893	2,51947	330,7
5,874	0,76893	$\bar{3}$,75062	5632,
0,5874	$\bar{1}$,76893	$\bar{3}$,18397	0,001527
0,05874	$\bar{2}$,76893	$\bar{2}$,43020	0,02693
0,005874	$\bar{3}$,76893	$\bar{1}$,85962	0,7238

83. A general rule to find the Index to the Log. of a given number.

To the left of the Logarithm, write that figure (or figures) which expreſſes the diſtance from unity, of the higheſt-place digit in the given number; reckoning the unit's place 0, *the next place* 1, *the next place* 2, *the next place* 3, &c.

When there are integers in the given number, the Index is always affirmative; but when there are no integers, the Index is negative, and is to be marked by a little line drawn above it: thus $\bar{1}$.

Thus a number having 1 . 2 . 3 . 4 . 5 &c. integer places.

The index of its Logarithm is 0 . 1 . 2 . 3 . 4 . &c.

And a fraction having a digit in the place of Primes, Seconds, Thirds, Fourths, &c.

Then the Index of its Logarithms will be $\bar{1}$. $\bar{2}$. $\bar{3}$. $\bar{4}$ &c.

By the above rule, the place of the fractional comma, or mark of diſtinction, in the number anſwering to a given Logarithm, will be always known.

84. The more places the Logarithms conſiſt of, the more accurate, in general, will be the reſult of any operation performed with them: But for the purpoſes of Navigation, as five places, excluſive of the Index, are ſufficient, therefore the logarithmic tables in this treatiſe are not extended any farther.

85. MUL-

85. MULTIPLICATION BY LOGARITHMS;

Or, Two or more numbers being given, to find their Product by Logarithms.

Rule. Add together the Logarithms of the Factors, and the ſum is a Logarithm, the correſponding number of which is the Product required.

Obſerving to add what is carried from the Logarithm to the ſum of the affirmative Indices.

And that the difference between the affirmative and negative Indices are to be taken for the Index to the Logarithm of the Product.

Ex. I. *Multiply* 86,25 *by* 6,48.

86,25 its Log. is	1,93576
6,48 its Log. is	0,81157
Product 558,9	2,74733

Ex. II. *Multiply* 46,75 *by* 0,3275.

46,75 its Log. is	1,66978
0,3275 its Log. is	$\bar{1}$,51521
Product 15,31	1,18499

Ex. III. *Multiply* 3,768 *by* 2,053 *and by* 0,007693.

3,768 its Log. is	0,57611
2,053	0,31239
0,007693	$\bar{3}$,88610
Product 0,05951	$\bar{2}$,77460

The 1 carried from the left hand column of the Logs. being affirmative, reduces $\bar{3}$ to $\bar{2}$.

Ex. IV. *Multiply* 27,63 *by* 1,859 *and by* 0,7258 *and by* 0,03591.

27,63 its Log. is	1,44138
1,859	0,26928
0,7258	$\bar{1}$,86082
0,03591	$\bar{2}$,55521
Product 1,339	0,12669

Here 2 being carried to the Index 1, makes 3; which takes off the $\bar{1}$ and $\bar{2}$.

86. DIVISION BY LOGARITHMS.

Or, Two numbers being given, to find how often the one will contain the other, by Logarithms.

Rule. From the Log. of the Dividend, ſubtract the Log. of the Diviſor; then the number agreeing to the Remainder, will be the Quotient required.

But obſerve to change the Index of the Diviſor from negative to affirmative, or from affirmative to negative: And then let the difference of the affirm. and neg. Indices be taken for the Index to the Log. of the Quotient.

When an unit is borrowed in the left-hand place of the Logarithm, add it to the Index of the Diviſor, if affirmative; but ſubtract it if negative; and let the Index ariſing be changed and worked with as before.

Ex. I. *Divide* 558,9 *by* 6,48.

Log. of Divid. 558,9 is	2,74733
Log. of Diviſor 6,48 is	0,81157
The Quotient is 86,25	1,93576

Ex. II. *Divide* 15,31 *by* 46,75.

Log. of Divid. 15,31 is	1,18497
Log. of Diviſor 46,75 is	1,66973
The Quotient is 0,3275	$\bar{1}$,51519

Ex. III. *Divide* 0,05951 *by* 0,007693.

Log. of Divid. 0,05951 is	$\bar{2}$,77459
Log. of Diviſor 0,007693 is	$\bar{3}$,88610
The Quotient is 7,735	0,88849

Ex. IV. *Divide* 0,6651 *by* 22,5.

Log. of Divid. 0,6651 is	$\bar{1}$,82289
Log. of Diviſor 22,5 is	1,35218
The Quotient is 0,02956	$\bar{2}$,47071

87. OF PROPORTION.

1st. State the terms of the question (by 46) and let them be written orderly under one another, prefixing to the first term the word *As*, to the second *To*, to the third *So*, and under them set the word *To*.

2d. Against the first term, write the arithmetical complement of its Logarithm. See Art. 88.

3d. Against the second and third terms, write their Logarithms.

4th. The sum of those three Logarithms, abating 10 in the Index, will be the Logarithm of the 4th term; which sought in the tables, the number answering to it is the answer or term sought.

88. The arithmetical complement of a Logarithm is thus found. Beginning at the Index, write down what each figure wants of 9, except the last, or right-hand figure, which take from 10.

But if the Index is negative, add it to 9; and proceed with the rest as before.

Ex. I. *Find a fourth proportional number to* 98,45 *and* 1,969 *and* 347,2

As 98,45 its * Ar. Co. Log.	8,00678
To 1,969	0,29425
So 347,2	2,54058
To 6,944	0,84161

Ex. II. *Find a third proportional number to* 9,642 *and* 4,821.

As 9,642 its Ar. Co. Log.	9,01583
To 4,821	0,68314
So 4,821	0,68314
To 2,411	0,38211

Ex. III. *What will a gunner's pay amount to in a year at* 2£. 12*s.* 6*d. a month of* 28 *days?*

As 28 days its Ar. Co. Log.	8,55284
To 365 days	2,56229
So 2£. 12*s.* 6*d.*=2,625£.	0,41913
To 34£. 4*s.* 5*d.*=34,22£.	1,53426

Ex. IV. *If* ¾ *of a yard of cloth cost* ⅔ *of a guinea: How many ells English for* 3£. 10*s.*?

As ⅔ Guin.=14*s.* Ar. Co.	8,85387
To 3£. 10*s.*=70*s.*	1,84510
So ⅗ ell =0,6	$\bar{1}$,77815
To 3 ells	0,47712

Ex. V. *What number will have the same proportion to* 0,8538 *as* 0,3275 *has to* 0,0131?

As 0,0131 its Ar. Co. Log.	11,88273
To 0,3275	$\bar{1}$,51521
So 0,8538	$\bar{1}$,93136
To 21,35	1,32930

Ex. VI. *How many yards of shalloon of* ¾ *ell wide will be enough to line a coat containing* 3½ *ells of* 1¾ *yards wide?*

As ¾ ×5/4 yd. w.=0,9375	10,02803
To 1¾ yd. w.=1,75	0,24304
So 3½×5/4 yd. l.=4,375	0,64098
To 8⅙ yd. long=8,167	0,91205

where w. stands for wide, l. for long.

* Ar. Co. Log. stands for the *Arithmetical Complement of the Logarithm.*

OF

OF POWERS AND THEIR ROOTS.

89. *A number being given, to find any proposed power of that Number.*

RULE 1st. Seek the Logarithm of the given number.

2d. Multiply this Logarithm by the Index of the proposed power.

3d. Find the number corresponding to the Product, and it will be the power required.

90. In multiplying a Logarithm having a negative Index, the Product of that Index is negative.

But the carriage from the Logarithm is affirmative.

Therefore the difference will be the Index of the Product.

And is to be of the same kind with the greater, or that which was made the minuend.

Ex. I. *What is the second power of the number* 3,874?

To 3,874 its Log. is	0,58816
The Index is	2
The power sought is 15,01	1,17632

Ex. II. *What is the 3d power of the number* 2,768?

The N° 2,768 its Log. is	0,44217
The Index is	3
The power sought is 21,21	1,32651

Ex. III. *What is the 12th power of the number* 1,539?

1,539 its Log. is	0,18724
The Index is	12
The power sought is 176.6	2,24688

Ex. IV. *What is the 365th power of the number* 2?

2 Its Log. is	0,30103
The Index is	365
	150515
	180618
	90309
	109,87595

In the IVth Ex. the Index of the Product being 109, shews that the required power will consist of 110 integer places; of which no more than 4 places are found in these tables; therefore the number sought may be thus expressed, 7515 [106]: That is, 7515 with 106 cyphers annexed.

Ex. V. *What is the 2d power of the number* 0,2857?

To 0,2857, its Log. is	$\bar{1}$,45591
The Index of 2d power	2
The power 0,08162	$\bar{2}$,91182

Here, there being no carriage from the Product of the Log. the whole Product of the negative Index is negative, *viz* $\bar{2}$.

Ex. VI. *What is the 3d power of the number* 0,7916?

To 0,7916, its Log. is	$\bar{1}$,89851
The Index of 3d power	3
The power is 0,4961	$\bar{1}$,69553

Here the carriage from the Product of the Log. is 2; then the Product of the negative Index $\bar{1}$, *viz.* $\bar{3}$, being lessened by 2, leaves $\bar{1}$, the Index of the Product.

91. *A*

91. *A number being given, to find any proposed Root of it.*

RULE 1st. Seek the Logarithm of the given number.

2d. Divide this Logarithm by the denominator of the Index of the proposed root.

3d. The number corresponding to the Quotient will be the root.

When the Index to the Logarithm to be divided is negative, and less than the Divisor, or Denominator of the root. Then

Increase the negative Index by as many units, borrowed, as shall be equal to the Divisor, and the Quotient will give $\bar{1}$ for the Index.

Carry the units borrowed as tens to the left-hand place of the Logarithm, and then divide that Logarithm as in whole numbers.

Ex. I. *What is the Square Root of the number* 1501?

2)3,17638

Root sought is 38,74 — 1,58819

Ex. II. *What is the Cube Root of the number* 2121?

3)3,32654

Root sought 12,85 — 1,10885

Ex. III. *What is the Root, of which* 176,6 *is the* 12*th power?*

12)2,24699

Root sought is 1,539 — 0,18725

Ex. IV. *What is the Root, of which* 2 *is the* 365*th power?*

365)0,30103

Root sought is 1,002 — 0,00082

Ex. V. *What is the Square Root of the number* 0,08162?

Log. of 0,08162, div. by 2)$\bar{2}$,91180

Gives Root 0,2857 to — $\bar{1}$,45590

Here the Divisor 2 can be taken in the Index $\bar{2}$, and gives for the Quotient $\bar{1}$.

Ex. VI. *What is the Cube Root of the number* 0,496?

Log. of 0,496 div. by 3)$\bar{1}$,69548

Gives Root 0,7916 to — $\bar{1}$,89849

Here the Divisor 3 cannot be taken in the Index $\bar{1}$; then $\bar{2}$ borrowed makes with $\bar{1}$, $\bar{3}$; in which the Divisor 3 will go $\bar{1}$: the 2 borrowed carried to the 6, &c. makes 269548, which divided by 3, gives 89849.

END OF BOOK I.

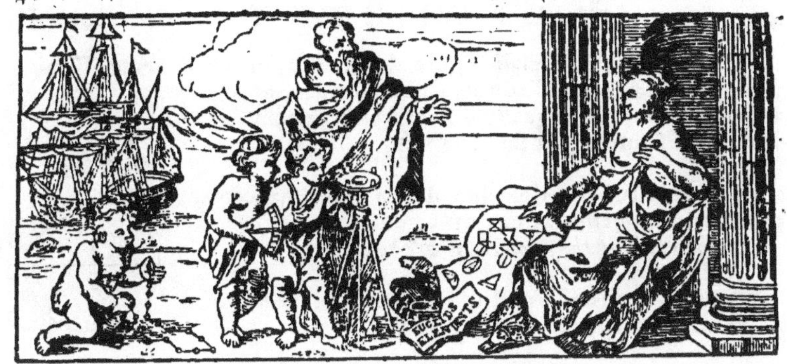

THE ELEMENTS OF NAVIGATION.

BOOK II.

OF GEOMETRY.

SECTION I.

Definitions and *Principles.*

1. GEOMETRY is a ſcience which treats of the deſcriptions, properties and relations of magnitudes in general: Or of ſuch things where length, or where length and breadth, or length, breadth, and thickneſs, are conſidered.

2. A POINT is that which is without parts or dimenſions.

A ——— B

3. A LINE is length without breadth: It is called a RIGHT LINE when it is the ſhorteſt diſtance between two points, as AB: Or a CURVED LINE when it is not the ſhorteſt diſtance, as CD.

A line is uſually denoted by two letters, viz. one at each end, as AB or CD.

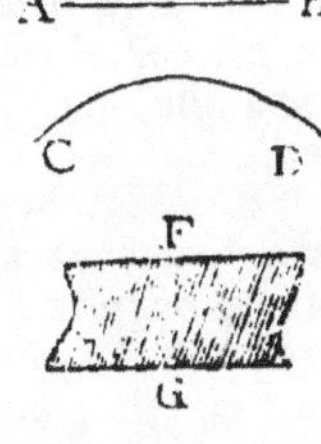

4. A SUPERFICIES or SURFACE is that magnitude which has only length and breadth, and is bounded by lines: as FG.

5. A SOLID is that magnitude which has length, breadth and thickneſs.

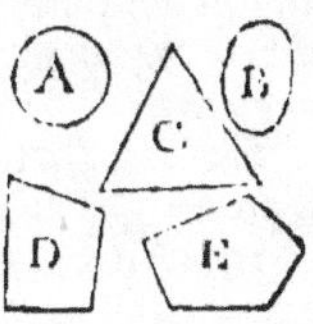

6. A FIGURE is a bounded ſpace, the limits or bounds of which may be either lines or ſurfaces.

7. A PLANE, or a PLANE FIGURE, is a ſuperficies which lies evenly, or perfectly flat, between its limits, and may be bounded by one curve line; but not with leſs than three right lines, as A, B, C, D, or E, &c.

8. A

8. A CIRCLE is a plain figure, bounded by an uniformly curved line, called the Circumference, as ABD, which is every where equally diſtant from one point, as C within the figure called the CENTER.

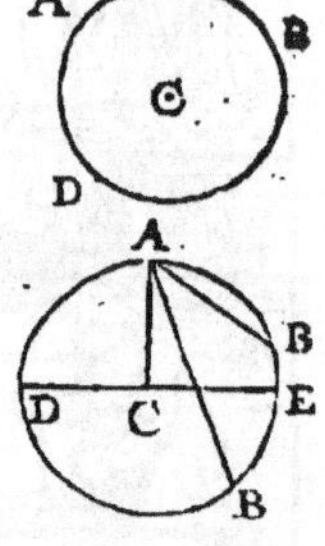

9. A RADIUS is a right line drawn from the center to the circumference as CA, CD or CE.

All the radii of the ſame circle are equal.

10. An ARC is any part of the circumference.

As the arc AB, *or the arc* AD.

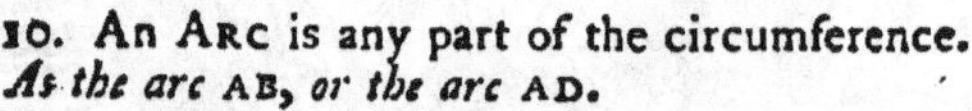

11. A CHORD is a right line joining the ends of an arc, as AB, and is ſaid to ſubtend that arc; it divides the circle into two parts, called SEGMENTS.

12. A DIAMETER is a chord paſſing through the center, as DE, and divides the circle into two equal parts, called SEMICIRCLES.

13. The CIRCUMFERENCE of every circle is ſuppoſed to be divided into 360 equal parts, called DEGREES; each degree into 60 equal parts, called MINUTES; each minute into 60 equal parts, called SECONDS, &c.

14. A PLANE ANGLE, is the inclination of two lines on the ſame plane meeting in a point, as ACB.

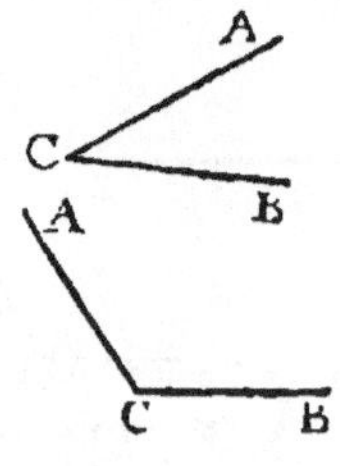

A right lined angle is formed by two right lines. The point where the lines meet is called the *angular point*, as C.

The lines which form the angle are called *legs*.

Thus CA *and* CB *are the legs of the angle* ACB.

An Angle is uſually marked by three letters, viz. one at the angular point, and one at the other end of each leg; but that at the angular point is always to be read the middle letter, as ACB, or BCA.

15. The meaſure of a right lined angle is an arc, as BA contained between the legs CB, CA, including the angle, the angular point C being the center of that arc.

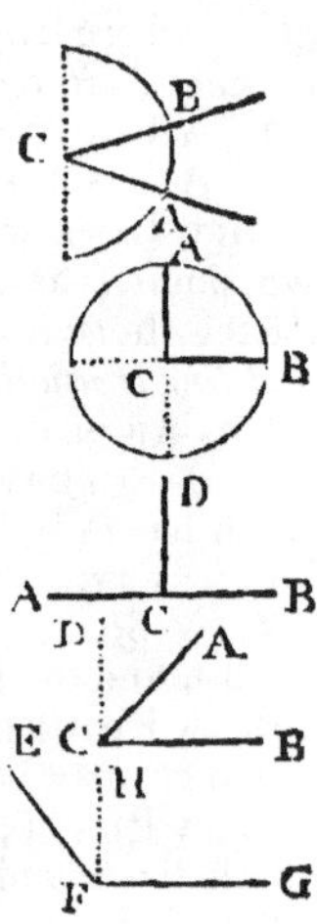

16. A RIGHT ANGLE is that, the meaſure of which is a fourth part of the circumference of a circle, or ninety degrees. *Thus the angle* ACB *is a right angle.*

17. A PERPENDICULAR is that right line which cuts another at right angles; or which makes equal angles on both ſides. *Thus* DC *is perpendicular to* AB, *when the angles* DCA *and* DCB *are equal, or are right angles.*

18. An ACUTE ANGLE, as ACB, is that which is leſs than a right angle DCB.

19. An OBTUSE ANGLE, as EFG, is that which is greater than a right angle HFG.

Acute and obtuſe angles are called OBLIQUE ANGLES.

20. PA-

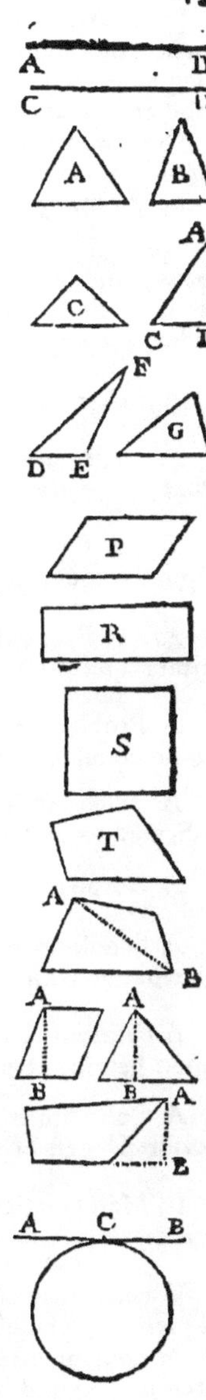

20. PARALLEL LINES, are right lines in the same plane, which do not incline to one another, as AB, CD.

21. A TRIANGLE is a plane figure bounded by three lines.

22. An EQUILATERAL TRIANGLE is that in which the three lines, or sides, are equal, as A.

23. An ISOSCELES TRIANGLE is that which has only two equal sides, as B or C.

24. A RIGHT ANGLED TRIANGLE, as ABC, is that which has one right angle B.

25. An OBTUSE ANGLED TRIANGLE, as DEF, has one obtuse angle E.

26. An ACUTE ANGLED TRIANGLE, as G, has all its angles acute.

27. A QUADRANGLE, or QUADRILATERAL, is a plane figure bounded by four right lines, or sides.

A Quadrangle is usually expressed by letters at the opposite angles.

28. A PARALLELOGRAM is a quadrangle the opposite sides of which are parallel and equal, as P.

29. A RECTANGLE is a parallelogram with right angles: and in which the length is greater than its breadth, as R.

30. A SQUARE is a parallelogram having four equal sides and right angles, as S.

31. A TRAPEZIUM is a quadrangle the opposite sides of which are not parallel, as T.

32. The DIAGONAL of a quadrangle, is a line, as AB, drawn from one angle, to its opposite angle.

33. The BASE of a figure, is the line it is supposed to stand on.

34. The ALTITUDE or HEIGHT of a figure, is the perpendicular distance AB, between the base and the vertex, or part most remote from the base.

35. CONGRUOUS FIGURES, are those which agree, or correspond, with one another, in every respect.

36. A TANGENT to a circle is a right line, as AB, touching its circumference, but not cutting; and the point C, where it touches, is called the *point of contact.*

37. An ANGLE, BAC, *in a Segment*, CADB, is, when the angular point is in the circumference of the segment, and the legs including the angle pass through the ends B and C, of the chord of the segment.

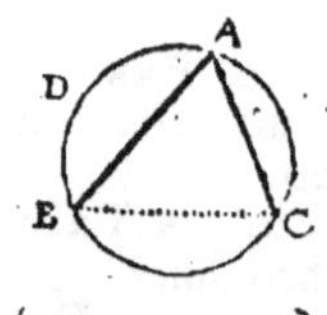

Such an angle is said to be in a circumference; and to stand on the arc, BC, *included between the legs*, AB *and* AC, *of the angle.*

38. Right lined figures, having more than four sides, are called *Polygons*; and have their names from the number of their angles, or sides; as those of five sides are called Pentagons; of six sides, Hexagons; of seven sides, Heptagons; of eight sides, Octagons, *&c.*

39. A regular Polygon is a figure with equal sides, and equal angles.

40. A figure is said to be inscribed in a circle, when all the angles of that figure are in the circumference of the circle.

41. A figure is said to circumscribe a circle, when every side of the figure is touched by the circumference of the circle.

42. A Proposition is something proposed to be considered; and requires either a solution or answer, or that something be made out, or proved.

A Problem is a practical proposition, in which something is proposed to be done, or effected.

A Theorem is a speculative proposition, or rule, in which something is affirmed to be true.

A Corollary is some conclusion gained from a preceding proposition.

A Scholium is a remark on some proposition; or an exemplification of the matter which it contains.

An Axiom is a self-evident truth, or principle, that every one assents to upon hearing it proposed.

A Postulate is a principle, or condition, requested; the simplicity or reasonableness of which cannot be denied.

In Mathematics, the following Postulates and Axioms, are some of the principal ones that are generally taken for granted.

When a proposition, from supposed premises, asserts such and such consequences; and subjoins, *And the contrary:* it is to be understood, that if the consequences be assumed as premises; then what were first taken as premises, would become consequences.

Thus, in Article 95, it is premised, *that if two parallel right lines are cut by another right line*, there results this consequence; *The alternate angles are equal.* And the contrary means; that *where equal alternate angles are made by a right line cutting two other right lines; the right lines so cut, are parallel lines.*

Postulates.

Poſtulates.

43. I. That a right line may be drawn from any given point to another given point.

44. II. That a given right line may be continued, or lengthened at pleaſure.

45. III. That from a given point, and with any radius, a circle may be deſcribed.

Axioms.

46. I. Things equal to the ſame thing, are equal to one another.

47. II. If equal things are added to equal things, the ſums or wholes will be equal. But if unequals be added, the ſums are unequal.

48. III. If equal things are taken from equal things, the remainders, or differences, are equal: but are unequal, when unequals are taken.

49. IV. Things are equal which are double, triple, quadruple, *&c.* or half, third part, &c. of one and the ſame thing, or of equal things.

50. V. Things which have equal meaſures, are equal. And the contrary.

51. VI. Equal circles have equal radii.

52. VII. Equal arcs in equal circles have equal chords, and are the meaſures of equal angles. And the contrary.

53. VIII. Parallel right lines have each the ſame inclination to a right line cutting them.

In what follows, it is to be underſtood, that right lines (*viz.* ſtraight lines) are drawn by the edge of a ſtraight ruler: circles or arcs, are deſcribed with one foot of a pair of compaſſes, the other foot reſting on the point which is taken for the center; and the diſtance of the feet, or points, of the compaſſes is taken as the radius: alſo, that the point marked out by a letter is to be underſtood, when the reference is made to that letter.

54. It is alſo taken for granted, that a line or diſtance can be taken between the compaſſes, and may be transferred or applied from one place to another. Alſo, that one figure can be applied to, or laid upon another, or conceived to be ſo applied.

In any problem, when a line, angle, or figure is ſaid to be given; that line, angle, or figure muſt be made, before any part of the operation is performed.

SEC-

SECTION II.

Geometrical Problems.

55. PROBLEM I.

To bisect, or divide into two equal parts, a given line AB.

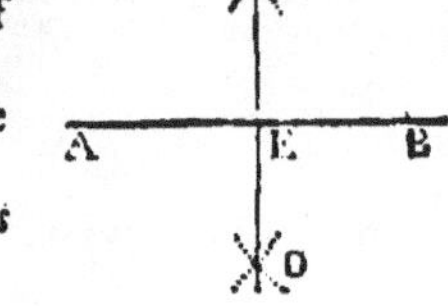

OPERATION. 1st. From the ends A and B *, with one and the same radius, greater than half AB, describe arcs cutting in C and D. (45)

2d. A ruler laid by C and D, gives E, the middle of AB, as required.

The proof of this operation depends on articles 101, 99.

56. PROBLEM II.

To bisect a given right lined angle ABC.

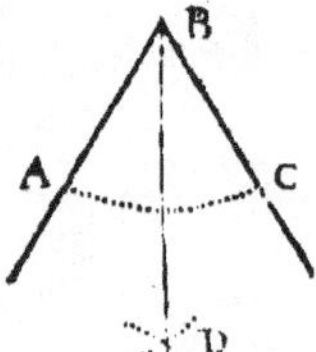

OPERATION. 1st. From B, describe an arc AC.

2d. From A and C*, with one and the same radius, describe arcs cutting in D. (45)

3d. A right line drawn through B and D will divide the angle into two equal parts, as required.

The proof depends on article 101.

57. PROBLEM III.

From a given point B, *in a given right line* AF, *to draw a right line perpendicular to the given line.*

CASE I. *When* B *is near the middle of the line.*

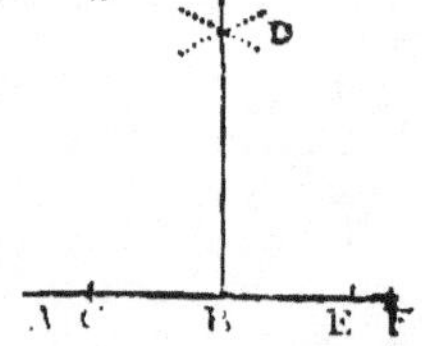

OPERATION. 1st. On each side of B, take the equal distances BC, and BE. (54)

2d. On C and E * describe, with one radius, arcs cutting in D. (45)

3d. A right line drawn through B and D will be the perpendicular required. (43)

The proof depends on article 103.

58. CASE II. *When* B *is at, or near the end of the given line.*

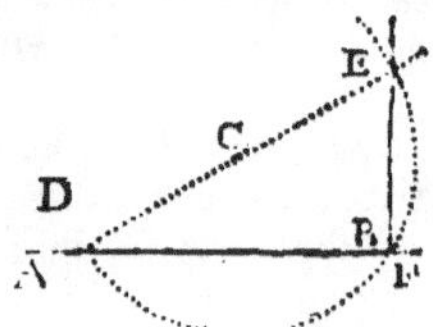

OPERATION. 1st. On any convenient point C, taken at pleasure, with the distance, or radius CB, describe an arc DBE, cutting AF in D, B. (45)

2d. A ruler laid by D and C will cut this arc in E.

3d. A right line drawn through B and E will be the perpendicular required.

This depends on article 130.

---

* That is, first describe an arc from one point; then describe an arc from the other point with the same opening of the compasses.

59. PRO-

59. PROBLEM IV.

To draw a line perpendicular to a given right line AB, *from a point* C *without that line.*

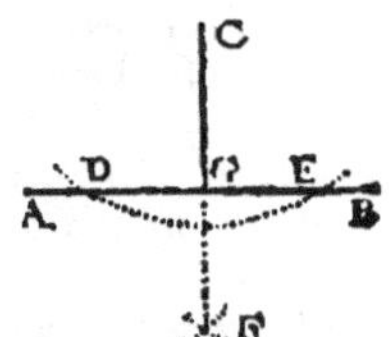

CASE I. *When the point* C *is nearly opposite to the middle of the given line.*

OPERATION. 1st. On C, with one radius, cut AB in D and E. (45)

2d. On D and E, with one radius, describe arcs cutting in F. (45)

A ruler laid by C and F gives G; then draw CG, and that will be the perpendicular required.

This depends on articles 101, 99.

60. CASE II. *When* C *is nearly opposite to one end of the given line* AB.

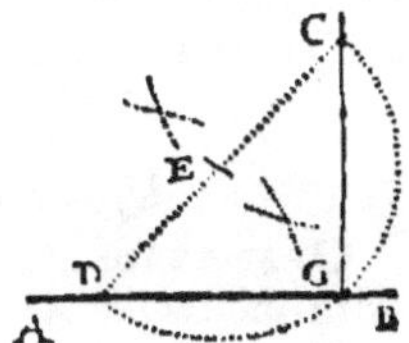

OPERATION. 1st. To any point D in AB, draw the line CD. (43)

2d. Bisect the line CD in E. (55)

3d. On E, with the radius EC, cut AB in G. Then CG being drawn, will be the perpendicular required.

This depends on article 130.

61. PROBLEM V.

To trisect, or divide into three equal parts, a right angle ABC.

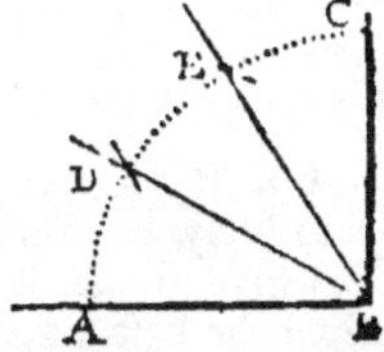

OPERATION. 1st. From B, with any radius BA, describe the arc AC, cutting the legs BA, BC, in A, C.

2d. From A, with the radius AB, cut the arc AC in E, and from C, with the same radius, cut AC in D.

3d. Draw BE, BD, and the angle ABC will be divided into three equal parts.

This depends on article 193.

62. PROBLEM VI.

At a given point D, *to make a right lined angle equal to a given right lined angle* ABC.

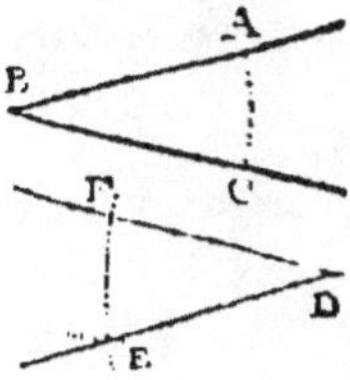

OPERATION. 1st. From D and B, with one radius describe the arcs EF, and AC, cutting the legs of the given angle in the points A, C.

2d. Transfer the distance AC to the arc EF, from F to E. (54)

3d. Lines drawn from D, through E and F, will form the angle EDF equal to the angle ABC.

This depends on article 101.

63. PROBLEM VII.

To draw a line parallel to a given right line AB.

CASE I. *When the parallel line is to pass through a given point*, C.

OPERATION. 1st. From C, with any convenient radius, describe an arc DF, cutting AB in D.

2d. Apply the radius CD from D to E; and from E, with the same radius, cut the arc DF in F.

3d. A line drawn through F and C will be parallel to AB.

This depends on article 101, 95.

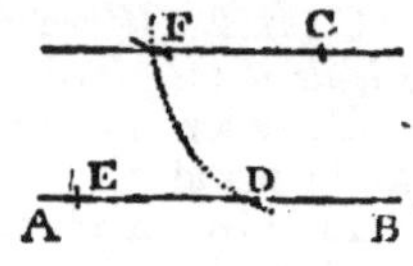

64. CASE II. *When the parallel line is to be at the given distance* C *from* AB.

OPERATION. 1st. From the points A and B, with the radius C, describe arcs D and E.

2d. Lay a ruler to touch the arcs D and E, and a line drawn in that position is the parallel required.

This operation is mechanical.

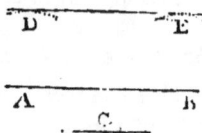

65. PROBLEM VIII.

Upon a given line AB, *to make an equilateral triangle.*

OPERATION. 1st. From the points A and B, with the radius AB, describe arcs cutting in C. (45)

2d. Draw CA, CB, and the figure ABC is the triangle required. (43.)

The truth of this operation is evident; for the sides are radii of equal circles.

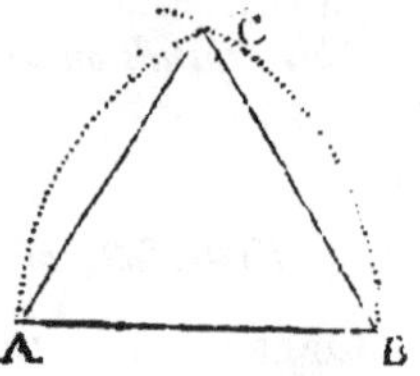

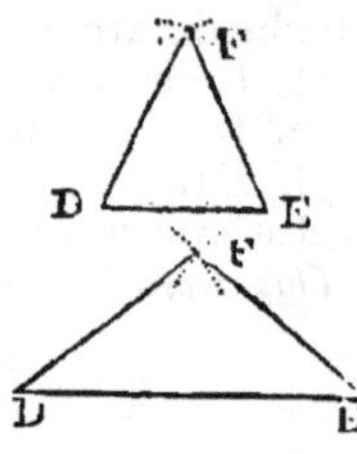

66. By a like operation, an Isosceles triangle DEF may be constructed on a given base DE, with the given equal legs DF, EF, either greater, or less, than the base DE.

67. PROBLEM IX.

To make a right lined triangle, the sides of which shall be respectively equal, [illegible] *those of a given triangle* ABC, *or to three given lines, provided any* [illegible] *them taken together are greater than the third.*

[illegible]TION. 1st. Draw a line DE equal to the [illegible] (54)

[illegible] with a radius equal to AC, describe [illegible] (45)

[illegible]th a radius equal to BC, describe [illegible] the former arc in F. (45)

[illegible]nd the triangle DFE will be

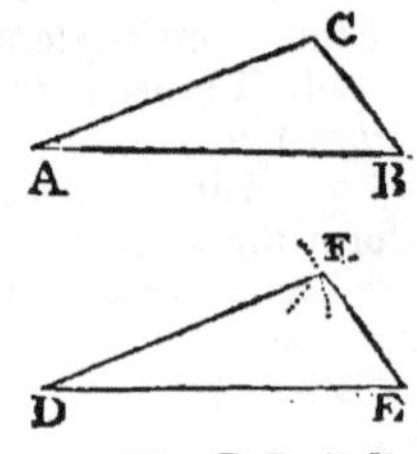

68. PROB-

68. PROBLEM X.

Upon a given line AB, *to deſcribe a ſquare.*

OPERATION. 1ſt. Draw BC perpendicular, and equal to AB. (58)

2d. On A and C, with the radius AB, deſcribe arcs cutting in D. (45)

3d. Draw DC, DA; and the figure ABCD is the ſquare required.

This depends on articles 101, 104, 95, 30.

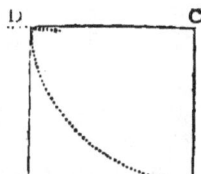

69. PROBLEM XI.

To deſcribe a rectangle whoſe length ſhall be equal to a given line EF, *and breadth equal to another given line* G.

OPERATION. 1ſt. At E and F erect two perpendiculars, EH and FI, each equal to the given line G.

2d. Draw HI, and the figure EFIH will be the rectangle required.

This depends on articles 29, 101, 104, 95.

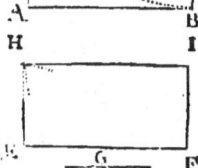

70. PROBLEM XII.

To find the center of a circle.

OPERATION. 1ſt. Draw any chord AB.

2d. Biſect AB with the chord CD. (55)

3d. Biſect CD with the chord EF, and their interſection G will be the center required.

This depends on article 125.

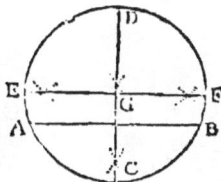

71. PROBLEM XIII.

To divide the circumference of a circle into two, four, eight, ſixteen, thirty-two, &c. equal parts.

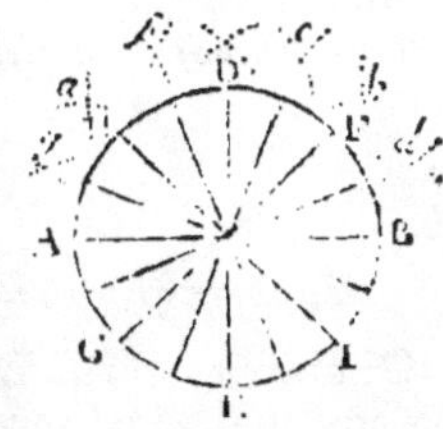

OPERATION. 1ſt. A diameter AB divides the circle into two equal parts. (12)

2d. A diameter DE, perpendicular to AB, divides the circumference into four equal parts.

3d. On A, D, B, deſcribe arcs cutting in *a*, *b*; then by the interſections *a*, *b*, and the center, the diameters FC, HI, being drawn, divide the circumference into eight equal parts; and ſo on by continual biſection.

For at each operation, the intercepted arcs are biſected, and the parts doubled.

72. PROBLEM XIV.

To deſcribe a circle, the circumference of which ſhall paſs through three given points A, B, C, *provided they do not lie in one right line.*

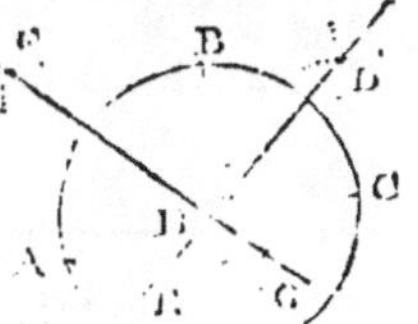

OPERATION. 1ſt. Biſect the diſtance CB with the line DE. (55)

2d. Biſect the diſtance AB with the line FG.

3d. On H, the interſection of theſe lines, with the diſtance to either of the given points, deſcribe the circle required.

This depends on article 125.

73. PROBLEM XV.

To draw a tangent to a given circle, that ſhall paſs through a given point A.

CASE I. *When* A *is in the circumference of the circle.*

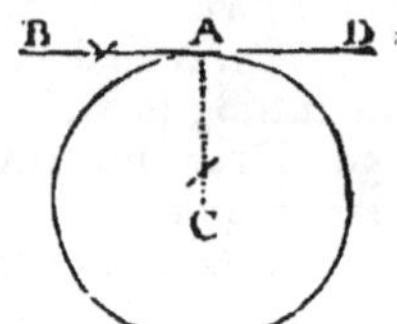

OPERATION. 1ſt. From the center C, draw the radius CA. (43)

2d. Through A draw BD perpendicular to CA (58), and BD is the tangent required.

This depends on article 126.

74. CASE II. *When the given point* A, *is without the given circle.*

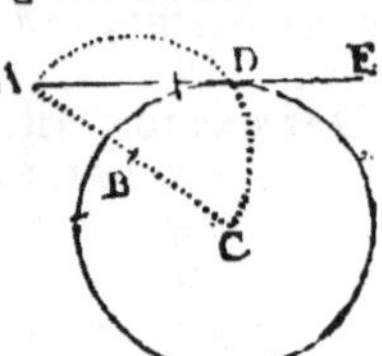

OPERATION. 1ſt. From the center C, draw CA, which biſect in B. (55)

2d. On B, with the radius BA, cut the given circumference in D.

3d. Through D, the line AE being drawn, will be the tangent required.

This depends on articles 130, 126.

75. PROBLEM XVI.

To two given right lines A, B, *to find a third proportional.*

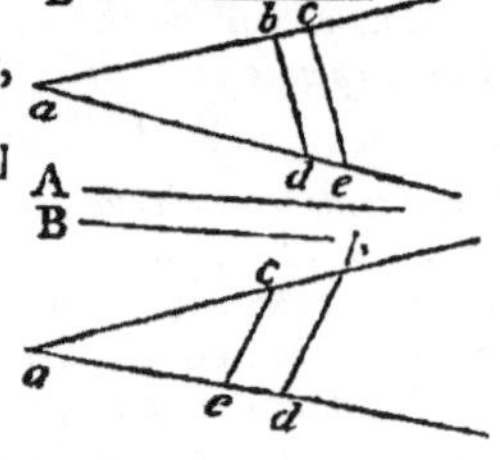

OPERATION. 1ſt. Draw two right lines making any angle, and meeting in *a*.

2d. In theſe lines, take *ab*=firſt term, and *ac*, *ad*, each equal to the ſecond term.

3d. Draw *bd*, and through *c*, draw *ce* parallel to *bd*; then *ae* is the third proportional ſought.

And *ab* : *ac* : : *ad* : *ae**.

This depends on article 165.

76. PROBLEM XVII.

To three given right lines A, B, C, *to find a fourth proportional.*

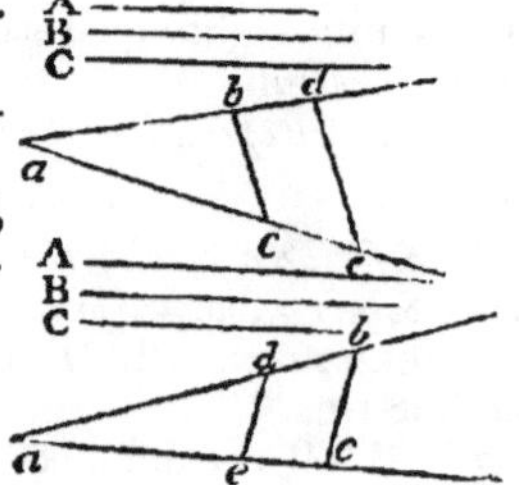

OPERATION. 1ſt. Draw two right lines making any angle, and meeting in *a*.

2d. In theſe lines take *ab*=firſt term, *ac*=ſecond term, and *ad*=third term.

3d. Draw *bc*, and parallel to it, through *d*, draw *de*; then *ae* is the fourth proportional required.

And *ab* : *ac* : : *ad* : *ae*.

This depends on article 165.

---

* And is thus read: *ab* is to *ac*, as *ad* is to *ae*.
The character (:) ſtanding for *is to*, and the character (: :) for *as*.

77. PROB-

77. ## PROBLEM XVIII.

Between two given right lines A, B, *to find a mean proportional.*

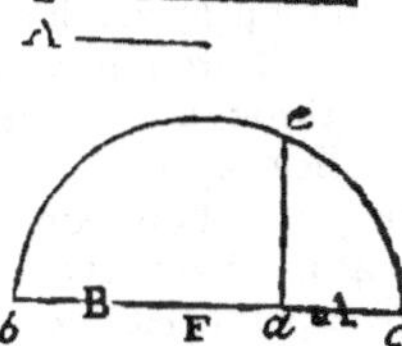

OPERATION. 1ſt. Draw a right line, in which take *ac*=A, *ab*=B.

2. Biſect *bc* in F (55); and on F, with the radius F*b*, deſcribe a ſemicircle *bec*.

3d. From *a* draw *ae* perpendicular to *bc* (57); then *ae* is the mean proportional required.

And *ac* : *ae* : : *ae* : *ab*.

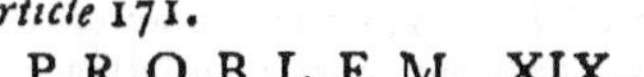

This depends on article 171.

78. ## PROBLEM XIX.

To divide a given line BC *in the ſame proportion as a given line* A *is divided.*

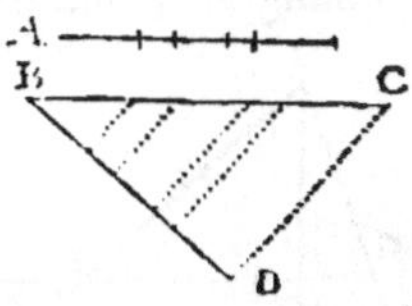

OPERATION. 1ſt. From one end B of BC draw BD, making any angle with BC.

2d. In BD apply from B the ſeveral diviſions of A; ſo BD will be equal to A, and alike divided.

3d. Draw CD; then lines drawn parallel to CD through the ſeveral diviſions of BD, will divide the line BC in the manner required.

This depends on article 165.

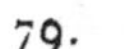

79. ## PROBLEM XX.

To divide a given right line AB *into a propoſed number of equal parts (ſuppoſe 7).*

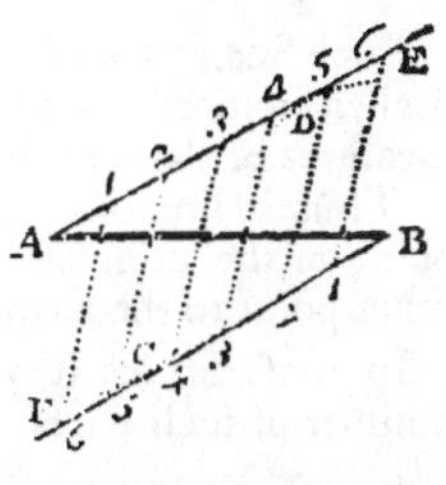

OPERATION. 1ſt. From A, one end of AB, draw AE to make any angle with AB; and from B, the other end, draw BF, making the angle ABF equal to the angle BAE. (62)

2d. In each of the lines AE, BF, beginning at A and B, take, of any length, as many equal parts, leſs one, as AB is to be divided into, *viz.* 1, 2, 3, 4, 5, 6.

3d. Lines drawn from 1 to 6, 2 to 5, 3 to 4, &c. will divide AB as was required.

This depends on article 165.

80. *Another Method.*

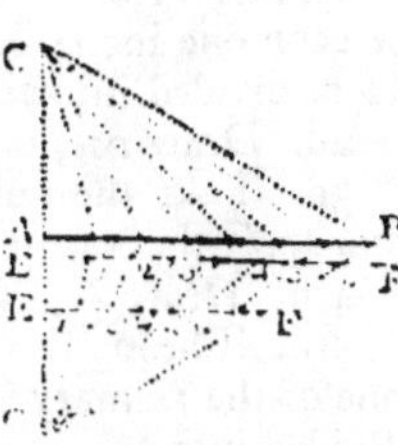

OPERATION. 1ſt. Through one end A, draw a line CC nearly perpendicular to AB.

2d. Draw EF parallel to AB, at any convenient diſtance.

3d. In EF take, of any length, as many equal parts as AB is to be divided into; as 1, 2, 3, 4, 5, 6, to F.

4th. Through B and F, where the diviſions terminate, draw BC, meeting CC in C.

5th. Lines drawn from C through the ſeveral diviſions of EF, will cut AB into the equal parts required.

Note, If the ſum of the diviſions from E to F chance to be leſs than AB, the point C, and the line EF, will be on the ſame ſide of AB; but if greater, C falls on the contrary ſide.

81. PROBLEM XXI.

To make Scales of equal parts.

Operation. 1ſt. Draw three lines, A, B, C, parallel to one another, and at convenient diſtances, ſuch as are here expreſſed.

2d. In the line C, take the equal parts *cb*, *bc*, *cd*, *da*, &c. each equal to ſome propoſed length.

3d. Through *c*, draw the line DE perpendicular to *ca*; and parallel to DE, through the ſeveral points *b*, *c*, *d*, *a*, &c. draw lines acroſs the three parallels A, B, C; then are the ſpaces or diſtances *cb*, *bc*, *cd*, &c. called the primary diviſions.

4th. Divide the left-hand ſpace into 10 equal parts (80), and through theſe points let lines, parallel to DE, be drawn acroſs the parallels BC; and the primary diviſion *cb* will be parted into 10 equal ſpaces, called ſubdiviſions.

5th. Number the primary diviſions from the left towards the right, beginning at *c*, and the ſcale is conſtructed.

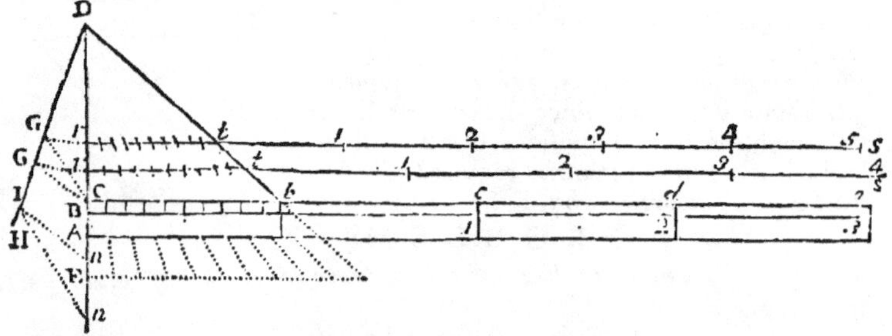

Such Scales are uſeful for conſtructing figures, the ſides of which are expreſſed in meaſures of length; as feet, yards, miles, &c. Or to find the meaſures of the length of lines in a given figure.

Thus a line of 36, or 360, feet, yards, &c. is taken by ſetting one point of the compaſſes on the third primary diviſion, and extending the other point to the ſixth ſubdiviſion: and ſo of others.

In theſe Scales it is uſually ſuppoſed, that an inch is divided into ſome number of ſuch parts, as are expreſſed by the ſubdiviſions.

82. *To find the diviſions of a Scale of equal parts, when any given number of them are to make an inch.*

Operation. 1ſt. Make a Scale *ca*, where the primary diviſions ſhall be each one inch; let DC be at right angles to *ca*, and the left-hand ſpace *cb* be divided into 10 equal parts, and draw D*b* from any point D.

2d. Draw DH, making with DC any angle; and make DI = *cb*.

3d. Take the number of parts propoſed in an inch, from the Scale *ca*, and apply them from D to *n*, in the line DC, continued if neceſſary.

4th. Draw *n*I, and CG parallel to *n*I; and make D*r* = DG.

5th. Through *r* draw *rs* parallel to *ca*, cutting D*b* in *t*; then *rt* will be one of the primary diviſions, containing 10 of the parts the inch was to be divided into.

6th. Lines drawn from D to the diviſions of *cb*, divide *rt* into 10 equal parts.

83. PROBLEM XXII.

To divide the circumference of a circle into degrees; and thence to make a Scale of chords.

OPERATION. 1ſt. Deſcribe the ſemicircle ABD, the center of which is C, and draw CD at right angles to AB.

2d. Triſect the angles ACD, DCB, in the points *a*, *b*; *c*, *d* (61): then by trials, divide the arcs A*a*, *ab*, *b*D, D*c*, *cd*, *d*B, each into three equal parts, and the ſemicircumference will be divided into 18 equal parts, of 10 degrees each.

3d. Theſe arcs being biſected, will give arcs of 5 degrees.

4th. And theſe arcs being divided into 5 equal parts, by trials, will give arcs of 1 degree each.

5th. The chords of the arcs A*d*, A*c*, AD, A*b*, A*a*, and of every other arc, being applied from A on the diameter AB, will divide AB into a Scale of chords; which are to be numbered from A towards B.

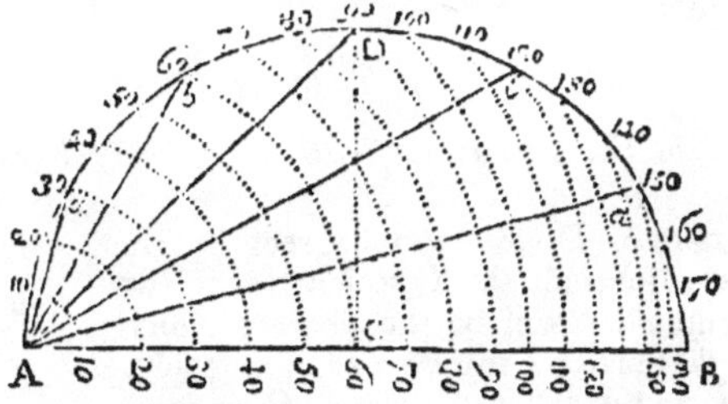

A Scale of chords is uſeful for conſtructing an angle of a given number of degrees: And for finding the meaſure of a given angle.

84. PROBLEM XXIII.

To make an angle of a propoſed number of degrees.

OPERATION. 1ſt. Take the firſt 60 deg. from the Scale of chords, and with this radius deſcribe an arc BC, the center of which is A.

2d. Take the chord of the propoſed number of degrees from the Scale, reckoning from its beginning, and apply this diſtance to the arc BC, from B to C.

3d. Lines drawn from A, through the points B and C, will form an angle BAC, the meaſure of which is the degrees propoſed.

With Scales of chords not exceeding 90 degrees, ſuch as are generally put on rulers, angles greater than 90 degrees, ſuppoſe of 138 deg. are to be taken at twice, *viz.* 69 and 69 ($\frac{1}{2}$ of 138), or 90 and 48.

When a given angle, BAC, *is to be meaſured.*

From the angular point A, with the chord of 60 degrees, deſcribe the arc BC, cutting the legs in the points B and C.

Then the diſtance BC, applied to the chords, from the beginning, will ſhew the degrees which meaſure the angle BAC.

85. PROBLEM XXIV.

In a given circle to inſcribe a regular polygon, the number of ſides being given.

OPERATION. 1ſt. Divide 360 degrees by the number of ſides, and the Quotient will be the degrees which meaſure the angle at the center of the circle, ſubtended by a ſide of the *polygon**.

2d. Draw the radius CB, make an angle BCD equal to thoſe degrees (84), and draw the chord DB; then will DB be the ſide of the polygon required; which applied to the circumference from B to *a*, *a* to *b*, *b* to *c*, &c. will give the points to which the ſides of the polygon are to be drawn.

If the polygon has an even number of ſides, draw the diameter AB; and divide half the circumference, as before; then lines drawn from theſe points through the center, as ED, will give the remaining points, in the other ſemicircumference.

86. PROBLEM XXV.

On a given right line AB, *to conſtruct a regular polygon of any aſſigned number of ſides.*

OPERATION. 1ſt. Divide 360 degrees by the number of ſides; ſubtract the Quotient from 180 degrees, the remainder will be the degrees which meaſure the angle made by any two adjoining ſides of that polygon, and is called the angle of the polygon †.

2d. At the ends A, B, of the line AB, make angles ABC, BAD, equal to the angle of the polygon.

3d. Make AD, BC, each equal to AB.

4th. At the points C, D, make angles equal to that of the polygon as before; and let the ſides including thoſe angles be each equal to AB; and thus proceed until the polygon is conſtructed.

In figures of any number of ſides, the two laſt ſides DE, CE; or EG, HG; are readieſt found by deſcribing arcs from C and D, or from E and H, with the radius AB, interſected in E, or in G.

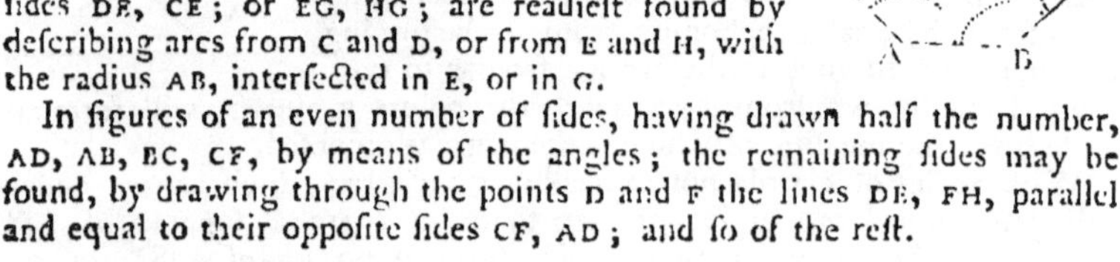

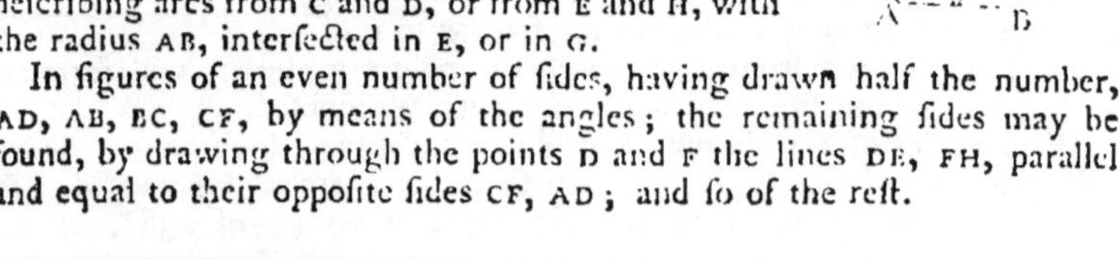

In figures of an even number of ſides, having drawn half the number, AD, AB, BC, CF, by means of the angles; the remaining ſides may be found, by drawing through the points D and F the lines DE, FH, parallel and equal to their oppoſite ſides CF, AD; and ſo of the reſt.

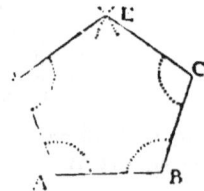

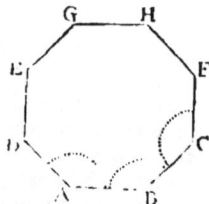

---

* *For there will be as many equal angles at the center as there are equal ſides. And the whole cirumference meaſures the ſum of all the angles at the center.*

† *For each ſide of the polygon with radii drawn to its ends form an Iſoſceles triangle.*

Then the angle of the polygon is derived from articles 85, 96, 104.

87. PROB.

87. PROBLEM XXVI.

About a given regular Polygon, to circumscribe a circle: or within that Polygon to inscribe a circle.

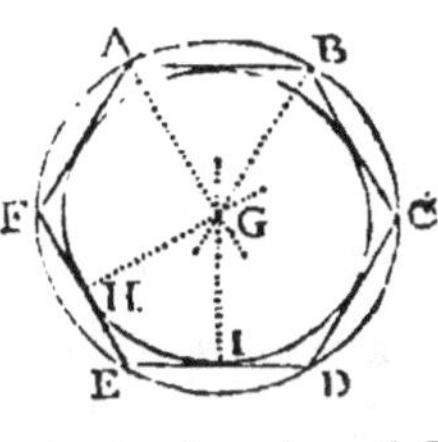

OPERATION. 1st. Bisect any two angles FAB, CBA, with the lines AG, BG, (56) and the point G, where they intersect one another, will be the center of the polygon.

2d. A circle described from G, with the radius GA, will circumscribe the given polygon.

This depends on article 85, 96, 104.

88. Again, 1st. Bisect any two sides FE, ED, in the points H and I (55); and draw HG, IG, at right angles to FE, ED (57); then the point G, where they intersect each other, will be the center of the Polygon.

2d. A circle described from G, with the radius GH, will be inscribed in the given Polygon.

This depends on article 126.

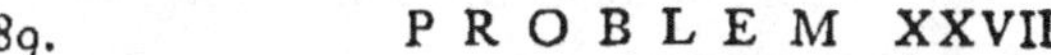

89. PROBLEM XXVII.

On a given right line AB, *to describe a segment of a circle, that shall contain an angle equal to a given right lined angle* C.

OPERATION. 1st. Make an angle BAF equal to the given angle C. (62)

2d. From H, the middle of AB, draw HI at right angles to AB (57), and from A draw AI at right angles to AF (58), cutting HI in I.

3d. From I, with the radius IA, describe a circle. Then will the segment AGB contain an angle AGB equal to the given angle C.

This depends on articles 125, 126, 132.

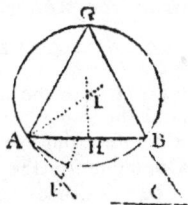

90. PROBLEM XXVIII.

To divide a right line in continued proportion, in the ratio of two given right lines AB, AC.

OPERATION. 1st. From B, with the radius AB (the antecedent) describe an arc Ac.

2d. In that arc apply (the consequent) AC from A to *c*; draw A*c*, and apply *c*A from *c* to D.

3d. Apply the following lines in the order directed, *viz.* AD from A to *d*, and from *d* to E; AE from A to *e*, and from *e* to F; AF from A to *f*, and from *f* to G; AG from A to *g*, and from *g* to H, &c. Then will the proportional lines be AB, AC, AD, AE, AF, AG, &c. And

AB : AC : : (A*c*=) AC : (A*d*=) AD.
AB : AC : : (A*d*=) AD : (A*e*=) AE.
AB : AC : : (A*e*=) AE : (A*f*=) AF.
&c.

This depends on articles 104, 95, 165.

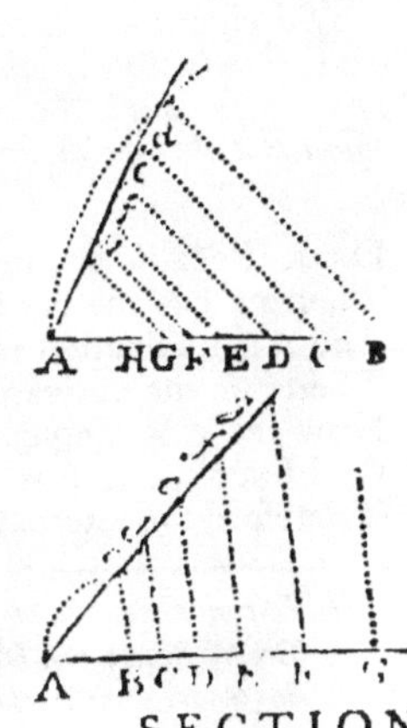

SECTION

SECTION III.

Geometrical Theorems.

Of Right Lines and Planes.

91. THEOREM I.

When one right line CD *ſtands upon another right line* AB, *they make two angles* BCD, ACD *which together are equal to two right angles.*

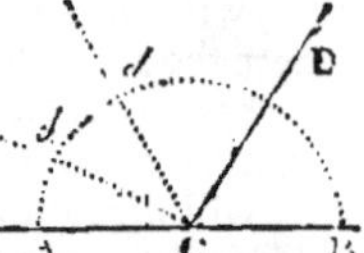

Demonstration. For deſcribing a ſemicircle ADB, on C. (45)
Then the arc DB meaſures the angle BCD. (15)
And the arc DA meaſures the angle ACD. (15)
But the arcs DB and AD together meaſure two right angles. (13, 16)
Therefore BCD and ACD together, are equal to two right angles (50)

92. Corollary. Hence if any number of right lines *cd* ſtands on one point C, on the ſame ſide of another right line AB; the ſum of all the angles are equal to two right angles; or are meaſured by 180 degrees.

93. THEOREM II.

If two right lines AC, EB *interſect each other in* D, *the oppoſite angles are equal, viz.*

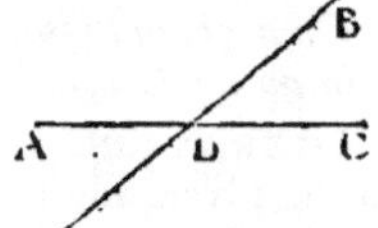

* ∠ CDE = ∠ ADE, and ∠ CDE = ∠ ADB.

† Dem. For the angles ADE and ADB together make two right angles. (91)
And the angles CDB and ADB together make two right angles. (91)
Therefore the ſum of ADE and ADB = ſum of CDB and ADB. (46)
Conſequently the ∠ CDB is equal to the ∠ ADE. (48)

94. ‡ Corol. Hence if any number of right lines croſs each other in one point, the ſum of all the angles which they make about that point, is equal to four right angles; or is meaſured by 360 degrees.

95. THEOREM III.

If a right line FE *cut two parallel right lines* AB, CD; *then is the outward angle a* ‖ *equal to the inward and oppoſite angle d; and the alternate angles c, d are equal: and the contrary.*

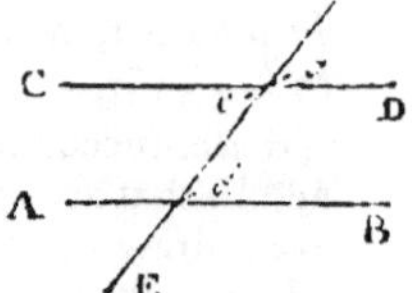

Dem. Becauſe CD and AB are parallel by ſuppoſition:
Then FE has the ſame inclination to CD and AB. (53)
And this inclination is expreſſed by the ∠ *a* or ∠ *d*: (14)
Therefore the outward ∠ *a* is equal to the inward and oppoſite ∠ *d*.
Now the ∠ *a* is equal to the ∠ *c*. (93)
And ſince the ∠ *a* is equal to the ∠ *d*;
Therefore the alternate angles *c* and *d* are equal. (46)

---

* *The mark* ∠ *ſtands for the word angle.*

† Dem. *ſtands for Demonſtration.* ‡ Corol. *ſtands for Corollary.*

‖ *Angles are ſometimes marked by a ſingle letter. Thus angle a is uſed for angle* FAD.

96. THEO-

96. THEOREM IV.

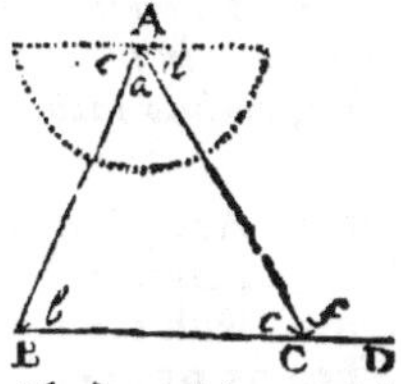

In any right lined triangle ABC, *the ſum of the three angles a, b, c, is equal to two right angles: And if one ſide* BC *be continued, the outward angle f is equal to the ſum of the two inward and oppoſite angles a, b.*

DEM. Through A, draw a right line parallel to BC, (63) making with AB the $\angle e$, and with AC the $\angle d$.

Now $\angle e = \angle b$; and $\angle d = \angle c$. being alternate. (95)
And two right angles meaſure the $\angle e + \angle a + \angle d$. (92)
Therefore $\angle b + \angle a + \angle c = \angle e + \angle a + \angle d$. (47)
Conſequently $\angle b + \angle a + \angle c =$ two right angles. (46)
Moreover $\angle c + \angle f =$ two right angles. (91)
Therefore $\angle b + \angle a = \angle f$. (46)

97. Hence, if one angle is right or obtuſe, each of the other is acute.

98. If two angles of one triangle are equal to two angles of another triangle, the remaining angles are equal. And if one angle in one triangle is equal to one angle in another triangle, then is the ſum of the remaining angles in one, equal to the ſum of the remaining angles in the other.

99. THEOREM V.

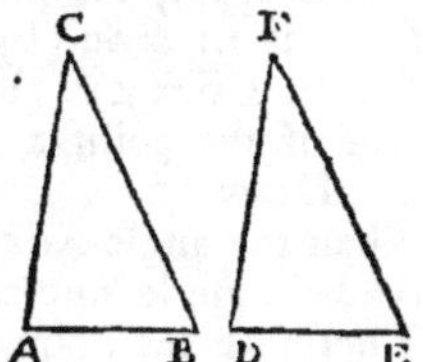

If two ſides AB, AC *and the included angle* A *in one triangle* ABC, *are reſpectively equal to two ſides* DE, DF *and the included angle* D *of another* DEF, *each to each; then are thoſe triangles congruous.*

DEM. Apply the point D to the point A, and the line DE to AB. (54)
Now as DE = AB (by ſuppoſition); therefore the point E falls on B.
But $\angle$D = $\angle$A (by ſup.); therefore DF will fall on AC.
And ſince DF = AC (by ſup.); therefore the point F falls on C.
Conſequently FE will fall on CB.
Therefore the triangles ACB, DFE, are congruous, ſince every part agrees.

100. THEOREM VI.

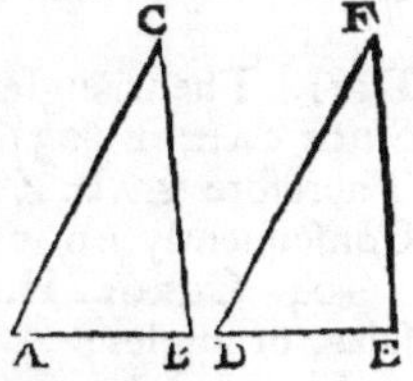

If two triangles ABC, DEF *have two angles* A, B *and the included ſide* AB *in one reſpectively equal to two angles* D, E *and the included ſide* DE *in the other, each to each; then are thoſe triangles congruous.*

DEM. Apply the point D to A, and the line DE to AB.
Now as DE = AB (by ſup.); therefore the point E falls on B.
And as $\angle$D = $\angle$A (by ſup.); therefore the line DF falls on AC.
Now if the line AC is leſs or greater than the line DF;
Then the line FE not falling on CB, makes the $\angle$B leſs or greater than $\angle$E.
But $\angle$B = $\angle$E (by ſup.); therefore AC is neither leſs nor greater than DF.
Or the line AC = DF; conſequently FE = CB.
Therefore the triangles are congruous,

101. THEO-

101. THEOREM VII.

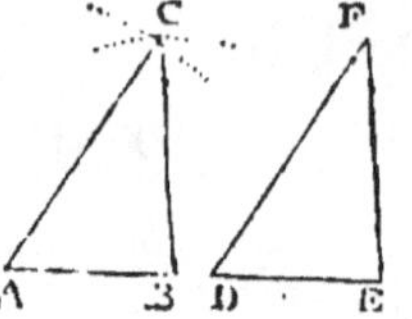

Two triangles ABC, DEF *are congruous, when the three ſides in the one are equal to the three ſides in the other, each to each.*

DEM. Apply the point D to A, and the line DE to AB. (54)
Now as DE=AB (by ſup.); therefore the point E falls on B.
On A, with the radius AC, deſcribe an arc.
Then as DF=AC, the point F will fall in that arc.
Alſo on B, with the radius BC, deſcribe another arc, cutting the former in C.
And ſince EF=BC, the point F will fall in this arc alſo.
But if the point F can fall in both theſe arcs, it can be only where they interſect, as in C.
Conſequently the triangles are congruous.

102. THEOREM VIII.

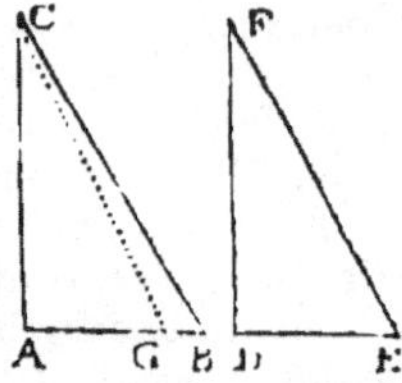

Two triangles ABC, DEF *are congruous, when two angles* A, B *and a ſide* AC *oppoſite to one of them, in one triangle, are reſpectively equal to two angles* D, E *and a ſide* DF *oppoſite to a like angle in the other triangle, each to each.*

DEM. Apply the point D to A, and the line DF to AC (54)
Now as DF=AC (by ſup.); therefore the point F falls on C.
And as ∠D=∠A (by ſup.); the line DE will fall on the line AB.
And if the point E does not fall on B, it muſt fall on ſome other point G. Draw CG.
Then the angle AGC is equal to the angle DEF. (99)
And the angle ABC=(DEF=) AGC, which is not poſſible. (96)
Therefore the point E can fall no where but on the point B.
Conſequently the triangles are congruous.

103. THEOREM IX.

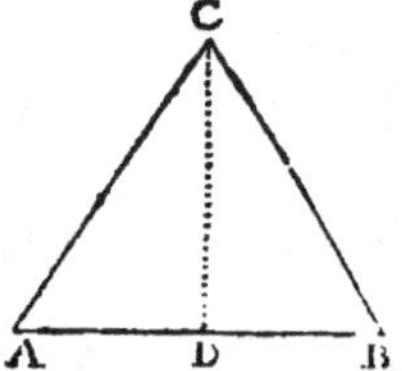

In the Iſoſceles, or equilateral triangle ACB; *a line drawn from the vertex* C *to the middle of the baſe* AB *is perpendicular to the baſe, and biſects the vertical angle: and the contrary* *.

DEM. The triangles ADC, BDC, are congruous.
Since CA=CB (23); CD=CD, and AD=DB by ſuppoſition:
Therefore ∠A=∠B, ∠ACD=∠BCD, ∠ADC=∠BDC. (101)
Conſequently CD is at right angles to AB. (17)

104. COROL. Hence in any right lined triangle where there are equal ſides, or angles;

The angles A, B, oppoſite to equal ſides BC, AC are equal.
And the ſides BC, AC, oppoſite to equal angles A, B, are equal.

* That is, if a line drawn perpendicular to the baſe of a triangle biſects the vertical angle; then that triangle muſt be Iſoſceles, and the perpendicular is drawn from the middle of the baſe.

105. THEO-

105. THEOREM X.

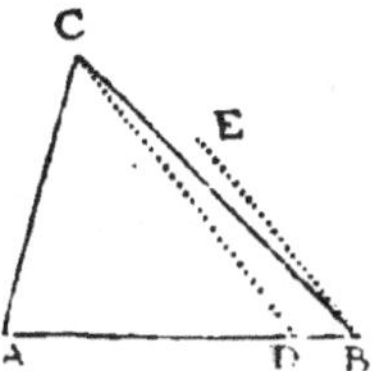

In every right lined triangle ABC *the greater angle* C *is opposite to the greater side* AB.

DEM. In the greater side AB, take AD=AC; draw CD, and through B draw BE parellel to CD. (63)
Then the angles ADC, ACD, are equal. (104)
And ∠ADC=∠ABE. (95)
Therefore ∠ACD=∠ABE. (46)
That is, a part of the angle ACB is greater than the angle ABC.
Consequently the ∠C is greater than the ∠B; and in the same manner, it may be proved to be greater than the ∠A, if the side AB be greater than CB.

106. COROL. Hence in every right lined triangle, the greater side is opposite to the greater angle.

107. THEOREM XI.

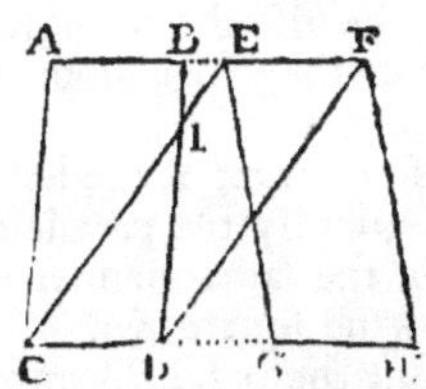

Parallelograms ACDB, ECDF, EGHF *standing on the same base* CD, *or on equal bases* CD, GH, *and between the same parallels*, CH, AF, *are equal.*

DEM. For AB=EF, being each equal to CD. (28, 46)
To each add BE, and AE=BF. (47)
Now AC=BD, and CE=DF. (28)
The triangles ACE, BDF, are therefore congruous. (101)
Now if from each of the triangles ACE and BDF, be taken the triangle BIE, the remaining trapeziums ABIC and FEID are equal. (48)
Then if to each of the trapeziums ABIC, FEID, be added the triangle CID, their sum will be the parallelograms AD and DE, which are equal. (47)

And in like manner it may be shewn, that the parallelogram EH is equal to the parellelogram ED=AD.

108. THEOREM XII.

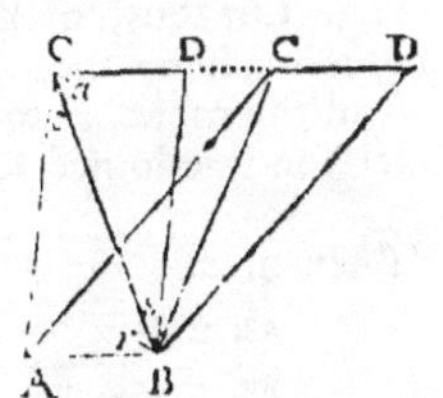

A triangle ABC *is the half of a parallelogram* AD, *when they stand on the same base* AB, *and are between the same parallels* AB, CD.

DEM. AC is equal to DB, and AB to DC. (28)
Also BC is a side common to both the triangles ABC and DCB.
These triangles are therefore congruous. (101)
Consequently the triangle ABC is half the parallelogram AD.

109. COROL. I. Hence every parallelogram is bisected by its diagonal.

110. COROL. II. Also, triangles standing on the same base, or on equal bases, and between the same parallels, are equal.
They being the halves of equal parallelograms under like circumstances.

111. THEO-

111. THEOREM XIII.

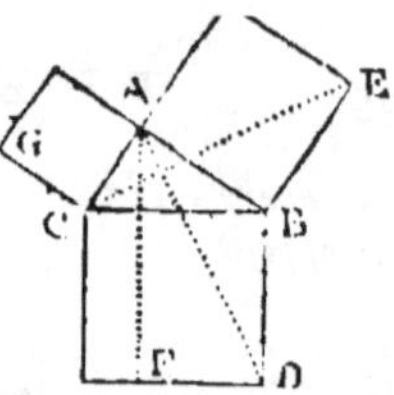

In every right angled triangle BAC *the ſquare on the ſide* BC *oppoſite to the right angle* A *is equal to the ſum of the ſquares of the two ſides* AB, AC *containing the right angle.*

DEM. On the ſides AB, AC, BC, conſtruct the ſquares AG, AE, CD (68): draw AD, CE; and draw AF parallel to BD. (63)
Then the triangles ABD, EBC, are congruous. (99)
For the ∠ABE=∠CBD, being right angles. (30)
To each add the angle ABC, then ∠EBC and ∠ABD are equal. (47)
Therefore EB, BC, ∠EBC are reſpectively equal to AB, BD, ∠ABD.
Alſo the triangle EBC is half the parallelogram AE (108)
For they ſtand upon the ſame baſe EB, and are between the ſame parallels EB and AC; BA making right angles with BE and CA continued.
Likewiſe the triangle ABD is half the parallelogram BF. (108)
For they ſtand upon the ſame baſe BD, and are between the ſame parallels BD, AF.
Therefore, as the halves of the parallelograms EA and BF are equal, conſequently the parallelogram BF is equal to the ſquare AE. (49)
In the ſame manner may it be ſhewn, that the parallelogram CF is equal to the ſquare AG.
But the parallelograms BF and CF together, make the ſquare CD,
Therefore the ſquare CD is equal to the ſquares EA and AG.

112. COROL. I. Hence if any two ſides of a right angled triangle are known, the other ſide is alſo known.

For BC=ſquare root of the ſum of the ſquares of AC and AB.
AC=ſquare root of the difference of the ſquares of BC and AB.
AB=ſquare root of the difference of the ſquares of BC and AC.

113. Or thus, making the quantities $\overline{BC}^2$, $\overline{AB}^2$, $\overline{AC}^2$, to ſtand for the ſquares made on thoſe lines.

And the mark $\surd$ to ſtand for the ſquare root of ſuch quantities as ſtand under the line joined to the top of this mark.

Then $BC=\sqrt{\overline{AC}^2+\overline{AB}^2}$;
$AC=\sqrt{\overline{BC}^2-\overline{AB}^2}$;
$AB=\sqrt{\overline{BC}^2-\overline{AC}^2}$.

Scholium. The lines of the lengths 5, 4, 3, (or their doubles, triples, &c.) will form a right angled triangle.

For $5^2=4^2+3^2$. Or $25=16+9$.

114. COROL.

114. Corol. II. Of all the lines drawn from a given point to a given line, the perpendicular is the ſhorteſt.

115. Corol. III. The ſhorteſt diſtance between two parallel right lines, is a right line drawn from one to the other perpendicular to both.

116. Corol. IV. Parallel right lines are equidiſtant; and the contrary. For two oppoſite ſides of a rectangular parallelogram are equal (28); and each is the ſhorteſt diſtance between the other ſides.

117. THEOREM XIV.

If a right line AB *be divided into any two parts* AC, CB; *then will the ſquare on the whole line be equal to the ſum of the ſquares on the parts, together with two rectangles under the two parts.*

That is $\overline{AB}^2 = \overline{AC}^2 + \overline{CB}^2 + 2 \times AC \times CB$.*

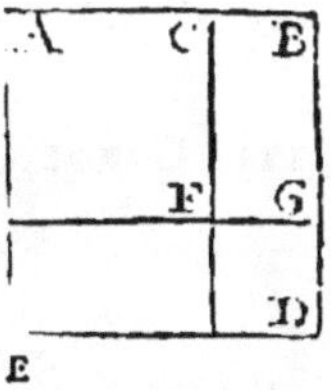

Dem. Let AD, AF, be ſquares on AB, AC. (68)
Then will FG, and GD, be each equal to CB. (48)
Hence FD is a ſquare on a line equal to CB. (30)
Alſo FB and FE are rectangles on lines equal to AC, CB.
But the ſquares AF, FD, and the rectangles FB, FE, fill up the ſquare AD, or are equal to AD.

118. Corol. I. Hence the ſquare of AC the difference between two lines AB, CB, is equal to the ſquare of the greater AB, leſſened by the ſquare of the leſs CB and by two rectangles under the leſſer line CB and the ſaid difference.

That is $\overline{AB-BC}^2 = \overline{AB}^2 - \overline{BC}^2 - 2BC \times AC$.
For $AB - BC = AC$.
Then $\overline{AC}^2 = \overline{AB}^2 - \overline{BC}^2 - 2BC \times AC$. (48)

119. Corol. II. The difference between the ſquares on two lines AB, AC is equal to the rectangle under the ſum AB+BC and difference AB—BC of thoſe lines.

That is $\overline{AB}^2 - \overline{AC}^2 = \overline{AB+BC} \times \overline{AB-AC}$.
For $\overline{AB}^2 - \overline{AC}^2 = \overline{CB}^2 + 2AC \times CB$. (117, 48)
$= \overline{CB+AC+AC} \times CB$.
$= \overline{AB+AC} \times (CB=)\overline{AB-AC}$.

---

* *The rectangle under two lines is generally expreſſed by 3 letters; the firſt two letters ſtand for one line, and the laſt two for the other line.*
Thus for AC × CB, *is written* ACB.
for AB × BC, *is written* ABC.
And for 2 × AC × CB, *is written* 2ACB.

120. THEOREM XV.

In every triangle, ADC *the square of a side* CD *subtending an acute angle* A, *is equal to the squares of the sides* AD, AC *about that angle, lessened by two rectangles under one of those sides* AC *and that part* AB *contained between the acute angle and the perpendicular* DB *drawn to that side* AC *from its opposite angle* D.

That is, $\overline{DC}^2 = \overline{AD}^2 + \overline{AC}^2 - 2CAB$.

DEM. $\overline{DC}^2 - \overline{BC}^2 = (\overline{DB}^2 =)\overline{AD}^2 - \overline{AB}^2$. (111)
And $\overline{AC}^2 = 2ABC + \overline{BC}^2 + \overline{AB}^2$. (117)
Then $\overline{DC}^2 - \overline{BC}^2 - \overline{AC}^2 = \overline{AD}^2 - \overline{BC}^2 - 2\overline{AB}^2 - 2ABC$. (48)

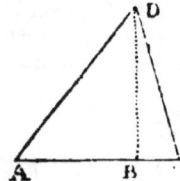

And $\overline{DC}^2 = \overline{AD}^2 + \overline{AC}^2 - 2\overline{AB}^2 - 2ABC$, by adding $\overline{BC}^2 + \overline{AC}^2$. (47)
$(-AB \times 2AB - BC \times 2AB)$
$(-\overline{AB + BC} \quad \times 2AB \quad)$
Then $\overline{DC}^2 = \overline{AD}^2 + \overline{AC}^2 - (AC \times 2AB =)2CAB$.

121. COROL. Hence $AB = \dfrac{\overline{AD}^2 + \overline{AC}^2 - \overline{DC}^2}{2CA}$.

122. THEOREM XVI.

In an obtuse angled triangle ACD, *the square of the side* AD *opposite to the obtuse angle* C *is equal to the sum of the squares of the sides* AC, CD *about the obtuse angle; together with two rectangles under one side* AC, *and the continuation* CB *of that side to meet a perpendicular* DB *drawn to it from the opposite angle* D.

That is, $\overline{AD}^2 = \overline{AC}^2 + \overline{CD}^2 + 2AC \times CB$.

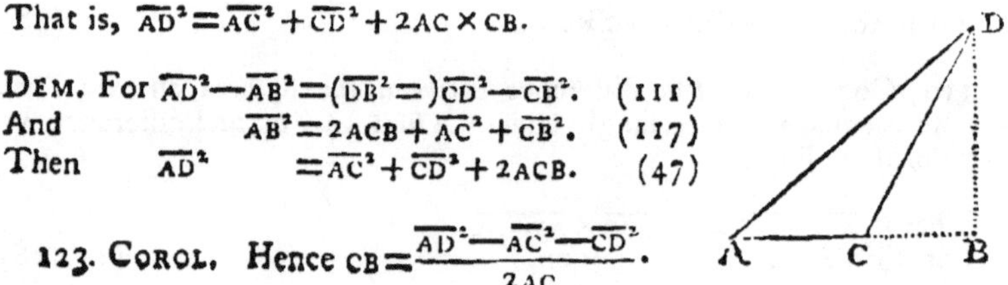

DEM. For $\overline{AD}^2 - \overline{AB}^2 = (\overline{DB}^2 =)\overline{CD}^2 - \overline{CB}^2$. (111)
And $\overline{AB}^2 = 2ACB + \overline{AC}^2 + \overline{CB}^2$. (117)
Then $\overline{AD}^2 = \overline{AC}^2 + \overline{CD}^2 + 2ACB$. (47)

123. COROL. Hence $CB = \dfrac{\overline{AD}^2 - \overline{AC}^2 - \overline{CD}^2}{2AC}$.

124. THEOREM XVII.

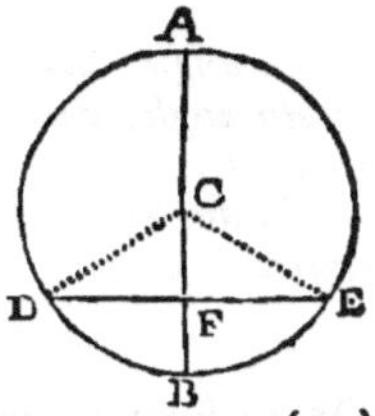

In any circle, a diameter, AB, *drawn perpendicular to a chord,* DE, *bisects that chord and its subtended arc* DBE.

DEM. From the center C, draw the radii CD, CE, to the extremities of the chord DE.
Then the triangles CFE, CFD, are congruous. (102)
For CF being at right angles to DE, the ∠CFD=∠CFE. (17)
And the triangle CDE being isosceles (23), the ∠D=∠E (104). Also CF is common.
Therefore DF=FE: And the arc DB=BE:
For those arcs measure the equal angles FCE, FCD. (15)

125. COROL. Hence, in a circle, a right line drawn through the middle of a chord at right angles to it, passes through the center of that circle; and the contrary.

126. THEOREM XVIII.

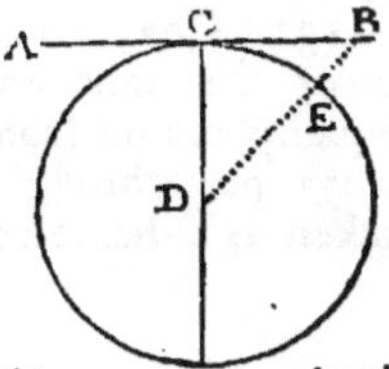

A tangent, AB, *to a circle is perpendicular to a diameter,* DC, *drawn to the point of contact,* C.

DEM. If it be denied that DC is perpendicular to AB.
Then from the center D, let some other line DE, cutting the circle in E, be drawn perpendicular to AB.
Now the angle DBC being right, the angle DCB is acute. (97)
Consequently DC is greater than DB. (106)
But DC=DE (9). Therefore DE is greater than DB, which is absurd.
Therefore no other line passing through the center can be perpendicular to the tangent, but that which meets it at the point of contact.

127. THEOREM XIX.

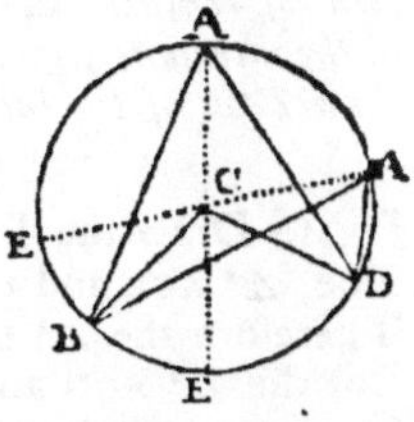

An angle, BCD, *at the center of a circle, is double of the angle,* BAD *at the circumference, when those angles stand on the same arc,* BD.

DEM. Through the point A draw the diameter AE.
Then the angle ECD=∠CAD+∠CDA. (96)
But the ∠CAD=∠CDA. (104)
Therefore the ∠ECD is equal to twice the angle CAD.
In the same manner it may be shewn, that the angle BCE is equal to twice the angle BAE.
Consequently the angle BCD (=∠ECD$\pm$* ∠BCE) is equal to twice the angle BAD (=∠EAD$\pm$∠BAE). (47, 48)

128. COROL. I. Hence an angle, BAD, at the circumference is measured by half the arc, BD, on which it stands.
For the angle at the center BCD is measured by the arc BD. (15)
Consequently the angle BAD=half the angle BCD, is measured by half the arc DB.

129. COROL. II. All angles in the circumference, and standing on the same arc, are equal.

* The mark $\pm$, signifies the sum or difference.

130. THEOREM XX.

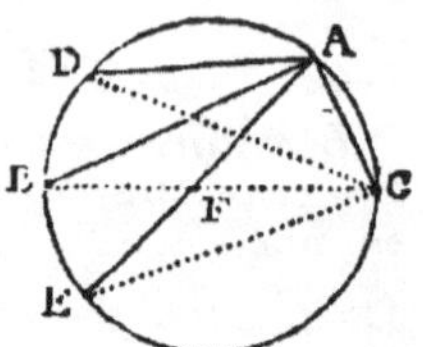

An angle, BAC, *in a ſemicircle, is a right one.*
An angle, DAC, *in a ſegment leſs than a ſemicircle, is obtuſe.*
An angle, EAC, *in a ſegment greater than a ſemicircle, is acute.*

DEM. For the angle BAC is meaſured by half the ſemicircular arc BEC, or is meaſured by half of 180 degrees; that is, by 90 degrees. (128, 16)
And ∠DAC is meaſured by half the arc DEC, greater than 180° *.
Alſo ∠EAC is meaſured by half the arc EC, leſs than 180°.
Therefore theſe angles are reſpectively equal to, greater, or leſs than 90 degrees.

131. COR. Hence in a right angled triangle BAC; the angular point A of the right angle, and the ends, B, C, of the oppoſite ſide, are equally diſtant from F, the middle of that ſide; that is, a circle will always paſs through the right angle, and the ends of its oppoſite ſide taken as a diameter.

132. THEOREM XXI.

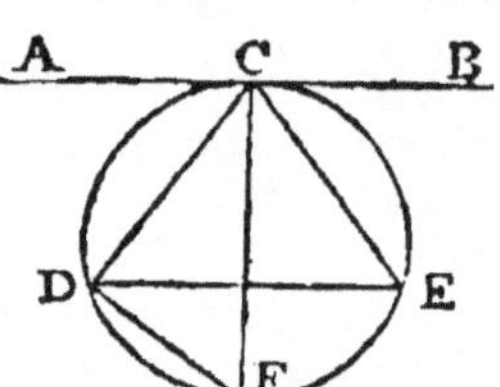

The angle ACD, *formed by a tangent* AB, *to a circle,* CDE, *and a chord,* CD, *drawn from the point of contact,* C, *is equal to an angle,* CED, *in the alternate ſegment; and is meaſured by half the arc* DC *of the included ſegment.*

DEM. Draw the diameter FC, and join DF.
The ∠ˢ ACF and CDF are both right. (126, 130)
Therefore the ∠ˢ DCF and DFC are together = a right ∠. (96)
But the ∠ˢ ACD and DCF are together = a right ∠.
Conſequently the ∠ DCF and DFC = the ∠ˢ ACD and DCF. (46)
Take the ∠ DCF from each, and the ∠ DFC = the ∠ ACD. (48)
But the ∠ˢ DFC and DEC are equal. (129)
Conſequently the ∠ˢ DEC and ACD are equal alſo. (46)

* A ſmall ° put above any figure, ſignifies degrees.

133. THEOREM XXII.

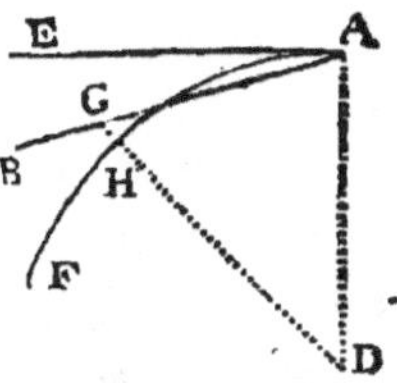

Between a circular arc AHF, *and its tangent* AE, *no right line can be drawn from the point of contact* A.

DEM. For if any other right line can be drawn, let it be the right line AB.
From D, the center of AHF, draw DG perpendicular to AB, cutting AB in G, and the arc in H.
Now as ∠ DGA is right; therefore DA is greater than DG. (106)
But DA=DH (9). Therefore DH is greater than DG, which is abfurd.
Confequently no right line can be drawn between the tangent AE and the arc AHF.

134. COROL. I. Hence the angle DAH, contained between the radius DA, and an arc AH, is greater than any right lined acute angle.

For a right line AB muft be drawn from A, between the tangent AE and radius AD, to make an acute angle.

But no fuch right line can be drawn between AE and the arc AH. (133)

135. COROL. II. Hence the angle EAH, between the tangent EA and arc AH, is lefs than any right lined acute angle.

136. COROL. III. Hence it follows, that at the point of contact the arc has the fame direction as the tangent, and is at right angles to the radius drawn to that point.

137. THEOREM XXIII.

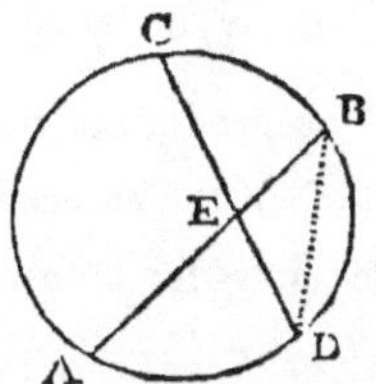

If two right lines, AB, CD, *interfect any how (in* E) *within a circle, their inclination,* AED, *or* CEB, *is meafured by half the fum of the intercepted arcs,* AD, CB.

DEM. For drawing DB; (43)
The ∠ AED=∠ EDB+∠ EBD. (96)
But the ∠EDB is meafured by $\frac{1}{2}$ arc CB. (128)
And the ∠EBD is meafured by $\frac{1}{2}$ arc AD. (128)
Confequently the ∠AED is meafured by half the arc CB, together with half the arc AD. (50)

SECTION IV.

Of Proportion.

DEFINITIONS and PRINCIPLES.

138. *One quantity* A, *is said to be measured or divided by another quantity* B, *when* A *contains* B *some number of times, exactly.*

Thus if A=20, and B=5; then A contains B four times.

A is called a multiple of B; and B is said to be part of A.

139. *If a quantity* A (=20) *contains another* B (=5) *as many times as a quantity* C (=24) *contains another* D (=6); *then*
A *and* C *are called like multiples of* B *and* D.
B *and* D *are called like parts of* A *and* C: *And*
A *is said to have the same relation to* B, *as* C *has to* D.

Or, like multiples of quantities are produced, by taking their Rectangle, or Product, by the same quantity, or by equal quantities.

The Rectangle or Product of quantities, A and B, is expressed by writing this mark × between them. Thus; A × B, or B × A, expresses the rectangle contained by A and B.

140 *When two quantities of a like kind are compared together, the relation which one of them has to the other, in respect to quantity, is called Ratio.*

The first term of a ratio, or the quantity compared, is called the Antecedent; and the second term, or the quantity compared to, is called the Consequent.

A ratio is usually denoted by setting the antecedent above the consequent with a line drawn between them.

Thus $\frac{A}{B}$ signifies, and is thus to be read, the ratio of A to B.

The multiple of a ratio $\frac{A}{B}$, is the product of each of its terms by the same quantity, or by equal quantities. Thus $\frac{A \times C}{B \times C}$ is the ratio $\frac{A}{B}$ taken C times.

The product of two or more ratios, $\frac{A}{B}$, $\frac{C}{D}$, is expressed by taking the product of the antecedents for a new antecedent, and the product of the consequents for a new consequent. Thus $\frac{A \times C}{B \times D} = \frac{A}{B} \times \frac{C}{D}$.

141. *Equal ratios are those where the antecedents are like multiples or parts of their respective consequents.*

Thus in the quantities A, B, C, D: Or 20, 5, 24, 6.

In the ratio of A to B, or of 20 to 5, the antecedent is a multiple of its consequent four times.

And in the ratio of C to D, or 24 to 6, the antecedent is a multiple of its consequent four times.

That is, the ratio of A to B is the same as the ratio of C to D.

And this equality of ratios is thus expressed, $\frac{A}{B} = \frac{C}{D}$.

142. *Ratio of equality is, when the antecedent is equal to the consequent.*

Thus when A=B, then $\frac{A}{B}$, or $\frac{A}{A}$, or $\frac{B}{B}$, is a ratio of equality.

143. *Four quantities are said to be proportional, which, when compared together by two and two, are found to have equal ratios.*

Thus, let the quantities to be compared be A, B, C, D: Or 20, 5, 24, 6.
Now in the ratio of A to B, or of 20 to 5; A contains B four times.
And in the ratio of C to D, or of 24 to 6; C contains D four times.

Then the ratios of A to B, and of C to D, are equal: Or $\frac{A}{B}=\frac{C}{D}$. (141)

And their proportionality is thus expressed, A:B::C:D. (75)
Also in the ratio of A to C, or of 20 to 24; C contains A, once and $\frac{1}{5}$.
And in the ratio of B to D, or of 5 to 6; D contains B, once and $\frac{1}{5}$.

Where the ratios are likewise equal, *viz.* $\frac{A}{C}=\frac{B}{D}$.

And these are also proportional, A:C::B:D.

144. *So that when four quantities of the same kind are proportional, the ratio between the first and second is equal to the ratio between the third and fourth; and this proportionality is called Direct.*

145. *Also the ratio between the first and third is equal to the ratio between the second and fourth; and this proportionality is called Alternate.*

146. *Similar, or like, right lined figures, are those which are equiangular,* (that is, the several angles of which are equal one to the other;) *and also, the sides about the equal angles proportional.*

Thus if the figures AC and EG are equiangular,
And AB : BC : : EF : FG; Or BC : CD : : FG : GH;
Then are those figures called similar, or like figures.
And the like in triangles, or other figures.

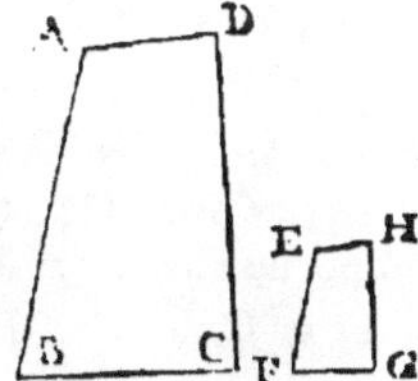

147. *Like arcs, chords, or tangents, in different circles, are those which subtend, or are opposite to, equal angles at the center.*

Let F be the center of two concentric arcs AEB, *aeb*, terminated by the radii FaA, FbB, produced; AB, *ab*, their chords, and CD, *cd*, their tangents. Then as the angle CFD is measured either by the arc AEB, or *aeb*, those arcs are said to be alike, or similar; that is, the arc *aeb* is the same part of its whole circumference, as the arc AEB is of its whole circumference.

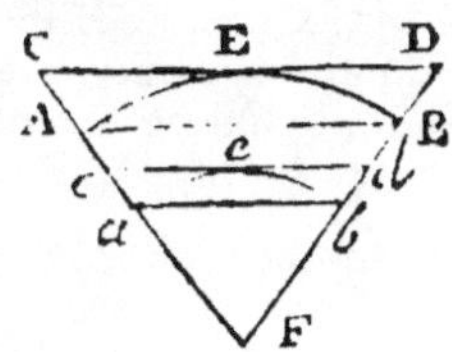

148. THEO.

148. THEOREM XXIV.

Quantities, and their like multiples, have the same ratio.

That is, the ratio of A to B is equal to the ratio of twice A to twice B, or thrice A to thrice B, &c. Or thus $\frac{A}{B}=\frac{2A}{2B}=\frac{3A}{3B}$, &c. $=\frac{C\times A}{C\times B}$; that is, equal to the ratio of C times A to C times B.

DEM. For the ratio of A to B must either be equal to the ratio of like multiples of A and B, or to the ratio of unlike multiples of them.
Now suppose the ratio of A to B is equal to the ratio of their unlike multiples, C times A, D times B; that is, $\frac{A}{B}=\frac{C\times A}{D\times B}$.
Then $A:B::C\times A:D\times B$ (143). And $A:C\times A::B:D\times B$. (145)
Therefore $\frac{A}{C\times A}=\frac{B}{D\times B}$ (144). Where the consequents are unequal multiples of their antecedents, by supposition.
But $\frac{A}{C\times A}$ is not equal to $\frac{B}{D\times B}$. (141)
Then $A:C\times A::B:D\times B$ is not true. Also $A:B::C\times A:D\times B$ is not true.
Consequently $\frac{A}{B}$ is unequal to $\frac{C\times A}{D\times B}$.
Therefore the ratio of unlike multiples of two quantities, is not equal to the ratio of those quantities.
Consequently the ratio of two quantities, and the ratio of their like multiples, are the same. Or $\frac{A}{B}=\frac{C\times A}{C\times B}$.

149. COR. I. In any ratio, if both terms contain the same quantity or quantities; the value of the ratio will not be altered by omitting, or taking away those quantities. For $\frac{C\times A}{C\times B}=\frac{A}{B}$, by taking away C.

150. COR. II. Quantities, and their like parts, have equal ratios. For A and B are like parts of $C\times A$ and $C\times B$.

151. COR. III. Quantities, and their like multiples, or like parts, are proportional. For $A:B::C\times A:C\times B$. And $C\times A:C\times B::A:B$ (148)

152. COR. IV. If quantities are equal, their like multiples, or like parts, are also equal. For if $A=B$; and $\frac{A}{B}=\frac{C\times A}{C\times B}$;
Then are the antecedents and consequents in a ratio of equality. (141)

153. COR. V. If the parts of one quantity are proportional to the parts of another quantity, they are like parts of their respective quantities.
For only like parts are proportional to their wholes. (151)

154. COR. VI. Ratios, which are equal to the same ratio, are equal to one another. For the ratio of $\frac{A}{B}=\frac{C\times A}{C\times B}=\frac{D\times A}{D\times B}$, &c. (148)

155. COR.

155. COR. VII. Proportions, which are the ſame to the ſame proportion, are the ſame to one another.
If A : B : : C : D ; and A : B : : E : F ; Then C : D : : E : F.

For $\frac{A}{B}=\frac{D}{C}$; and $\frac{A}{B}=\frac{E}{F}$ (144). Then $\frac{C}{D}=\frac{E}{F}$. (46)

156. COR. VIII. If two ratios or products are equal, their like multiples, either by the ſame or by equal quantities, or by equal ratios, are alſo equal.

That is, if $\frac{A}{B}=\frac{C}{D}$: Then $\frac{A\times E}{B\times E}=\frac{C\times}{D\times E}$.

And if E=F : Then $\frac{A\times E}{B\times E}=\frac{C\times F.}{D\times F}$

And if $\frac{E}{F}=\frac{G}{H}$: Then $\frac{A\times E}{B\times F}=\frac{C\times G}{D\times H}$.

For in either caſe, the ratios may be conſidered as quantities.

157. THEOREM XXV.

Equal quantities, A *and* B, *have the ſame ratio or proportion to another quantity* C. *And any quantity has the ſame ratio to equal quantities.*

That is, if A=B : Then A : C : : B : C. And C : A : : C : B.

DEM. Since A=B ; then C is the like multiple, or part of B, as it is of A.
And A : B : : C : C (151). Therefore A : C : : B : C. (145)
Alſo C : C : : A : B (151). Therefore C : A : : C : B. (145)

158. COR. I. Hence, when the antecedents are equal, the conſequents are equal ; and the contrary.

159. COR. II. Quantities are equal, which have the ſame ratio to another quantity : or to like multiples or parts of another quantity.
Thus, if A : C : : B : C. Then A=B.

160. COR. III. Since A : C : : B : C ; and C : A : : C : B. Therefore, when four quantities are in proportion, As antecedent is to conſequent, ſo is antecedent to conſequent : Then ſhall the firſt conſequent be to its antecedent, as the ſecond conſequent to its antecedent : and this is called *the inverſion of ratios.*

161. THEOREM XXVI.

In two, or more, ſets of proportional quantities, the rectangles under the like terms are proportional.

That is, if A : B : : C : D ; and E : F : : G : H.
Then A×E : B×F : : C×G : D×H.

DEM. Since $\frac{A}{B}=\frac{C}{D}$; and $\frac{E}{F}=\frac{G}{H}$. (144)

Therefore $\frac{A\times E}{B\times F}=\frac{C\times G}{D\times H}$. (156)

Conſequently A×E : B×F : : C×G : D×H. (143)

 162. THEO-

162. THEOREM XXVII.

In four proportional quantities A : B : : C : D. *Then the Rectangle or Product of the two extremes is equal to the Rectangle or Product of the two means.* That is, $A \times D = B \times C$.

DEM. Since A : B : : C : D by ſuppoſition. Therefore $\frac{A}{B} = \frac{C}{D}$. (144)

And $\frac{A}{B} = \frac{A \times D}{B \times D}$ (156). Alſo $\frac{C}{D} = \frac{C \times B}{D \times B}$. (156)

Therefore $\frac{A \times D}{B \times D} = \frac{C \times B}{D \times B}$ (46), where the conſequents are equal.

Conſequently $A \times D = C \times B$. (158)

163. Hence, if the Rectangle or Product of two quantities is equal to the Rectangle or Product of other two quantities; thoſe four quantities are proportional.

Thus, ſuppoſe the two Rectangles, X, Z, are equal;
Where A, C, are their lengths, and B, D, their breadths.

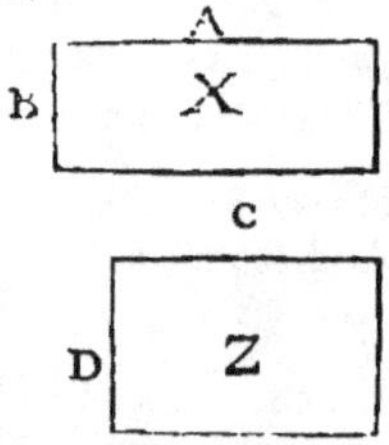

Then $A \times B = C \times D$ by ſuppoſition.
Therefore A : C : : D : B,
That is, As the length of X is to the length of Z.
So the breadth of Z is to the breadth of X.

In ſuch caſes, the lengths are ſaid to be to one another reciprocally, as their breadths.
Or that proportion A : C : : D : B is reciprocal, when $A \times B = C \times D$.

164. THEOREM XXVIII.

If four quantities are proportional; then will either of the extremes, and the ratio of the product of the means to the other extreme, be in the ratio of equality: And either mean, and the ratio of the product of the extremes to the other mean, will be alſo in a ratio of equality.

That is, if A : B : : C : D. Then $A = \frac{B \times C}{D}$. And $B = \frac{A \times D}{C}$.

DEM. Since A : B : : C : D by ſuppoſition.
Therefore $A \times D = B \times C$. (162)

And $\frac{A \times D}{C} = \frac{B \times C}{C}$ (157). Alſo $\frac{B \times C}{D} = \frac{A \times D}{D}$. (157)

But $B = \frac{B \times C}{C}$ (149). And $A = \frac{A \times D}{D}$. (149)

Therefore $\frac{A \times D}{C} = B$. And $\frac{B \times C}{D} = A$. (46)

165. THEO-

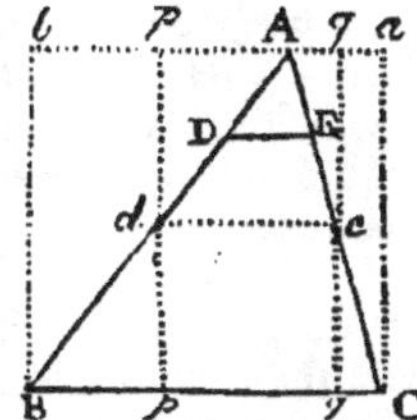

165. THEOREM XXIX.

In any plane triangle, ABC, *any two adjoining ſides,* AB, AC, *are cut proportionally by a line* DE, *drawn parallel to the other ſide* BC, *viz.*
AD : DB : : AE : EC.

DEM. Through B and C draw B*b*, C*a*, at right angles to BC, meeting *ba*, drawn through A, parallel to BC: Through *p*, *q*, the middles of A*b*, A*a*, draw *pp*, *qq*, parallel to B*b* or C*a*, meeting AB, AC, in the points *d*, *c*; and join *dc*.
Now the triangles A*dp*, B*dp*, and A*cq*, C*cq*, are congruous. (95,100)
Therefore A*d*=B*d*, A*c*=C*c*, *pd*=*pd*, *qc*=*qc*.
But *pp*=*qq* (116): Therefore *pd*=*qc*. (49)
And *dc* is parallel to BC. (116)

In the ſame manner it may be ſhewn, that lines parallel to B*b*, drawn through the middles of A*p*, *pb*; A*q*, *qa*; will alſo biſect A*d*, B*d*; A*c*, C*c*; and that lines joining theſe points of biſection will alſo be parallel to BC: And the ſame may be proved at any other biſections of the ſegments of the lines AB, AC: Alſo the like may be readily inferred at any other diviſions of the lines A*b*, A*a*.
Therefore lines parallel to BC, cut off like parts from the lines AB, AC.
Then AB : AC : : AD : AE. And AB : AC : : BD : CE. (151)
Therefore AD : AE : : BD : CE. (155)
And by Alternation AD : BD : : AE : CE. (145)

166. COR. Hence, when the ſides AB, AC, of a triangle are cut proportionally, in D, E, the ſegments AD, AE; DB, EC; of thoſe ſides are proportional to the ſides: And the line DE, drawn to thoſe ſections, is parallel to the other ſide BC.

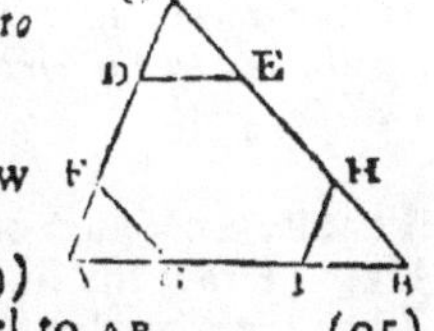

167. THEOREM XXX.

In equiangular triangles, ABC, *abc, the ſides about the equal angles are proportional; and the ſides oppoſite to equal angles are alſo proportional.*

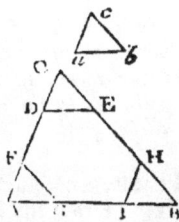

DEM. In CA, CB, take CD=*ca*, CE=*cb*; and draw DE.
Then the triangles CDE, *cab*, being congruous. (99)
The ∠CDE=(∠*a*=) ∠A. Therefore DE is parallel to AB. (95)

In the ſame manner, taking AF=*ac*, AG=*ab*; alſo BH=*bc*, BI=*ba*; and drawing FG, HI, the triangles AGF, IBH, *abc*, are congruous; therefore FG is parallel to CB, and HI is parallel to CA.

Then (CD=) *ca* : CA : : (CE=) *cb* : CB.
(AF=) *ca* : CA : : (AG=) *ab* : AB. } (165)
(BH=) *bc* : BC : : (BI=) *ab* : AB.

168. COR. Hence, Triangles have one angle in each equal, and the ſides about thoſe equal angles proportional, thoſe triangles are equiangular and ſimilar.

169. THEO-

169. THEOREM XXXI.

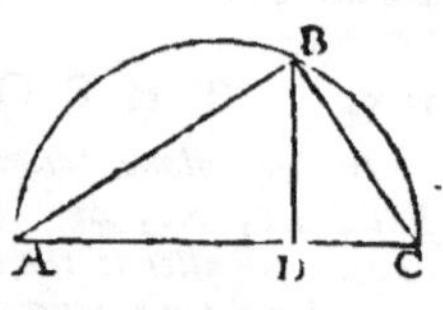

In a right angled triangle, ABC, *if a line,* BD, *be drawn from the right angle* B, *perpendicular to the opposite ſide,* AC; *then will the triangles* ABD, BCD, *on each ſide the perpendicular, be ſimilar to the whole* ABC, *and to one another.*

DEM. For in the triangles ABC, ADB, the ∠A is common;
And the right angle ABC = right angle ADB.
Therefore the remaining ∠C = ∠ABD. (98)
In the ſame manner it will appear, that the triangles ABC, BDC, are like.
Therefore the triangles ABD, BCD, are alſo ſimilar.

170. COR. I. Hence, AC : AB :: AB : AD.
AC : BC :: BC : DC.
AD : DB :: DB : DC. (167)

171. COR. II. Hence a right line BD, drawn from a circumference of a circle perpendicular to the diameter AC, is a mean proportional between the ſegments AD, DC, of the diameter.
And AD × DC = DB^2. (162)
For a circle, the diameter of which is AC, will paſs through A, B, C. (131)

Scholium. This corollary includes what is uſually called one of the chief properties of the circle, namely;
The ſquare of the Ordinate is equal to the rectangle under the two Abſciſſas.
Here, the ordinate is the perpendicular BD; and the two Abſciſſas are the two ſegments AD, DC, of the diameter AC.

172 THEOREM XXXII.

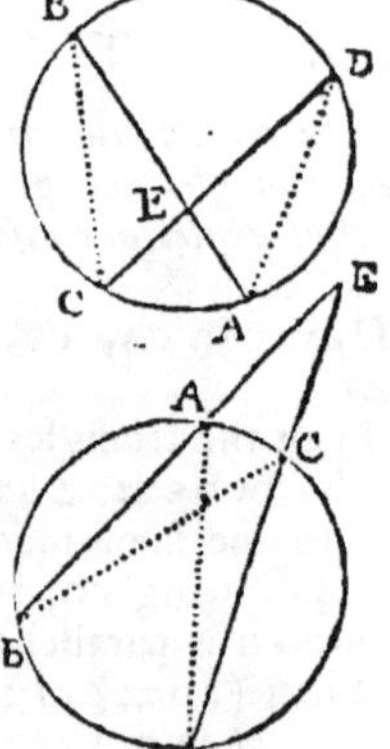

In a circle, if two chords, AB, CD, *interſect each other in* E, *either within the circle, or without, by prolonging them; then the rectangle under the ſegments, terminated by the circumference and their interſection, will be equal.*

That is, AE × EB = CE × ED.
DEM. Draw the lines BC, DA.
Then the triangles DEA, BEC, are ſimilar.
For the angle at E is equal (93), or common.
And the ∠D = ∠B, as ſtanding on the ſame arc AC (129). Then the other angles are equal. (98)
Therefore AE : CE :: ED : EB. (167)
Conſequently AE × EB = CE × ED. (162)

173. THEO-

173. THEOREM XXXIII.

If with the least side AB *of a given triangle* ABC, *a semicircle be described from the angular point* A; *meeting the side* AC, *produced in the points* D, E; *and from* B, *the lines* BE, BD, *be drawn, and also* BG *perpendicular to* DE: *Then the values of the several lines* AG, CG, GE, GD, BE, BD, BG, *may be expressed in terms of the sides of the triangle* ABC, *as follow.*

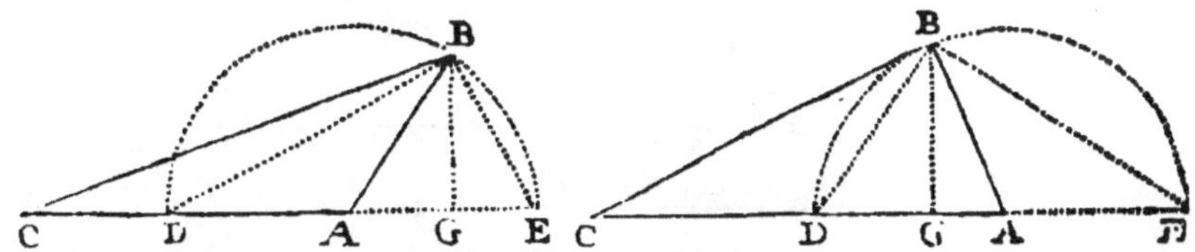

174. $AG = \frac{\overline{BC}^2 - \overline{AC}^2 - \overline{AB}^2}{2AC}$. (123)

Or $AG = \frac{\overline{AC}^2 + \overline{AB}^2 - \overline{BC}^2}{2AC}$. (121)

175. $CG = \frac{\overline{AC}^2 - \overline{AB}^2 + \overline{BC}^2}{2AC}$. For $CG = AC + AG$, or to $AC - AG$.

And $AC + AG = AC \pm \frac{\overline{BC}^2 - \overline{AC}^2 - \overline{AB}^2}{2AC}$. (174)

$= \frac{2\overline{AC}^2 + \overline{BC}^2 - \overline{AC}^2 - \overline{AB}^2}{2AC}$. (149)

176. $GE = \frac{2H \times \overline{H - CB}}{2AC}$: Here $2H = AC + AB + BC$.

For $GE = AB(AE) \pm AG = AB + \frac{\overline{AC}^2 + \overline{AB}^2 - \overline{CB}^2}{2AC}$. (174)

$= \frac{2AC \times AB + \overline{AC}^2 + \overline{AB}^2 - \overline{BC}^2}{2AC}$. (149)

But $2AC \times AB + \overline{AC}^2 + \overline{AB}^2 = (\overline{AC + AB}^2 =)\overline{CE}^2$. (117)

Then $GE\left(= \frac{\overline{CE}^2 - \overline{BC}^2}{2AC}\right) = \frac{\overline{CE + BC} \times \overline{CE - BC}}{2AC}$. (119)

$= \frac{\overline{CA + AB + BC} \times \overline{CA + AB - BC}}{2AC}$.

$= \frac{2H \times \overline{2H - 2BC}}{2AC} = \frac{2H \times \overline{H - BC}}{AC}$.

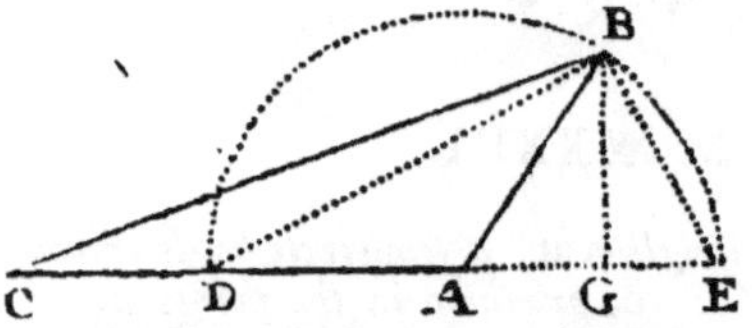

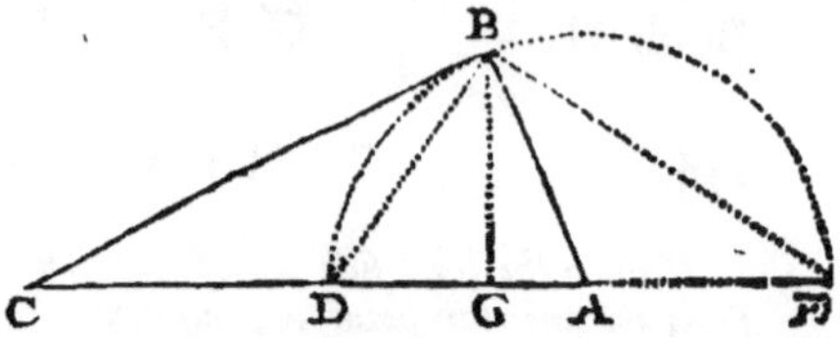

C D A G E C D G A E

177. $GD=\frac{\overline{H-AC}\times\overline{2H-2AB}}{AC}$. Here $2H=AC+AB+BC$.

For $GD=AD\mp AG=AB\mp AG=AB-\frac{\overline{AC}^2-\overline{AB}^2+\overline{BC}^2}{2AC}$. (174)

$$=\frac{2AC\times AB-\overline{AC}^2-\overline{AB}^2+\overline{BC}^2}{2AC}.$$

$$=\frac{\overline{BC}^2-\overline{AC-AB}^2}{2AC}=\frac{\overline{BC}^2-\overline{CD}^2}{2AC}. \quad (118)$$

$$=\frac{\overline{BC-CD}\times\overline{BC+CD}}{2AC}. \quad (119)$$

$$=\frac{\overline{BC+AB-AC}\times\overline{BC+AC-AB}}{2AC}.$$

$$=\frac{\overline{2H-2AC}\times\overline{2H-2AB}}{2AC}.$$

178. $BE=\sqrt{\frac{AB}{AC}\times 2H\times\overline{H-CB}}$.

For $\overline{BE}^2=DE\times CE$. (170)

$$=2AB\times\frac{\overline{CE}^2-\overline{BC}^2}{2AC}. \quad (176)$$

Therefore $BE=\sqrt{\frac{2AB}{2AC}\times\overline{CE}^2-\overline{BC}^2}=\sqrt{\frac{AB}{AC}\times 2H\times\overline{H-CB}}$. (176)

179. $BD=\sqrt{\frac{AB}{AC}\times\overline{H-AC}\times\overline{2H-2AC}}$.

For $\overline{BD}^2=DE\times GD$. (170)

$$=2AB\times\frac{\overline{BC}^2-\overline{CD}^2}{2AC}. \quad (177)$$

Therefore $BD=\sqrt{\frac{2AB}{2AC}\times\overline{BC}^2-\overline{CD}^2}$. (177)

180. $BG=\frac{2}{AC}\times\sqrt{H\times\overline{H-CB}\times\overline{H-AC}\times\overline{H-AB}}$.

For $\overline{BG}^2=GE\times GD$. Therefore $BG=\sqrt{GE}\times\sqrt{GD}$. (170)

And $GE=\frac{2}{AC}\times H\times\overline{H-CB}$. (176) $GD=\frac{2}{AC}\times\overline{H-AC}\times\overline{H-AB}$. (177)

181. Corol. Hence is derived the Rule uſually given for finding the area, or ſuperficial content, of a Triangle, the three ſides being known.

Rule. 1. From half the ſum of the three ſides, ſubtract each ſide ſeverally, noting the three remainders.

2d. Multiply the ſaid half ſum, and the three noted remainders continually.

3d. The ſquare root of the product is the area of the Triangle.

182. THEO-

182. THEOREM XXXIV.

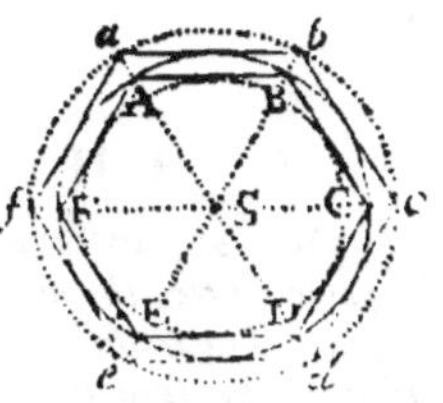

If a regular polygon, ABCDEF, *be inscribed in a circle; and parallel to these sides if tangents to the circle be drawn, meeting one another in the points a, b, c, d, e, f; then shall the figure formed by these tangents circumscribe the circle, and be similar to the inscribed figure.*

DEM. Since the circle touches every side of the figure *abcdef*, by construction; therefore the circle is circumscribed by that figure. (41)
Through A and B, draw the radii SA, SB, prolonged till they meet the tangent *ab*, in *a*, *b*.
Then the triangles ASB, *asb*, are equiangular.
For the ∠ at S is common; and the other angles are equal, because AE and *ab* are parallel, by supposition.
Also *sa*=*sb*: For the triangles ASB, *asb*, are isosceles. (104)
And the same may be proved of the other triangles; and also, that they are equal to one another.
Therefore the figure *abcdef* has equal sides, and is equiangular to the figure ABCDEF.
Now SA : *sa* : : AB : *ab*; and SA : *sa* : : AF : *af*. (167)
Therefore AB : *ab* : : AF : *af*. And the like of the other sides. (155)
Consequently the figures ABCDEF, *abcdef*, are similar. (145)

183. COR. I. If two figures are composed of like sets of similar triangles, those figures are similar.

184. COR. II. Hence, if from the angles *a*, *b*, of a regular polygon circumscribed a circle, lines *as*, *bs*, be drawn to the center S; the chords AB of the intercepted arcs will be the sides of a similar polygon, inscribed in the circle: and the sides AB, *ab*, of the inscribed and circumscribing polygons will be parallel.

185. COR. III. The chords or tangents of like arcs in different circles, are in the same proportion as the radii of those circles.
For if a circle circumscribe the polygon *abcdef*; then the sides of the polygons *abcdef*, ABCDEF, are chords of like arcs in their respective circumscribing circles.
And if a circle be inscribed in the polygon ABCDEF, the sides AB, *ab*, &c. are tangents of like arcs also: And these have been shewn to be proportional to their radii SA, *sa*.

186. COR. IV. The Perimeters of like polygons (or the sum of their sides) are to one another as the radii of their inscribed or circumscribed circles.
For SA : *sa* : : AB : *ab*. (182)
And AB, *ab*, are like parts of the perimeters of their polygons.
Therefore SA : *sa* : : perimeter ABCDEF : perimeter *abcdef*. (151)

187. THEO-

187. THEOREM XXXV.

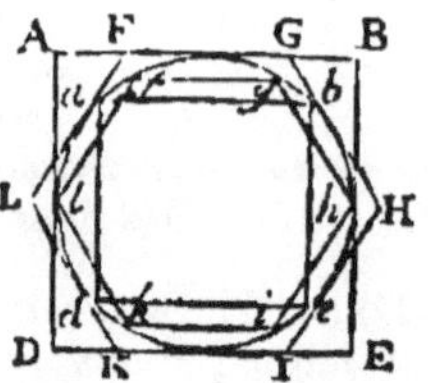

If there be two regular and like polygons applied to the ſame circle, the one inſcribed and the other circumſcribed: Then will the circcumference of that circle, and half the ſum of the perimeters of thoſe polygons, approach nearer to equality, as the number of ſides in the polygons increaſe.

DEM. It is evident at ſight, that the circumſcribing hexagon FGHIKL is leſs than the circumſcribing ſquare ABED.

And alſo that the inſcribed hexagon *fghikl* is greater than the inſcribed ſquare *abed*.

And in both caſes, the difference between the hexagon and the circle is leſs than the difference between the circle and the ſquare.

Therefore the polygon, whether inſcribed or circumſcribed, differs leſs from the circle, as the number of its ſides is increaſed.

And when the number of ſides in both is very great, the perimeters of the polygons will nearly coincide with the circumference of the circle; for then the difference of the polygonal perimeters becomes ſo very ſmall, that they may be eſteemed as equal.

And yet ſo long as there is any difference between theſe polygons, though ever ſo ſmall, the circle is greater than the inſcribed, and leſs than the circumſcribed polygons: Therefore half their ſums may be taken for the circumference of the circle, when the number of thoſe ſides is very great.

Hence, the circumferences of circles are in proportion to one another, as the radii of thoſe circles, or as their diameters.

For the perimeters of the inſcribed and circumſcribing polygons are to one another, as the radii of the circles. (186)

And theſe perimeters and circumferences continually approach to equality.

189. THEOREM XXXVI.

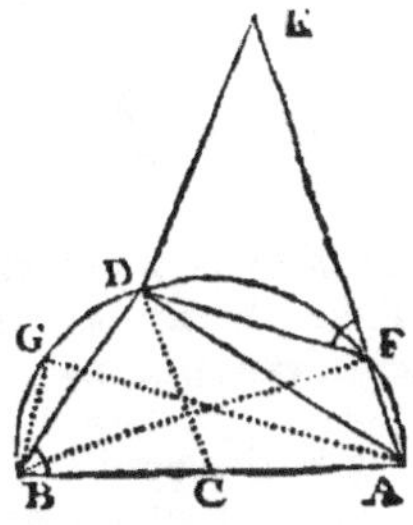

In a circle AFB, *if lines*, BA, DA, FA, *be drawn from the extremities of two equal arcs*, BD, DF, *to meet in that point* A *of the circumference determined by one of them*, BA, *paſſing through the center; then ſhall the middle line* AD, *be a mean proportional between the ſum* AB + AF *of the extreme lines, and the radius* BC *of that circle.*

DEM. On D, with the diſtance DA, cut AF produced in E.
Then drawing DE, DF, DB, the triangles ADB, EDF, are congruous. (102)
For ∠EFD = (∠FDA + ∠FAD (96) =) ∠DBA (128). Becauſe the arc DFA = DF + FA.
And ∠E = ∠FAD (104) = ∠DAB, by conſtruction; and DE = DA.
Therefore EF = AB; and AE = AB + AF.
Draw CD; then the triangles ACD, ADE, are ſimilar.
For they are Iſoſceles and equiangular.
Therefore AC : AD :: AD : (AE =) AB + AF. (167)

190. Hence, whence the radius of the circle is expreſſed by 1, and one of the extreme lines, or chords, paſſes through the center; then if the number 2 be added to the other extreme chord, the ſquare root of that ſum will be equal to the length of the mean chord.
For ſince AC : AD :: AD : AB + AF (189.) Th. $\overline{AD}^2 = AC \times \overline{AB \times AF}$. (162)
Now if AC = 1, then AB = 2; And $\overline{AD}^2 = 2 + AF$; becauſe multiplying by 1 is uſeleſs here. Therefore $AD = \sqrt{2+AF}$.

As the arcs BD and DFA make a ſemicircle, they are called the ſupplements of one another: Therefore if the arc BD is any part (as, $\frac{1}{3}$, $\frac{1}{6}$, $\frac{1}{12}$, &c.) of the ſemicircumference; then is the line DA called the ſupplemental chord of that part.

191. REMARK. In the poſthumous works of the Marquis *de le Hoſpital*, (page 319, Engliſh edition) this principle is applied to the doctrine of angular ſections; that is, to the dividing of a given arc into any propoſed number of equal parts: Or the finding of the chord of any propoſed arc.

For if BF was any aſſumed arc, the chord of which had a known ratio to the given radius BC; then as BFA is a right angled triangle (130), the ſide $AF = \sqrt{\overline{AB}^2 - \overline{BF}^2}$ (113) will alſo be known. And by this Theorem the mean chord AD will be known; and alſo DB $(= \sqrt{\overline{AB}^2 - \overline{AD}^2})$ the chord of half the arc BF will alſo be known.

And by biſecting the arc DB in G, and drawing AG, GB, the mean chord AG is known (189); and GB $(= \sqrt{\overline{AB}^2 - \overline{AG}^2})$ is alſo given.

And in this manner, by a continual biſection, the chord of a very ſmall arc may be obtained; the practice of which is facilitated by article (190) deduced from page 330 of the ſaid work.

192. Ex-

192. Example. *Required the chord of the $\frac{1}{3072}$ part of the circumference of a circle, the radius of which is 1. Or, required the side of a regular polygon of 3072 sides, inscribed in a circle, the diameter of which is 2.*

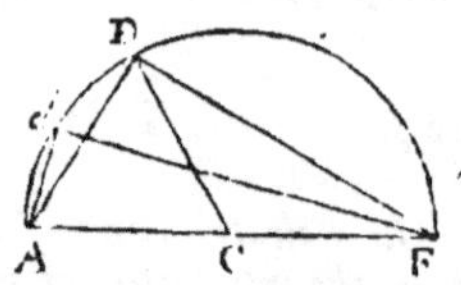

Let ADF be a semicircle, the diameter AF=2, and center C. Take the arc AD=$\frac{1}{3}$ of the semicircumference, or equal to 60 degrees; and draw DC, DA, DF.

Let *d* represent the point where the arc is bisected; *d*F the supplemental chord to that bisection: and let the marks d, d'', d''', d^{iv}, &c. express the bisected points agreeable to the number of bisections.

193. Now since ∠ACD=60°.
Therefore ∠CAD+∠ADC=(180°—60°=)120°. (98)

But ∠CAD=∠ADC (104); then ∠CAD=($\frac{120°}{2}$=) 60°.
Therefore DA=(DC=AC=) 1.

And as the triangle ADF is right angled at D. (130)
Then $DF=(\sqrt{\overline{AF}^2-\overline{AD}^2}\ (113)=\sqrt{4-1}=)\sqrt{3}=1,7320508075688773$
Therefore the supplemental chord of the arc AD, or of

$\frac{1}{3}$ of the semicircumference is	FD	$=\sqrt{3}$	=1,7320508075688773
$\frac{1}{6}$ of the same (190) is	Fd'	$=\sqrt{2+FD}$	=1,9318516525781366
$\frac{1}{12}$	Fd''	$=\sqrt{2+Fd'}$	=1,9828897227476208
$\frac{1}{24}$	Fd'''	$=\sqrt{2+Fd''}$	=1,9957178464772070
$\frac{1}{48}$	Fd^{iv}	$=\sqrt{2+Fd'''}$	=1,9989291749527313
$\frac{1}{96}$	Fd^{v}	$=\sqrt{2+Fd^{iv}}$	=1,9997322758191236
$\frac{1}{192}$	Fd^{vi}	$=\sqrt{2+Fd^{v}}$	=1,9999330678348022
$\frac{1}{384}$	Fd^{vii}	$=\sqrt{2+Fd^{vi}}$	=1,9999832668887013
$\frac{1}{768}$	Fd^{viii}	$=\sqrt{2+Fd^{vii}}$	=1,9999958167178004
$\frac{1}{1536}$	Fd^{ix}	$=\sqrt{2+Fd^{viii}}$	=1,9999989541791767

Now Fd^{ix} the supplemental chord of $\frac{1}{1536}$ being known, the chord Ad^{ix} of $\frac{1}{1536}$, part of the semicircumference, or of $\frac{1}{3072}$, part of the whole circumference, is also known.

That is $Ad^{ix}=(\sqrt{\overline{AF}^2-\overline{Fd^{ix}}^2}=)\ \sqrt{4-2+Fd^{viii}}=0,0020453073606764$

194. Consequently, the side of a regular polygon of 3072 sides, inscribed in a circle whose diameter is 2, is 0,0020453073606764

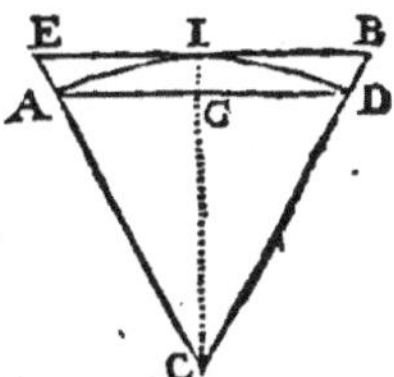

195. *The side of a similar polygon circumscribing the same circle, the center of which is* C, *may be thus found.*

Let BE be the side of the circumscribed polygon; and draw BC, EC, cutting the circle in D and A.

Draw DA, and it will be the side of the inscribed polygon; and is parallel to BE. (184)

Draw CI bisecting the angle ECE, and it will bisect BE and DA at right angles (103). And $DG = (\frac{1}{2}DA =) \frac{1}{2}Ad^{ix}$.

Then $CG = \sqrt{\overline{CD}^2 - \overline{DG}^2} = \sqrt{1 - \frac{1}{2}\overline{Ad^{ix}}^2}$.

But $\frac{1}{2}Ad^{ix} = 0{,}001022653680338$. And its square is 0,00000104582055

Which subtracted from 1 leaves 0,99999895417945

Whose square root, or CG, is equal to 0,99999947708959

Now the triangles CBI, CDG, are similar.

Then CG : CI : : 2DG : 2BI. (167, 151)

Therefore $(2BI =)\ BE = (\frac{2DG \times CI}{CG}(164) =) \frac{DA}{CG}$; For IC = 1.

Or $BE = \frac{0{,}0020453073606764}{0{,}9999994770895883} = 0{,}0020453084301895$

which is the side of a regular polygon of 3072 sides, circumscribing a circle the diameter of which is 2.

196. SCHOLIUM. The side of a regular polygon of 3072 sides, inscribed in a circle, the diameter of which is 2, is 0,0020453073606764. (194). Which multiplied by 3072, will give the perimeter of that polygon, which is 6,2831842119979622.

The side of a similar polygon, circumscribing the same circle is 0,0020453084301895. (195)

Which multiplied by 3072, will give for the perimeter of that polygon 6,2831874973420925.

The sum of these perimeters is 12,5663717093400547.

The half sum is 6,28318585, &c.

Which is very nearly equal to the circumference of a circle, the diameter of which is 2 (187), the difference between it

{ and the inscribed polygon being only 0,00000164, &c.
{ and the circumscribed polygon being only 0,00000164, &c.

197. Now the circumferences of circles being in the same proportion, as their diameters. (188)

Therefore the diameter of a circle being 1,

The circumference will be 3,141592, &c. which agrees with the circumference as found by other methods.

SECTION V.

Of Planes and Solids.

DEFINITIONS and PRINCIPLES.

198. A line is said to be in a plane, when it passes through two or more points in that plane; and the common section of two planes is a line which is in both of them.

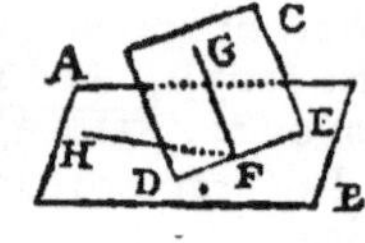

199. The inclination of two meeting planes AB, CD, is measured by an acute angle GFH, made by two right lines FG, FH, one in each plane, and both drawn perpendicular to the common section DE, of these planes from F, some point in it.

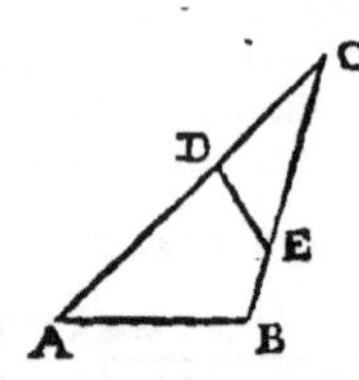

200. A right line DE intersecting two sides AC, BC, of a triangle ABC, so as to make angles CDE, CED, within the figure, equal to the angles CBA, CAB, at the base AB, but with contrary sides of the triangle, is said to be in a subcontrary position to the base.

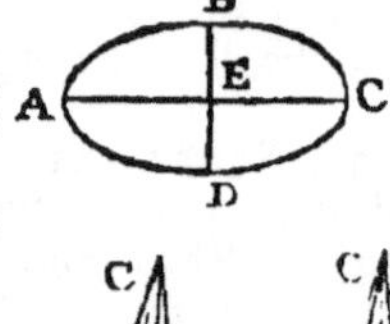

201. If a circle in an oblique position be viewed, it will appear of an oval form, as ABCD; that is, it will seem to be longer one way, as AC, than another, as DB; nevertheless the radii EA, EB, are to be esteemed as equal. And the same must be understood in viewing any regular figure, when placed obliquely to the eye.

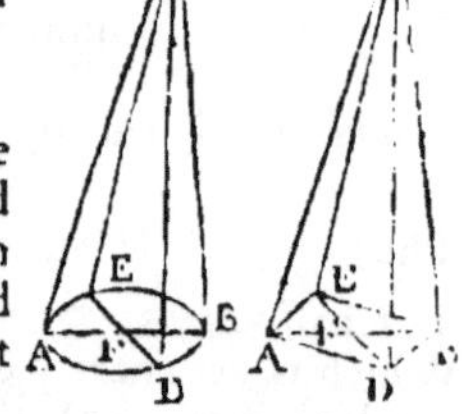

202. If a line be fixed to any point C above the plane of a circle ADBE, and this line while stretched be moved round the circle, so as always to touch it; then a solid which would fill the space passed over by the line, between the circle and the point C, is called a CONE.

203. If the figure ADBE had been a polygon, and the stretched line had moved along its sides, the figure which would then have been described, is called a PYRAMID.

So that Cones and Pyramids are solids which regularly taper from a circle, or polygon, to a point.

The circle or polygon is called the *Base*; and the point C the *Vertex*.

When the vertex is perpendicularly over the middle or center of the base, then the solid is called a RIGHT CONE, or a RIGHT PYRAMID; otherwise an OBLIQUE CONE, or OBLIQUE PYRAMID.

204. If a Cone or Pyramid be cut by a plane passing through the vertex C, and center of the base F, the section ABC, or EDC, is a triangle.

205. A right line AB, is perpendicular to a plane CD, when it makes right angles ABE, ABF, ABG, with all the right lines BE, BF, BG, drawn in that plane to touch the ſaid right line AB.

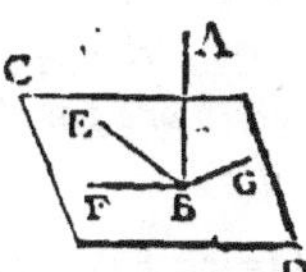

206. So that from the ſame point B, in a plane, only one perpendicular can be drawn to that plane on the ſame ſide.

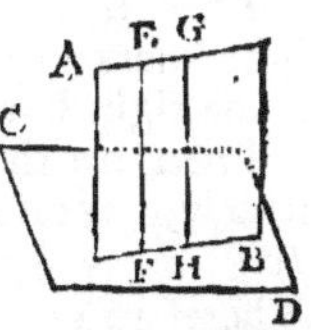

207. A plane AB, is perpendicular to a plane CD, when the right lines EF, GH, drawn in one plane AB, at right angles to FB, the common ſection of the two planes, are alſo at right angles to the other plane CD.

208. So that a line EF, perpendicular to a plane CD, is in another plane AB, and at right angles to FB, the common ſection of the two planes.

209. THEOREM XXXVII.

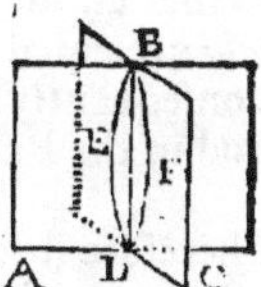

If two planes AB, CD, *cut each other, their common ſection* BD, *will be a right line.*

DEM. For if it be not, draw a right line DEB in the plane AB, from the point D to the point B; alſo draw a right line DFB in the plane BC.

Then two right lines DEB, DFB, have the ſame terms, and include a ſpace or figure, which is abſurd. (7)

Therefore DEB and DFB are not right lines: Neither can any other lines drawn from D to B, beſides BD, be right lines.

Conſequently the line DB, the common ſection of the planes, is a right line.

210. THEOREM XXXVIII.

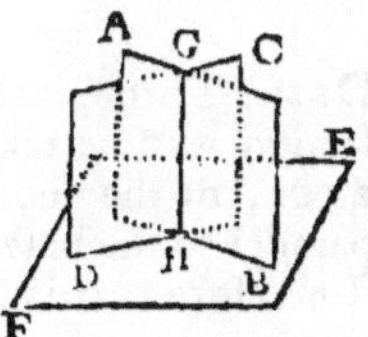

If two planes AB, CD, *which are both perpendicular to a third plane* EF, *cut one another; their interſection* HG *is at right angles to that third plane* EF.

DEM. For the common ſection of AB and CD is a right line GH. (209)
Alſo HB, HD, are the common ſections of AB, CD, with the plane EF.

Now from the point H, a line HG drawn perpendicular to the plane EF, muſt be at right angles to HB, HD. (205)

But HG muſt be in both planes AB, CD. (208)

Therefore it muſt be in the common ſection of thoſe planes.

Conſequently the ſection HG of the planes AB, CD, is at right angles to the plane EF.

211. THEOREM XXXIX.

The sections, aebd, of a Cone or Pyramid CAEBD, *which are parallel to the base* AEBD, *are similar to that base.*

DEM. For let AFBC, DFEC, be sections through the vertex C, and center F of the base.

Then these sections will cut one another in the right line FC (209), and the transverse section *abde*, in the right lines *ab*, and *ed*, intersecting in *f*.

Then are the following sets of triangles similar; namely, AFC, *afc*; BFC, *bfc*; DFC, *dfc*; EFC, *efc*.

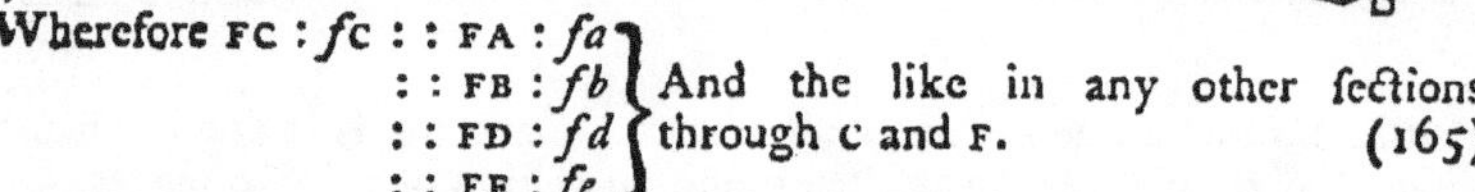

Wherefore FC : *fc* : : FA : *fa*
: : FB : *fb* And the like in any other sections
: : FD : *fd* through C and F. (165)
: : FE : *fe*

Now in the Cone, FA = FB = FD = FE; therefore *fa* = *fb* = *fd* = *fe*. (152)
So that all the right lines drawn from *f* to the circumference of the figure *adbe* are equal to one another.
Consequently the figure *adbe* is a circle. (9)
And in the Pyramid, FC : *fc* : : DC : *dc* : : DB : *db* : : DA : *da*.
FC : *fc* : : EC : *ec* : : EA : *ea* : : EB : *eb*.
Therefore in each pair of corresponding triangles in the base and transverse section, the sides are respectively proportional.
Consequently, as the base and transverse section are composed of like sets of similar triangles; therefore they are also similar. (183)

212. THEOREM XL.

If a Cone ABLCK, *the base of which is a circle* CBLCK, *be cut by a plane in a subcontrary position to the base, the section* DIEH *will be a circle.*

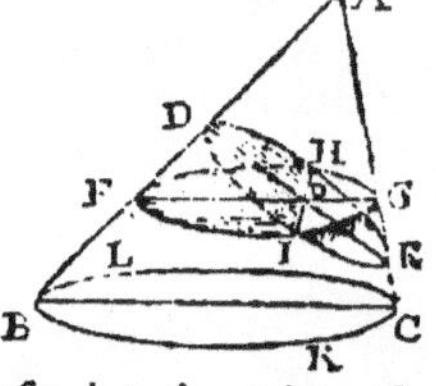

DEM. Through the vertex A, and center of the base, let the triangular section ABC be taken, so as to be at right angles to the planes of the base BKCL, of the subcontrary section DIEH, and of the section FIGH, taken parallel to the base, and cutting the subcontrary section in the line IOH.
Therefore IOH is perpendicular to DE and FG (210) cutting one another in O.
Now the section FIGH is a circle (211). Therefore FO × OG = OI². (171)
Again the triangles GOE, FOD, are similar.
For ∠GEO = ∠DFO = ∠ABC by constr. And ∠GOE = ∠DOF. (93)
Therefore EO : OG : : FO : DO (167.) And EO × DO = FO × OG (162) = OI².
So that OI is a mean proportional, either between FO and OG, or DO and EO. But as the same would happen wherever FG cuts DE; therefore all the lines OI, both in the sections FIGH and DIEH, are lines in a circle.
Consequently the section DIEH is a circle.

213. If

213. If the ſection cut both ſides of the cone not in a ſubcontrary poſition to BC, the diameter of the baſe, then the ſection (ſuppoſe it ſtill) DIEH, is called an ELLIPTIC SECTION, which though not a circle, will be a bounded curve, longer one way than the other; and, like a circle, return into itſelf.

The curve DIEH is called an Ellipſis.

214. The line DE, the TRANSVERSE DIAMETER or AXIS.

The line OH or OI, is called an ORDINATE.

215. The ordinate through the middle of DE, is called the CONJUGATE AXIS.

The interſection of the Tranſverſe and Conjugate Axes, is called the CENTER of the Ellipſis.

216. If a circular arc be deſcribed, with a radius equal to half the Tranſverſe Axis, from one end of the Conjugate Axis, its interſections with the Tranſverſe Axis, are called FOCI, one on each ſide of the center of the Ellipſis.

217. Every right line paſſing through the center of the Ellipſis, and terminated at each end by the curve, is called a DIAMETER.

218. The radius that would deſcribe a circular arc of the ſame curvature with the ellipſis at any point of it, is called the RADIUS OF CURVATURE.

A TANGENT to any point in the Ellipſis, is a right line perpendicular to the radius of curvature at that point.

219. Two Diameters being ſo drawn, that one is parallel to a tangent, and the other paſſes through the point of contact; thoſe two Diameters are ſaid to be CONJUGATE DIAMETERS; and have certain relations to their Ordinates, Tangents, Radii of Curvature, and other lines belonging to the Ellipſis.

220. A third proportional to any two Conjugate Diameters, is called the PARAMETER.

SECTION VI.

Of the Spiral.

221. *Suppose the radius of a circle to revolve with an uniform motion round its center, and while it is so revolving, let a point move along the radius; then will the successive places of that point be in a curve, which is called a spiral.*

This will be readily conceived by imagining a fly to move along the spoke of a wheel, while the wheel is turning round.

If while the radius revolves once, the point has moved the length of the radius; then the spiral will have revolved but once round the center, or pole; consequently the motion in the circumference is to the motion in the radius, as the circumference is to the radius: And if the wheel revolves twice, thrice, or in any proportion to the motion in the radius; then the spiral will make so many turns, or parts of a turn, round the center.

222. *Now suppose, while the radius revolves equably, a point from the circumference moves towards the center, with a motion decreasing in a geometric progression; then will a spiral be generated, which is called a proportional spiral.*

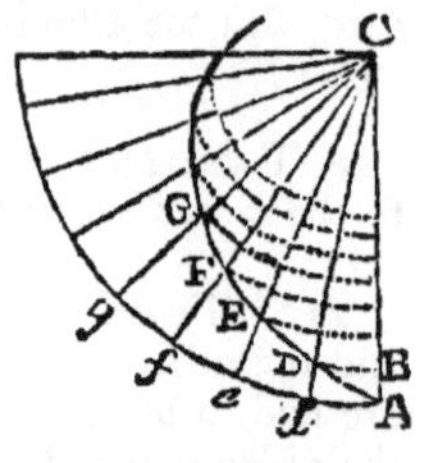

Let the radius CA be divided in any continued decreasing geometric progression (90), as of 10 to 8; then the series of terms will be 10; 8; 6,4; 5,12; 4,096; 3,2768; 2,62144, &c. Also let the circumference be divided into any number of equal parts, in the points *d*, *e*, *f*, *g*, &c. Then if the several divisions of the radius CA be successively transferred from the center C, cutting the other radii in the points D, E, F, G, &c. and a curved line be evenly drawn through those points, it will be a spiral of the kind proposed.

223. From the nature of a decreasing geometric progression, it is easy to conceive that the radius CA may be continually divided; and although each successive division becomes shorter than the next preceding one, yet if ever so great a number of divisions, or terms, be taken, there will still remain a finite magnitude.

224. Hence it follows, that this spiral winds continually round the center, and does not fall into it till after an infinite number of revolutions.

Also, that the number of revolutions decrease, as the number of the equal parts, into which the circumference is divided, increases.

225. THEO-

225. THEOREM XLI.

Any proportional ſpiral cuts the intercepted radii at equal angles.

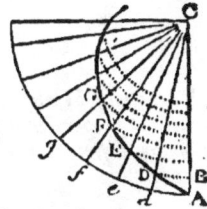

Dem. If the diviſions A*d*, *de*, *ef*, *fg*, &c. of the circumference were very ſmall, then would the ſeveral radii be ſo cloſe to one another, that the intercepted parts AD, DE, EF, FG, &c. of the ſpiral, might be taken as right lines.

And the triangles CAD, CDE, CEF, &c. would be ſimilar, having equal angles at the point C, and the ſides about thoſe angles proportional. (168) Therefore the angles at A, D, E, F, &c. being equal, the ſpiral muſt neceſſarily cut the radii at equal angles.

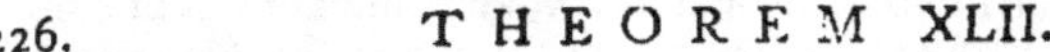

226. THEOREM XLII.

If the radii of any proportional ſpiral be taken as numbers, then will the correſponding arcs of the circle, reckoned from their commencement, be as the logarithms of thoſe numbers.

Dem. As the lines CA, CD, CE, CF, CG, &c. are a ſeries of terms in geometric progreſſion; and the arcs A*d*, A*e*, A*f*, A*g*, &c. are a ſeries of terms in arithmetic progreſſion; therefore theſe arcs may ſerve (I. 66) as the indices to the geometric terms, and be thus placed;

Radii of the ſpiral CA, CD, CE, CF, CG, &c. Geometric terms.
Correſponding arcs 0, A*d*, A*e*, A*f*, A*g*, &c. Arithm. terms, or indices.

In this diſpoſition, the firſt term CA is not diſtant from itſelf, therefore its index is repreſented by 0.
Then if the diſtance of the ſecond term CD from the firſt term CA be expreſſed by the arc A*d*; the diſtance of the third term CE, from CA, will be expreſſed by the arc A*e*; and ſo of the reſt.
Conſequently, if the terms in the geometric ſeries be repreſented by numbers, taken as parts of the radius, then the numbers of the ſame kind, expreſſing the meaſures of the arcs, or indices, will be as the logarithms of the geometric terms. (I. 73)

227. Corol. If the difference between CA and CB was indefinitely ſmall, or CA and CB were nearly in a ratio of equality; then might the number of proportional lines into which CA could be divided, be ſo many, that any propoſed number might be found among the terms of this ſeries; and if the number of parts in the circumference was increaſed in like manner, then would every term of the proportional diviſion of the radius CA have its correſponding index among the equal diviſions of the circumference; and conſequently would exhibit the logarithms of all numbers.

228. THEOREM XLIII.

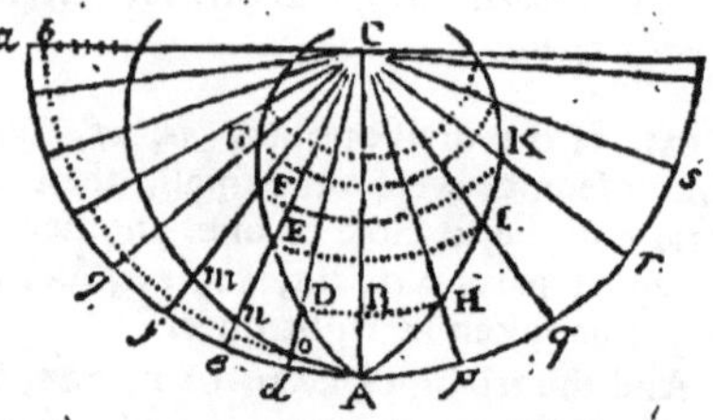

There may be almoſt an infinite variety of proportional ſpirals, and as many different kinds of logarithms.

DEM. For with the ſame equal diviſions A*d*, *de*, *ef*, &c. of the circumference, every variation in the ratio of CA to CB, as of C*a* to C*b*, will produce a different ſpiral, A*onm*.

And with the ſame diviſions of the radius CA, and different ſets of equal parts, A*d*, *de*, *ef*, &c. and A*p*, *pq*, *qr*, &c. of the circumference, may be formed different ſpirals ADEF, AHIK.

Alſo, varying at the ſame time both the diviſions of the radius and circumference, different ſpirals will be produced.

But the variations in theſe three caſes may be almoſt infinite: Therefore the number of ſuch ſpirals are almoſt infinite.

Now it is evident, that there is a peculiar relation between the rays of any ſpiral, and the correſponding arcs of the circle; that is, between the terms of a geometric progreſſion, and its indices: Therefore there may be as many kinds of logarithms, as there are proportional ſpirals.

229. THEOREM XLIV.

That proportional ſpiral which interſects equidiſtant rays at an angle of 45 *degrees, produces logarithms that are of* Nepier's *kind.*

DEM. Suppoſe AB, the difference between CA and CB, the firſt and ſecond terms of the geometric progreſſion, to be indefinitely ſmall, and take A*p*, the logarithm of CB, equal to AB; then may the figure ABH*p* be taken as a ſquare, whoſe diagonal AH would be part of the ſpiral AHIK, and the angle BAH would be half a right one, or 45 degrees.

Therefore that ſpiral which cuts its rays CA, CH, &c. at angles of 45 degrees, has a kind of logarithms belonging to it, ſo related to their correſponding numbers, that the ſmalleſt variation between the firſt and ſecond numbers is equal to the logarithm of the ſecond number.

But of this kind were the firſt logarithms made by Lord *Nepier*.

Therefore the logarithms to the ſpiral which cuts its equidiſtant rays at an angle of 45 degrees, are of the *Nepierian* kind.

END OF BOOK II.

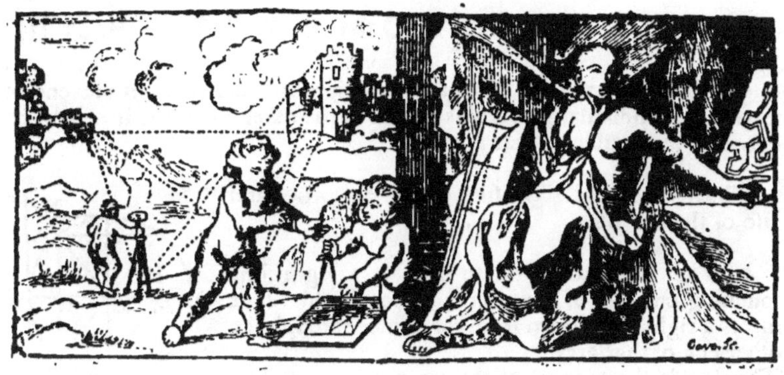

THE

ELEMENTS

OF

NAVIGATION.

BOOK III.

OF PLANE TRIGONOMETRY.

SECTION I.

Definitions and *Principles*.

1. PLANE TRIGONOMETRY is an art which ſhews how to find the meaſures of the ſides and angles of plane Triangles, ſome of them being already known.

It will be proper for the learner, before he reads the following Articles, to turn to the definitions relative to a circle and angle, contained in the Articles 8, 9, 10, 11, 12, 13, 14, 15, 16, 17, 18, 19, and 36, of Book II.

2. A Triangle conſiſts of ſix parts; namely, three ſides and three angles.

The ſides of plane triangles are denoted, or eſtimated by meaſures of length; ſuch as Feet, Yards, Fathoms, Furlongs, Miles, Leagues, &c.

The angles of triangles are eſtimated by circular meaſures, that is, by arcs containing Degrees, Minutes, Seconds, &c. (II. 15); and for convenience theſe circular meaſures are repreſented by right lines, called right ſines, tangents, ſecants, and verſed ſines.

3. The

3. The RIGHT SINE of an arc, is a right line drawn from one end of the arc perpendicular to a radius drawn to the other end: Or it is half the chord of the double of that arc.

Thus AH is the right ſine of the arc AG; and alſo of the arc DBA.

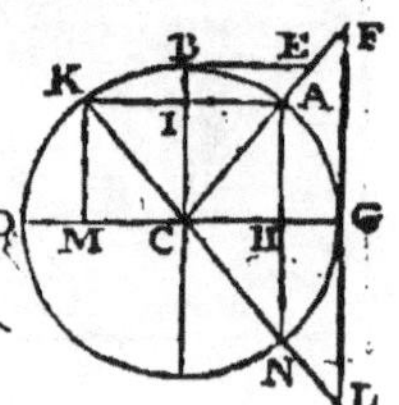

4. The TANGENT of an arc, is a right line touching one end of the arc, and continued till it meets a right line drawn from the center through the other end of that arc.
Thus GF is the tangent of the arc GA.

5. The SECANT of an arc, is a right line drawn through the center and one end of the arc, and produced till it meets the tangent drawn from the other end.
Thus CF is the ſecant of the arc AG.

6. The VERSED SINE of an arc, is that part of the radius intercepted between the arc and its right ſine.
Thus HG is the verſed ſine of the arc AG.

7. The COMPLEMENT of an arc, is what that arc wants of 90 degrees.

Thus if the arc GB = 90°. Then AB is called the complement of AG; and AG is the complement of AB.

8. The SUPPLEMENT of an arc, is what that arc wants of 180 degrees.
Thus the arc ABD is the ſupplement of AG; and AG of ABD.

9. The CO-SINE of an arc, is the right ſine of the complement of that arc.

The CO-TANGENT of an arc, is the tangent of that arc's complement.

The CO-SECANT of an arc, is the ſecant of its complement.

The CO-VERSED SINE of an arc, is the verſed ſine of its complement.

Thus AI, BE, CE, BI, being reſpectively the ſine, tangent, ſecant, and verſed ſine of the arc AB, which is the complement of AG; therefore AI is called the co-ſine; BE the co-tangent, CE the co-ſecant, BI the co-verſed ſine, of the arc AG.

The right lines, called ſines, tangents, ſecants, and verſed ſines, are uſed as well for the meaſures of angles, as for the arcs which meaſure theſe angles: And it is as common to ſay the ſine, tangent, &c. of an angle, as the ſine, tangent, &c. of an arc.

10. The

10. The greatest right sine, is the sine of 90°; and the sines to arcs less than 90°, serve equally for arcs as much greater than 90°.

Thus the sines of 80° and 100°; of 60° and 120°; of 40° and 140°, &c. are respectively equal.

11. The same tangent and secant will serve to arcs equally distant from 90 degrees; that is, to any arc and its supplement.

Thus if the arc BAG=90°, and BK=BA; then the arcs GN, GA, DK, are equal; and the arcs GAK and GN, or DK, are supplements to one another: Then the sine KM, the tangent GL, the secant CL, of the arc GBK, are respectively equal to the sine AH, the tangent GF, the secant CF of the arc GA.

12. When an arc is greater than 90°, the sine, tangent, secant, of the supplement is to be used.

13. The chord of an arc is equal to twice the co-sine of half the supplemental arc.

Thus AN, the chord of the arc AGN,=2CI, the co-sine of the arc AB, and AB is half of the arc ABK, the supplement of AGN.

14. The versed sine and co-sine together, HG+CH of any arc AG, is equal to the radius; CH being equal to AI.

15. The sines, tangents, secants, or versed sines of similar arcs in different circles, are in the same proportion to one another, as the radii of those circles. (II. 185)

16. The angles of two triangles may be respectively equal, although their sides may be unequal.

Therefore in a triangle among the things given, in order to find the rest, one of them must be a side.

In Trigonometry, the three things given in a triangle must be either,

1st. Two sides and an angle opposite to one of them.

2d. Two angles and a side opposite to one of them.

3d. Two sides and the included angle.

4th. The three sides.

In either case, the other three things may be found by the help of a few Theorems, and a *Triangular Canon*, which is a table where is orderly inserted every degree and minute in a quadrant or arc of 90 degrees; and against them, the measures of the lengths of their corresponding sines, tangents, and secants, estimated in parts of the radius, which is usually supposed to be divided into a number of equal parts, as 10, 100, 1000, 10000, 100000, &c.

SECTION II.

Of the Triangular Canon.

PROPOSITION I.

17. *To find the lengths of the Chords, Sines, Tangents, and Secants to arcs of a circle of a given radius.*

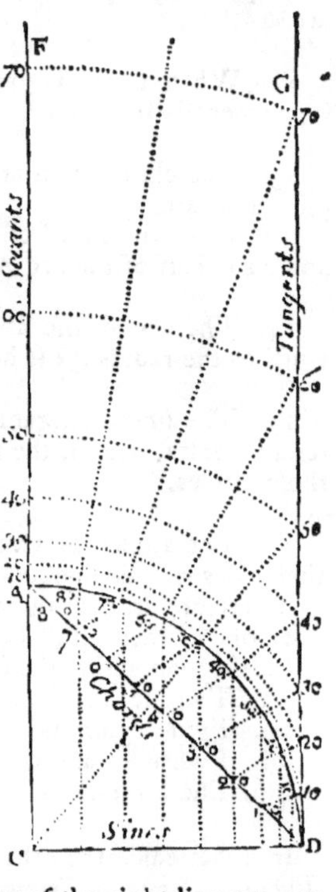

CONSTRUCTION. Through each end of the given radius CD, and at right angles to it (II. 60) draw the lines CF, DG: On C, with the radius CD, deſcribe the quadrantal arc DA, and draw the chord DA.

18. FOR THE CHORDS. Triſect the arc AD (II. 61.), and (by trials) triſect each part; then the arc AD will be divided into 9 equal parts of 10 degrees each; if theſe arcs are divided each into 10 equal parts, the quadrant will be divided into 90 degrees: But, in this ſmall figure, the diviſions to every 10 degrees only are retained, as in (II. 83).

From D, as a center, with the radius to each diviſion, cut the right line DA; and it will contain the chords of the ſeveral arcs into which the quadrantal arc AD was divided.

For the diſtances from D to the ſeveral diviſions of the right line DA, are thus made reſpectively equal to the diſtances or chords of the ſeveral arcs reckoned from D.

19. FOR THE SINES. Through each of the diviſions of the arc AD, draw right lines parallel to the radius AC; theſe parallel lines will be the right ſines of their reſpective arcs, and CD will be divided into a line of ſines, which are to be numbered from C to D, for the right ſines; and from D to C for the verſed ſines.

For the diſtance from C to the ſeveral diviſions of the right line CD, are reſpectively equal to the ſines of the ſeveral arcs beginning from A.

20. FOR THE TANGENTS. A ruler on C, and the ſeveral diviſions of the arc AD, will interſect the line DG; and the diſtances from D to the ſeveral diviſions of DG, will be the lengths of the ſeveral tangents.

21. FOR THE SECANTS. From the center C, with radii to the diviſions of the tangents DG, cut the line CF; and the diſtances from C to the ſeveral diviſions of CF, will be the lengths of the ſecants to the ſeveral arcs.

For theſe lengths are made reſpectively equal to the ſecants reckoned from C to the ſeveral diviſions of the tangent DG.

22. If the figure was ſo large, that the quadrantal arc could contain every degree and minute of the quadrant, or 5400 equal parts; then the chord, ſine, tangent, and ſecant to each of them could be drawn. Now a ſcale of equal parts being conſtructed (II. 81), 1000 of which parts are equal to the radius CD; then the lengths of the ſeveral ſines, tangents, and ſecants may be meaſured from that ſcale, and entered in a table called the triangular canon, or the table of ſines, tangents, and ſecants.

But as theſe meaſures cannot be taken with ſufficient accuracy to ſerve for the computation to which ſuch tables are applicable; therefore the ſeveral lengths have been calculated for a radius divided into a much greater number of equal parts; as is ſhewn in the following articles.

23. PROP. II.

In any circle the chord of 60 degrees, is equal to the radius: and the ſine of 30 degrees is equal to half the radius.

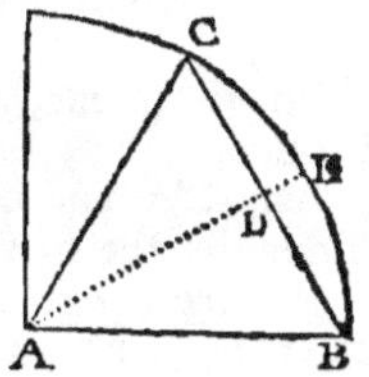

DEM. Let the arc CB, or ∠ CAB = 60 degrees;
and draw the chord CB.
Now ſince the radii AC and AB are equal; (II. 9)
Therefore ∠C = ∠B. (II. 104)
And the ∠C + ∠B = (180° — (∠A =) 60° =) 120° (II. 96)
Therefore ∠ C, or ∠ B = (half 120°; or =) 60° = ∠A
Conſequently CB = AB = AC.
From A, draw the radius AE perpendicular to CB.
Then AE biſects the arc CB, and its chord. (II. 124)
And CD = ſine of (the arc CE = half of 60° =) 30°. (3)
Conſequently CD is equal to half the radius AB.

24. Hence, *Twice the co-ſine of 60 degrees is equal to the radius.* For 30° is the complement of 60°, and twice the ſine of 30° is equal to the radius.

25. PROP. III.

To find the ſine of one minute of a degree.

It is evident (II. 187), that the leſs the arc is, the leſs is the difference between the arc and its ſine, or half chord; ſo that a very ſmall arc, ſuch as that of one minute, may be reckoned to differ from its ſine, by ſo ſmall a quantity, that they may be eſteemed as equal; and conſequently may be expreſſed by the ſame number of ſuch equal parts of which the radius is ſuppoſed to contain 1,00000, &c. which is readily found by the following proportion.

As the circumference of the circle in minutes	21600
To the circumf. in equal parts of the radius (II. 196)	6,283185
So is the arc of one minute	1,
To the corresponding parts of the radius	0,0002908882
So that for the ſine of one minute, may be taken	0,0002908882

26. PROP.

In a series of arcs in arithmetic progression, the sine of any one of them, taken as a mean, and the sum of the sines of any other two, taken as equidistant extremes, are ever in a constant ratio, of radius to twice the co-sine of the common difference of those arcs.

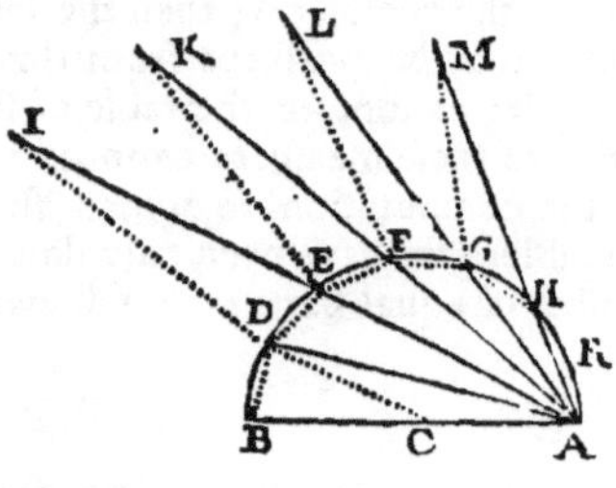

Dem. For in a circumference, the center of which is C, and diameter AB, let there be taken a series of arcs, ARB, ARD, ARE, ARF, ARG, ARH, &c. the common difference of which is the arc BD.

Then drawing the chords AB, AD, AE, AF, AG, AH, &c. their halves will be the sines of half the arcs ARB, ARD, &c. (3)

Also half the arc BD, is the common difference of half the arcs ARB, ARD, ARE, &c. (II. 150)

And the chord AD is twice the co-sine of half the supplemental arc BD. (13)

From the points, D, E, F, G, &c. with the radii DA, EA, FA, GA, &c. cut AE, AF, AG, AH, &c. produced in I, K, L, M, &c. draw ID, KE, LF, MG, &c. and BD, DE, EF, FG, GH, &c.

Then by the first part of the demonstration (II. 189), the following triangles are congruous, namely,

ABD, IED; ADE, KFE; AEF, LGF; AFG, MHG, &c.

Therefore IE = AB; KF = AD; LG = AE; MH = AF, &c.

Also the triangles IDA, KEA, LFA, MGA, &c. being each of them isosceles, and their angles respectively equal, are similar to DCA. (II. 167)

Therefore CA : AD : : (AD : (AI =)AB + AE : :) $\frac{1}{2}$AD : $\frac{1}{2}$AB + $\frac{1}{2}$AE.
: : (AE : (AK =)AD + AF : :) $\frac{1}{2}$AE : $\frac{1}{2}$AD + $\frac{1}{2}$AF.
: : (AF : (AL =)AE + AG : :) $\frac{1}{2}$AF : $\frac{1}{2}$AE + $\frac{1}{2}$AG.
&c. &c.

The halves being in the same ratio as the wholes. (II. 150)

27. Consequently, in a series of arcs in arithmetic progression, *viz.* $\frac{1}{2}$ARB, $\frac{1}{2}$ARD, $\frac{1}{2}$ARE, &c. the common difference of which is half the arc BD, it will be, (II. 164)
As (AC) radius.
To (AD) twice the co-sine of the common difference;
So is the sine of either arc taken as a mean,
To the sum of the sines of two equidistant extremes.

28. Hence, *The sine of either extreme, subtracted from the product of the sine of the mean by twice the co-sine of the common difference, will give the sine of the other extreme.* (II. 164)

29. When

29. When the common difference of three arcs is 60 degrees; then twice the co-sine of that difference is equal to the radius. (24)

And with any such three arcs, as 30, 90, 150; or 25, 85, 145; or 20, 80, 140, &c. it will be (27).

			(10)
As R : (2 cos. 60 =) R	: : s, 90°	: (s, 30° + s, 150° =) s, 30° + s, 30°.	
	: : s, 85	: (s, 25° + s, 145° =) s, 25° + s, 35°.	
	: : s, 80	: (s, 20° + s, 140° =) s, 20° + s, 40°.	
	: : s, 75	: (s, 15° + s, 135° =) s, 15° + s, 45°.	
	&c.	&c.	

Here the first and second terms in the proportions being equal, the third and fourth terms are also equal.

30. Hence, *The sine of an arc greater than 60 degrees, is equal to the sine of an arc as much less than 60 degrees, added to the sine of its difference from 60 degrees.*

Therefore the sines of arcs above 60 degrees are readily obtained from those under 60 degrees.

31. PROP. V.

The right sine of an arc being known, to find its co-sine; and from these to find the tangent, secant, versed sine; and also the co-tangent, co-secant, and co-versed sine.

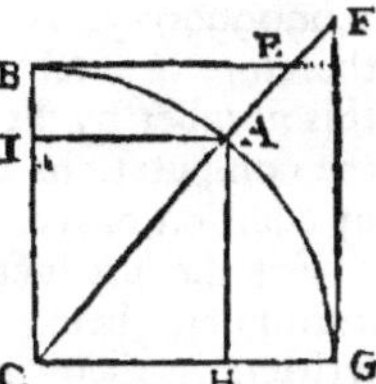

Let AG be any arc, and let AH be its sine, AI its co-sine; GF the tangent, BE the co-tangent; CF the secant, CE the co-secant; HG the versed sine, BI the co-versed sine.

Now if the sine AH be given, then the co-sine AI or CH, will be known (II. 113): For $CA^2 - AH^2 = CH^2$. Therefore *the square root of the difference between the squares of the radius and sine, will be the co-sine.*

32. Then the versed sine HG = CG — CH; and co-versed sine IB = CB — CI.
And since the triangles CHA, CGF, CBE, are similar,

33. Therefore (II. 167) CH : HA : : CG : GF, the tangent.
That is, *As the co-sine to the sine, so is radius to the tangent.*

34. And CH : CA : : CG : CF, the secant.
That is, *As the co-sine to the radius, so is radius to the secant.*

35. And CI : CA : : CB : CE, the co-secant.
That is, *As the sine to radius, so is radius to the co-secant.*

36. Also CI : IA : : CB : BE, the co-tangent.
That is, *As the sine to the co-sine, so is radius to the co-tangent.*
Or GF : CG : : CB : BE; that is, *As tangent : rad. : : rad. : co-tangent.*

37. Hence it is evident, that *the tangent and co-tangent of an arc of 45° are equal to one another, and to the radius, or sine of 90 degrees.*

And as the square of radius is equal to the rectangle of any tangent and its co-tangent,

Therefore tan. × cot. = *tan.* × *cot.* Therefore tan. : *tan.* : : *cot.* : cot. (II. 163)

Or the tangents of different arcs are reciprocally as their co-tangents.

38. The

38. The principles by which the lengths of the ſines, tangents, ſecants, &c. may be conſtructed, being delivered, the following examples are annexed to illuſtrate this doctrine.

Required the co-ſine of one minute.

The ſine of 1 minute being	0,0002908882 (25)
Its ſquare is	0,00000008461594
Which ſubtracted from the ſquare of radius	1,
Leaves	0,99999991538406
Whoſe ſquare root	0,9999999577 is the

co-ſine of 1 minute; or the ſine of 89° 59′.

Now having the ſine and co-ſine of 1 minute, the other ſines may be found in the following manner. (28)

twice the coſ. 1 min. × ſine of 1 m. = ſum of the ſines of 0′ & 2′.
twice the coſ. 1 min. × ſine of 2 m. = ſum of the ſines of 1′ & 3′.
twice the coſ. 1 min. × ſine of 3 m. = ſum of the ſines of 2′ & 4′.
twice the coſ. 1 min. × ſine of 4 m. = ſum of the ſines of 3′ & 5′.
twice the coſ. 1 min. × ſine of 5 m. = ſum of the ſines of 4′ & 6′.

Proceeding thus in a progreſſive order from each ſine to its next, all the ſines may be found.

But as twice the co-ſine of 1 minute, *viz.* 1,9999999154 is concerned in each operation, therefore if a table be made of the products of this number by the nine digits, as here annexed, the computations of the ſines may be performed by addition only.

Multipliers.	Products.
1	1,9999999154
2	3,9999998308
3	5,9999997462
4	7,9999996616
5	9,9999995770
6	11,9999994924
7	13,9999994078
8	15,9999993232
9	17,9999992386

For the products by the digits in the given multiplier, being taken from the table, and written in their proper order, will prevent the trouble of multiplication.

And even this operation may be very much ſhortened, by ſetting under the right hand place (*viz.* 4.) of the double co-ſine of one minute, the unit place of the ſine uſed as a multiplier, and reverſing or placing in a contrary order, all its other figures; then the right-hand figure of each line ariſing by the multiplication, is to be ſet under one another; and in theſe lines, the firſt figure to be ſet down, is what ariſes from the figure ſtanding over the preſent multiplying one; obſerving to add what would be carried from the places omitted.

Now if the products of the figures in the multiplier, thus inverted, be taken from the above table of products, it is neceſſary to remark what number of places will ariſe from each digit uſed in the multiplier; then in the products of thoſe digits in the table, take only the like number of places, obſerving to add 1 to the right-hand place, if the next of the omitted figures exceed 5.

Required

Required the sine of two minutes.

1,9999999154
2888092000,0
4000000
1800000
16000
1600
160
4
0,0005817764

The sine of 1 min. placed in an inverted order under the double cos. of 1 min. as in the margin; the right-hand figure 2 stands under the 9 in the 6th decimal place, therefore the first 6 decimal places of the product against 2 in the table, are to be used; but 1 being added, because the 7th place 8, exceeds 5, makes the product 4000000: Also for 9 the next figure in the multiplier, standing under the 5th decimal place, take 17,99999 from the table of products, and 1 being added to the 5th place, because the 6th exceeds 5, make it 18,00000: In like manner the product by 8, adding 1, is 16000, &c. and the sum of these products 0,0005817764 is the sine of 2 minutes, as required.

This kind of operation will be very easily conceived without farther illustration, by comparing the process in this and the following operations, with what has been already said.

Required the sines of 3′, 4′, 5′, and 6 minutes.

For 3 min.	For 4 min.	For 5 min.	For 6 min.
1,9999999154	1,9999999154	1,9999999154	1,9999999154
4677185000,0	5466278000,0	6255361100,0	7044454100,0
10000000	16000000	20000000	20000000
1600000	1400000	2000000	8000000
20000	40000	1200000	1000000
14000	12000	60000	80000
1400	1200	10000	8000
120	80	1000	800
8	10	40	10
		12	
0,0011635528	0,0017453290	0,0023271052	0,0029088810
0,0002908882	0,0005817764	0,0008726645	0,0011635526
0,0008726646	0,0011635526	0,0014544407	0,0017453284

In each example, the sine of an arc which is 2 minutes less than that required, (28) is subtracted.

The sines being made, the tangents, secants, &c. are to be constructed as before shewn. (33, 34)

39. There are many methods by which the triangular canon may be made; but that which is here delivered was chosen as the most easy, the best adapted to this work, and what would give the learner a sufficient notion how these numbers are to be found: For at this time there is no occasion to construct new tables of sines, and rarely to examine those already extant; they having passed through the hands of a great many careful examiners, and for a long time have been received by the learned as a work sufficiently correct.

These lines were first introduced into mathematical computations by *Hipparchus* and *Menelaus*, whose methods of performance were contracted by *Ptolemy*, and afterwards perfected by *Regiomontanus*; and since his time *Rheticus*, *Clavius*, *Petiscus*, and many other eminent men, have treated largely on this subject, and greatly exemplified the use of this triangular Canon, or Tables; which are now, by way of distinction, called Tables of *natural* sines, tangents, &c. But the greatest improvement ever made in this kind of mathematical learning, was by the Lord *Nepier*, Baron of *Merchiston* in *Scotland*; who, being very fond of such studies, where calculations by the sines, tangents, &c. did frequently occur, judged it would be of vast advantage if these long multiplications and divisions could be avoided; and this he effected by his happy invention of computing by certain numbers, considered as the indices of others (I. 63), which he called logarithms; this was about the year 1614.

The tables now chiefly used in Trigonometrical computations, are the logarithms of those numbers which express the lengths of the sines, tangents, &c. and therefore to distinguish them from the *natural* ones, they are called *Logarithmic* sines, tangents, &c. (or by some artificial sines, &c.) Only those of the logarithmic sines and tangents are annexed to this treatise, because the business of Navigation may be performed by them; neither are these tables carried to more than five places beside the index, that being sufficiently exact for all nautical purposes: But it must be allowed that, for general use, such tables are the most esteemed, as consist of most places.

40. These tables are at the end of Book IX. and are so disposed, that each opening of the book contains eight degrees; four of which are numbered at the top, and four at the bottom of the page; and those at the top proceed from left to right, or forwards, from 0 degrees to 45; and those at the bottom, from right to left, or backwards, from 45 to 90 degrees: To each degree there are four columns, titled sines, co-sines, tangents, co-tangents; and the minutes are in the marginal column of each page, signed with M; those on the left side of the page belong to the degrees which are at the top, and those on the right-hand side, to the degrees which are at the bottom of the page.

41. A sine, tangent, co-sine, co-tangent, to a given number of degrees, is found as follows:

For an arc less than 45 degrees,

Seek the degree at the top, and the minutes in the column signed M at the top; against which, in the column signed at the top with the proposed name, stands the sine, or tangent, &c. required.

But when the arc is greater than 45 degrees,

Seek the degrees at the bottom, the minutes in the column with M at the bottom, and the proposed name at the bottom.

EXAMPLE

EXAMPLE I. *Required the logarithmic ſine of* 28° 37′.

Find 28 deg. at the top of the page; and in the ſide column, marked with M at the top, find 37; againſt which, in the column ſigned at the top with the word ſine, ſtands 9,68029, the log. ſine of 28° 37′, as required.

EXAMPLE II. *Required the logarithmic tangent of* 67° 45′.

Find 67 deg. at the bottom of the page; and in the ſide column, titled M at the bottom, find 45; then againſt this, in the column marked tangent at the bottom, ſtands 10,38816, which is the log. tangent required.

42. But when a logarithmic ſine or tangent is propoſed, to find the degrees and minutes belonging to it, then,

Seek in the table, among the proper columns, for the neareſt logarithm to the given one; and the correſponding degrees and minutes will be found; obſerving to reckon them from the top or bottom, according as the column is titled, where the neareſt logarithm to the given one is found.

43. It may ſometimes happen that a log. ſine or log. tang. may be wanted to degrees, minutes, and parts of minutes; which may be thus found.

Take the difference between the logs. of the degrees and minutes next leſs, and thoſe next greater than the given number.

Then for $\frac{1}{4}$, take a quarter of this difference; for $\frac{1}{3}$, take a third; for $\frac{1}{2}$, take a half; for $\frac{2}{3}$ take two thirds; for $\frac{3}{4}$, take three quarters, &c.

Add the parts taken of this difference to the right-hand figures of the log. belonging to the deg. and min. next leſs, and the ſum will be the log. to the deg. min. and parts propoſed.

EXAMPLE I. *Required the log. tang. to* 60° 56′$\frac{1}{2}$.

Log. tang. 60° 57′ is		10,25535
Log. tang. 60 56 is		10,25506
The diff. is		29
Its half is		14
Add it to tang. 60° 56′		10,25506
Gives tang.	60 56$\frac{1}{2}$	10,25520

EXAMPLE II. *Required the log. ſine to* 32° 15′$\frac{3}{4}$.

Log. ſine 32° 16′ is		9,72743
Log. ſine 32 15 is		9,72723
The diff. is		20
Its three fourths is		15
Add it to ſine 32° 15′		9,72723
Gives ſine	32 15$\frac{3}{4}$	9,72738

In moſt moſt caſes the work may be done by inſpection.

44. And if a given log. ſine or log. tangent falls between thoſe in the tables: then the degrees and minutes anſwering may be reckoned $\frac{1}{4}$, or $\frac{1}{3}$, or $\frac{1}{2}$, &c. minutes more than thoſe belonging to the neareſt leſs log. in the tables, according as its difference from the given one is $\frac{1}{4}$, or $\frac{1}{3}$, or $\frac{1}{2}$, &c. of the difference between the logarithm next greater and next leſs than the given log.

SECTION III.

Of the Solution of Plain Triangles.

45. PROBLEM I.

In any plain triangle, ABC, if among the things given there be a ſide and its oppoſite angle, to find the reſt.

Then ſay, *As a given ſide,*	(AB)
To the ſine of its oppoſite angle ;	(C)
So is another given ſide,	(AC)
To the ſine of its oppoſite angle.	(B)

Therefore, to find an angle, begin with a ſide oppoſite to a known angle.

Alſo, *As the ſine of a given angle,*	(B)
To its oppoſite ſide ;	(AC)
So is the ſine of another given angle,	(C)
To its oppoſite ſide.	(AB)

Therefore, to find a ſide, begin with an angle oppoſite to a known ſide.

DEM. Take BD=CF=radius of the tables.

Draw DE, AH, FG, each perpendicular to BC. (II. 59)

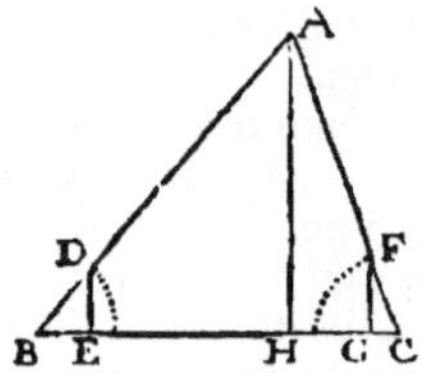

Then DE and FG are the ſines of the angles B and C. (3)

Now the triangles BDF, BAH, are ſimilar, and ſo are the triangles CFG, CAH.

Therefore BD : DE : : BA : AH. (II. 167)

And (CF=)BD : FG : : CA : AH. (II. 167)

But (BD × AH=) DE × BA=FG × CA. (II. 162)

Therefore DE : CA : : FG : BA. Or, s, ∠B : AC : : s, ∠C : BA. (II. 163)

SCHOL. Or, by circumſcribing the triangle with a circle, it will readily appear, that the half of each ſide is the ſign of its oppoſite angle. And halves have the ſame proportion as the wholes.

46. PROBLEM II.

In a right-angled plane triangle, ABC, if the two ſides containing the right angle B are known, to find the reſt.

Then, *As one of the known ſides,*	(AB)
To the radius of the tables (or tangent of 45°) ;	(AD)
So is the other known ſide,	(BC)
To the tangent of its oppoſite angle.	(DE)

DEM. Take AD=radius of the tables.

Then DE, perpendicular to AD, is the tangent of the angle A. (4)

And the triangles ADE, ABC, are ſimilar.

Therefore AB : AD : : BC : DE. (II. 167)

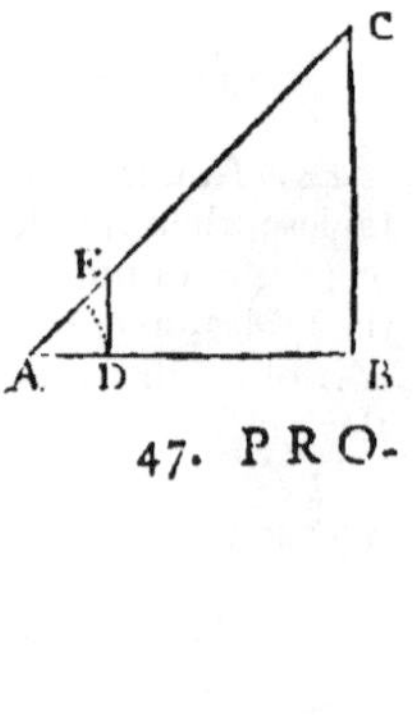

47. PRO-

47. PROBLEM III.

In any two quantities, *their half difference added to their half sum, gives the greater.*

The half diff. subtracted from the half sum, gives the less.

And if half the sum be taken from the greater, the remainder will be the half difference of those quantities.

DEM. Let AB be the greater, and BC the less, of two quantities.
Take AD = BC; then BD is their difference.
Bisect DB in E; then DE = EB, is the half diff.
And AD + DE = BC + BE (II. 47); therefore AE is the half sum.
Now AE + EB = AB, is the greater.
And AE − ED = (AD =) BC, is the less.
Also AB − AE = BE, is the half diff.

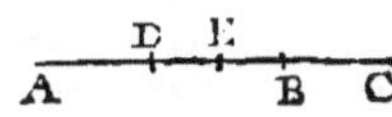

48. PROBLEM IV.

In any plane triangle, ABC; if the three things known, be two sides, AC, CB, and their contained angle C, to find the rest.

Find the sum and difference of the given sides.

Take half the given angle from 90 degrees, and there remains half the sum of the unknown angles. Then say,

As the sum of the given sides,	AC + CB
To the difference of those sides;	AC − CB
So is the tangent of half the sum of the unknown angles,	t. $\frac{1}{2}\overline{B+A}$
To the tangent of half the difference of those angles.	t. $\frac{1}{2}\overline{B-A}$

Add the half difference of the angles to the half sum, and it will give the greater angle = B.

Subtract the half difference of the angles from the half sum, and it will give lesser angle = A.

DEM. On C, with the radius CB, describe a circle, cutting AC, produced, in E and D; draw EB, and BD; also draw DF parallel to EB.
Then AE = AC + CB, is the sum of the sides.
And AD = AC − CB, is the difference of the sides.
Now ∠CDB = ∠CBD. (II. 104)
And (CDB + CBD =) 2CDB = ∠CBA + ∠A. (II. 98)

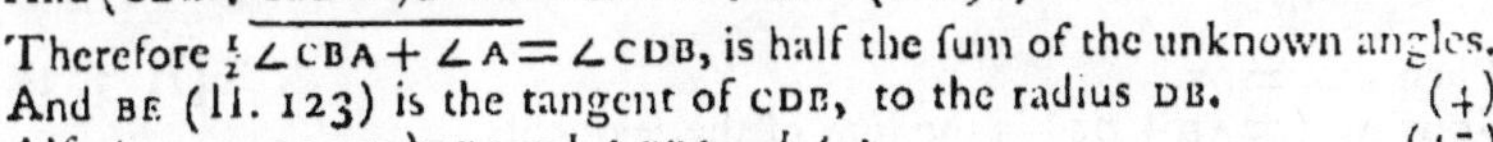

Therefore $\frac{1}{2}\overline{\angle CBA + \angle A}$ = ∠CDB, is half the sum of the unknown angles.
And BE (II. 123) is the tangent of CDB, to the radius DB. (4)
Also (CBA − CBD =) DBA = $\frac{1}{2}$∠CBA − $\frac{1}{2}$∠A (47)
Therefore $\frac{1}{2}\overline{\angle CBA - \angle A}$ = ∠DBA, is half the difference of the unknown angles.
And DF is the tangent of DBA, to the radius DB. (4)
Now the triangles AEB, ADF, are similar, DF being parallel to EB.
Therefore AE : AD : : BE : DF. (II. 167)
Or AC + CB : AC − CB : : t. $\frac{1}{2}\overline{\angle CBA + \angle A}$: t. $\frac{1}{2}\overline{\angle CBA - \angle A}$.

49 PROBLEM V.

In a plane triangle, ABC, if the three fides are known, and the angles required.

From the greateſt angle, B, *ſuppoſe a line* BD *drawn perpendicular to its oppoſite ſide, or baſe, dividing it into two ſegments,* AD, CD, *and the given triangle into two right-angled triangles,* ADB, CDB: Then ſay,

As the baſe, or ſum of the ſegments,	AC
Is to the ſum of the other two ſides;	AB + BC
So is the difference of thoſe ſides,	AB — BC
To the difference of the ſegments of the baſe.	AD — DC

Add half the difference of the ſegments to half the baſe, gives the greater ſegment AD. (47)

Subtract half the difference of the ſegments from half the baſe, there remains the leſſer ſegment DC. (47)

Then, in each of the triangles, ADB, CDB, *there will be known two ſides, and a right angle oppoſite to one of them; therefore the angles will be found by Problem* I. (45)

When two of the given ſides are equal; *then a line drawn from the included angle, perpendicular to the other ſide, biſects the ſide.* (II. 103)

And the angles being found in one of the right-angled triangles, will alſo give the angles of the other.

DEM. of the foregoing proportion.
In the triangle ABC, the line BD, perpendicular to AC, divides AC into the ſegments AD, DC.
On B with the radius BC, deſcribe a circle GCE, cutting AB, continued, in G, E; and AC in F; draw BF.

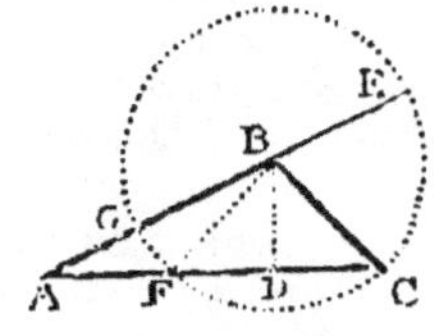

Then DC = DF. (II. 103)
Now AC (= AD + DC) is the ſum of the ſegments.
And AF (= AD — FD) is the difference of the ſegments.
Alſo AE (= AB + BC) is the ſum of the other ſides.
And AG (= AB — BC) is the difference of thoſe ſides.
But AC × AF = AE × AG. (II. 172)
Therefore AC : AE : : AG : AF. (II. 163)
Or AC : AB + BC : : AB — BC : AD — DC; or = AD — DF.

50. PRO-

In any plane triangle, ABC, the three ſides being known, to find either of the angles.

Put E *and* F *for the ſides including the angle ſought.*
G for the ſide oppoſite to that angle.
D for the difference between the ſides E *and* F.
Find half the ſum of G *and* D.
And half the difference of G *and* D.
Then write theſe four logarithms under one another, namely,
The Arithmetical complement of the logarithm of E ; (I. 88)
The Arithmetical complement of the logarithm of F ;
The logarithm of the aforeſaid half ſum of G *and* D ;
The logarithm of the aforeſaid half difference of G *and* D.
Add them together, take half their ſum ; which ſeek among the log. ſines.
And the degrees and minutes anſwering, being doubled, will give the meaſure of the angle ſought.

DEM. In the triangle, ABC, let A be the angle ſought.

Take AH = AB, draw BH ; and through K, the middle of BH, draw AP, which biſects the angle A, and is perpendicular to BH. (II. 103)

Through K draw KL, KQ, parallel, to BC, AC ; which will biſect HC, BC, in L and I ; then KL = IC, KI = LC. (II. 28, 163)

And the difference between AC and AB is HC = D ; then KI = $\frac{1}{2}$D.

From I, with the radius IK, deſcribe a circle cutting AP, BH, KQ, BC, in P, O, Q, M, N, and join CQ ; now IQ = IK = LC = LH ; therefore KQ = HC, and CQ = KH, as the triangles CQI, KHL, are congruous. (II. 99)

Therefore CQ parallel to KH (II. 28.) being produced, will meet AP at right angles (II. 53), in the point P, by the reverſe of (II. 130).

Then PQ = KO, as the triangles KQP, QOK, are congruous. (II. 95, 100)

Now BM = (BI + IM = $\frac{1}{2}$BC + $\frac{1}{2}$HC =) $\frac{1}{2}\overline{G+D}$: And BN = $\frac{1}{2}\overline{G-D}$.

Alſo BO = CP : For BK = (KH =) CQ, and KO = PQ.

Let A*r* = radius of the tables ; then *rn* (parallel to BH) = ſine of $\frac{1}{2}\angle$A. (3)

Then the triangles A*nr*, AKB, APC, are ſimilar.

And A*r* : *rn* : : AB : BK ; alſo A*r* : *rn* : : AC : (CP =) BO. (II. 167)

Therefore Ar^2 : rn^2 : : AC × AB : (BK × BO =) BM × BN. (II. 161, 172)

Or (ſq. rad. = R^2 : ſq. ſine $\frac{1}{2}\angle$A : : AC × AB : $\frac{1}{2}\overline{G+D} \times \frac{1}{2}\overline{G-D}$.

Therefore the ſquare of the ſine $\frac{1}{2}\angle A = \frac{\frac{1}{2}\overline{G+D} \times \frac{1}{2}\overline{G-D}}{AC \times AB} \times R^2$. (II. 164)

Therefore ſine $\frac{1}{2}\angle A = \sqrt{\frac{\frac{1}{2}\overline{G+D} \times \frac{1}{2}\overline{G-D}}{E \times F}}$; (II. 113)

And R, the radius of the tables, being 1,

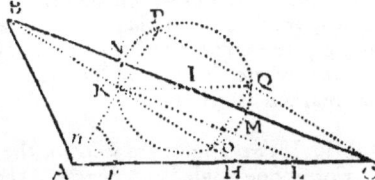

$$\text{Or Log.s,}\tfrac{1}{2}\angle A = \frac{\text{Log.}\tfrac{1}{2}\overline{G+D} + \text{Log.}\tfrac{1}{2}\overline{G-D} - \text{Log. E} - \text{Log. F}}{2}$$

$$\text{Or Log.s,}\tfrac{1}{2}\angle A = \frac{\text{l. E} + \text{l. F} + \text{L.}\tfrac{1}{2}\overline{G+D} + \text{L.}\tfrac{1}{2}\overline{G-D}}{2}$$

} 85, 86, 91 } I.

Where L. ſtands for logarithm, and l. for Arith. comp. of the logarithm.

51. Every poſſible caſe in plane Trigonometry may be readily ſolved by the preceding Problems, obſerving the following Precepts.

I. Make a rough draught of the triangle, and put the letters A, B, C, at the angles.

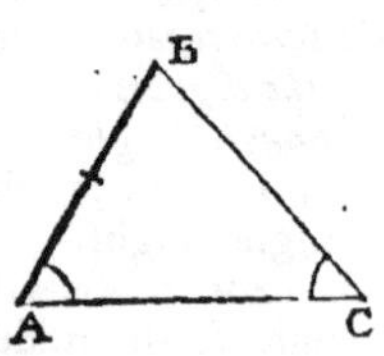

II. Let ſuch parts of this triangle be marked, as repreſent the things which are given in the queſtion. Thus, mark a given ſide with a ſcratch acroſs it; and a given angle by a little crooked line; as in the figure; where the ſide AB, and the angles A and C, are marked as given.

III. If two angles are known, the third is always known.

For if one angle is 90 degrees, the other given angle (which (II. 97) will be acute) taken from 90 degrees, leaves the third angle.

And if both the given angles are oblique; their ſum taken from 180 degrees, gives the other angle. (II. 96)

IV. Compare the given things together, and determine to which Problem the queſtion propoſed belongs.

V. Then according as the Problem directs, perform the preparatory work; and write down, under one another, in four lines, (or more if neceſſary), the *literal ſtating*; expreſſing each angle by a letter, or by three; each line by two letters; and the ſums, or differences, of lines, by proper marks.

VI. Againſt ſuch terms as are known, write their numeral value, as given in the queſtion, or as found in the preparatory work; and againſt theſe numbers write their logarithms; thoſe for the lines being found (by I. 81) in the table of the logarithms of numbers; and thoſe for the angles, found (by 41) in the table of logarithmic ſines and tangents: Obſerving that an Arithmetical complement (ſee I. 88) is always uſed in the firſt term: And that when an angle is greater than 90 degrees, its ſupplement is uſed.

VII. Add theſe logarithms together, and ſeek the ſum (I. 81) in the log. numbers, when a line is wanted; or (42) in the log. ſines or tangents, when an angle is wanted. Then the number or degree, anſwering to that logarithm which is the neareſt to the ſaid ſum, will be the thing required.

A SYNOPSIS.

Of the Rules in Plane Trigonometry.

Prob.	*Given.*	*Required.*	SOLUTION.
	All the angles and one ſide.	Either of the other ſides.	Since two angles are known, the third is known. And, As ſin. of ∠ opp. to ſide given, is to that opp. ſide; So ſin. of another angle, to its opp. ſide.
I. ſee art, 45	Two ſides and an ∠ oppoſ. to one ſide.	The angle oppoſ. to the other given ſide.	As one given ſide is to the ſine of its opp. angle; So is the other given ſide, to the ſide of its opp. angle. Then two angles being known, the third is known. And the other ſide is found as before.
II. art. 46	Two ſides and the included right ∠.	Either of the other angles.	As one of the given ſides, is to the Radius; So is the other given ſide, to the tangent of its opp. ∠ Then two ∠s being known, the third is known. The other ſide is found by opp. ſides and ∠s.
III. art. 48	Two ſides and the included oblique angle.	The other angles.	Find the ſum and diff. of the given ſides. Take ½ given ∠ from 90° leaves ½ ſum of the other ∠s. Then, As ſum ſides, is to diff. of ſides; So tan. ½ ſum other ∠s, to tan. ½ diff. thoſe ∠s. The ½ ſum ∠s $\left\{ \begin{matrix} + \\ - \end{matrix} \right\}$ ½ diff. ∠s, gives $\left\{ \begin{matrix} \text{greater } \angle. \\ \text{leſſer } \angle. \end{matrix} \right.$ Find the other ſide by opp. ſides and angles.
IV. art. 49	The three ſides.	All the angles.	Draw a line perpend. to the greateſt ſide, from the opp. ∠, dividing that ſide into two parts. Then, As the longeſt ſide is to ſum other two ſides; So is the diff. thoſe ſides, to the diff. p[ts] of longeſt. Then ½ long. ſide $\left\{ \begin{matrix} + \\ - \end{matrix} \right\}$ ½ dif. p[ts] gives the $\left\{ \begin{matrix} \text{great.} \\ \text{leſſer} \end{matrix} \right\}$ part. Now the ſaid perp. cuts the triangle into 2 right ∠d ones. In both, are known the Hyp. a Leg. and the right ∠. The angles are found by Problem I.
V. art. 50	The three ſides.	Either Angle.	Having choſe which angle to find; call the ſides including that angle E and F. The ſide opp. that ∠, call G. Put D for the difference between E and F. Find the half ſum, and half diff of G and D. Then write theſe four Logs. under one another; *Viz.* $\left\{ \begin{matrix} \text{The Ar. Co. Log. of E, The Ar. Co. Log. of F,} \\ \text{The Log. of ½ ſum, And the Log. of ½ difference.} \end{matrix} \right.$ Add the four logs. together, take half their ſum. Seek it among the log ſines; and the correſponding deg. and min. doubled, is the angle ſought.

53. **Example I.** *In the plane Triangle* ABC.

Given AB=195 Poles.
∠B= 90° 00′
∠A= 47 55.
Required the other parts.

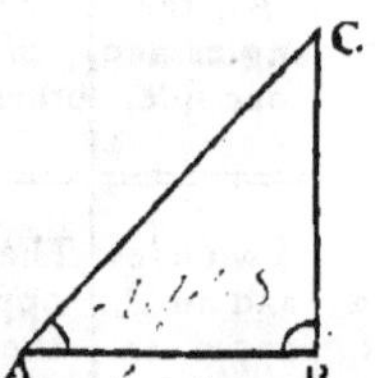

For the linear Solution.

1st. Draw AB equal to 195 poles, taken from a scale of equal parts.
2d. From B, draw BC, making with AB an angle of 90°. (II. 84)
3d. From A, draw AC, making with AB an angle of 47° 55′; and meeting BC in the point C.
Then is the triangle ABC such, the parts of which correspond with the things given; and the sides CA, CB, being applied to the scale that AB was taken from, their measures will be found, *viz.* AC=291; and BC=216.

For the numeral Solution, or Computation.

Since two angles are known; Therefore,

From	90° 00′
Take	47 55=∠A
Remains	42 05=∠C

Now in this triangle, there are known all the angles and one side; therefore among the known things, there is a side and its opposite angle; which belongs to the first problem.
Then to find the side AC, begin with the angle C opposite AB.

As the sine of ∠ C,	Or thus, As s, ∠C=42° 05′		0,17379 Ar. Co.
To the opposite side AB;	To	AB=195 po.	2,29003
So the sine of the ∠ B,	So s, ∠B=90° 00′		10,00000
To the opposite side AC.	To	AC=291 po.	2,46382

And to find the side BC, begin with the angle C opposite AB.

As the sine of the ∠ C,	Or thus, As s, ∠C=42° 05′		0,17379 Ar. Co.
To the opposite side AB;	To	AB=195 po.	2,29003
So the sine of the ∠ A,	So s, ∠A=47° 55′		9,87050
To the opposite side BC.	To	BC=216 po.	2,33432

So that AC is 291 poles, and BC is 216 poles.
The letters Ar. Co. standing on the right of the first line, signify the arithmetical complement of the log. sine of 42° 05′. (I. 88)

54. **EXAMPLE II.** *In the plane Triangle* ABC.

Given AB=117 miles.
∠B=134° 46′
∠A= 22 37.
Required the other parts.

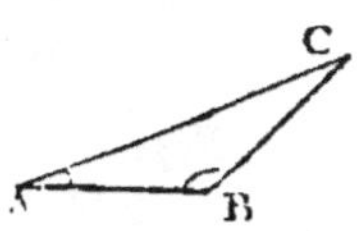

FOR THE LINEAR SOLUTION, OR CONSTRUCTION.

Make AB=117 equal parts; at A make an angle=22° 37′ (II. 84); and at B make an angle of 134° 46′; then the lines which make with AB those angles, will meet in C, and form the triangle proposed. And the measure of BC will be 117, and of AC 216.

BY COMPUTATION. See art. 45.

Since two angles are known,

Namely,		Now from		And from	
∠B=	134° 46′		180° 00′		180° 00′
∠A=	22 37	Take	157 23	Take	134 46
Their sum =	157 23	Leaves ∠C=	22 37	The sup^t ∠B=	45 14

Since the angle C=∠A
Therefore BC=AB (II. 104)

To find the side AC.

As s, ∠C=	22° 37′	0,41503	Ar. Co.
To AB=	117 M.	2,06819	
So s, ∠B=	134° 46′	9,85125	sup.
To AC=	216 M.	2,33447	

55. **EXAMPLE III.** *In the plane Triangle* ABC.

Given AB=408 yards.
∠B=22° 37′
∠A=58 07.
Required the other parts.

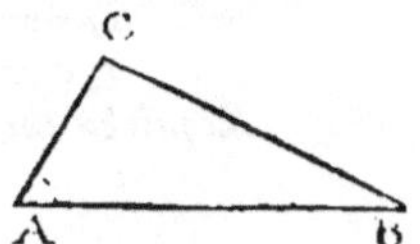

CONSTRUCTION.

Make AB=408 yards, or equal parts; make the angle A=58° 07′; and the ∠B=22° 37′; then the lines forming these angles will meet in C; and the measure of AC is 159 yards, and of BC is 351.

COMPUTATION. See art. 45.

Two angles being known, *viz*		From	
∠A=	58° 07′		180° 00′
∠B=	22 37	Take	80 44
Their sum =	80 44	Leaves	99 16=∠C.

To find the side AC.

As s, ∠C=	99° 16′	0,00570	Ar. Co.
To AB=	408 Y.	2,61066	
So, s, ∠B=	22° 37′	9,58497	
To AC=	159 Y.	2,20133	

To find the side BC.

As s, ∠C=	99° 16′	0,00570	Ar. Co.
To AB=	408 Y.	2,61066	
So s, ∠A=	58° 07′	9,92897	
To BC=	351 Y.	2,54533	

In these operations the supplement of the angle C is used.

(I 3)

56. Ex-

56. EXAMPLE IV. *In the plane Triangle* ABC.

Given AB=195 } Furlongs.
AC=291 }
∠B=90° 00′.
Required the rest.

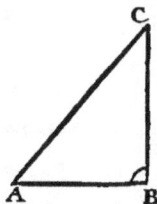

CONSTRUCTION.

Make AB=195 equal parts; draw BC, making an angle at B=90° 00′. From A with 291 equal parts cut BC in C, and draw AC.

Then the ∠A measured on the scale of chords will be about 48 degrees, and ∠C about 42°: Also BC, on the equal parts, measures about 216.

COMPUTATION.

Here being two sides, and an angle opposite to one of them, the solution falls under problem the first. See art. 45.

To find the angle C.

As	AC=291 F.	7,53611 Ar. Co.
To s, ∠B=90° 00′		10,00000
So	AB=195 F.	2,29003
To s, ∠C=42° 05′		9,82614

From	90° 00′
Take	42 05 =∠C,
Leaves	47 55=∠A.

To find the side BC.

As s, ∠B=90° 00′	10,00000
To AC=291 F.	2,46389
So s, ∠A=47° 55′	9,87050
To BC=216 F.	2,33439

Here the sine of 90° 00′ or radius being the first term, its Arith. Comp. being 0, is not taken.

57. EXAMPLE V. *In the plane Triangle* ABC.

Given AC=216 } Yards.
AB=117 }
∠C=22° 37′.
Required the rest.

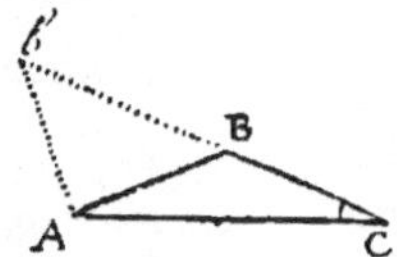

CONSTRUCTION.

Make AC=216 yards; the ∠C=22° 37′; and draw CB: Then from A, with 117 yards, cut CB in *b* or in B; and either of the triangles AC*b* or ACB will answer the conditions proposed: But the triangle to be used is generally determined by some circumstances in the question it belongs to. Thus if the angle opposite to AC is to be obtuse, the triangle is ABC.

COMPUTATION.

The solution belongs to problem the first. See art. 45.

To find the angle B

As	AB=117 Y.	7,93181
To s, ∠C=22° 37′		9,58497
So	AC=216 Y.	2,33445
To s, ∠B=134° 46′		9,85123
∠C+∠B=157 23		

From	180° 00′
Take	157 23=∠C+∠B,
Leaves	22 37∠A.

And as ∠A=∠C,
Therefore BC=AB, (II. 104)

If the angle required be obtuse, subtract the deg. and min. corresponding to the fourth log. from 180; the remainder is the ∠B For the fourth log. gives the ∠*b*, which is the supplement to the angle B. (II. 104, 96).

58. **Example VI.** *In the plane Triangle* ABC.

Given AC=408 } Fathoms.
AB=159 }
∠C=22° 37′.
Required the rest.

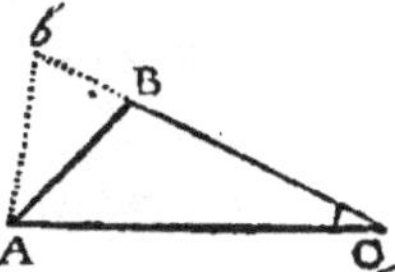

Construction.

Make AC=408 fathoms; the ∠C=22° 37′; and draw C*b*; from A, with 159 fathoms, cut C*b* in *b*, or in B, and draw A*b* or AB:
Then if the angle opposite to AC is to be acute, the triangle AC*b* is that which is required; but if the angle is to be obtuse, ACB is the triangle sought.

Computation. See art. 45.

Here being a side and its opposite angle known, the solution falls under problem the first; the ∠B is to be obtuse.

To find the angle B *obtuse.*		*To find* BC.	
As AB=159 F.	7,79860	As s,∠C=22° 37′	0,41503
To s,∠C=22° 37′	9,58497	To AB=159 F.	2,20140
So AC=408 F.	2,61066	So s,∠A=58° 04′	9,92874
To s,∠B=99° 19′	9,99423	To BC=350,9 F.	2,54517

∠C+∠B=121 56
Taken from 180 00

Leaves ∠A=58 04

59. **Example VII.** *In the plane Triangle* ABC.

Given AB=195 } Furlongs.
BC=216 }
∠B=90° 00′.
Required the rest.

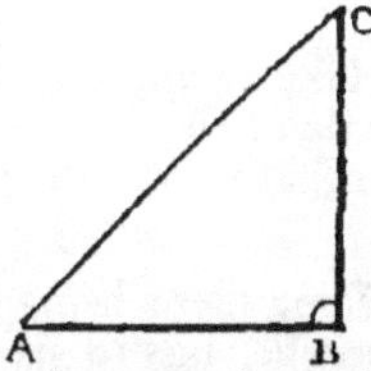

Construction.

Make the angle ABC=90°; take BA=195 equal parts, and BC=216; and draw AC; then ABC is the triangle proposed; where the parts required may be measured by the proper scales.

Computation. See art. 46.

As two sides and the contained right angle are known, the solution belongs to problem the second.

To find the angle A		*To find* AC.	
As AB=195 F.	7,70997	As s,∠A=47° 55′	0,12950
To Rad. or tang. 45° 00′	10,00000	To BC=216 F.	2,33445
So BC=216 F.	2,33445	So s, ∠B=90° 00′	10,00000
To t.∠A=47° 55′	10,04442	To AC=291 F.	2,46395

90 00

∠C= 42 05

60. Ex-

60. **Example VIII.** *In the plane Triangle* ABC.

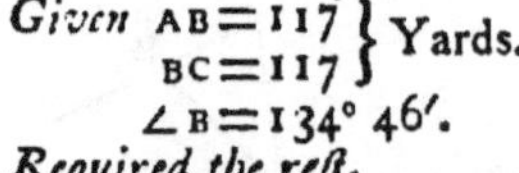

Given AB=117 } Yards.
BC=117 }
∠B=134° 46′.
Required the rest.

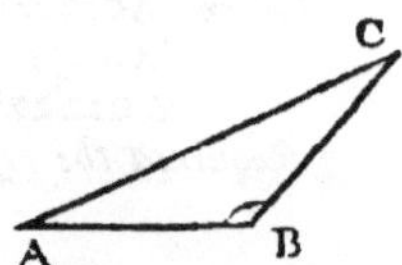

Construction.

Make the ∠ABC=134° 46′; take BA and BC, each equal to 117 equal parts, from the same scale, and draw AC; then is the triangle ABC equal to that proposed; and the parts required, measured on their proper scales, will give their values.

Computation. See art. 48.

Now as AB and BC are equal; therefore the angles A and C are also equal.

From	180° 00′	
Take	134 46	=∠B.
Leaves	45 14	=∠A+∠C.
The half	22 37	=∠A=∠C.

To find AC.

As	s,∠A=22° 37′	0,41503
To	BC=117 Y.	2,06818
So	s,∠B=134° 46′	9,85125
To	AC=216 Y.	2,33446

61. **Example IX.** *In the plane Triangle* ABC.

Given AB=408 } Yards.
AC=159 }
∠A=58° 07′.
Required the rest.

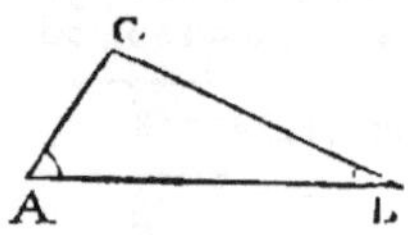

Construction.

Make an angle CAB=58° 07′; take AC=159, AB=408, from the same scale of equal parts; and draw CB; then will the triangle ACB be equal to that which was proposed.

Computation.

Here, there being two sides and their contained angle known, the solution belongs to art. 48.

AB=408
AC=159

AB+AC=567=sum of sides.

AB−AC=249=diff. of sides.

The half of	58° 07′	
Is	29 03½,	which
Taken from	90 00	
Leaves	60 56½	=½∠C+½∠B.

To find the angles.

As	AB+AC=567		7,24642
To	AB−AC=249		2,39620
So	t.½∠C+∠B=60° 56½′	(See 43)	10,25520
To	t.½∠C−∠B=38 19½		9,89781
Then (47)	99 16=∠C.		(II. 105)
And	22 37=∠B.		

To find BC.

As	s,∠C=99° 16′	0,00570
To	AB=408 Y.	2,61066
So	s,∠A=58° 07′	9,92897
To	BC=351 Y.	2,54533

62. Ex-

62. EXAMPLE X. *In the plane Triangle* ABC.

Given AB = 195
BC = 216
AC = 291
Required the angles.

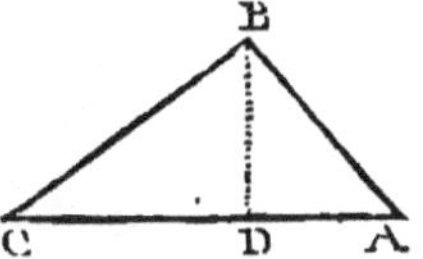

CONSTRUCTION.

Make CA = 291 equal parts; from C, with 216, describe an arc B; from A with 195 cut the arc B in B; draw BC, BA, and the triangle is constructed, then the angles may be measured by the help of a scale of chords.

COMPUTATION.

The three sides being given, the solution falls under either Problem V. or Problem VI. But that the use of these Problems may be sufficiently illustrated, the solutions according to both of them are here annexed.

Solution by Problem V. (49)

From the angle B, draw BD perpendicular to CA, which will be divided into the segments CD, DA, the sum of which AC is known.

	To find the diff. of the segments.		
Now BC = 216	As AC = 291	—	7,53611
And AB = 195	To BC + AB = 411	—	2,61384
BC + AB = 411 = sum of sides.	So BC — AB = 21	—	1,32222
BC — AB = 21 = diff. of the sides.	To CD — AD = 29,66	—	1,47217

Now the half of 291 is 145,5
And the half of 29,66 is 14,83

Therefore (47) the sum 160,33 = CD; or CD = 160,3

the difference 130,67 = AD; or AD = 130,7.

Then in the triangle CDB.			*And in the triangle* ADB.		
As BC	= 216	7,66555	As AB	= 195	7,70997
To s, ∠CDB	= 90° 00′	10,00000	To s, ∠ADB	= 90° 00′	10,00000
So CD	= 160,3	2,20493	So AD	= 130,7	2,11628
To s, ∠CBD	= 47° 55′	9,87048	To s, ∠ABD	= 42 05	9,82625
Wh. taken from	90 00		Wh. taken from	90 00	
Leaves ∠C	= 42 05		Leaves ∠A	= 47 55, & ∠B = 90° 0′.	

Solution by Problem VI. (50)

To find the angle C.		
Put E = 291 = AC	Then To Ar. Co. log. E. = 291	7,53611
F = 216 = BC	Add Ar. Co. log. F. = 216	7,66555
	And the log. $\frac{1}{2}\overline{G+D}$ = 135	2,13033
	Also the log. $\frac{1}{2}\overline{G-D}$ = 60	1,77815
D = 75 = E — F		
G = 195 = AB	The half of this sum	2)19,11014
2)270(135 = $\frac{1}{2}\overline{G+D}$	Is the log. sine of 21° 02′½ (43)	9,55507
2)120(60 = $\frac{1}{2}\overline{G-D}$.	Which doubled, gives 42° 05′ = ∠C.	

The angle C being known, the other angles may be found by Prob. I.

63. Ex-

63. EXAMPLE XI. *In the plane Triangle* ABC.

Given AC=408
BC=351
AB=159
Required the angles.

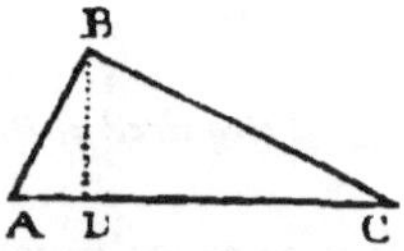

CONSTRUCTION.

The construction and mensuration is performed as in the last EXAMPLE.

COMPUTATION BY PROB. V. art. 49.

From the ∠ B draw the perpendicular BD; and find the segments AD, DC; which may be done without logarithms.

Thus BC=351 AB=159	Then (I. 46), As 408 : 510 :: 192 : 240=DC—DA. For 192×510=97920; which divided by 408 gives 240.
BC+AB=510	Now half of 408=204; and half of 240 is 120.
BC—AB=192	Then 204+120=324=DC; and 204—120=84=DA.

In the triangle ADB.		*In the triangle* BDC.	
As AB=159	7,79860	As BC=351	7,45469
To s, ∠D=90° 00′	10,00000	To s, ∠D=90° 00′	10,00000
So AD=84	1,92428	So DC=324	2,51054
To s, ∠ABD=31° 53′	9,72288	To s, ∠CBD=67° 23′	9,96523
And ∠A =58 07		And ∠C=22 37	

Then ∠ABD+∠CBD= ∠ABC=99° 16′

COMPUTATION BY PROB. VI. art. 50.

To find the angle C.

Put E=408=AC
F=351=BC

D= 57=E—F.
G=159=AB

2)216(108=$\frac{1}{2}\overline{G+D}$

2)102(51 =$\frac{1}{2}\overline{G-D}$

Then, to Ar. Co. log. E	=408	7,38934
Add Ar. Co. log. F	=351	7,45469
And the log.	$\frac{1}{2}\overline{G+D}$=108	2,03342
Also the log.	$\frac{1}{2}\overline{G-D}$= 51	1,70757
The half of this sum		2)18,58502
Is the log. sine of 11° 18′½		9,29251
Which doubled, is 22° 37′=∠C.		

Now the angle C being known, the other angles may be found by Prob. I. But for a farther illustration of Prob. VI. the work for another angle is here repeated.

To find the angle B.

Put E=351=BC
F=159=AB

D=192=E—F.
G=408=AC

2)600(300=$\frac{1}{2}\overline{G+D}$

2)216(108=$\frac{1}{2}\overline{G-D}$

Then, to Ar. Co. log. E	=351	7,45469
Add Ar. Co. log. F	=159	7,79860
And the log.	$\frac{1}{2}\overline{G+D}$=300	2,47712
Also the log.	$\frac{1}{2}\overline{G-D}$=108	2,03342
The half of this sum		2).9,76383
Is the log. sine of 49° 38′		9,88191
Which doubled, is 99° 16′=∠B.		

64. Ex-

Given AB = 117 }
BC = 117 } Miles.
AC = 216 }
Required the angles.

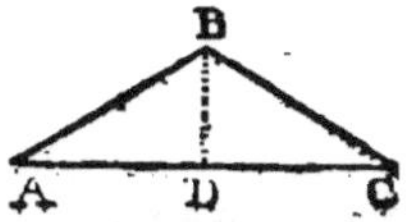

CONSTRUCTION.

The conſtruction of this triangle, and the meaſuring of the angles, is performed as in the Xth and XIth Examples.

COMPUTATION.

In the triangle ABC, as AB = BC ; therefore the angles A and C are equal (II. 104) ; and the perpendicular BD biſects the ſide AC ; ſo that the right angled triangles ADB, CDB, are congruous ; conſequently, the angles being found in one triangle, will give thoſe of the other.

Now in the triangle ADB, the ſide AB = 117 ; the ſide AD, = ½AC, is 108 ; and the ∠D is 90° 00′ : Here, therefore, being a ſide and its oppoſite angle given, the ſolution belongs to Prob. I.

To find the angle ABD.

As AB	= 117	7,93181
To s, ∠ D	= 90° 00′	10,00000
So AD	= 108	2,03342
To s, ∠ABD	= 67° 23′	9,96523
Wh. taken from	90° 00′	
Leaves	22° 37′ = ∠A = ∠C.	

And 67° 23′ doubled

Gives 134° 46′ = ∠ABC.

A like proceſs is to be uſed in every triangle, in which are two equal ſides.

The foregoing examples contain all the variety that can poſſibly happen in the ſolutions of plane triangles, conſidered only with regard to their ſides and angles ; but beſides the methods ſhewn of reſolving ſuch triangles by conſtruction and computation, there is another way to find theſe ſolutions, called Inſtrumental ; and this is of two kinds, *viz.* either by a ruler called a Sector, or by one called the Gunter's ſcale : The method by the ſector, the curious reader may ſee in many books, particularly in a treatiſe on Mathematical Inſtruments publiſhed in the year 1775, 3d edition * : But the other method by the Gunter's ſcale being in great uſe at ſea, it will be proper in this place to treat of it.

* By the author of theſe Elements.

SECTION IV.

Description and Construction of the Gunter's Scale.

65. Mr. *Edmund Gunter*, Professor of Astronomy at *Gresham* College, sometime about the year 1624, applied the Logarithms of Numbers to a flat ruler: This he effected by taking the lengths expressed by the figures in those logarithms from a scale of equal parts, and transferring them to a line, or scale, drawn on such a ruler; and this is the line which, from his name, is called the *Gunter's line:* He also, in like manner, constructed lines containing the logarithms of the sines and tangents; and since his time there have been contrived other logarithmic scales adapted to various purposes.

The Gunter's scale is a ruler, commonly two feet long; having on one of its flat sides several lines or logarithmic scales; and on the other side various other scales; which, to distinguish them from the former, may be called natural scales.

While the reader is perusing what follows, it is proper he should have a Gunter's scale before him.

66. *Of the Natural Scales.*

The half of one side is filled with different scales of equal parts, for the convenience of constructing a larger, or smaller figure: The other half contains scales of Rhumbs, marked Rhu; Chords, marked Ch; Sines, marked Sin; Tangents, marked Tan; Secants, marked Sec; Semi-tangents, denoted by S. T. and Longitude distinguished by M. L. The descriptions and uses of these scales will be considered hereafter, in the places where they will be wanted.

67. *Of the Logarithmic Scales.*

On the other side of the scale are the following lines.

I. A line marked S. R. (sine rhumbs), which contains the logarithmic sines of the degrees to each point and quarter point of the compass.

II. A line signed T. R. (tan. rhumbs), the divisions of which correspond to the logarithmic tangents of the said points and quarters.

III. A line marked Num. (numbers), where the logarithms of numbers are laid down.

IV. A line marked Sin. containing the log. sines.

V. A line of log. versed sines, marked V. S.

VI. A line of log. tangents, marked Tan.

VII. A meridional line signed Mer.

VIII. A line of equal parts, marked E. P.

The whole length of this line, or ſcale, is divided into two equal ſpaces, or intervals: the beginning, or left-hand end of the firſt, is marked 1; the end of the firſt interval, and beginning of the ſecond, is alſo marked 1; and the end of the ſecond interval, or end of the ſcale, is marked with 10; Both theſe diſtances are alike divided, beginning at the left-hand ends, by laying down in each the lengths of the logarithms of the numbers 20, 30, 40, 50, 60, 70, 80, 90; taken from a ſcale of equal parts, ſuch that 10 of its primary diviſions make the length of one interval: And the intermediate diviſions are found, by taking the logarithms of like intermediate numbers.

From this conſtruction it is evident, that when the firſt 1 ſtands for 1, the ſecond 1 ſtands for 10, and the end 10 denotes 100;

And if the firſt 1 is called	the 2d 1 ſtands for	And the 10 at the end ſtands for
10,	100,	1000;
100,	1000,	10000;
&c.	*&c.*	*&c.*;
$\frac{1}{10}$,	1,	10;
$\frac{1}{100}$,	$\frac{1}{10}$,	1;
&c.	*&c.*	*&c.*;

And the primary and intermediate diviſions in each interval muſt be eſtimated according to the values ſet on their extremities, *viz.* at the beginning, middle, and end of the ſcale.

Now the examples moſt proper to be worked by this ſcale, are ſuch where the numbers concerned do not exceed 1000, and then the firſt 1 ſtands for 10, the middle 1 for 100, and the 10 at the end for 1000: The primary diviſions in the firſt interval, *viz.* 2, 3, 4, 5, 6, 7, 8, 9, ſtands for 20, 30, 40, 50, 60, 70, 80, 90, and the intermediate diviſions ſtand for units. In the ſecond interval, the primary diviſions ſigned 2, 3, 4, 5, 6, 7, 8, 9, ſtand for 200, 300, 400, 500, 600, 700, 800, 900; each of theſe diviſions are alſo divided into ten parts, which repreſent the intermediate tens. Between 100 and 200 the diviſions for tens are each ſubdivided into five parts; ſo that each of theſe leſſer diviſons ſtand for two units. The tens between 200 and 500 are divided into two parts, each ſtanding for five units: The units between the tens from 500 to 1000 are to be eſtimated by the eye; which by a little practice is readily done.

From this deſcription it will be eaſy to find the diviſion repreſenting a given number not exceeding 1000: Thus the number 62 is the ſecond ſmall diviſion from the 6, between the 6 and 7 in the firſt interval: The number 435 is thus reckoned; from the 4 in the ſecond interval, count towards the 5 on the right, three of the larger diviſions, and one of the ſmaller; and that will be the diviſion expreſſing 435. And the like of other numbers.

69. II. *For the Line of Sines.*

This ſcale terminates at 90 degrees, juſt againſt the 10 at the end of the line of numbers; and from this termination the degrees are laid backwards, or from thence towards the left: Now ſeeking in a table of logarithmic ſines, for the numbers expreſſing their arithmetic complements, without the index, take thoſe numbers from the ſcale of equal parts the logs. the numbers were taken from, and apply them to the ſcale of ſines from 90°, and they will give the ſeveral diviſions of this ſcale.

Thus the arith. comp. of the log. ſines (or the co-ſecants) abating the index, of 10°, 20°, 30°, 40°, &c. are the numbers 76033, 46595, 3010, 19193, &c. then the equal parts to thoſe numbers, laid from 90°, will give the diviſions for 10°, 20°, 30°, 40°, &c. and the like for the intermediate degrees.

Proceeding in this manner, the arith. comp. of the ſine of 5° 45′ will be about equal to 10 of the primary diviſions of the ſcale of equal parts, or to one interval in the log. ſcale; ſo that a decreaſe of the index by unity, anſwers to one interval; then a decreaſe of the index by 2 anſwers to two intervals, or the whole length of the log. ſcale; and this happens about the ſine of 35 min. and the diviſions anſwering to the ſine of a little above 3 min. *viz.* 3′ 26″. will be equal to 3 intervals; and the ſine of about 26″ will be 4 intervals, &c. ſo that the ſine of 90° being fixed, the beginning of the ſcale is vaſtly diſtant from it.

It is uſual to inſert the diviſions to every 5 minutes, as far as 10 degrees; from 10° to 30°, the ſmall diviſions are of 15 minutes each; from 30° to 50°, contains every half degree; from 50° to 70°, are only whole degrees; the reſt are eaſily reckoned.

70. III. *For the Line of Tangents.*

As the tangent of 45 degrees is equal to the radius, or ſine of 90°; therefore 45° on this ſcale, is terminated directly oppoſite to 90 on the ſines; and the ſeveral diviſions of this ſcale of log. tangents are conſtructed in the ſame manner as thoſe of the ſines, by applying their arith. comp. backwards from 45°, or towards the left-hand.

The degrees above 45, are to be counted backwards on the ſcale: Thus the diviſion at 40° repreſents both 40° and 50°; the diviſion 30 ſerves for 30° and 60°; and the like of the other diviſions, and their intermediates.

71. IV. *For the Line of Verſed Sines.*

This line begins at the termination of the numbers, ſines, and tangents: But as the numbers on thoſe lines deſcend from the right to the left, ſo theſe aſcend in the ſame direction: Now having a table of logarithmic verſed ſines to 180 degrees, let each log. verſed ſine be ſubtracted from that of 180 degrees; then the remainders being ſucceſſively taken from the ſaid ſcale of equal parts, and laid on the ruler backwards from the common termination, the ſeveral diviſions of this ſcale will be obtained.

The

The numbers for each 10 deg. are in the following table.

D.	Numb.	D.	Numb.	D.	Numb.	Deg.	Numb.	Deg.	Numb.	Deg.	Numb.
10	0,0033	40	0,0540	70	0,1733	100	0,3839	130	0,7481	160	1,5207
20	0,0133	50	0,0854	80	0,2315	110	0,4828	140	0,9319	170	2,2194
30	0,0301	60	0,1219	90	0,3010	120	0,6021	150	1,1740	180	10,3010

The other scales will be described in their proper places.

72. *Demonstration of the foregoing constructions.*

That of the log. numbers, is evident from the nature of logarithms.

For the Sines and Tangents.

Now co-sine : rad. : : rad. : secant (34). Then co-s. × secant = 1 II. 162
sine : rad. : : rad. : co-sec. (35). sine × co-sec. = 1
tan. : rad. : : rad. : co-tan. (36). tan. × co-tan. = 1

The radius of the tables being supposed equal to 1.

Hence it is evident, that in either case, one of the quantities will be equal to the quotient of unity divided by the other.

But division is performed by subtraction with logarithms.

And to subtract a log. is the same as to add its arith. comp.

Consequently, the logarithmic co-sine and secant of the same degrees are the arithmetical complements of one another.

And so are the logarithmic sines and co-secants: Also the logarithmic tangents and co-tangents are the arith. comp. of one another.

73. Now as the arith. comp. of any number is what that number wants of unity in the next superior place;

Therefore every natural sine and its arith. comp. together make the radius.

And the sines begin at one end of a radius, and end in 90° at the other end.

Therefore in a scale of sines, the arith. comp. of any sine, or its co-secant, laid backwards from 90°, gives the division for that sine. And the like must happen in a scale of log. sines.

74. Also, as the logarithmic tangents and co-tangents are the arith. comp. of one another; therefore in a scale of log. tangents, the divisions to the degrees both under and above 45, are equally distant from the division of 45°.

Consequently the divisions serving to the degrees under 45, will serve, by reckoning backwards, for those above 45.

75. *For the Versed Sines.*

Although the numbers in the line of versed sines ascend from right to left, yet they are only the supplements of the real versed sines, which are numbered in the same order as the sines, that is, from left to right: But as the beginning of the versed sines falls without the *ruler*, therefore it is most convenient to lay down the divisions from the point where the versed sines terminate at 180 degrees, that is, against 90° on the sines.

Now it is evident that the divisions laid off from this termination must be the differences between the log. versed sines of the several degrees, &c. and that of 180 degrees.

SECTION V.

The use of the Gunter's Scale in Plane Trigonometry.

76. When a Trigonometrical Question is to be solved by the Gunter's scale, it must first be stated by the precepts to that problem under which the question falls, whether it be by opposite sides and angles, or by two sides and their included angle, or by three sides.

77. In all proportions wrought by the Gunter's scale, when the first and second terms are of the same kind, then

The extent from the first term to the second will reach from the third term to the fourth.

Or, when the first and third terms are of the same kind.

The extent from the first term to the third will reach from the second term to the fourth.

That is, set one point of the compasses on the division expressing the first term, and extend the other point to the division expressing the second (or third) term; then, without altering the opening of the compasses, set one point on the division representing the third term (or second term), and the other point will fall on the division shewing the fourth term or answer.

In working by these directions, it is proper to observe,

78. First. The extent from one side to another side, is to be taken from the scale of numbers; and the extent from one angle to another is to be taken from the scale of sines, in working by opposite sides and angles; or from the scale of tangents, in working by two sides and the included angle.

Secondly. When the extent from the first term to the second (or third) is decreasing, or is from the right to the left, then the extent from the third term (or second) must be also decreasing; that is, applied from the right towards the left: And the like caution is necessary when the extent is from the left towards the right.

These precepts being carefully attended to, what follows will be readily understood.

79. In EXAMPLE I. See article 53.

As s,∠C : AB : : s,∠B : AC. Or s,42° 05′ : 195 : : s, 90° 00′ : Q, where Q stands for the number sought.

Now the extent from 42° 05′ to 90° 00′, taken on a scale of sines, and applied to the scale of numbers, will reach from 195 to 291. See art 69.

Also. As s,∠C : AB : : s,∠A : BC. Or s, 42° 05′ : 195 : : s,47° 55′ : Q.

Then the extent from 42° 05′ to 47° 55′ on the sines, being applied to the numbers, will reach from 195 to 216. See art. 68.

In each of these operations, the first extent was from the left to the right, or increasing; therefore the second extent must be from left to right also.

80. In EXAMPLE IV. See art. 56.

As AC : s,∠B : : AB : s,∠C. Or 291 : s,90° 00′ : : 195 : Q.

Here the extent from 291 to 195, taken on the numbers, and applied to the sines, will reach from 90° 00′ to 42° 05′.

The first extent being from the right towards the left, or decreasing; therefore the second extent must be also from the right to the left.

In EXAMPLE VII. See art. 59.

As AB : Rad. : : BC : t,∠A. Or 195 : t, 45° 00′ : : 216 : Q.

Then the extent from 195 to 216 on the numbers, will reach from 45° 00′ to 47° 55′ on the tangents.

Here the first extent being from left to right, or increasing, therefore the second extent must also be increasing: Now on the tangents, this increase above 45° does not proceed from left to right, but from right to left, the same way that the decrease proceeds (70); consequently the division which the point falls on for the fourth term, must be estimated according as the first extent is increasing or decreasing.

Thus had the proportion been,

As BC : Rad. : : AB : t,∠C. Or, 216 : t,45° 00′ : : 195 : Q.

Then the extent from 216 to 195 on the numbers, will reach from 45° 00′ to 42° 05′, estimated as decreasing.

81. When two sides and the included angle are given, and the tangent of half the difference of the unknown angles is required.

Then, on the line of numbers take the extent from the sum of the given sides to their difference; and on the line of tangents apply this extent from 45° downwards, or to the left; let the point of the compasses rest where it falls, and bring the other point (from 45°) to the division answering to the half sum of the unknown angles; then this extent applied from 45° downwards, will give the half difference of the unknown angles: Whence the angles may be found. (47)

In EXAMPLE IX. See the art. 61.

As AB + AC : AB — AC : : t, $\frac{1}{2}\overline{\angle C + \angle B}$: t, $\frac{1}{2}\overline{\angle C - \angle B}$.
Or 567 : 249 : : t, 60° 56′ : Q.

Now the extent from 567 to 249 on the numbers, being applied to the tangents, will reach from 45° to about 23° 40′: Let one point of the compasses rest on this division, and bring the other to 60° 56′; then this extent will reach from 45° to 38° 19′, the half difference sought.

And this method will always give the half difference, whether the half sum of the angles is greater or less than 45°.

82. But when the half sum and half difference are greater than 45°; then the extent from the sum of the sides to their difference on the scale of numbers, will (on the tangents) reach from the half sum of the angles to their half difference, reckoning from left to right.

And when the half sum and half difference are both less than 45; then the extent from the sum of the sides to their difference, taken from the numbers and applied to the tangents, will reach from the half sum of the angles downwards to their half difference.

83. When the three sides are given to find an angle, and a perpendicular is drawn from an angle to its opposite side. See Ex. X. art. 62.

As AC : BC + AB : : BC — AB : CD — AD.
Or 291 : 411 : : 21 : Q.

Now the extent from 291 to 411 on the scale of numbers, will reach from 21 to 29,6 on the numbers also.

Then the extent for the angles is performed in the same manner as shewn in Ex. I. (78)

84. Or an angle may be found by Problem VI. as follows.

In the scale of numbers, take the extent from the half sum (of G and D) to either of the containing sides (as E); apply this extent from the other containing side (as F), to a fourth term: Let one point of the compasses rest on this fourth term, and extend the other to the half difference (of G and D); then this extent applied to the versed sines from the beginning, will give the supplement of the angle sought.

In EXAMPLE X. See art. 62.

E = 291; F = 216; half sum = 135; half diff. = 60.

Then on the numbers, the extent from 135 to 291, will reach from 216 to 465; let the point rest there, and extend the other to 60; then this extent applied to the versed sines, will reach from the beginning to 137° 56′; which taken from 180°, leaves 42° 04′ for the angle sought.

85. In

85. In Example XI. See art. 63.

Here E=408; F=351; half ſum of G and D=108; half diff.=51. Then on the numbers, the extent from 108 to 408, will reach from 351 in the ſecond interval, to a fourth number: But as the point of the compaſſes falls beyond the end of the ſcale, therefore let the extent from 108 to 408 be applied in the firſt interval, which will reach from 35,1 to 132,6; let one point reſt on 132,6, and extend the other point of the compaſſes to 51. Now as this extent of the compaſſes is leſs than it ought to be, by one interval, or half the length of the ſcale of numbers; therefore the laſt extent, when applied to the verſed ſines, muſt be from that diviſion, on the verſed ſines, oppoſite to the middle of the ſcale of numbers, which is nearly at 143°; and it will reach from thence to the verſed ſine of 157° 23′; which taken from 180°, leaves 22° 37′ for the angle ſought.

86. Moſt of the writers on Plane Trigonometry treat of right angled, and of oblique angled triangles ſeparately; making ſeven caſes in the former, and ſix caſes in the latter: But as every one of theſe thirteen caſes fall under one or other of the foregoing Problems, therefore ſuch diſtinctions are here avoided, it being conceived, that they rather tend to perplex than inſtruct a learner: Alſo in the generality of the treatiſes on this ſubject, it is uſually ſhewn how the ſolutions of right angled triangles are performed, by making (as it is called) each ſide radius; that is, by comparing each ſide of the triangle with the radius of the tables: And although theſe conſiderations are here omitted, yet the inquiſitive reader will find them in Book VII. near the beginning.

87. Beſide the demonſtration of Problem IV. at art. 48. it has been thought proper to give another demonſtration; becauſe there ariſes from it a Theorem uſeful on ſome occaſions: Moreover, there is alſo added methods of deriving other rules for the ſolution of the caſe where the three ſides are given to find an angle; which, if they ſhould be found of no other uſe, will perhaps be agreeable exerciſes of Geometry to thoſe who are delighted with theſe ſtudies.

SECTION

SECTION VI.

Properties of Plane Triangles.

88. In any plane triangle ABC,
Given CA, CB, and ∠C.
Required the angles B and A.

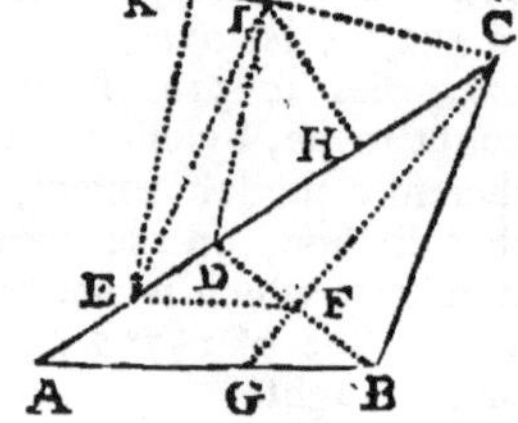

SOLUTION. Take CD=CB, and draw DB. Bisect DB in F, DA in E, draw CFG, and EF, which is parallel to AB. (II. 165)
Now DE or AE is equal to half the difference of CA and CB.
And CE (=CA—AE) is equal to the half sum of CA and CB. (47)

The sum of the equal angles CBD, CDB (II. 104) is equal to the sum of the unknown angles CBA, CAB. (II. 98)

Then the angle CBD is the half sum, and the angle ABD is the half difference of the unknown angles CBA, CAB. (47)
And as CFG is at right angles to DB (II. 103); CF is the tangent of ∠CBD, and GF is the tangent of ∠ABF to the rad. BF. (4)
Then CE : EA : : CF : GF (II. 165) : Or 2CE : 2EA : : CF : FG. (II. 151)

That is, CA+CB : CA—CB : : tan. $\frac{1}{2}$∠$\overline{\text{CBA+CAB}}$: tan. $\frac{1}{2}$∠$\overline{\text{CBA—CAB}}$.

89. AGAIN. From H, the middle of CD, draw HI at right angles, and equal to CH; draw DI, and EK parallel to DI, meeting CI produced in K; and join IE.
Now HE=($\frac{1}{2}$CD+$\frac{1}{2}$DA)$\frac{1}{2}$CA; and CH=$\frac{1}{2}$CB.
And HE=tangent of the angle HIE to the radius, HI=HC.
Then CB : CA : : (2HC : 2HE : : HC : HE : :) Radius : tan. ∠HIE.
And ∠HIE— (∠HID=) 45°=∠DIE=∠KEI (II. 95) is known.

Then rad. : tan. ∠KEI : : EK : KI : : CK : KI; because ∠KCE=∠KEC.
But : : CK : KI : : CE : ED. (II. 166)
: : 2CE : 2ED. (I. 151)
: : CA+CB : CA—CB : : *t*, $\frac{1}{2}$ sum ∠*s* : *t*, $\frac{1}{2}$ diff. ∠*s* (48)

Consequently rad. : tan. ∠KEI : : tan. $\frac{1}{2}$∠$\overline{\text{CBA+CAB}}$: tan. $\frac{1}{2}$∠$\overline{\text{CBA—CAB}}$.

This rule is often useful in Astronomical calculations, when the logarithms of the sides AB, BC are only known, and the angles BAC, BCA, are required, without finding, from those logarithms, the sides themselves.

For the difference between the logarithms of the sides, increased by radius, gives the tangent of an arc; which arc lessened by 45° leaves a second arc.

Then as rad. : tan. second arc : : tan. $\frac{1}{2}$ sum ∠*s* : tan. $\frac{1}{2}$ diff. ∠*s*.

90. In

90. In any plane triangle ABC, where the three ſides are known, the meaſure of either angle (as the angle A, included between the ſides AB, AC) may be found ſeveral ways, as ſhewn in the following articles.

The letters s, t, v, ſtand for ſine, tangent, verſed ſine.
s', t', ſtand for co-ſine, co-tangent.
v', ſtands for the verſed ſine of the ſupplement.
Alſo ss, tt, ſtand for the ſquares of the ſine and tangent.
Alſo $s's'$, $t't'$, ſtand for the ſquares of the co-ſine and co-tangent.
Radius $= R = AB = AE = AD$; and $H = \frac{1}{2}AB + \frac{1}{2}AC + \frac{1}{2}BC$.

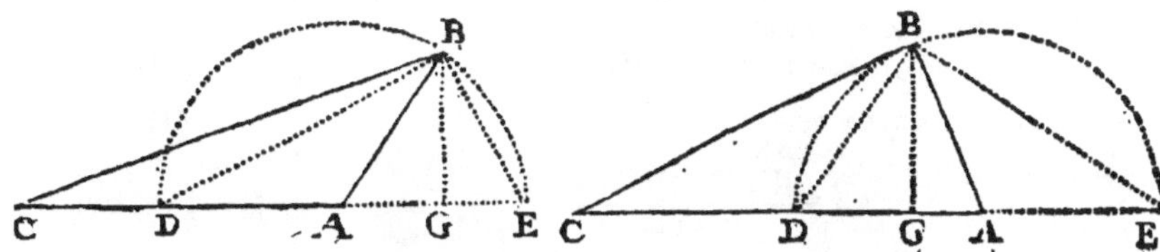

91. $s,\frac{1}{2}\angle A = R \times \sqrt{\frac{\overline{H-AC} \times \overline{H-BC}}{AC \times AB}}$. Here $\angle E = \frac{1}{2}\angle A$.

For $R : s, \frac{1}{2}\angle A :: (DE=)2AB : BD$. (45)
And $RR : ss, \frac{1}{2}\angle A :: 4AB^2 : BD^2$. (II. 161)

Now $ss,\frac{1}{2}\angle A = RR \times \frac{BD^2}{4AB^2}$. (II. 164)

$= \frac{2AB}{4AB^2} \times \frac{\overline{2H-2AC} \times \overline{2H-2BC}}{2AC} \times RR$. (II. 179)

Then $s, \frac{1}{2}\angle A = R \times \sqrt{\frac{\overline{H-AC} \times \overline{H-AB}}{AC \times AB}}$.

92. $s,\angle A = \frac{2R}{AB \times AC} \times \sqrt{H \times \overline{H-CB} \times \overline{H-AC} \times \overline{H-AB}}$.

For $AB : BG :: R : s,\angle A$. (45)
And $AB^2 : BG^2 :: RR : ss, \angle A$. (II. 161)

Now $ss, \angle A = \frac{RR}{AB^2} \times BG^2$. (II. 164)

$= \frac{RR}{AB^2} \times \frac{4}{AC^2} \times H \times \overline{H-CB} \times \overline{H-AC} \times \overline{H-AB}$. (II. 180)

93. $s',\frac{1}{2}\angle A = R \times \sqrt{\frac{H \times \overline{H-CB}}{AC \times AB}}$. Here $\angle E = \frac{1}{2}\angle A$; and $\angle D =$ comp. $\angle E$.

For $R : s', \frac{1}{2}\angle A :: (DE=)\ 2AB : BE$. (45)
And $RR : s's', \frac{1}{2}\angle A :: 4AB^2 : BE^2$. (II. 161)

Now $s's', \frac{1}{2}\angle A = RR \times \frac{BE^2}{4AB^2}$. (II. 164)

$= RR \times \frac{2AB \times 4 \times H \times \overline{H-CB}}{4AB^2 \times 2AC}$. (II. 178)

94. $t,\frac{1}{2}$

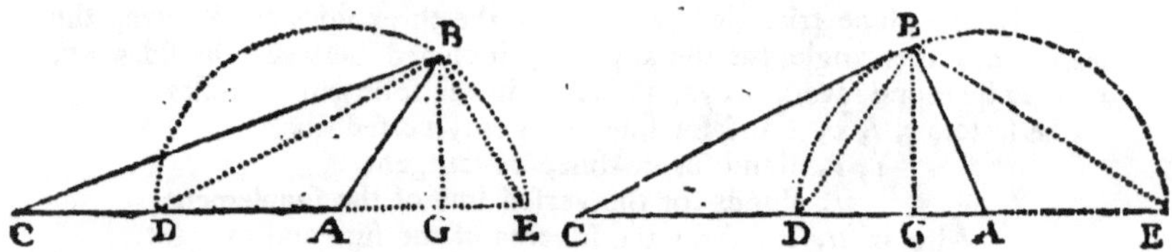

94. $t, \frac{1}{2}\angle A = R \times \frac{\sqrt{\overline{H-AC} \times \overline{H-AB}}}{H \times \overline{H-CB}}$.

For $R : t, \frac{1}{2}\angle A :: BE : BD$. (46)

And $RR : tt, \frac{1}{2}\angle A :: BE^2 : BD^2$. (II. 161)

Now $tt, \frac{1}{2}\angle A = RR \times \frac{BD^2}{BE^2}$. (II. 164)

$= RR \times \frac{\overline{H-AC} \times \overline{H-AB}}{H \times \overline{H-BC}}$. (II. 178, 179)

95. $t', \frac{1}{2}\angle A = R \times \sqrt{\frac{H \times \overline{H-CB}}{\overline{H-AC} \times \overline{H-AB}}}$.

For $BD^2 : BE^2 :: (tt, \frac{1}{2}\angle A : RR ::)\ RR : t't', \frac{1}{2}\angle A$. (36)

Then $t't', \frac{1}{2}\angle A = RR \times \frac{BE^2}{BD^2}$. (II. 178, 179)

96. $v, \angle A = 2R \times \frac{\overline{H-AC} \times \overline{H-AB}}{AC \times AB}$.

For $R : v, \angle A :: AB : GD$. (45)

Then $v, \angle A = R \times \frac{GB}{AB} = R \times \frac{2 \times \overline{H-AC} \times \overline{H-AB}}{AC \times AB}$ (II. 177)

97. $v' \angle A = 2R \times \frac{H \times \overline{H-CB}}{AC \times AB}$.

For $R : v', A :: AB : GE$. (45)

Then $v', \angle A = R \times \frac{GE}{AB} = R \times \frac{2 \times H \times \overline{H-CB}}{AC \times AB}$. (II. 176)

98. $s' \angle A = \frac{1}{2} R \times \frac{CB^2 - AC^2 - AB^2}{AC \times AB}$

For $R : s', \angle A :: AB : AG$. (45)

Then $s', \angle A = R \times \frac{AG}{AB} = R \times \frac{BC^2 - AC^2 - AB^2}{2AC \times AB}$. (II. 174)

END OF BOOK III.

THE

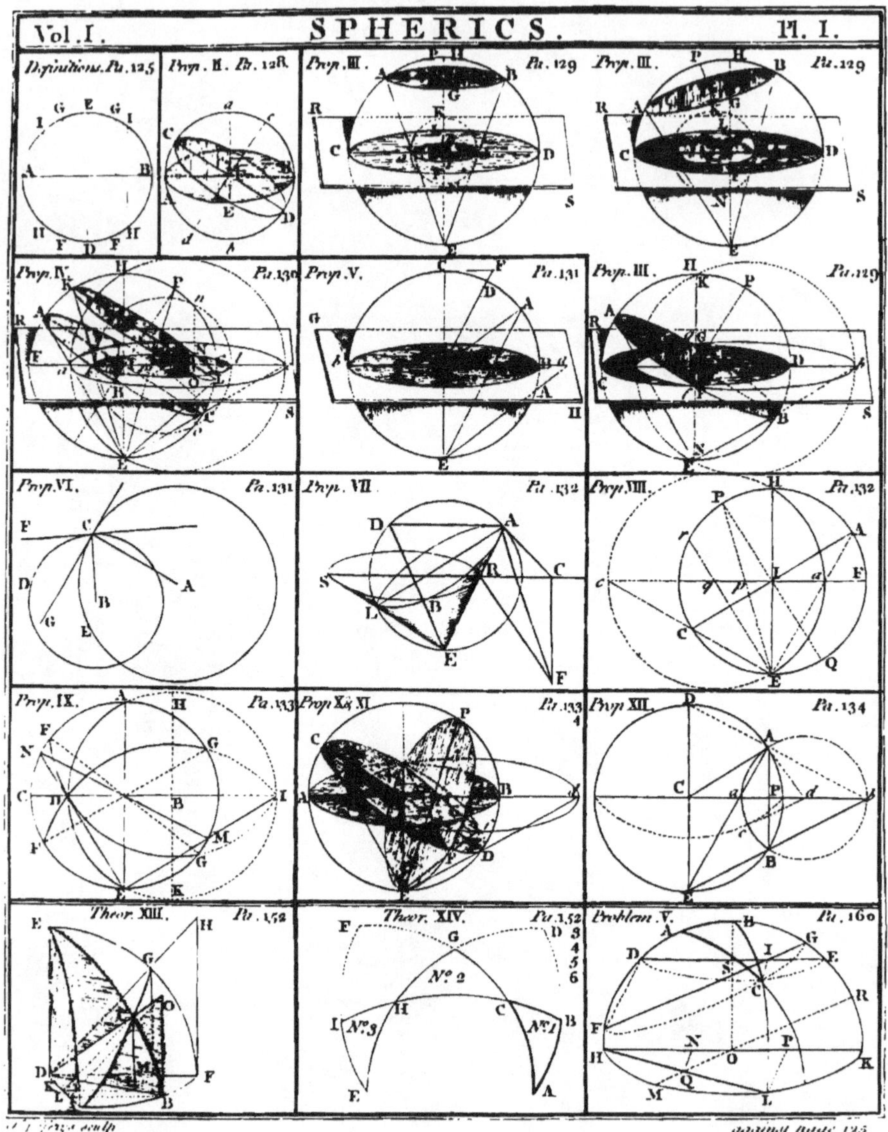
Vol. I.
SPHERICS.
Pl. I.
Definitions. Pa. 125
Prop. II. Pa. 128
Prop. III. Pa. 129
Prop. III. Pa. 129
Prop. IV. Pa. 130
Prop. V. Pa. 131
Prop. III. Pa. 129
Prop. VI. Pa. 131
Prop. VII. Pa. 132
Prop. VIII. Pa. 132
Prop. IX. Pa. 133
Prop. X & XI Pa. 133
Prop. XII. Pa. 134
Theor. XIII. Pa. 152
Theor. XIV. Pa. 152
Problem. V. Pa. 160
opposite page 125

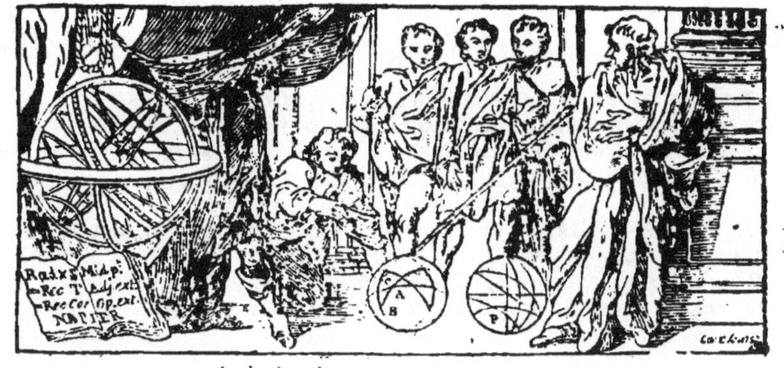

THE

ELEMENTS

OF

NAVIGATION.

BOOK IV.

OF SPHERICS.

SECTION I.

Definitions and *Principles.*

1. SPHERICS is that part of the Mathematics which treats of the poſition and magnitude of arcs of circles deſcribed on the ſurface of a ſphere.

2. A SPHERE is a ſolid contained under one uniform round ſurface, ſuch as would be formed by the revolution of a circle about its diameter, that diameter being immoveable during the motion of the circle.

Thus the circle AEBD *revolving about the diameter* AB, *will generate a ſphere, the ſurface of which will be formed by the circumference* AEBD. See Plate I.

3. The CENTER and AXIS of a ſphere are the ſame as the center and diameter of a generating circle: And as a circle has an indefinite number of diameters, ſo a ſphere may be conſidered as having alſo an indefinite number of axes, round any one of which the ſphere may be conceived to be generated.

4. CIRCLES OF THE SPHERE are thoſe circles deſcribed on its ſurface by the motion of the extremities of ſuch chords in the generating circle as are at right angles to the diameter, or to the axis of the ſphere.

Thus by the motion of the circle AEBD *about the diameter* AB, *the extremities of the chords* ED, GF, IH, *at right angles to* AB, *will deſcribe circles the diameters of which are equal to thoſe chords reſpectively.* Plate I.

5. The

5. The POLES of a circle on the sphere, are those points on its surface equally distant from the circumference of that circle.

Thus A *and* B *are the poles of the circles described on the sphere by the ends of the chords* ED, GF, IH. Plate I.

6. A GREAT CIRCLE of the sphere, is that circle which is equally distant from both its poles.

Thus the circle described by the extremities E, D, *of the diameter* ED, *at right angles to* AB, *being equally distant from its poles* A *and* B, *is called a great circle.*

7. LESSER CIRCLES of the sphere, or small circles, are those circles which are unequally distant from both their poles.

Thus the circles of which FG, HI, *are diameters, having their poles* A *and* B *unequally distant from them, are called lesser circles.*

8. PARALLEL CIRCLES of the sphere, are those circles, the planes of which are considered as parallel to the plane of some great circle.

Thus the circles having the diameters FG, HI, *are called parallel circles in respect of the great circle of which* ED *is the diameter.*

9. A SPHERIC ANGLE is the inclination of two great circles of the sphere meeting one another.

10. A SPHERIC TRIANGLE is a figure formed on the surface of a sphere by the mutual intersections of three great circles.

11. The STEREOGRAPHIC PROJECTION of the sphere, is such a representation of its circles, upon the plane of one of them passing through the center, and called the PLANE OF PROJECTION, as would appear to an eye placed in one of the poles of that great circle, and thence viewing the circles on the sphere.

12. The place of the Eye is called the PROJECTING POINT, or lower pole: and the point diametrically opposite is called the remotest, or opposite, or upper pole.

Also, the projection of any point on the sphere, is that point in the plane of projection, through which the visual ray passes to the eye.

13. The PRIMITIVE CIRCLE is that great circle, on the plane of which the representations of all the other circles are supposed to be drawn.

14. An OBLIQUE CIRCLE is one which has its plane oblique to the eye.

15. A RIGHT CIRCLE is that which is perpendicular to the plane of the primitive circle, and if it be a great circle, its plane passes through the eye, and it is seen edgewise; consequently it is represented by a straight line drawn through the center of the primitive circle.

AXIOMS.

AXIOMS.

16. The diameter of every great circle passes through the center of the sphere; but the diameters of small circles do not pass through the same center: Also the center of the sphere is the common center of all its great circles.

17. Every section of a sphere, by a plane passing though its circumference, is a circle.

18. A sphere is divided into two equal parts by the plane of every great circle; and into two unequal parts by the plane of every small circle.

19. The pole of every great circle is at 90 degrees distance from it on the surface of the sphere: And no two great circles can have a common pole.

20. The poles of a great circle are the extremities of that diameter, or axis, of the sphere, which is perpendicular to the plane of that circle.

21. Lines flowing to the projecting point, or place of the eye, from every point in the circumference of a circle which it views, form the convex surface of a Cone.

22. A plane passing through three points on the surface of a sphere, equally distant from the pole of a great circle, will be parallel to the plane of that circle.

23. The shortest distance between two points on the surface of a sphere, is the arc of a great circle passing through those points.

24. If one great circle meets another, the angles on either side are supplements to one another; and every spheric angle is less than 180 degrees.

25. A spheric angle is measured by an arc of a great circle intercepted between the legs of that angle, 90 degrees distant from the angular point.

26. If two circles intersect one another, the opposite angles are equal.

27. Two spheric triangles are congruous, if two sides and their contained angle in one, are equal to two sides and their contained angle in the other, each to each: Or if two angles and the contained side in the one, are equal to two angles and their contained side in the other, each to each: Or if the three sides in the one are respectively equal to the three sides in the other.

28. All parallel circles have the same pole, and may be conceived to be concentric to the great circle which they are parallel to.

29. All parallel circles on the sphere, having the same pole, are cut into similar arcs by two great circles passing through that pole.

SECTION

30. PROPOSITION I.

Great circles of a ſphere mutually cut one another into two equal parts.

Dem. Any two great circles have the ſame common center. (16)
And their planes interſect in a right line. (II. 209)
Now the center muſt lie in the line of their interſection.
Therefore this right line is a diameter common to both.
But every circle is biſected by its diameter.
Therefore the circles mutually biſect one another.

31. Corol. I. The circumferences of any two circles interſecting one another twice, make the angles at both ſections equal.

For the planes of thoſe circles have the ſame inclination at both ends of their interſection, or where the circumferences interſect.

32. Corol. II. Two great circles of the ſphere will cut each other twice at the diſtance of 180 degrees, or in oppoſite points of the ſphere.

33. PROP. II.

The diſtance of the poles of two great circles, is equal to the angle formed by the inclination of thoſe circles. Plate I.

Dem. Let AEB, CED, be two great circles of the ſphere, their planes paſſing through its center F; and let a, b, be the poles of the circle AEB, and c, d, the poles of the circle CED.
Then is the arc Aa=arc Cc=90°. (19)
And the arc Ca is common to both the arcs Aa and Cc.
Therefore the arc AC, meaſuring the inclination CFA of the circles, is equal to the arc ac meaſuring the diſtance of the poles. (II. 48.)

34. Corol. I. Two great circles are at right angles to one another, when they paſs through each other's poles.

35. Corol. II. The pole of a great circle is 90 degrees diſtant from it, taken in another great circle, or in an arc of it, drawn perpendicular to the former circle.

36. Corol. III. Two or more great circles, at right angles to another great circle, interſect one another 90° diſtant from it, or in the pole of the latter circle. And the like of arcs of great circles.

37. Corol. IV. If ſeveral great circles interſect one another in the pole of another great circle; then are the former circles perpendicular to the latter.

38. PROP.

38. PROP. III.

In the stereographic projection of the sphere, the representations of all circles, not passing through the projecting point, will be circles. Plate I. three figures.

Let ACEDB represent a sphere, cut by a plane RS, passing through the center I, at right angles to the diameter EH, drawn from E, the place of the eye.

And let the section of the sphere (17) by the plane RS, be the circle CFDL, its poles being H, and E.

Suppose AGB is a circle on the sphere to be projected, its pole, most remote from the eye, being P: And the visual rays from the circle AB meeting in E, form the cone AGBE (21) of which the triangle AEB is a section through the vertex E, and diameter of the base AB. (II. 204)

Then will the figure *agbf*, which is the projection of the circle BGA, be a circle.

DEMONSTRATION. Since the ∠E*ab* is measured by ½ arc AC + (½ arc ED =) ½ arc CE. (II. 137)
And the ∠EBA is measured by ½ arc AC + ½ arc CE. (II. 128)
Therefore the angle EBA = angle E*ab*. (II. 50)
And so the triangles EAB, E*ba* are similar, the ∠E being common.
Therefore *ab* cuts the sides EA and EB of the cone, in a subcontrary position to AB; and consequently the section *afbg* is a circle. (II. 213)

Now suppose the plane RS to revolve on the line CD, till it coincides with the plane of the circle ACEB;

Then it is evident, that the point L will fall in H, the point F in E, and the circle CFDL will coincide with the circle CEDH, which now becomes the primitive circle, where the point F, or E, is the projecting point: Also the projected circle *afbg* will become the circle *aNb*K.

39. COROL. I. Hence the middle of the projected diameter is the center of the projected circle, whether it be a great circle or a small one.

40. COROL. II. Hence in all circles parallel to the plane of projection, their centers and poles will fall in the center of the projection.

41. COROL. III. The centers and poles of circles, inclined to the plane of projection, fall in that diameter of the primitive circle which is at right angles to the diameter drawn through the projecting point; but at different distances from its center.

42. COROL. IV. All oblique great circles cut the primitive circle in two points diametrically opposite.

43. PROP. IV.

The measure of the angle which the projected diameter of any circle subtends at the eye, is equal to the distance of that circle from its pole, which is most remote from the projecting point, taken on the surface of the sphere. And that angle is bisected by a right line joining the projecting point and that pole. Plate I.

Let the plane RS cut the sphere HFEG, as in the last.
And let ABC be any oblique great circle, the diameter of which AC is projected into *ac*; and KOL any small circle parallel to ABC, the diameter of which KL is projected into *kl*.

The distances of those circles from the pole P, being the arcs AHP, KHP, and the angles *aEc*, *kEl*, are angles at the eye subtended by their projected diameters *ac*, *kl*.

Then is the angle *aEc* measured by the arc AHP, the angle *kEl* is measured by the arc KHP; and those angles are bisected by EP.

DEM. For arc PHA = arc PC; and arc PHK = arc PL. (5)
And the ∠ AEC is measured by $\frac{1}{2}$ arc APC = arc PHA. (II. 128)
Also the ∠ KEL is measured by $\frac{1}{2}$ arc KPL = arc PHK. (II. 128)
Therefore the angles AEC, KEL, are respectively measured by the arcs PHA, PHK.
And it is evident those angles are bisected by the line EP.

44. COROL. I. Hence as the line EP projects the pole P in *p*; so the same line refers a projected pole to its place on the sphere, in the circumference of the primitive circle.

45. COROL. II. Hence, on the plane of the primitive circle, may be described the representation of any circle whose distance from its pole, and the projected place of that pole, are given.

For PA and PC are projected into *pa* and *pc*; and the bisection of *ac* gives the center of the circle sought.

46. COROL. III. Hence every projected oblique great circle cuts the primitive circle in an angle equal to the inclination of the plane of that oblique circle to the plane of projection.

For F*a* is equivalent to FA the inclination.
And F*a* measures the angle FH*a*, since FH, H*a*, are each 90°. (9)

47. COROL. IV. The distance between the projections of a great circle and any of its parallels is equivalent to their distance on the sphere.
Thus the projection *ak* is equivalent to AK.

48. PROP. V.

Any point of a sphere stereographically projected, is distant from the center of projection, by the tangent of half the arc intercepted between that point and the pole opposite to the eye: The semidiameter of the sphere being made radius. Plate I.

Let c*b*EB be a great circle of the sphere, the center of which is *c*, GH the plane of projection cutting the diameter of the sphere in *b*, B; E, C, the poles of the section by that plane; and *a* the projection of A.
Then is *ca* equal to the tangent of half the arc AC.

DEM. Draw CF, a tangent to the arc CD=½ arc CA, and join *c*F.
Now the triangles CF*c*, *ca*E, are congruous: For C*c*=*c*E, ∠ C=∠ E*ca* =right ∠, ∠ C*c*F=*c*E*a* (II. 128): Therefore *ca*=CF.
Consequently *ca* is equal to the tangent of half the arc CA.

49. PROP. VI.

The angle made by the intersection of the circumferences of two circles in the same plane, is equal to the angle made by tangents to those circles in the point of section; and also is equal to the angle made by their radii drawn to that point. Plate I.

Let CE, CD, be two arcs of circles in the same plane cutting in the point C; AC, BC, their radii; GC, FC, tangents at the point C.
Then is the curve-lined angle ECD=∠GCF=∠ACB.

DEM. Since the radii AC, BC, are at right angles to their tangents GC, FC (II. 126); and are also at right angles to the arcs CE, CD. (II. 136)
Therefore the position of the tangents and arcs at the point C are the same; and consequently the ∠ECD=∠GCF.
Also the ∠ACB+∠BCG=(right∠=)∠FCG+∠BCG.
Therefore the angle ACB is equal to the angle FCG, by taking away the common angle BCG. (II. 48)
Consequently ∠ECD=GCF=∠ACB.

50. SCHOLIUM. If the arcs CE, CD, were in different planes, the same would hold true with regard to their tangents.

For suppose the circle CD to revolve on the fixed radius BC, still cutting the circle CE in C: Then the tangent CF revolving with it, has still the same inclination to BC: And as the inclination of the planes of the circles vary, so much will the inclination of the tangents vary.

Therefore the angle made by the tangents, in all positions of the circular planes, is the same as the angle made by their circumferences.

51. COROL. Hence if a plane touches a sphere, at the point where two circles of it intersect one another, the tangents to both circles will lie in that plane; and consequently, in all oblique positions, a right line perpendicular to one tangent will cut the other tangent.

52. PROP. VII.

The angle which any two circles make, when stereographically projected, is equal to the angle which those circles make on the sphere. Plate I.

Suppose DAEL a sphere to be projected on the plane SBRCF, and ALDE a great circle passing through the projecting point E. Let LBA be any other circle, cutting the former in L and A, under the angle BAE, which will be represented by the circle SBR, (38) as the circle ELDA is by the right line SC (15). The angle BAE is equal to the angle BRC.

From the point A draw AC, AF, to touch the circles AEL, ABS in A, and meet the plane of projection in C and F; also draw RF and CF, which will be in that plane; and, in the plane of the great circle AEL, draw AD parallel to SC, and join ED.

DEM. The angular point A is projected into R; (12) consequently AC is projected into RC, and AF into RF. And since SC is the common section of the plane of projection with that of the great circle ELDA (II. 210) the lines AC, SC, AD, ED, AE, lie all in the plane of that circle: Also because AD is parallel to SC, the ∠ARC=∠DAE=∠ADE=∠RAC (II. 94, 104, 132) consequently AC=RC (II. 104). Now the plane passing through AC and AF touches the sphere in A, (51) it is therefore perpendicular to the plane of the circle AED; and FC its common section with the plane of projection, is at right angles to that plane (II. 210); FC is therefore at right angles both to the lines AC and CR (II. 205): Hence, the triangles ACF, RCF, being right angled at C, having the side FC common, and AC=CR, are congruous (II. 99), and the ∠CAF=∠CRF. Consequently the ∠EAB=∠FAC (51) =∠FRC. Now it is manifest that as AF touches the base, ABL, of the cone EABL, in the point A, a plane passing through AF and AE will touch the side of the cone in the line AE; but AF is also in that plane (II. 198); therefore AR touches the cone in the line AE; and as AR lies also in the plane of the circle SBR, it must touch that circle also; consequently (50) BRC=∠FRC=∠FAC=∠ABE.

53. PROP. VIII.

The distance between the poles of the primitive circle and an oblique great circle, in stereographic projections, is equal to the tangent of half the inclination of those circles; and the distance of their centers is equal to the tangent of their inclination: The semidiameter of the primitive circle being made radius. Plate I.

Let AC be the diameter of a circle, the poles of which are P and Q, and inclined to the plane of projection in the angle AIF.

And let *a*, *c*, *p*, be the projections of the points A, C, P.

Also let H*a*E be the projected oblique circle, the center of which is *q*.

Now when the plane of projection becomes the primitive circle, the pole of which is I,

Then is I*p*=tangent of half ∠AIF, or of half the arc AF.

And I*q*=tangent of AF, or of the ∠FH*a*=AIF.

DEM. For AH+HP=AH+AF. Therefore HP=AF.

But I*p*=tangent of half HP, or of half AF. (48)

Again.

Again. As AC is projected in ac, then q, the middle of ac, is the center of the projected circle, and of its representative HaE. (45)
Draw Eq produced to r: Then as qa=qE; the ∠qEA=∠qaE. (II. 104)
But the ∠qaE is measured by half the arc EFA. (II. 137)
Therefore the arc AHr=arc AFE (II. 50): And as the arc AHP=FQE;
Therefore Pr=AF=HP; and HPr=twice the arc AF.
Therefore (II. 127) the ∠IEq=AIF, the inclination of the circles.
But Iq is the tangent of the ∠IEq, EI being the radius.

54. COROL. Hence the radius of an oblique circle is equal to the secant of the obliquity of that circle to the primitive.
For Eq is the secant of the angle IEq, to the radius EI.

55. PROP. IX.

If through any given point in the primitive circle an oblique circle be described; then the centers of all other oblique circles passing through that point, will be in a right line drawn through the center of the first oblique circle at right angles to a line passing through the given point, and the center of the primitive.

Let GACE be the primitive circle, ADEI a great circle described through D, its center being B.

HK is a right line drawn through B, perpendicular to a right line CI passing through D, and the center of the primitive circle.

Then the centers of all other great circles FDG passing through D will fall in the line HK.

DEM. For if E be the projecting point, the circle EDAI will be the projection of a circle, the diameter of which is NM. (38)

Therefore D and I are the projections of N, M, which are opposite points on the sphere; or of points at a semicircle's distance.

Therefore all circles passing through D and I must be the projections of great circles on the sphere.

But DI is a chord in every circle passing through the points D, I.

Consequently the centers of all those circles will be found in HK drawn perpendicularly through B, the middle of DI. (II. 125)

56. PROP. X.

Equal arcs of any two great circles of the sphere, will be intercepted between two other circles drawn on the sphere through the remotest poles of those great circles. Plate I.

Let PBEA be a sphere, on which AGB, CFD, are two great circles, the remotest poles of which are E, P; and through these poles let the great circle PBEC, and small circle PGE, be drawn, intersecting the great circles AGB, CFD, in the points B, G, and D, F.
Then are the intercepted arcs BG and DF equal to one another.

DEM. For the arcs ED+DB=arcs PB+DB; therefore ED=PB.
And the arcs EF+FG=arcs PG+FG (19); therefore EF=PG.
For the points F and G are equally distant from their poles P, E.
Also the ∠DEF=BPG; for intersecting circles make equal angles at the sections. (31)
Therefore the triangles EFD and PGB are congruous. (27)
Therefore the arc BG=arc DF.

57. PROP. XI.

If lines be drawn from the projected pole of any great circle, cutting the peripheries of the projected circle and plane of projection, the intercepted arcs of those circumferences are equal. Plate I.

On the plane of projection, AGB, let the great circle CFD be projected into *cfd*, and its pole P in *p*; moreover, draw the lines *pd*, *pf*: the arcs GB and *fd* are equal.

Since *pd* lies both in the plane AGB and APBE it is their common section. (II. 198)
But the point B is in their common section: (56)
Therefore *pd* passes through the point B.
And in this manner it may be proved that *pf* passes through G.
Now the points D and F are projected into *d* and *f*. (38)
Therefore the arc *fd* is equivalent to the arc FD.
But the arc FD is equal to the arc GB: (56)
Therefore the arc GB is equivalent to the arc *fd*. (II. 46)

58. PROP. XII.

The radius of any small circle, the plane of which is perpendicular to that of the primitive circle, is equal to the tangent of that lesser circle's distance from its pole; and the secant of that distance, is equal to the distance of the centers of the primitive and lesser circle. Plate I.

Let P be the pole, and AB the diameter of a lesser circle, the plane being perpendicular to the plane of the primitive circle, the center of which is C: Then *d* being the center of the projected lesser circle, *d*A is equal to the tangent of the arc PA, and *dc* = secant of PA.

DEM. Draw the diameter ED parallel to AB, and through P draw C*b*. Now E being the projecting point, the diameter AB is projected in *ab*. (22)
And *d*, the middle of *ab*, is the center of a circle on *ab*. (39)
Then a right line drawn from D through A, will meet *b*: (II. 130)
And draw CA, *d*A.
Now the right-angled triangles DC*b*, DAE, having the angle D common; the ∠D*b*C = ∠DEA. (II. 98)
But ∠DEA = ½∠DCA; and ∠D*b*C = ½∠A*dc*: (II. 127)
Therefore ∠DCA = ∠A*dc*.
Now ∠DCA + ∠AC*d* = a right angle.
Then ∠A*dc* + ∠ACD = a right angle: Therefore ∠CA*d* is right. (II. 96)
Consequently *d*A, = radius of the circle A*a*B, is the tangent of the arc PA, to the radius CA. (II. 126)
And *dc*, the distance of the centers, is the secant of the arc AP. (III. 5)

59. COROL. Hence the tangent and secant of any arc of the primitive circle, belongs also to an equal arc of any oblique circle; those arcs being reckoned from their intersection.

For the arc P*c* of every oblique circle intercepted between P and the arc of the small circle A*a*B, is equivalent to the arc PA of the primitive circle: Because the arc A*a*B is equally distant from its pole P. (5)

SECTION

SECTION II.

Spherical Geometry.

Spheric Geometry, or ſpheric projection, is the art of deſcribing, or repreſenting, ſuch circles or arcs of circles as are uſually drawn upon a ſphere on the plane of any one of them; and of meaſuring ſuch arcs, and their poſitions to one another, when projected.

60. PROBLEM I.

To deſcribe a great circle that ſhall paſs through two given points in the primitive circle, or plane of projection.

Let the given points be A, B; and C the center of the prim. circle.

CASE 1. *When one point,* A, *is the center of the primitive circle.*

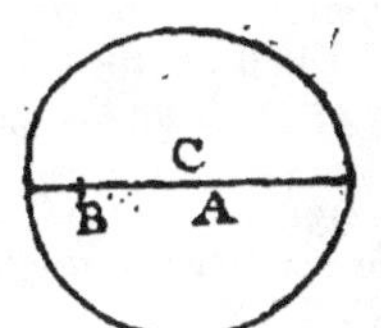

CONST. A diameter drawn through the given points A, B, will be the great circle required. (15)

CASE 2. *When one point* A, *is in the circumference of the primitive circle.*

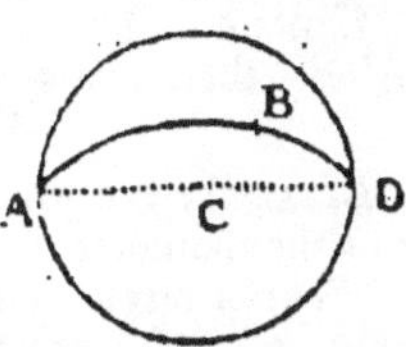

CONST. Through A draw a diameter AD.
Then an oblique circle deſcribed through the three points A, B, D, (II. 72) will be the great circle required. (42)

61. CASE 3. *When neither point is at the center, or circumference of the primitive circle.*

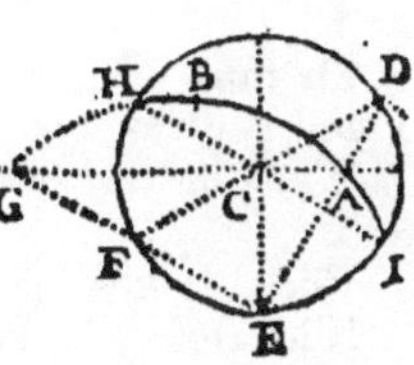

CONST. Through one point A, and the center C, draw AG, and draw CE at right angles to AG.
A ruler by E and A gives D; by D and C gives F; and by E and F gives G, in AC continued.
Through the three points G, E, A, deſcribe a circumference (II. 72) cutting the primitive circle in H and I.

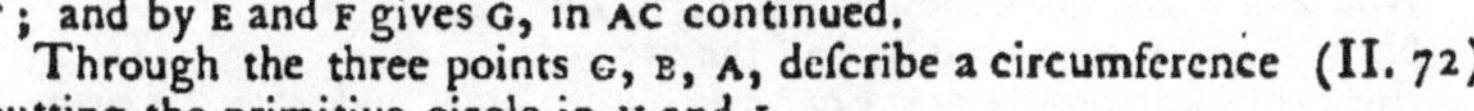

Then the oblique circle HBAI will be the great circle required.
For AG may be taken as the projection of the great circle FD. (12)
Therefore A and G are the projections of oppoſite points on the ſphere. (32)
Conſequently, all circles paſſing through G and A will be the repreſentatives of great circles on the ſphere.

62. PROBLEM II.

About any given point as a pole, to describe a great circle in a given primitive circle.

Let P be the given point, and I the center of the primitive circle,

CASE I. *When the given pole,* P, *is in the center of the primitive circle.*

CONST. The primitive circle will be the great circle required, (13)

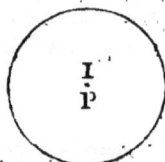

CASE 2. *When the given pole,* P, *is in the circumference of the primitive circle.*

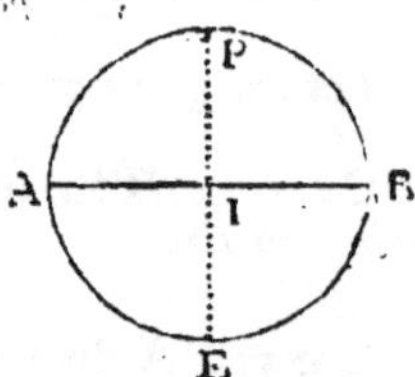

CONST. Through the given pole P, draw PE a diameter to the primitive circle.

Then another diam. AB, drawn at right angles to PE, will be the great circle required. (20, 15)

63. CASE 3. *When the given pole,* P, *is neither in the center or circumference of the primitive circle.*

CONST. Through P draw a diameter *bd*, and another BE at right angles to *bd*; then a ruler by E and P gives *p*.

Make the arc *p*A=90°; a ruler by E and A gives *a* in the diameter *bd*.

Then a circle described through the three points B, *a*, E, is the great circle required.

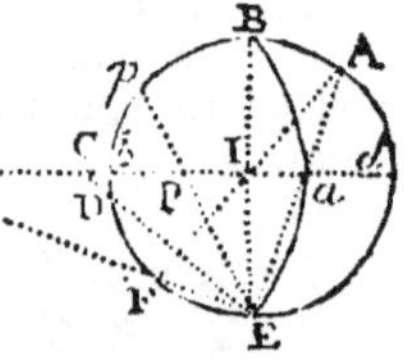

Or thus. Make the arc *p*D=arc *p*B; a ruler on E and D gives C in *db* produced.

Then on C, with the radius C*a* describe B*a*E.

For, As E is the projecting point, and P the projected pole;
Therefore *p* is the pole of the circle AF to be projected. (44)
And B*a*E is the projection of the circle AF. (38)
Now ∠C*a*E is measured by half the arc A*d*E. (II. 137)
But arc ABD=arc A*d*E: For A*p*=(B*d*=)*d*E; and *p*D=A*d* by construction,
Therefore ∠AEC=∠C*a*E; and CE=C*a*. (II. 104)
Consequently C is the center required.

64. PROB.

64. PROBLEM III.

A projected circle being given; to find its poles.

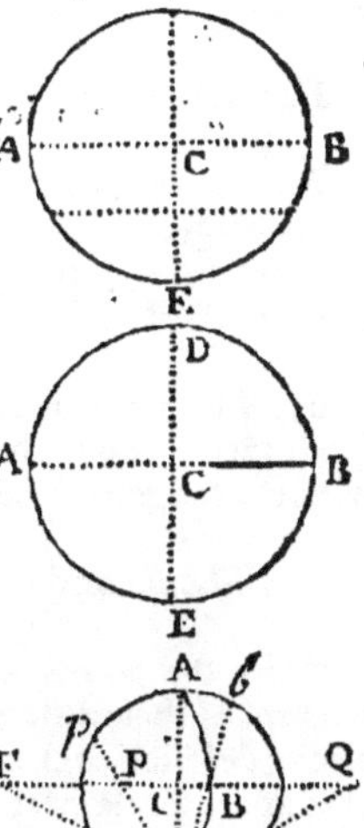

CASE 1. *When the given circle* AEB *is the primitive.*

CONST. Find the center C, (II. 70) and it is the pole fought.

CASE 2. *When the given circle* ACB *is a right circle.*

CONST. Draw a diameter ED at right angles to AB, and the ends or points, D, E, of that diameter are the poles required.

65. CASE 3. *When the given circle* ABE *is oblique.*

CONST. Through the interfections of the primitive and oblique circles draw a diameter AE, and another at right angles to AE, cutting the given oblique circle in B.

A ruler by E and B gives *b*; make *bp*, *bq*, each = an arc of 90°.

A ruler by E and *p* gives, in the diameter through B, the point P, which is the pole required.

And a ruler by E and *q* gives, in CB continued, the point Q for the other, or oppofite or exterior pole.

Make *p*D = *p*A; then a ruler by E and D gives, in BC continued, the point F, which is the center of the oblique circle ABE.

THE reafon of this operation is evident from that of the laft Problem.

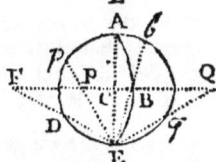

66. PROBLEM IV.

About any given projected pole, to defcribe a circle at a given diftance from that pole.
Or, at a propofed diftance from a given great circle, to defcribe a parallel circle.

Let P be the given pole, belonging to the given great circle DFE.

GENERAL SOLUTION. Through the given pole P, and C the center of the primitive circle, draw a diameter, and another DE at right angles to it,

A ruler on E and P gives *p* in the primitive circle.

Make *p*A and *p*B, each equal to the propofed diftance from the pole.

A ruler on E and A, and then on E and B, will cut the diameter CP in *a* and *b*.

Bifect *ab* in *c*; and on *c* as a center defcribe a circle paffing through *a* and *b*, which will be the circle required.

But

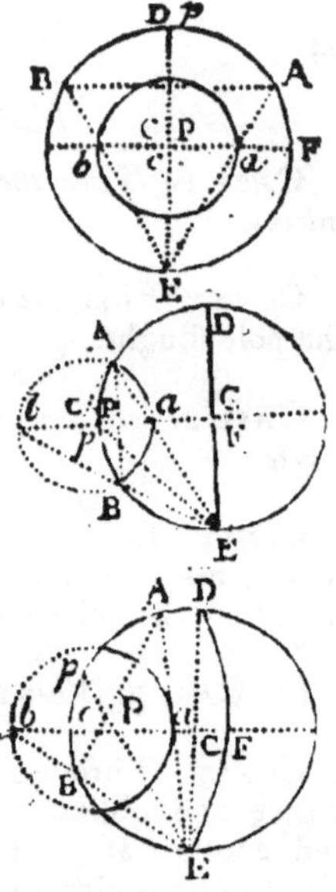

But when the parallel-circle is to be at a proposed distance from the given great circle DFE,

Find p as before; and make $pA = pB$, equal to the complement of the proposed distance; the rest as before.

For p is the pole, the projection of which is P. (44)

But p is the pole of a circle, the diameter of which AB is projected in ab. (12)

Therefore c, the middle of ab, is the center of the projected circle. (39)

67. The first case is readily done, by describing the small circle about the center of the primitive circle with the tangent of half its distance from the pole P.

68. The second case is soonest performed thus.

From the points A, B, (found as above) with the tangent of their distance from P, the pole of the right circle, describe arcs cutting in c, which is the center of a small circle parallel to the right circle DFE.

For Ap is the tangent of the arc AP. (58)

69. PROBLEM V.

The primitive circle, and the projection of a small circle, being given; to find the pole of that small circle.

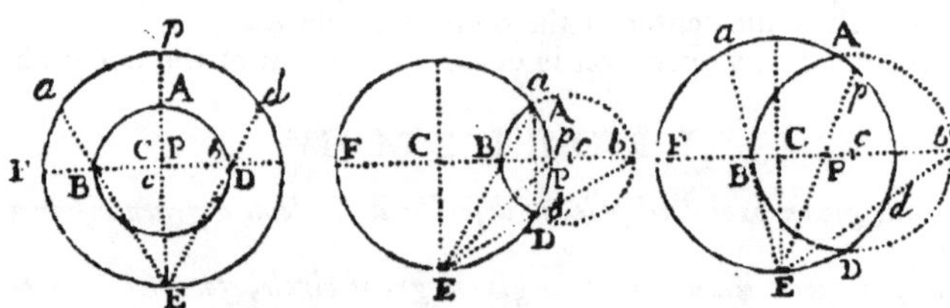

Let C be the center of the primitive circle, and ABD a projected small circle, the center of which is c, and radius cB.

General Solution. Through c the center of the small circle, and C the center of the primitive, draw a diameter CF, and another, CE, at right angles to it.

Find the projected diameter Bb = 2cB.

Lines drawn from E through B and b, cut the primitive circle in a, d; then bisect the arc ad in p.

A ruler by E and p cuts the diameter Bb in P, the pole sought.

The truth of this construction is evident by that of the last Prob.

70. PROBLEM VI.

To measure any arc of a projected great circle: Or, in a given projected great circle, to take an arc of a given number of degrees.

General Solution. Find the pole of the given circle. (64)

From that pole draw lines through the ends of the proposed arc, cutting the primitive circle.

Then the intercepted arc of the primitive circle applied to the scale of chords will give the measure sought.

Thus, if AB be the arc to be measured, and P the pole of the given circle DAF.

Then lines drawn from P through A and B, give the arc *ab* in the primitive circle, corresponding to AB in the projected circle.

Now if an arc of a given number of degrees was to be taken from a given point A, in the given projected circle DAF.

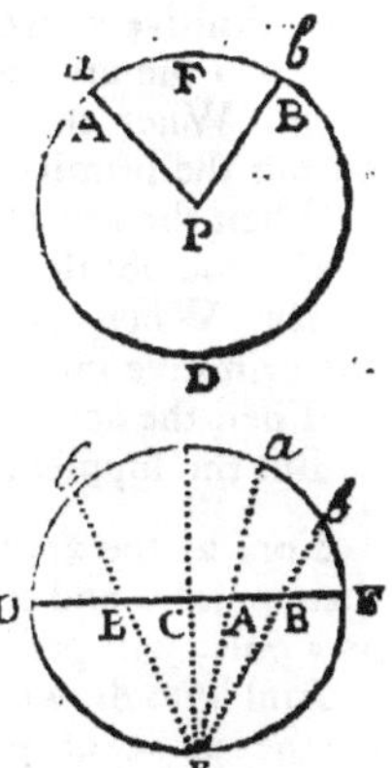

Draw, from the pole P, through A, the line P*a* to the primitive circle.

Apply the given number of degrees from *a* to *b*.

Draw P*b*, and the intercepted arc AB will contain the degrees proposed.

71. Any number of degrees is readily applied to a right circle by the scale of half-tangents. Thus

When the distance of the point A from the center C is known, and the given quantity of the arc is to be laid from A towards F;

To the known distance CA add the proposed arc AB, the degrees in the sum taken from the scale of half-tangents, and laid from C to B, will make the arc AB equal to the degrees proposed.

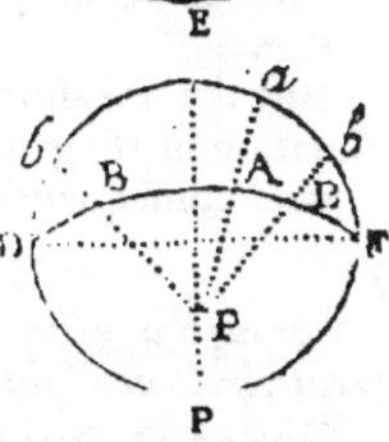

But when the arc AB is to be laid from A towards D;

Then the difference between the arcs AB and AC, taken from the scale of half-tangents and laid towards D from C to B, will make the arc AB equal to the degrees proposed.

The reason of all these operations is evident from art. 57.

Note, The half, or semi-tangents, are only the tangents of half the arcs the scale of tangents is made to; their construction depends on art. 48. On the *plane scale* they are put under the Tangents, and marked S. T.

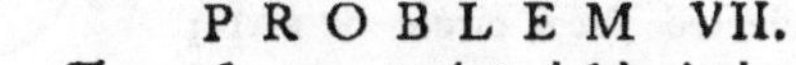

72. PROBLEM VII.

To measure any projected spherical angle.

General Solution. Find the poles of the two circles which form the angle (64); and from the angular point draw lines through those poles to cut the primitive circle.

Then the measure of that angle, if acute, will be the intercepted arc of the primitive circle; or the supplement of that arc will be the measure of the angle when obtuse.

Let the proposed angle DAB, formed by the great circles AD, AB, the poles of which are C and P; and lines drawn from the angular point A, through the poles C and P, cut the primitive circle in E and *p*.

1st.

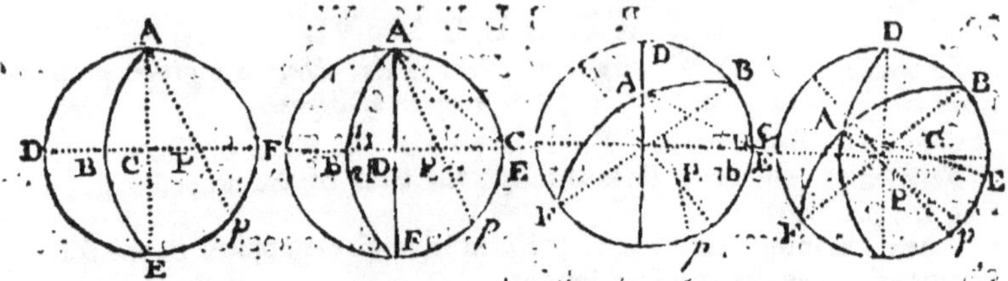

1ſt. When the angle is formed by the primitive and oblique circles.

Then the arc pE meaſures the acute angle DAB.

But the obtuſe angle BAF is meaſured by the ſupplement of pE.

2d. When the angle is formed by right and oblique circles meeting in the primitive's circumference.

Then the arc pE meaſures the angle DAB.

3d. When the angle is formed by right and oblique circles meeting within the primitive circle.

Then the arc pE meaſures the acute angle DAB.

But the obtuſe angle DAF is meaſured by the ſupplement of pE.

4th. When the angle is formed by two oblique circles meeting within the primitive circle;

Then the acute angle DAB is meaſured by the arc pE.

But the ſupplement of pE meaſures the obtuſe angle DAF.

For, as the angular point A is in both circles, and 90° diſtant from their poles C and P (19). Therefore a great circle deſcribed about A, as a pole, will paſs through the poles C and P.

And lines drawn from A through C and P, cut off, in the circumference of the plane of projection, an arc equal to the diſtance of the poles C and P. (57)

But the meaſure of the diſtance of the poles C, P, is equal to the inclination of the planes of the circles AD, AB; (33)

And conſequently meaſures the angle DAB.

73. PROBLEM VIII.

Through a given point in any projected great circle, to deſcribe another great circle at right angles to the given one.

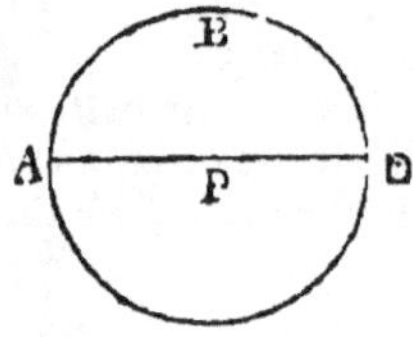

GENERAL SOLUTION. Find the pole of the given circle. (64)

Then a great circle deſcribed through that pole and the given point will be at right angles to the given circle.

Let the given projected great circle be BAD; and A the given point.

1ſt. *When* BAD *is the primitive circle, the pole of which is* P.

A diameter through A will be perpendicular to BAD. (II. 136)

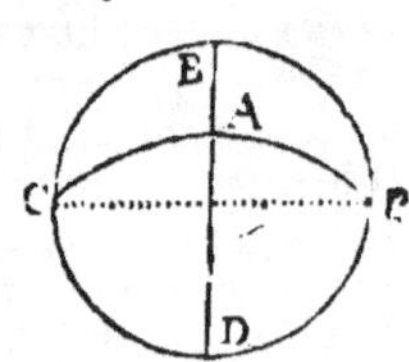

2d. *When* BAD *is a right circle, the poles of which are* P *and* C.

An oblique circle deſcribed through the points C, A, P, (II. 72) will be at right angles to BAD.

3d. When

3d. *When* BAD *is an oblique circle, the pole of which is* P.

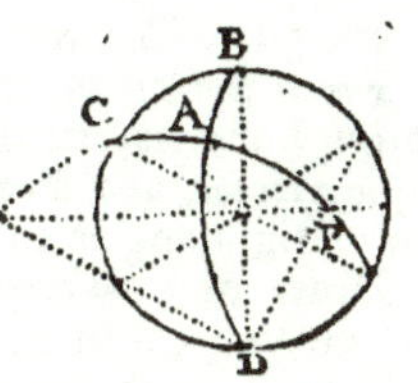

Through the points P and A, a great circle PAC being described (61), will be at right angles to BAD.

The truth of these operations is evident from art. 34.

74. PROBLEM IX.

Through any assigned point in a given projected great circle, to describe another great circle cutting the former in an angle of a given number of degrees.

Let P be a given point in any great circle APB.

1st. *When* APB *is the primitive circle.*

Through the given point P draw a diameter PE, and draw the diameter AB at right angles to PE.

Draw PD cutting AB in D, so that the angle CPD be equal to the angle proposed.

On D with the radius DP describe the great circle PFE.

Then will the angle APF contain the given degrees.

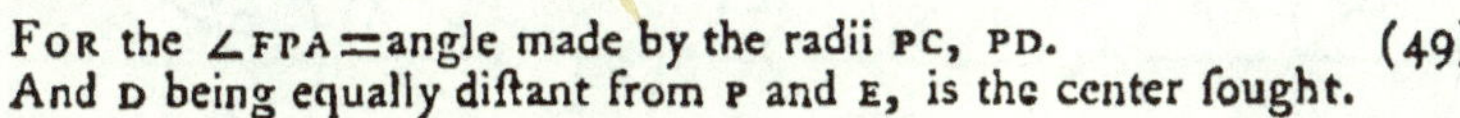

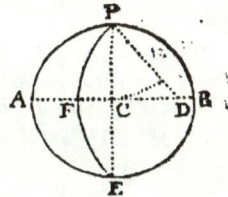

For the ∠FPA = angle made by the radii PC, PD. (49)

And D being equally distant from P and E, is the center sought.

75. Or thus. Make CD equal to the tangent of the given angle to the radius CP.

Or, Make PD equal to the secant of that angle.

76. 2d. *When* APB *is a right circle.*

Draw a diameter GH at right angles to APB.

Then a ruler by G and P gives *a* in the primitive circle.

Make H*b* = 2A*a*; a ruler by G and *b* gives C in AB.

Draw CD at right angles to AB.

Draw PD cutting CD in D, so that the ∠CPD = complement of the degrees given. (II. 84)

On D with the radius DP describe a circle FPE, which will be a great circle making with APB the angle APF as required.

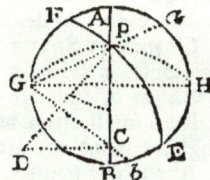

For, C is the center of a great circle GPH, by the demonstration to art. 63.

And the centers of all great circles through P, will be in CD. (55)

Now ∠DPE = 90°. (II. 136)

Therefore ∠APF or ∠BPE (26), the compl. of CPD, is the angle sought.

77. 3d.

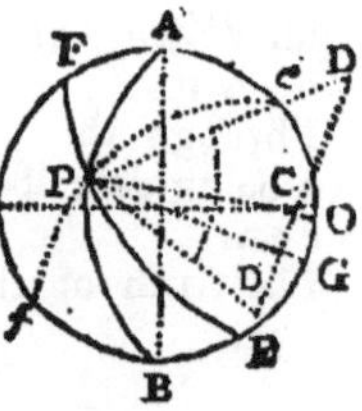

77. 3d. *When* APB *is an oblique circle.*

From the given point P, draw the lines PG, PC, through the centers of the primitive and given oblique circles, and through C the center of APB draw CD at right angles to PG. (II. 59)

Draw PD, making the ∠CPD = given degrees, and cutting CD in D. (II. 84)

From D with the radius DP, a circle FPE being described, will be a great circle cutting APB in the angle proposed.

For C, the center of APD, is in a line perpendicular to PG, drawn through P and the center of the primitive, by construction.

And the centers of all great circles through P will be in CD. (55)

Now the ∠CPD made by the radii PC, PD, contains the given degrees.

Therefore the angle APF is equal to the angle required. (49)

78. PROBLEM X.

Through any point in the plane of projection, or primitive circle, to describe a great circle that shall cut a given great circle in any angle proposed: Provided the measure of that proposed angle is not less than the distance between the given point and circle.

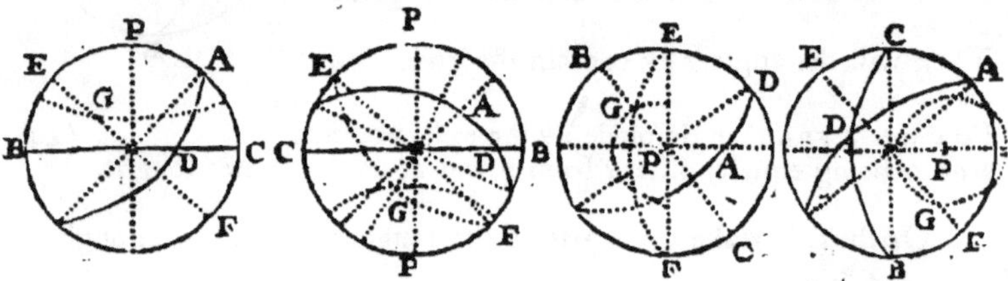

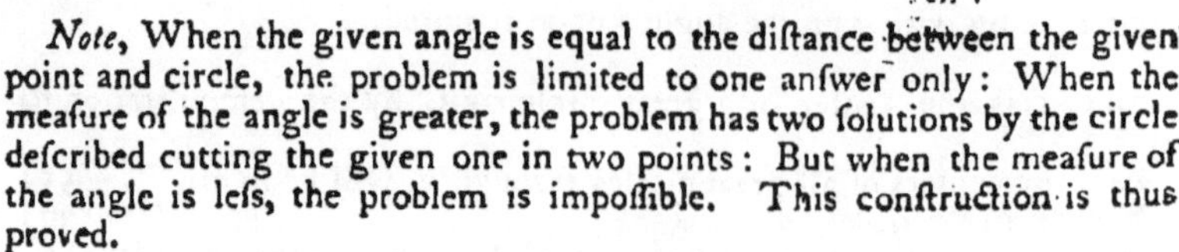

Let the given point be A, through which a circle is to be described to cut a given great circle BDC, the pole of which is P, in an angle equal to a proposed number of degrees.

General Solution. About the given point A, as a pole, describe a great circle EGF. (62)

About P, the pole of the given circle BDC, describe a small circle at a distance equal to the given angle, cutting the great circle EGF in G. (66)

About the point G, as a pole (62), describe a great circle cutting the given circle BDC in D. Then will ADC be the angle required.

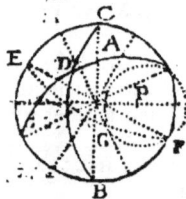

Note, When the given angle is equal to the distance between the given point and circle, the problem is limited to one answer only: When the measure of the angle is greater, the problem has two solutions by the circle described cutting the given one in two points: But when the measure of the angle is less, the problem is impossible. This construction is thus proved.

P and G are the poles of BC and AD.

And

And the diſtance of P and G is equal to the degrees in the propoſed angle, by conſtruction. But ∠ADC = diſtance of P and G. (33)
Therefore the ∠ADC is the angle required.

79. *When the required circle is to make a given angle with the primitive.*

Then, from the center of the primitive, with the tang. of the given angle, deſcribe an arc; and from the given point A, with the ſecant of the given angle, cut the former arc.

On this interſection, a circle being deſcribed through the given point A, will cut the primitive circle in the angle propoſed.

THIS depends on art. 75.

80. PROBLEM XI.

Any great circle, cutting the primitive, being given, to deſcribe another great circle, which ſhall cut the given one in a propoſed angle, and have a given arc intercepted between the primitive and given circles.

Let ABC be the primitive circle, the center of which is P; and the given great circle be ADC, the center of which is E.

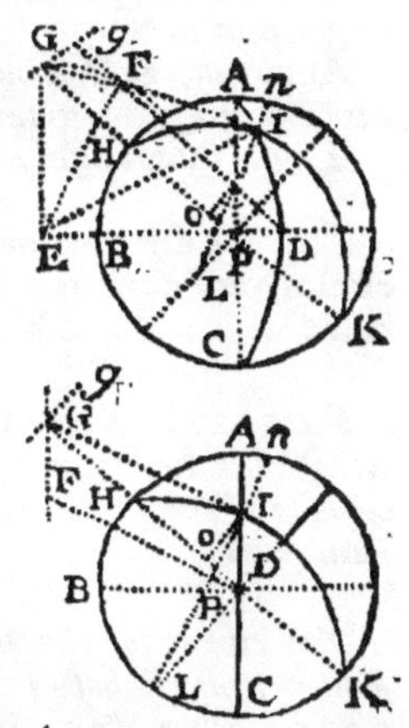

SOLUTION. Draw a diameter EBD at right angles to ADC; and make the angle BDF equal to the complement of the given angle; ſuppoſe = complement of 35°.

Make DF equal to the tangent of the given arc (ſuppoſe 58°); and from P, with the ſecant of that arc, deſcribe an arc *Gg*.

Now when ADC is an oblique circle; from E the center of ADC, with the radius EF, cut the arc *Gg* in G.

But when ADC is a right circle; through F draw FG parallel to ADC, cutting the arc *Gg* in G.

From G, with the tangent DF, deſcribe an arc, *no*, cutting ADC in I; and draw GI.

Through G and the center P draw GK, cutting the primitive circle in H, K; draw PL perpendicular to GK; and IL at right angles to IG, cutting PL in L.

And L will be the center of a circle paſſing through H, I, K, which will be the great circle required.

Then the ∠AIH = 35°; and arc IH = 58°, as was propoſed.

For GP is the ſecant, and GI is the tang. of the arc HI. (59)

And as the triangles EGI, EFD, are congruous; the ∠EIG = ∠EDF. (II. 101)

But the ∠EIG made by the tangent of the arc HI and the radius of the arc AI, is the complement of the angle made by thoſe arcs. (49)

Conſequently the ∠AIH is the complement of the ∠EDF.

The center of the right circle AC being ſuppoſed at an infinite diſtance, therefore any circle FG deſcribed from that center, will be parallel to AC.

When the given arc is more than 90°, the tangent and ſecant of its ſupplement is to be applied on the line DF the contrary way, or towards the right; the former conſtruction being reckoned to the left.

81. PROBLEM XII.

Any great circle in the plane of projection being given; to deſcribe another great circle, which ſhall make given angles with the primitive and given circles.

Let the given great circle be ADC, and its pole Q.

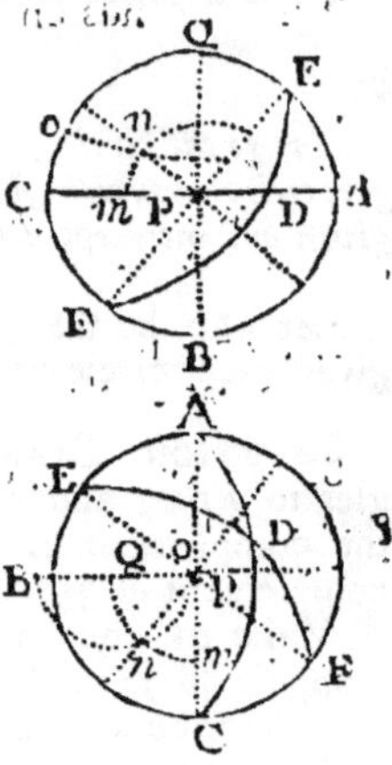

SOLUTION. About P, the pole of the primitive circle, deſcribe an arc *mn*, at the diſtance of as many degrees as are in the angle which the required circle is to make with the primitive: Suppoſe 62°. (67)

About Q, the pole of the other given circle, and at a diſtance equal to the meaſure of the angle which the required circle is to make with the given circle ADC (ſuppoſe 48°), deſcribe an arc *on*, cutting *mn* in *n*. (66)

About *n*, as a pole, deſcribe the great circle EDF, cutting the given circles in E and D. (62)

Then is the angle AED = 62°; and ADE = 48°.

FOR the diſtance of the poles of any two great circles, is equal to the angle which thoſe circles make with one another. (33)

REMARK. The 11th Problem, which is particularly uſeful in conſtructing a ſpherical triangle, *in which are given two angles and a ſide oppoſite to one of them*, includes only two caſes of a more general Problem, viz.

Any two great circles being given in poſition; to deſcribe a third, which ſhall cut one of thoſe given in an angle propoſed, and have a given arc intercepted between the given circles.

Alſo the 12th Problem, uſed when *the three angles are given*, contains only two caſes of another Problem; viz.

Any two great circles being given in poſition, to deſcribe a third which ſhall cut the given circles in given angles.

The ſolution of theſe two general Problems not being wanted in any part of this work; it was not thought neceſſary here to annex them; more having been already delivered in the preceding pages than it is uſual to meet with on this ſubject. However, their ſolution is recommended as exerciſes to ſpeculative learners.

SECTION IV.

Spheric Trigonometry.

DEFINITIONS.

82. SPHERIC TRIGONOMETRY is the art of computing the meaſures of the ſides and angles of ſuch triangles as are formed on the ſurface of a ſphere, by the mutual interſections of three great circles deſcribed thereon.

83. A SPHERIC TRIANGLE conſiſts of three ſides and three angles.

The meaſures of unknown ſides or angles of ſpheric triangles are eſtimated by the relations between the ſines, or the tangents, or the ſecants, of the ſides or angles known, and of thoſe that are unknown.

84. A RIGHT ANGLED SPHERIC TRIANGLE has one right angle: The ſides about the right angle are called Legs; and the ſide oppoſite to the right angle is called the Hypothenuſe.

85. A QUADRANTAL SPHERIC TRIANGLE has one ſide equal to ninety degrees.

86. An OBLIQUE SPHERIC TRIANGLE has all its angles oblique.

87. The CIRCULAR PARTS of a triangle, are the arcs which meaſure its ſides and angles.

88. Two ſpheric triangles are ſaid to be ſupplements to one another, when the ſides and angles of the one are reſpective ſupplements of the angles and ſides of the other: And one, in regard to the other, is called the ſupplemental triangle.

89. Two arcs or angles, when compared together, are ſaid to be alike, or of the ſame kind, when both are acute, or leſs than 90°, or when both are obtuſe, or greater than 90°: But when one is greater and the other leſs than 90°, they are ſaid to be unlike.

The leſſer circles of the ſphere do not enter into Trigonometrical computations, becauſe of the diverſity of their radii.

SECTION V.

Spherical Theorems.

90. THEOREM I.

In every ſpheric triangle, ABC, *equal angles,* B, C, *are oppoſite to equal ſides,* AC, AB: *And equal ſides,* AB, AC, *are oppoſite to equal angles,* C, B.

DEM. Since AB = AC, make AE = AD; and draw BD, CE.
Then is BD = CE; and ∠AEC = ∠ADB. (27)
For the triangles AEC, ADB are congruous,
Since AB = AC; AD = AE; ∠A common.
Alſo, the triangles BEC, CDB are congruous; (27)
Therefore ∠EBC = ∠DCB.
For EC = BD; EB = (AB − AE =) DC (= AC − AD). (II. 48)
And ∠BEC = ∠CDB, they being the ſuppl. of equal angles AEC, ADB.
Again, if ∠ABC = ∠ACB: Then is AB = AC.
For take BE = CD; and deſcribe the arcs CE, BD.
Then is EC = DB, ∠BEC = ∠CDB; ∠BCE = ∠CBD. (27)
For △* BCE = △CBD; ſince BC is common, BE = CD, ∠EBC = ∠DCB.
Alſo the triangles ABD, ACE are congruous;
Since EC = DB, ∠ACE = (∠BCA − BCE =) ∠ABD (= ∠CBA − CBD). (II. 48)
And ∠AEC = (ſup. ∠BEC =) ∠ADB (= ſup. ∠CDB). (II. 48)
Therefore AE = AD; and AB = (AE + EB =) AC (= AD + DC). (II. 47)

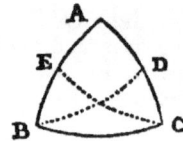

91. COROL. A line drawn from the vertex of an iſoſceles ſpheric triangle, to the middle of the baſe, is perpendicular to the baſe.
This is eaſily proved from art. 90, 27.

92. THEOREM II.

Either ſide of a ſpheric triangle is leſs than the ſum of the other two ſides.

DEM. For on the ſurface of the ſphere, the ſhorteſt diſtance between two points, is an arc of a great circle paſſing through thoſe points. (23)
But each ſide of a ſpheric triangle is an arc of a great circle. (10)
Therefore either ſide being the ſhorteſt diſtance between its extremities, is leſs than the ſum of the other two ſides.

93. THEOREM III.

Each ſide of a ſpheric triangle is leſs than a ſemicircle, or 180 degrees.

DEM. Two great circles interſect each other twice at the diſtance of 180 degrees. (32)
The ſides about any ſpheric angle are arcs of two great circles. (10)
But a ſpheric triangle has three ſides.
Therefore every two ſides before their ſecond meeting muſt be interſected by the third ſide.
Conſequently each ſide is leſs than a ſemicircle.

* The mark △ ſtands for the word triangle.

94. THEOREM IV.

In every spheric triangle, ABC, *the greatest side,* BC, *is opposite the greatest angle,* A.

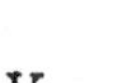

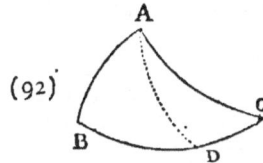

DEM. Make ∠BAD = ∠ABC.
Then AD = BD (90); and BC = AD + DC.
But AD + DC is greater than AC. (92)
Therefore BC is greater than AC.

95. THEOREM V.

If from the three angles of a spheric triangle, ABC, *as poles, be described three arcs of great circles, forming another spheric triangle,* EDF; *then will the sides of the latter, and the opposite angles of the former, be the supplements of one another: Also the angles in the latter, and their opposite sides in the former, are the supplements of one another.*

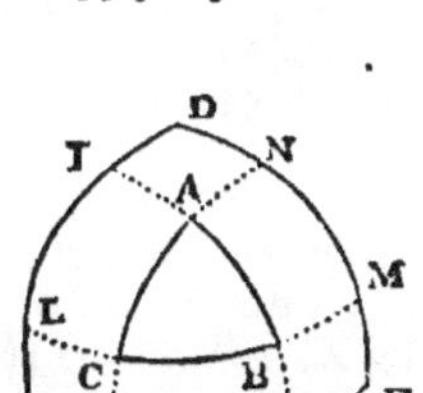

That is, FE and ∠CAB, FD and ∠ABC, DE and ∠ACB, are supplements to one another.
Also ∠E and AC, ∠D and CB, ∠F and AB, are the supplements to one another.
DEM. The intersection E of the arcs about the poles A and C, being 90° distant from them, is the pole of the arc AC. (19)
And for the same reason, D is the pole of CB, and F of AB.

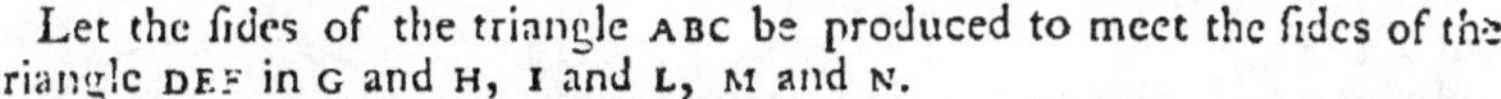

Let the sides of the triangle ABC be produced to meet the sides of the triangle DEF in G and H, I and L, M and N.
Then FI = DL = 90°: Therefore (DL + FI = DL + FL + LI =) DF + LI = 180°. (II. 47)
Therefore DF and LI are supplements to one another.
But LI measures the angle ABC. (9)
Therefore ∠ABC and DF are the supplements to one another.
And in the same manner it may be demonstrated, that the ∠BAC and FE, ∠ACB and DE, are the supplements of one another.
Again, since BI = AH = 90 degrees; (19)
Therefore (IB + AH = IB + BH + AB =) IH + AB = 180 degrees.
But IH measures the angle F; (9)
Therefore AB and ∠F are the supplements of one another.
And the same may be shewn of AC and ∠E, CB and ∠D.

96. THEOREM VI.

The sum of the three sides of every spheric triangle, ABC, *is less than a circumference, or 360 degrees.*

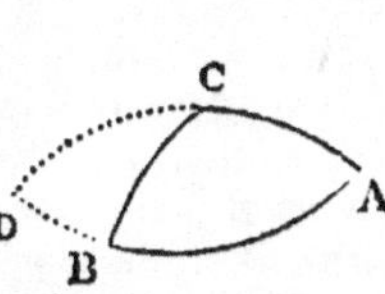

DEM. Continue the sides AC, AB, till they meet in D.
Then the arcs ACD, ABD, are each 180°. (32)
But DC + DB is greater than BC. (92)
Therefore AC + AB + DC + DB is greater than AC + AB + BC.
Or the semicircles ACD + ABD is greater than AC + AB + BC.
That is, 360° is greater than the three sides of the triangle ABC.

97. THEOREM VII.

The ſum of the three angles of a ſpheric triangle, ABC, *is greater than two right angles, and leſs than ſix; or will always fall between* 180 *and* 540 *degrees.*

DEM. Since ∠A and FE, ∠B and FD, ∠C and DE, are ſupplements to one another. (95)

Therefore the three angles A, B, C, together with the three ſides FE, FD, DE make thrice 180°, or 540°.

Now the ſum of the three ſides FE + FD + DE, is leſs than twice 180°. (96)

Therefore the ſum of the three angles A + B + C is greater than 180°.

Again, as a ſpheric angle is ever leſs than 180; (24)

Therefore the ſum of any three ſpheric angles is ever leſs than thrice 180°, or 540 degrees.

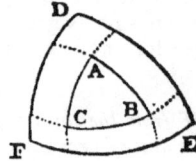

98. THEOREM VIII.

If one ſide, AB, *of a ſpheric triangle,* ABC, *be produced, then the outward angle,* CBD, *is either equal to, leſs, or greater than the inward oppoſite angle* A, *adjacent to that ſide; according as the ſum of the other two ſides,* CA + CB, *is equal to, greater, or leſs than* 180 *degrees.*

DEM. Produce AC, AB, to meet in D.

Then arc ACD = arc ABD = 180°. (32)

And ∠D = ∠A. (31)

Now if AC + CB is equal to 180°; then CB = CD.

And ∠CBD = (∠D =) ∠A. (90)

If AC + CB is greater than 180°; then CB is greater than CD.

And ∠CBD is leſs than (∠D =) ∠A. (94)

If AC + CB is leſs than 180°; then CB is leſs than CD. (94)

And ∠CBD is greater than (∠D =) ∠A.

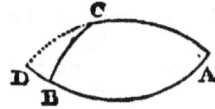

99. THEOREM IX.

In right angled ſpheric triangles, the oblique angles and their oppoſite ſides are of the ſame kind: That is, if a leg is leſs or greater than 90°, *its oppoſite angle is alſo leſs or greater than* 90°.

In the right angled ſpheric triangle ABC, right angled at A.

If AC is greater than 90°; then ∠ABC is greater than 90°.

If AC is leſs than 90°; then ∠ABC is leſs than 90°.

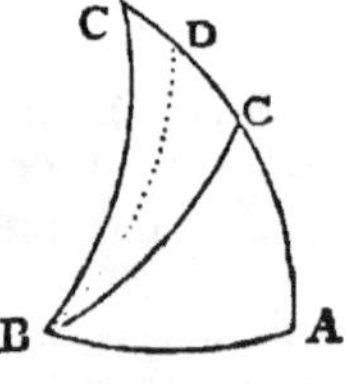

DEM. Let the leg AC be leſs, AD equal, AC greater, than 90°, and deſcribe the arc DB.

Now D being the pole of AB (37). Therefore ∠DBA is right.

Conſequently if AC is leſs than AD, the ∠CBA is leſs than ∠DBA.

But if AC is greater than AD, the ∠CBA is greater than ∠DBA.

And the ſame may be proved of the leg AB and its oppoſite angle.

100. THEOREM X.

In right angled ſpheric triangles, BAC, *the hypothenuſe,* BC, *is leſs than* 90°, *when the legs,* AB, AC, *are of a like kind: But the hypothenuſe is greater than* 90°, *when the legs are of different kinds.*

1ſt. When the legs AB, AC, are both leſs than 90°.

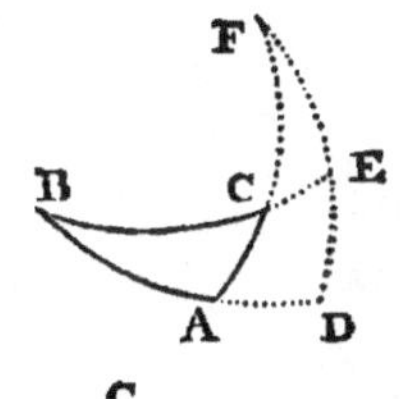

DEM. In BA, AC produced, take BD, AF equal to quadrants; through F and D deſcribe an arc FD meeting BC produced in E.

Now F being the pole of BD (19). Therefore B is the pole of ED.

Conſequently BC is leſs than (BE =) 90°.

2d. When the legs AB, AC, are both greater than 90°.

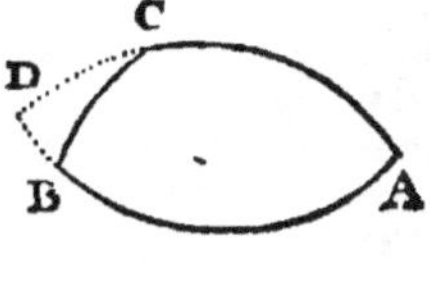

Produce AC, AB, till they meet in D.

Now the hypothenuſe CB is common to both the right angled triangles BAC and BDC.

And the legs DC, DB, being both leſs than 90°.

Therefore the hypothenuſe BC is leſs than 90°, by the firſt caſe of this Theorem.

3d. When the legs AB, AC, are one greater, the other leſs than 90°.

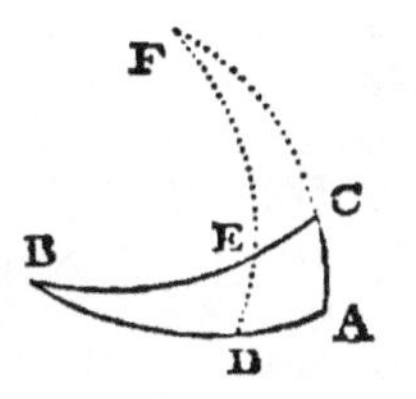

In AB, and AC produced, take BD, AF each of 90°, and deſcribe the arc FED.

Then B is the pole of FD; and ſince F is the pole of BA, and FD is at right angles to BD. Therefore BE = 90°. (37)

Conſequently BC is greater than 90 degrees.

101. COROL. I. The hypothenuſe is leſs or greater than 90°, according as the oblique angles are of a like, or different kinds.

For if legs are like, or unlike, the angles are like or unlike. (99)

And if legs are like, or unlike, the hypoth. is acute or obtuſe. (100)

Therefore if the angles are like, the hypothenuſe is acute, or leſs than 90°; but if unlike, the hypothenuſe is obtuſe, or greater than 90°.

102. COROL. II. The legs and their adjacent angles are like, or unlike, as the hypothenuſe is leſs, or greater than 90 degrees.

For like legs, or like angles, make the hypothenuſe acute (by 1ſt and 2d of 100).

And unlike legs, or unlike angles, make the hypothenuſe obtuſe (by 3d of 100 and by 101).

103. COROL. III. A leg and its oppoſite angle are both acute, or both obtuſe, according as the hypothenuſe and other leg are like, or unlike.

This is evident from the three caſes of this Theorem.

104. COROL. IV. Either angle is acute, or obtuſe, as the hypothenuſe and the other angle are like, or unlike.

This follows from caſe 1ſt and 2d of this Theorem.

105. **THEOREM XI.**

In every spheric triangle, ABC, if the angles adjacent to either side, AB, be alike, then a perpendicular, CD, drawn to that side from the other angle, will fall within the triangle: But the perpendicular CD falls without the triangle, when the angles adjacent to the side AB it falls on are unlike.

DEMONST. Since in all right angled triangles the perpendicular and its opposite angle are of the same kind. (99)

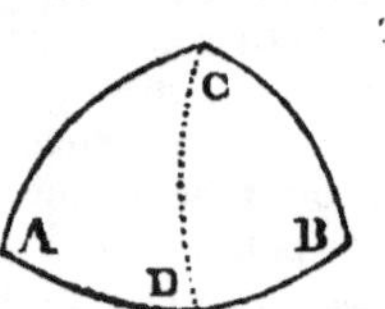

Therefore the ∠s CAD, CBD, are each like CD.

Now in Fig. 1. the angles CAD, CBD, or CAB, CBA, are angles adjacent to the base AB within the triangle, and are therefore alike.

Therefore the perpendicular falling between A and B, falls within the triangle.

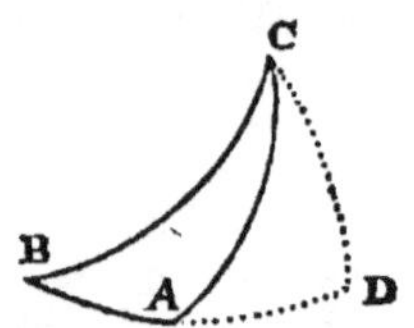

In Fig. 2. the angles CAD and CAB are the supplements of each other, and are therefore unlike, as CA falls obliquely on AB.

Therefore ∠CAB is unlike to ∠CBA.

Consequently the perpendicular CD cannot fall between A and B: Therefore it must fall without.

106. **THEOREM XII.**

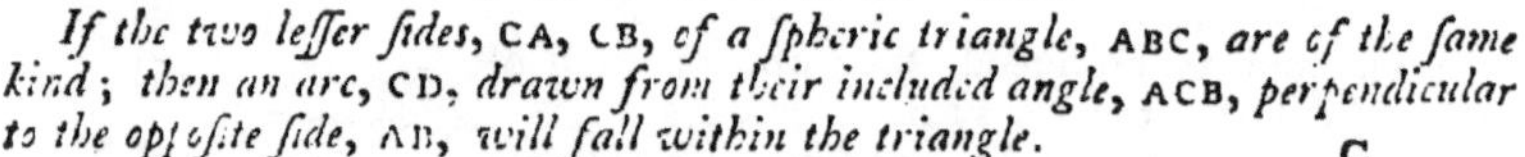

If the two lesser sides, CA, CB, of a spheric triangle, ABC, are of the same kind; then an arc, CD, drawn from their included angle, ACB, perpendicular to the opposite side, AB, will fall within the triangle.

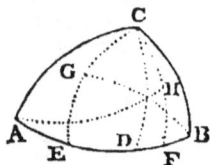

DEMONST. In AB take AF=AC; draw CF and AH at right angles to CF.

Then CH=HF (91) are each less than 90°. (93)

Also take BE=BC; draw CE and BG at right angles to CE.

Then CG=GE (91) are each less than 90°. (93)

Now in the right angled triangles FHA, EGB; if the hypothenuses AF (=AC), and BE (=BC), are acute, or like FH and EG;

Then the angles AFH and BEG are acute, and like AC and BC; (103)

Therefore the perpendicular CD falls on EF, within the triangle. (105)

Also if the hypothenuses AF and BE are obtuse, or unlike to FH and GE;

Then the angles AFH and BEG are obtuse, and also like CA and CB. (103)

Consequently the perpendicular will fall on EF. (105)

Therefore in either case the perpendicular falls within the triangle.

107. **THEOREM XIII.**

In all right angled spheric triangles,

As sine hypoth. : Rad : : sine of a leg : sine of its opposite angle.

108. *And sine a leg : Rad. : : tan. other leg : tan. of its opposite angle.* Pl. I.

DEMONST. Let EDAFG represent the eighth part of a sphere, where the quadrantal planes EDFG, EDBC, are both perpendicular to the quadrantal plane ADFB; and the quadrantal plane ADGC is perpendicular to the quadrantal plane EDFG: and the spheric triangle ABC is right angled at B, where CA is the hypothenuse, and BA, BC, are the legs.

To the arcs GF, CB, draw the tangents HF, OB, and the sines GM, CI, on the radii DF, DB; also draw BI, the sine of the arc AB, and CK, the sine of AC; then join IK and OL.

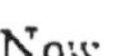

Now

Now HF, OB, GM, CI, are all perpendicular to the plane ADFB.

And HD, CK, OL, lie all in the same plane ADGC.

Also FD, IK, BL, lie all in the same plane ADFB.

Therefore the right angled triangles HFD, CIK, OBL, having the equal angles HDF, CKI, OLB, (II. 199) are similar. (II. 167)

Therefore CK : DG :: CI : GM.

That is, As sin. hyp. : Rad. :: sin. of a leg : sin. opp. angle.

For GM is the sine of the arc GF, which measures the angle CAB. (9)

Also, As LB : DF :: BO : FH.

That is, As sin. of a leg : Rad. :: tan. of other leg : tan. opp. angle.

109. THEOREM XIV.

In right angled spheric triangles, ABC, *if about the oblique angles,* A, C, *as poles, at* 90° *distance, there be described arcs,* DE, FE, *cutting one another in* E; *and the sides* AB, AC, BC, *of the triangle be produced to cut those arcs in* D; G, F; H, I; *there will be constituted two other triangles,* CGH, HIE, *the parts of which are either equal to, or are the complements of, the parts of the given triangle,* ABC. Pl. I.

DEMONST. Now since A is the pole of ED (19). Therefore AD, AG are at right angles to ED; and so is ED to AD. (37)

And since BI and DE are at right angles to AD, their intersection H is the pole of AD (36). Therefore HB, HD are quadrants. (35)

Then in the triangle CGH, right angled at G.

CG = complement of AC.

HG = comp. ∠A; For HG is the comp. of GD, which mea. ∠A. (9)

HC the hypoth. is the comp. of CB.

The ∠HCG = ∠ACB. (26)

The ∠CHG = comp. AB: For BD, the comp. of AB, measures ∠CHG.

Also in the triangle EIH, right angled at I: Because CF, CI are at right angles to EF; and EF, EG being also at right angles to AF; therefore E is the pole of AF; (36) consequently EF and EG are quadrants. (35)

Then the hypoth. EH = ∠A; For GH = comp. of EH and GD; and GD measures the angle A.

HI = CB; for HC = comp. of HI and CB.

EI = comp. ∠C; For EI = comp. of IF, which measures ∠C.

The ∠H = comp. AB; For BD, the comp of AB, measures ∠H.

The ∠E = AC; For GF, the measure of ∠E, is equal to ∠AC.

110. THEOREM XV.

In every spheric triangle, it will be,
As the sine of either angle, is to the sine of its opposite side;
So is the sine of another angle, to the sine of its opposite side.

Let ABC be a spheric triangle, where BD is perpendicular to AC produced; forming the two right angled triangles ADB, CDB.

DEM. Now sin. AB : rad. :: sin. BD : sin ∠A. (167)

And sin. BC : rad. :: sin. BD : sin. ∠C.

Therefore sin. AB × sin. ∠A = rad. × sin. BD. (II. 162)

And sin. BC × sin. ∠C = rad. × sin. BD. (II. 162)

Therefore sin. AB × sin. ∠A = sin. BC × sin. ∠C. (II. 46)

Therefore sin. ∠A : sin. BC :: sin. ∠C : sin. AB. (II. 163)

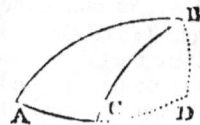

SECTION VI.

Of the Solution of right angled ſpheric Triangles.

In every caſe of right angled ſpheric triangles, three things beſide the radius enter the proportion, of which two are given, and the third is ſought.

Now the ſolution of every caſe will be obtained by the application of the two following rules to Theorem XIII. and XIV. (107, 108, 109.)

111. RULE I. If of the three things concerned, or their complements, two are oppoſite to one another, and the third is oppoſite to the right angle, in one of the triangles marked 1, 2, 3, in the fig. to Theo. XIV. Pl. I. Then the thing ſought will be found by the firſt proportion (107) either directly, or by inverſion.

112. RULE II. If of the three things concerned, or their complements, two are ſides, and the third is an oblique angle, in either of the three triangles marked 1, 2, 3, in fig. to Theo. XIV. Pl. I. Then the thing ſought will be found by the ſecond proportion (108) either directly, or by inverſion.

113. PROBLEM I.

In the right angled ſpheric triangle ABC, Plate I. Theorem XIV.

Given the hypothenuſe AC and one of the legs AB } required the reſt.

1ſt. *To find the angle* ACB *oppoſite the given leg* AB.

Here the things concerned are AC, ∠B, AB, ∠C; which are found in the triangle, N° 1, to be oppoſite; and ſo fall under Rule I. (111)

Then ſin. AC : rad. : : ſin. AB : ſin. ∠ACB. (107)

Or ſin. hyp. : rad. : : ſin. g. leg : ſin. op. ∠. Like the g. leg. (99)

2d. *To find the angle* CAB *adjacent to the given leg* AB.

Here the things concerned are AC, ∠B, AB, ∠A.

Now trying in the triangle, N° 1, I find the things concerned will fall under neither of the Rules.

But trying in the triangle, N° 2, the things concerned, or their complements, fall under Rule II. (112)

Then ſin. HG : rad. : : tan. GC : tan. ∠CHG. (108)

Or co-ſ. ∠CAB : rad. : : co-t. AC : co-t. AB.

Or co-ſ. ∠CAB : co-t. AC : : (rad. : co-t. AB) : : tan. AB : rad. (III. 36)

Therefore rad. : co-t. hyp. : : tan. g. leg : co-ſ. adj. angle. (II. 145)

Like, or unlike the given leg; as the hyp. is acute, or obtuſe. (102)

3d. *To find the other leg* BC.

Here the things concerned are AC, ∠B, AB, BC; which in the triangle, N° 1, do not fall under either Rule: But in N° 2 they will be found to fall under the firſt Rule. (111)

Then ſin. HE : rad. : : ſin. CG : ſin. ∠CHG. (107)

Or co-ſ. CB : rad. : : co-ſ. AC : co-ſ. AB.

Therefore co-ſ. g. leg, AB, : rad. : : co-ſ. hyp. AC, : co-ſ. req. leg CB.

And is acute, if hyp. and given leg are like; but obtuſe, if unlike. (103)

114. PROB.

114. ## PROBLEM II.

In the right angled ſpheric triangle ABC. Pl. I. Theorem XIV.
Given the hypothenuſe AC
And one of the oblique angles A } Required the reſt.

1ſt. *To find the leg* CB *oppoſite to the given angle* A.
In the triangle, N° 1. the things concerned fall under Rule I. (111)
Then rad. : ſin. AC : : ſin. ∠CAB : ſin. CB. (107)
Or rad. : ſin. hyp. : : ſin. given angle : ſin. opp. ſide.
And is like the given angle. (99)

2d. *To find the leg* AB *adjacent to the given angle* A.
In the triangle, N° 2. the things concerned fall under Rule II. (112)
Then ſin. HG : rad. : : tan. CG : tan. ∠CHG. (108)
Or coſ. ∠BAC : rad. : : (co-t. AC : co-t. AB : :) tan. AB : tan. AC. (III. 37)
Therefore rad. : tan. AC : : co-ſ. ∠BAC : tan. AB.
Or rad. : tan. hyp. : : co-ſ. given angle : tan. adjacent leg.
And is acute, if hyp. and given angle are alike; but obtuſe if unlike. (104)

3d. *To find the other angle* ACB.
In the triangle, N° 2, the things concerned fall under Rule II. (112)
Then ſin. CG : rad. : : tan. GH : tan. ∠HCG. (108)
Or co-ſ. AC : rad. : : co-t. ∠ BAC : tan. ∠BCA : :) co-t. ∠ BCA. : tan. ∠BAC. (III. 37)
Therefore rad. : tan. ∠BAC : : co-ſ. AC : co-t. ∠BCA. (II. 145)
Or rad. : co-ſ. hyp. : : tan. given angle : co-t. req. angle.
And is acute, if hyp. and given angle are alike; but obtuſe, if unlike. (104)

115. ## PROBLEM III.

In the right angled ſpheric triangle ABC. Plate I. Theorem XIV.
Given one of the legs AB
And its oppoſite angle ACB } Required the reſt.

1ſt. *To find the hypothenuſe* AC.
In the triangle, N° 1. the things concerned fall under Rule I. (111)
Then ſin. ∠ACB : ſin. AB : : rad. : ſin. AC. (107)
Or ſin. given angle : ſin. given leg : : rad. : ſin. hyp.
And is either acute or obtuſe.

2d. *To find the other leg* CB.
In the triangle, N° 1. the things concerned fall under Rule II. (112)
Then ſin. CB : (rad. : :) tan. AB (: tan. ∠ ACB) : : co-t. ∠ ACB : rad. (III. 36)
Or rad. : co-t. given angle : : tan. given leg : ſin. req. leg.
And is either acute or obtuſe.

3d. *To find the other angle* CAB.
In the triangle, N° 3. the things concerned fall under Rule I. (111)
Then ſin. EH : rad. : : ſin. EI : ſin ∠IHE. (107)
Or ſin. ∠BAC : rad. : : co-ſ. ∠ ACB : co-ſ. AB.
Or co-t. given leg : co-t. given angle : : rad. : ſin. required angle.
And is either acute or obtuſe.

116. PROB-

116. PROBLEM IV.

In the right angled ſpheric triangle ABC, Plate I. Theorem XIV.
Give one of the legs AB
And its adjacent angle BAC } Required the reſt.

1ſt. *To find the other angle* BCA.
In the triangle N° 3. the things concerned fall under Rule I. (111)
Then rad. : ſin. EH : : ſin. ∠EHI : ſin. EI. (107)
Or rad. : ſin. ∠BAC : : co-ſ. AB : co-ſ. ∠ACB.
Therefore rad. : co-ſ. given leg : : ſin. given angle : co-ſ. req. angle.
And is like the given leg. (99)

2d. *To find the other leg* BC.
In the triangle, N° 1. the things concerned fall under Rule II. (112)
Then ſin. AB : rad. : : tan. BC : tan. ∠CAB. (108)
Or rad. : ſin. AB : : tan. ∠CAB : tan. BC.
Therefore rad. : ſin. given leg : : tan. given angle : tan. req. leg.
And is like the given angle. (99)

3d. *To find the hypothenuſe* AC.
In the triangle, N° 2. the things concerned fall under Rule II. (112)
Then ſin. GH : rad. : : tan. CG : tan. ∠CHG. (108)
Or co-ſ. ∠CAB : rad. : : co-t. AC : co-t. AB.
Therefore rad. : co-ſ. given angle : : co-t. given leg : co-t. hypothenuſe.
And is acute, if the given leg and angle are alike; but obtuſe, if unlike. (102)

117. PROBLEM V.

In the right angled ſpheric triangle ABC, Plate I. Theorem XIV.
Given both the legs AB, BC.
Required the reſt.

1ſt. *To find either of the oblique angles, as* BAC.
In the triangle, N° 1. the things concerned fall under Rule II. (112)
Then, as ſin. AB : rad. : : tan. BC : tan. ∠BAC. (108)
Or rad. : ſin. AB : : (tan. ∠BAC : tan. BC : :) co-t. BC : co-t. ∠BAC. (III. 37)
Therefore rad. : ſin. one leg : : co-t. oth. leg : co-t. opp. angle.
And is like its oppoſite leg. (99)

2d. *To find the hypothenuſe* AC.
In the triangle, N° 2. the things concerned fall under Rule I. (111)
Then, As rad. : ſin. HC : : ſin. ∠CHG : ſin. CG. (107)
Or rad. : co-ſ. BC : : co-ſ. AB : co-ſ. AC.
Therefore rad. : co-ſ. one leg : : co-ſ. oth. leg : co-ſ. hypothenuſe.
And is acute, if the legs are alike; but obtuſe, if unlike. (100)

118. PROBLEM VI.

In the right angled ſpherical triangle ABC, Plate I. Theorem XIV.
Given both the angles BAC, BCA.
Required the reſt.

1ſt. *To find either of the legs, as* BC.
In the triangle, N° 2 or 3. the things concerned fall under Rule I. (111)
Then, rad. : ſin. HC : : ſin. ∠HCG : ſin. HG. (107)
Or rad. : co-ſ. BC : : ſin. ∠ACB : co-ſ. ∠BAC.
Therefore ſine of one angle : rad. : : co-ſ. oth. angle : co-ſ. oppoſite ſide.
And is like its oppoſite angle. (99)

2d. *To find the hypothenuſe* AC.
In the triangle, N° 2. the things concerned fall under Rule II. (112)
Then, As ſin. CG : rad. : : tan. GH : tan. ∠HCG. (108)
Or co-ſ. AC : (rad. : :) co-t. ∠BAC (: tan. ∠BCA) : : co-t. ∠BCA : rad. (III. 36)
Therefore rad. : co-t. one angle : : co-t. oth. angle : co-ſ. hypothenuſe.
And is acute, if the angles are like. - (101)
But obtuſe, if unlike.

In theſe ſix Problems are contained ſixteen proportions, which are applicable to the like number of caſes uſually given to right angled ſpheric triangles; and theſe proportions being collected and diſpoſed in a Table, will readily ſhew, by inſpection, how any of the caſes are to be ſolved.

The celebrated Lord NEPIER, the inventor of logarithms, contrived a general rule, eaſy to be remembered, by which the ſolution of every caſe in right angled ſpheric triangles is readily obtained, where the table of proportions is wanting; which rule is as follows.

GENERAL RULE.

119. *Radius multiplied by the ſine of the middle part, is either equal to the product of the tangents of extremes conjunct.*

Or to the product of the co-ſines of extremes disjunct.

Obſerving ever to uſe the complements of the hypoth. and angles.

Lord *Nepier* called the five parts of every right angled ſpheric triangle, omitting the right angle, circular parts; which he thus diſtinguiſhed; the *two legs*, the *complements of the two angles*, and the *complement of the hypothenuſe*; and any two of theſe circular parts being given, the others are to be found by this rule, as is ſhewn in what follows.

Now, In all the proportions about right angled ſpheric triangles, there are, beſides the radius, three things concerned; one of which may be called the middle term in reſpect of the other two; and theſe two, in reſpect of the middle term, may be called extremes.

When the two extremes are joined to the middle, they are called extremes conjunct: But when each of them is disjoined from the middle, by an intermediate term (not concerned), they are then called extremes disjunct; taking notice that the right angle does not disjoin the legs.

If the three parts under conſideration do all join, the middle one of thoſe three is readily ſeen, and the other two are extremes conjunct.

But if only two of the three parts are joined, theſe two are extremes disjunct, and the other term is the middle part.

These

Thefe things duly obferved, the practice of the Rule will appear in the following examples.

Example I. *When the hypothenufe and the angles are concerned.*

The hypoth. is the middle term, and the two angles are extremes conjunct; then by the rule.

Rad. × fin. hyp. = tan. one angle × tan. other angle.

But the comp. of the hypoth. and angles are always to be ufed.

Therefore rad. × co-f. hyp. = co-t. one angle × co-t. other angle.

Hence rad. : co-t. one angle : : co-t. other angle : co-f. hypoth. (II. 163)

From whence are deduced the 6th and 15th cafes.

Exam. II. *When the hypothenufe and legs are under confideration.*

The hypothenufe is the middle term, and the two legs are extremes disjunct, having the angles between them and the hypothenufe.

Then by the rule. Rad. × fin. hyp. = co-f. one leg × co-f. other leg.

But the complement of the hypothenufe is to be ufed.

Therefore rad. × co-f. hypoth. = co-f. one leg × co-f. other leg.

Hence rad. : co-f. one leg : : co-f. other leg : co-f. hypoth. (II. 163)

From whence are deduced the 3d and 13th cafes.

Exam. III. *The legs and an angle under confideration.*

Here the angle and its oppofite leg are extremes conjunct; and the other leg is the middle part.

And thefe being refolved into a proportion by the rule, will produce the 8th, 11th, and 14th cafes.

Exam. IV. *The angles and a leg under confideration.*

Here one angle is the middle, and the other angle and leg are extremes disjunct, the hypothenufe and other leg intervening.

Now thefe being refolved into a proportion, give the 9th, 12th, and 16th cafes.

Exam. V. *The hypothenufe, a leg, and the angle between them, being under confideration.*

Here the angle is the middle term, and the hypothenufe and leg are extremes conjunct.

And thefe being refolved into a proportion, will give the 2d, 4th, and 10th cafes.

Exam. VI. *The hypothenufe, a leg, and its oppofite angle, being under confideration.*

Here the leg is the middle term, and the hypothenufe and angle are extremes disjunct, the other leg and other angle falling between them and the middle.

And thefe being converted into a proportion, from thence the 1ft, 5th, and 7th cafes are deduced.

SECTION

SECTION VII.

Of the Solution of oblique angled ſpheric Triangles.

120. All the caſes in oblique angled ſpheric triangles, except where the three ſides, or the three angles are given, are moſt conveniently reſolved by drawing a perpendicular from one of the angles to its oppoſite ſide, continued if neceſſary; which perpendicular will either divide the given triangle into two right angled triangles, or make two that are right angled, by joining a right angled one to the given triangle.

In drawing this perpendicular, obſerve,

1ſt. It muſt be drawn from the end of a given ſide, and oppoſite to a given angle.

2d. It muſt be ſo drawn, that two of the given things in the oblique triangle may remain known in one of the right-angled triangles.

3d. This perpendicular is to be uſed as a known quantity; and being drawn as here directed, will either fall within or without the triangle, as the angles, next the ſide on which it falls, are of the ſame or of different kinds. (105)

121. PROBLEM I.

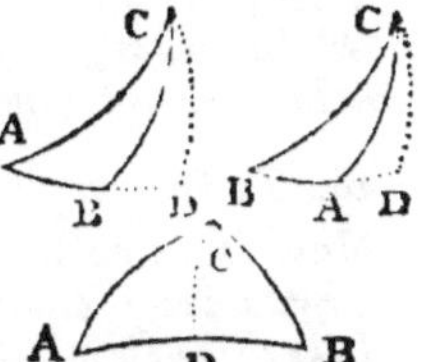

In the oblique angled ſpheric triangle ABC.
Given two ſides CA, CB } Requir. the reſt
And the angle opp. to one, ∠CAB }

1ſt. *To find the angle oppoſite to the other given ſide* (∠CBA).
As ſin. BC : ſin. ∠CAB : : ſin. AC : ſin. ∠CBA. (110)

Or, *As ſin. one ſide : ſin. oppoſite angle : : ſin. other ſide : ſin. oppoſite angle.*
Which may be either acute or obtuſe.

2d. *To find the angle between the given ſides* (∠ACB).
Now rad. : tan. ∠CAB : : co-ſ. AC : co-t. (ACD, call it) m. (3d 114)
Or rad. : tan. given ∠ : : *co-ſ. adj. ſide : co-t. (of a fourth*=) *m.*
And is acute, if AC *and* ∠CAB *are like; but obtuſe, if unlike.*
But rad. : tan. CD : : co-t. AC : co-ſ. (ACD=) m. (2d 113)
rad. : tan. CD : : co-t. CB : co-ſ. (BCD, call it) n
Therefore co-t. AC : co-t. CB : : co-ſ. m : co-ſ. n. (II. 155)
Or co-t. ſide adj. given ∠ : *co-t. other ſide : : co-ſ. m : co-ſ. n.*
And is like the ſide oppoſite the given angle, if that angle is acute.
But unlike that ſide, if the given angle is obtuſe.
Then the angle ſought, viz. ∠ACB= { *ſum of m and n, if* ⊥* *falls within* / *diff. of m and n, if* ⊥ *falls without.* }

* The mark ⊥ ſignifies the perpendicular.

3d. *To find the other side* AB.

Now rad. co-s. ∠CAB : : tan. AC : tan. (AD, call it) M. (2d 114)
Or rad. : co-s. given angle : : tan. adj. side : tan. (of a fourth =) M.
Acute, if the angle and its adj. side are like; but obtuse, if unlike.
But co-s. CD : rad. : : co-s. AC : co-s. (AD =) M.
co-s. CD : rad. : : co-s. CB : co-s. (DB call it) N. (3d 113)
Therefore co-s. AC : co-s. CB : : co-s. M. : co-s. N. (II. 155)
Or co-s. side adj. given angle : co-s. other side : : co-s. M. : *co-s.* N.
Like the side opposite the given angle, if that angle be acute;
But unlike that side, if the angle be obtuse.

Then the side sought AB = { *sum of* M *and* N, *if the* ⊥ *falls within.* / *diff. of* M *and* N, *if the* ⊥ *falls without.* }

But if CA = CB, or if CA = 180° − CB, or if CA is between BC and 180 − BC;
Then ∠B is like BC only.
And if BC is { like / unlike } ∠A; { Then ∠ACB = m ± n only; and AB = M ± N only. }

122. PROBLEM II.

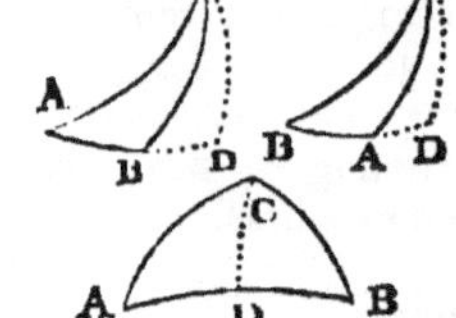

In the oblique angled spheric triangle ABC.
Given two angles CAB, CBA } Required
And a side opposite one of them AC } the rest.

1st. *To find the side opposite the other given angle, viz.* CB.

Then, As sin. ∠CBA : sin. AC : : sin. ∠CAB : sin. CB. (110)
Or sin. one angle : sin. opposite side : : sin. other angle : sin. opposite side.
Which may be either acute or obtuse.

2d. *To find the side included by the given angles, viz.* AB.

Now rad. : co-s. ∠CAB : : tan. AC : tan. (AD, call it) M. (II. 114)
Or rad. : co-s. ∠adj. given side : : tan. the given side : tan. (of a fourth =) M.
Like the angle adj. the side given, if that side is acute; but unlike, if obtuse.
But rad. : tan. CD : : co-t. ∠CAB : sin. (AD =) M
rad. : tan. CD : : co-t. ∠CBD : sin. (DB, call it) N. (2d 115)
Therefore co-t. ∠CAB : co-t. ∠CBD : : sin. M : sin. N. (II. 155)
Or co-t. ∠adj. given side : co-t. other angle : : sin. M : *sin.* N.
Which may be either acute or obtuse.

Then the side sought AB = { *sum of* M *and* N, *if the given angles are alike.* / *diff. of* M *and* N, *if the given angles are unlike.* }

3d. *To find the other angle, viz.* ∠ACB.

Now rad. : tan. ∠CAD : : co-s. AC : co-t. (∠ACD, call it) m. (3d 114)
Or rad. : tan. ∠adj. side given : : co-s. of given side : co-t. (of a fourth =) m.
Like ∠adj. side given, if that side is acute; but unlike, if obtuse.
But co-s. CD : rad. : : co-s. ∠CAB : sin. (∠ACD =) m.
co-s. CD : rad. : : co-s. ∠ABC : sin. (∠BCD, call it) n. (3d 115)
Therefore co-s. ∠CAB : co-s. ∠ABC : : sin. m. to sin. n. (II. 155)
Or co-s. ∠adj. side given : co-s. other angle : : sin. m : *sin.* n.
Which may be either acute or obtuse.

Then

Then ∠ ſought ABC = { *ſum of m and n, if the given angles are alike.* / *diff. of m and n, if the given angles are unlike.* }

But if AC = BC, or to 180° — BC, or is between BC and 180° — BC.
Then BC cannot be unlike its oppoſite angle.
Neither can DB, or the ∠ BCD be obtuſe.

123. PROBLEM III.

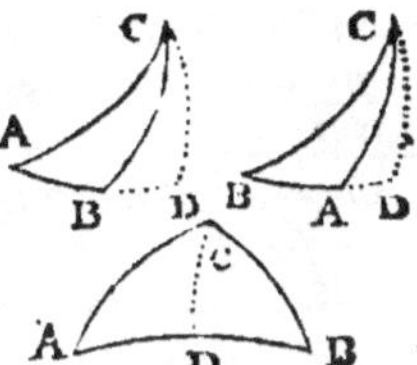

In the oblique angled ſpheric triangle ABC.
Given two ſides AC, AB }
And their contained angle BAC } Required the reſt.

1ſt. *To find either of the other angles, as* ∠ ABC.

As rad. : co-ſ. ∠ CAB : : tan. AC : tan. (AD, call it) M. (2d 114)
Or rad. : co-ſ. given ∠ : : tan. ſide oppoſit ∠ ſought : tan. (of a fourth =) M.
Like the ſide oppoſite ∠ ſought, if the given ∠ is acute;
But unlike that ſide, if the given ∠ is obtuſe.
Take the diff. between AB, *ſide adj. ∠ ſought, and* (AD =) M; *call it* N.
Now rad. : co-t. CD : : ſin. (AD =) M : co-t. ∠ CAB. (1ſt 117)
rad. : co-t. CD : : ſin. (DB =) N : co-t. ∠ ABC.
Therefore ſin. N : ſin M. : : co-t. ∠ ABC : co-t. ∠ CAB. (II. 155)
: : tan. ∠ CAB : tan. ∠ CBA. (III. 37)
Or ſin. N : *ſin.* M : : *tan. given ∠ : tan. ∠ ſought.*
Like the given angle, BAC, *if* M *is leſs than* AB, *the ſide adjacent the angle ſought; but unlike, if* M *is greater.*

2d. *To find the other ſide* CB.

As rad : co-ſ. ∠ CAB : : tan. AC : tan. (AD, call it) M. (2d 114)
Or rad. : co-ſ. given ∠ : : tan. of either given ſide : tan. (of a fourth =) M.
Like the ſide uſed in this proportion, if the given ∠ is acute;
But unlike that ſide, if the angle is obtuſe.
Take the difference between the other ſide, AB, *and* (AD =) M; *call it* N.
Now rad. : co-ſ. CD : : co-ſ. (AD =) M : co-ſ. AC. (2d 117)
rad. : co-ſ. CD : : co-ſ. (DB =) N : co-ſ. CB.
Therefore co-ſ. M : co-ſ. N : : co-ſ. AC : co-ſ. CB. (II. 155)
Or co-ſ. M : *co-ſ.* N : : *co-ſ. ſide uſed in firſt proportion : co-ſ. ſide required.*
Like N, *if the given ∠ is acute; but unlike* N, *if that ∠ is obtuſe.*

124. PROBLEM IV.

In the oblique angled ſpheric triangle ABC.
Given two angles ∠ CAB, ∠ ACB }
And their included ſide AC } Required the reſt.

1ſt. *To find either of the other ſides, as* CB.

As rad. : co-ſ. AC : : tan. ∠ CAB : co-t. (∠ ACD, call it) m. (3d 114)
Or rad. : co-ſ. given ſide : : tan. ∠ oppoſite ſide ſought : co-t. (of a fourth =) m.
Like the angle oppoſite ſide ſought, if the given ſide is acute;
But unlike that angle, if the given ſide be obtuſe.
Take the diff. between ∠ ACB, adj. ſide ſought, and (∠ ACD =) m, call it n.
Then rad. : co-t. CD : : co-ſ. (∠ ACD =) m : co-t. AC. (3d 116)
rad. : co-t. CD : : co-ſ. (∠ BCD =) n : co-t. CB.

Therefore

Therefore co-ſ. n. : co-ſ. m : : co-t. CB : co-t. AC. (II. 155)
: : tan. AC : tan. CB. (III. 37)

Or co-ſ. n : co-ſ. m. : : tan. given ſide : tan. ſide required.
Like n, if the angle oppoſite the ſide ſought be acute;
But unlike n, if the angle is obtuſe.

2d. *To find the other angle* ABC.

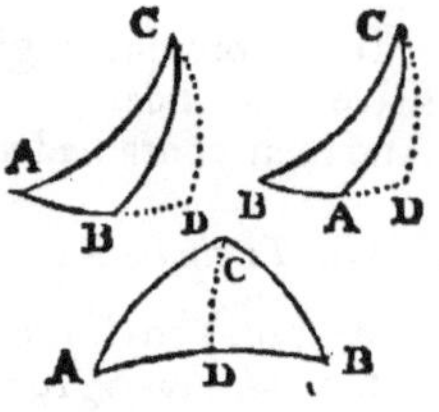

As rad. : co-ſ. AC : : tan. ∠CAB : co-t. (∠ACD, call it) m. (3d 114)

Or rad.:co-ſ. given ſide : : tan. either given ∠: co-t. (of a fourth =) m.

Like ∠ uſed in this proportion, if the given ſide, AC, *is acute;*
But unlike that ∠, if the given ſide is obtuſe.
Take the difference between the other ∠, ACB, *and ∠(ACD =) m, call it n.*

Now rad. : co-ſ. CD : : ſin. (∠ACD =) *m* : co-ſ. ∠CAB. (1ſt 116)
rad. : co-ſ. CD : : ſin. (∠BCD =) *n* : co-ſ. ∠ABC.
Therefore ſin. m : ſin. n : : co-ſ. ∠CAB : co-ſ. ∠ABC. (II. 155)

Or ſin. m : *ſin.* n : : *co-ſ. ∠ uſed in firſt prop. : co-ſ. ∠ ſought.*
Like the ∠ uſed in both proportions, if m *is leſs than the other ∠;*
But unlike, if m *is greater than the other angle.*

125. PROBLEM V.

In the oblique angled ſpheric triangle ABC. Plate I. Problem V.
Given the three ſides AB, BC, AC; Required the angles.
To find the angle ABC.

Let HBKLM repreſent the quarter of a ſphere, the center of which is O. Where the ſemicircular ſections HBK, HLK, are at right angles to one another; and OB is perpendicular to HK.

Then, continuing the ſide BC to L, the arc HML meaſures ∠ABC. (9)
And HQ = $\frac{1}{2}$ chord HL, will be the ſine of $\frac{1}{2}$ (arc HMC = $\frac{1}{2}$) ∠ABC.
Draw the radius OQM; and draw LP, QN at right angles to HK.
Then LP = ſine, HP = verſed ſine, of ∠ ABC; And HN = NP. (II. 165)
But as HQO is a right-angled triangle; OQ being perp. to HL. (II. 125)
Therefore OH : HQ : : HQ : HN. (II. 170)
And OH × HN = $\overline{HQ}^2$ (II. 162) = ſquare of the ſine of $\frac{1}{2}$ ∠ABC.
Make BD = BE = BC; and AF = AG = AC.

Then the ſemicircular plane DCE, which is parallel to HLK (23), will be cut by the ſemicircular plane FCG, drawn at right angles to the plane HBK, in the line CI (II. 209) at right angles to DE. (II. 210)

And the arc DC, and its verſed ſine DI, are ſimilar to the arc HL and its verſed ſine HP. (29. III. 15)

Then rad. CH : rad. DS : : PH : ID = $\left(\frac{PH}{OH} \times DS = \right) \frac{2HN}{OH} \times DS$.

Draw OR parallel to FG; then arc AR = (90° =) arc BK, and RK = AB.
Therefore ∠DIF = (∠KOR = arc RK =) arc AB.
Now DS = (SE = ſine arc DE =) ſine arc BC.
And AD = (BD − BA = BC − BA) = diff. ſides about ∠ ſought.
Alſo ∠DFI = $\frac{1}{2}$ arc(DG = AG + AD =) $\overline{AC+AD}$, the ſine of which is $\frac{1}{2}$ ID. Schol. to art. III. 45.
And arc FD = (AF − AD =) AC − AD, the ſine of which is $\frac{1}{2}$ DF.

 Now

Now ſin. $\angle DIF$: ſin. $\angle DFI$: : ($FD : ID$: :) $\frac{1}{2} FD : \frac{1}{2} ID$. (Schol. III. 45)

Or ſin. $\angle DIF$: ſin. $\angle DFI$: : $\frac{1}{2} FD : \frac{HN}{OH} \times DS$.

Therefore ſin. $\angle DIF \times DS \times \frac{HN}{OH} =$ ſin. $\angle DFI \times \frac{1}{2} FD$. (II. 163)

Therefore ſin. $\angle DIF \times DS \times \frac{HN}{OH} \times OH =$ ſin. $\angle DFI \times \frac{1}{2} FD \times OH$ (II. 156)

Or ſin. $\angle DIF \times DS \times HN =$ ſin. $\angle DFI \times \frac{1}{2} FD \times OH$. (II. 149)

Theref. ſin. $\angle DIF \times DS$: ſin. $\angle DFI \times \frac{1}{2} FD$: : $OH : HN$. (II. 163)

: : $OH \times OH : (HN \times OH =) \overline{HQ}^2$. (II. 155)

Therefore ſin. $\angle DIF \times DS$: ſin. $\angle DFI \times \frac{1}{2} FD$: : $\overline{OH}^2 : \overline{HQ}^2$.

Or ſin. $AB \times$ ſin. BC : ſin. $\frac{1}{2}\overline{AC+AD} \times$ ſin. $\frac{1}{2}\overline{AC-AD}$: : $\overline{\text{Rad}^2}$: $\overline{\text{ſin. } \frac{1}{2}\angle ABC^2}$

$$\text{Theref. ſqu. ſin.} \tfrac{1}{2}\angle ABC = \frac{\text{ſin. } \frac{1}{2}\overline{AC+AD} \times \text{ſin. } \frac{1}{2}\overline{AC-AD}}{\text{ſin. } AB \times \text{ſin. } BC} \times \text{ſqu. Rad.} \quad \text{(II. 164)}$$

Now ſuppoſing Rad. $= 1$, and L. to ſtand for logarithm.

Then 2L, ſin. $\frac{1}{2} \angle ABC =$ L. ſin. $\frac{1}{2}\overline{AC+AD}$ + L, ſin. $\overline{AC-AD}$ — L. ſin. AB — L. ſin. BC. (I. 90, 85, 86)

And putting *l* for the arithmetic complement of a logarithm.

$$\text{Then L, ſin.} \tfrac{1}{2}\angle ABC = \frac{l.\ \text{ſin. } AB + l.\ \text{ſin. } BC + \text{L. ſin. } \frac{1}{2}\overline{AC+AD} + \text{L. ſin. } \frac{1}{2}\overline{AC-AD}}{2}$$

That is, having determined which angle to find,
To the arithmetic complement of log. ſin. of one containing ſide,
Add the arithmetic complement of log. ſin. of the other containing ſide,
And the log. ſin. of the ½ ſum of 3d ſide and difference of the containing ſides,
Alſo the log. ſin. of the ½ difference of 3d ſide and diff. of the containing ſides,
Then the degrees anſwering to half the ſum of theſe four logarithms, found among the ſines, being doubled, will give the angle ſought.

126. PROBLEM VI.

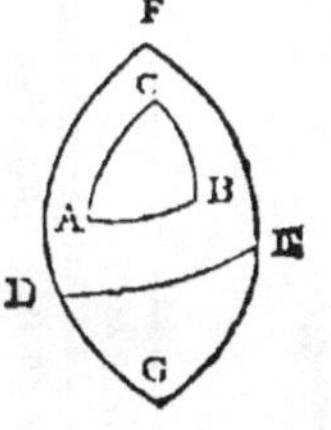

In the oblique angled ſpheric triangle ABC.
Given the three angles A, B, C; Requ. the ſides.
To find the ſide AB.

About the given angles as poles, deſcribe arcs of great circles meeting one another, and forming the triangle FDE.

Then are the ſides of FDE, the ſupplements of the angles A, B, C. (95)

Continue FD, FE, the ſupplements of the angles B, A, adjacent to the ſide AB required, till they meet in G.

Then in the triangle DGE, the ſides GD, GE, are the meaſures of the angles B and A, adjacent to the ſide ſought.

The ſide DE is the ſupplement of $\angle$ C oppoſite the ſide AB.

Now $\angle$ G ($= \angle$ F, by 31) is the ſupplement of AB.

Therefore the $\angle$ G being found in the triangle DGE by PROB. V. (125) will give the ſupplement of the ſide AB required.

That is, Let the given angles be taken as the ſides of another triangle, obſerving to uſe the ſupplement of that angle oppoſite to the ſide required.

In this new triangle find (by PROB. V.*) the angle oppoſite to that ſide where the ſupplement is uſed.*

Then will the ſupplement of the angle thus found be the ſide required.

A Table *containing all the cases of right angled, or Quadrantal, spheric Triangles, with the Solutions and Determinations.*

	Pr.	Given.	Required.	SOLUTION.				Determination.
127.	I.	Hyp. and a leg	∠ op. gn. leg	sin. Hyp.	: Rad.	: : sin. gn. leg	: sin. op. ∠	Like given leg.
128.			∠ ad. gn. leg	Rad.	: co-t. Hyp.	: : tan. gn. leg	: co-s. adj. ∠	{ ac. or ob. as hyp. is like or unl. gn. leg.
129.			other leg	co-s. gn. leg :	Rad.	: : co-s. Hyp.	: co-s. req. leg	{ ac. or ob. as hyp. is like or unl. gn. leg.
130.	II.	Hyp. and an angle	leg. op. gn. ∠	Rad.	: sin. Hyp.	: : sin. gn. ∠	: sin. op. leg	Like given angle.
131.			leg. ad. gn. ∠	Rad.	: tan. Hyp.	: : co-s. gn. ∠	: tan. adj. leg	{ ac. or ob. as hyp. is like or unl. gn. ∠.
132.			other angle	Rad.	: co-s. Hyp.	: : tan. gn. ∠	: co-t. req. ∠	{ ac. or ob. as hyp. is like or unl. gn. ∠.
133.	III.	A leg and its op. ∠	Hypoth.	sin. gn. ∠	: sin. gn. leg	: : Rad.	: sin. Hyp.	either ac. or ob.
134.			other leg	Rad.	: co-t. gn. ∠	: : tan. gn. leg	: sin. req. leg	either ac. or ob.
135.			other angle	co-s. gn. leg	: co-s. gn. ∠	: : Rad.	: sin. req ∠	either ac. or ob.
136.	IV.	A leg. and its adj. ∠	other angle	Rad.	: co-s. gn. leg	: : sin. gn. ∠	: co-s. req. ∠	Like given leg.
137.			other leg	Rad.	: sin. gn. leg	: : tan. gn. ∠	: tan. req. leg	Like given angle.
138.			Hypoth.	Rad.	: co-s. gn. ∠	: : co-t. gn. leg	: co-t. Hyp.	{ ac. or ob. as gn. leg like or unlike gn. ∠.

139.	V.	Both legs	either angle	Rad.	: ſin. either leg	: : co-t. oth. leg	: co-t. op. ∠	Like oppoſite leg.
140.			Hypoth.	Rad.	: co-ſ. either leg	: : co-ſ. oth. leg	: co-ſ. Hyp.	ac. or ob. as legs are like or unlike.
141.	VI.	Both angles	either leg	ſin. eith. ∠	: Rad.	: : co-ſ. other ∠	: co-ſ. op. leg	Like oppoſite angle.
142.			Hypoth.	Rad.	: co-t. either ∠	: : co-t. oth. ∠	: co-ſ. Hyp.	ac. or ob. as ∠s are like or unlike.

143. In a quadrantal triangle, if the quadrantal ſide be called radius; the ſupplement of the angle oppoſite to that ſide be called hypothenuſe; the other ſides be called angles, and their oppoſite angles be called legs: Then the ſolution of all the caſes will be as in this table; obſerving, that where the kind of a ſide or angle is determined by the hypothenuſe; or the hypothenuſe is to be determined; to uſe unlike inſtead of like, and like inſtead of unlike.

In this table, beſide the contractions for ſine, tangent, co-ſine, co-tangent; *op.* ſtands for oppoſite; *adj.* for adjacent; *oth.* for other; *cith.* for either; *ac.* for acute; *ob.* for obtuſe; *gn.* for given; *lik. unl.* for like, unlike; *req.* for required; *ang.* or ∠, for angle.

A TABLE *containing all the cases of Oblique angled Spheric Triangles, with the Solutions and Determinations.*

	[illegible]	*Given.*	*Required.*	SOLUTION.	*Determination.*
144.	I.	Two sides and an angle op. to one	∠ op. oth. sid.	sin. one side : sin. op. ∠ : : sin. other side : sin. op. ∠	either acute or obtuse.
145.			∠ bet. gn. sid.	Rad. : tan. given ∠ : : co-s. adj. side : co-t. m co-t. sid. adj. gn. ∠ : co-t. other side : : co-s. m : co-s. n Then req. angle is either equal to sum, or diff. of m and n	{ acute or obtuse as given angle and its adjacent side are like or unlike. { like or unlike side op. given angle as that angle is acute or obtuse. as given sides are like or unlike.
146.			other side	Rad. : co-s. given ∠ : : tan. adj. side : tan. M. co-s. S. adj. gn. ∠ : co-s. other S. : : co-s. M : co-s. N Then required side = sum or difference of M and N	{ acute or obtuse as given angle and its adjacent side are like or unlike. { like or unlike side op. given angl. as that angle is acute or obtuse. as the given sides are like or unlike.
147.	II.	Two angles and a side op. to one	S. op. other ∠	sin. one angle : si. opposite S. : : sin. other ∠ : sin. op. S.	either acute or obtuse.
148.			S. bet. gn. ∠s	Rad. : co-s. ∠ adj. gn. S. : : tan. given S. : tan. M co-t. ∠ adj. gn. S : co-t. other angle : : sin. M : sin. N Then required side = sum or difference of M and N	{ like or unlike ang. adj. given side, as that side is acute or obtuse. either acute or obtuse. { as the given angles are like or unlike.
149.			other angle	Rad. : tan. ∠ adj. gn. S : : co-s. given side : co-t. m co-t. ∠ adj. gn. S. : co-s. other angle : : sin. m : sin. n Then required angle = sum or difference of M and N	{ like or unlike ang. adj. given side, as that side is acute or obtuse. either acute or obtuse. { as the given angles are like or unlike.
150.	III.	Two sides	either of other angles	Rad. : co-s. given angle : : tan. S. op. req. ∠ : tan. M Take the difference between side adj. req. angle and M, call it N sine N : sine M : : tan. given ∠ : tan. req. ∠	{ like or unlike side op. req. angle, as given angle is acute or obtuse. { like or unlike given angle as M is less or greater than S. adj. req. ∠.

		Given	Sought	Solution	Species
151.		and their included ∠	other side	Rad. : co-s. given angle : : tan. eith. gn. S. : tan. M Take the difference between the other side and M, call it N co-s. M : co-s. N : : co-s. S. 1st used : co-s. req. S.	like or unlike side used, as given angle is acute or obtuse. like or unlike N, as given angle is acute or obtuse.
152.	IV.	Two angles and their included side	either of other sides	Rad. : co-s. given side : : tan. ∠ op. req. S : co-t. m Take the difference between ∠ adj. required side and m, call it n co s. n : co-s. m : : tan. given side : tan. req. S	like or unlike angle op. req. side, as given side is acute or obtuse. like or unlike n, as the angle opposite req. side is acute or obtuse.
153.			other angle	Rad. : co-s. given side : : tan. eith. gn. ∠ : co-t. m Take the difference between the other angle and m, call it n sine m. : sine n : : cos. ∠ 1st used : co-s. req. ∠	like or unlike angle used, as given side is acute or obtuse. like or unlike angle here used, as m is less or greater than other ang.
154.	V.	Three sides	either angle	Call the sides including the angle sought E and F; the opposite side call G. Put D equal to difference between E and F; find the half sum and half difference of G and D. Then. To the Ar. Co. of Log. sine of E, add the Ar. Co. of Log. sine of F, And the Log. sine of ½ sum of G and D; Also the Log. sine of ½ difference of G and D. Take half the sum of these four Logarithms, which seek among the Log. sines; And the degrees and minutes answering being doubled, will give the angle sought.	
155.	VI.	Three angles	either side	Let the given angles be taken as the sides of another triangle, observing to use the supplement of that angle opposite the side required. In this new triangle, find the angle opposite to that side where the supplement is used, by the precepts in Problem V. Then will the supplement of the angle thus found be the side required.	

 SECTION

SECTION VIII.

The Construction and numerical Solution of the cases of right angled spheric Triangles.

156. EXAM. I. In the right-angled spheric triangle ABC.

Given the hypoth. AC=64° 40′ } Required the rest.
And one leg BC=42 12 }

CONSTRUCTIONS.

1st. *To put the given leg on the primitive circle.*

Describe the primitive circle, and draw the right circle AB.

Apply the given leg (42° 12′) to the primitive circle from B to C.

About C, as a pole, at a distance equal to the hypothenuse (64° 40′) describe (68) a small circle *aa*, cutting the right circle AB in A; and draw the right circle CD.

Through C, A, D, describe an oblique circle. (II. 72)

And ABC is the triangle sought.

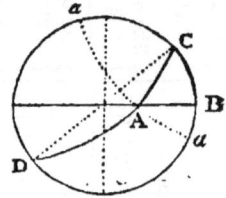

2d. *To put the required leg on the primitive circle.*

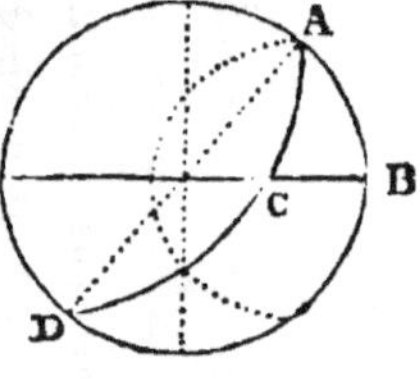

Describe the primitive circle, and draw the right circle CB; on which lay the given leg (42° 12′) to C. (70)

About C, as a pole (66), at a distance equal to the hypothenuse (64° 40′) describe a small circle cutting the primitive in A; and draw AD.

Through A, C, D, describe an oblique circle. (II. 72)

Then ABC is the triangle required: Whose sides and angles are measured by art. 70, 72.

COMPUTATION.

To find ∠ oppos. the given leg.			(127)
As sin. hyp.	=64°	40′	0,04391
To Rad.	=90	00	10,00000
So sin. gn. leg	=42	12	9,82719
To sin. op. ∠	=48	00	9,87110

This angle is acute, because it is to be like the given leg, which is acute.

To find ∠ adj. the given leg.			(128)
As Rad.	=90°	00′	10,00000
To co-t. hyp.	=64	40	9,67524
So tan. gn. leg.	=42	12	9,95748
To co-s. adj ∠	=64	35	9,63272

This angle is acute, because the hyp. and given leg are of like kinds.

To find the other leg.			(129)
As co-s. gn. leg	=42°	10′	0,13030
To Rad.	=90	00	10,00000
So co-s. hyp.	=64	40	9,63133
To co-s. req. leg	=54	43	9,76163

This leg is acute, because the hyp. and given leg are of like kinds.

NOTE, In these operations, and in all the following ones, although the word co-sine, or co-tangent, is used in the proportions, yet the degrees and minutes set down, are not the complements, but the real sides or angles.

157. Ex-

157. EXAMPLE II. In the right-angled ſpheric triangle ABC.

Given the hyopth. AC = 64° 40′ } Required the reſt.
And one angle ACB = 64 35 }

CONSTRUCTIONS.

1ſt. *To put the leg adjacent to the given angle on the primitive circle.*

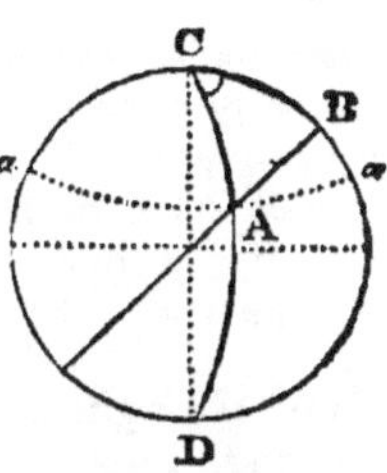

Through any point C, in the primitive circle, deſcribe (75) the oblique circle CAD, making with the primitive circle the angle BCA, equal to the given angle 64° 35′.

In the oblique circle CAD, take CA equal to the given hypothenuſe 64° 40′. (70)

Through A deſcribe the right circle AB.

And CAB is the triangle required.

2d. *To put the leg oppoſite the given angle on the primitive circle.*

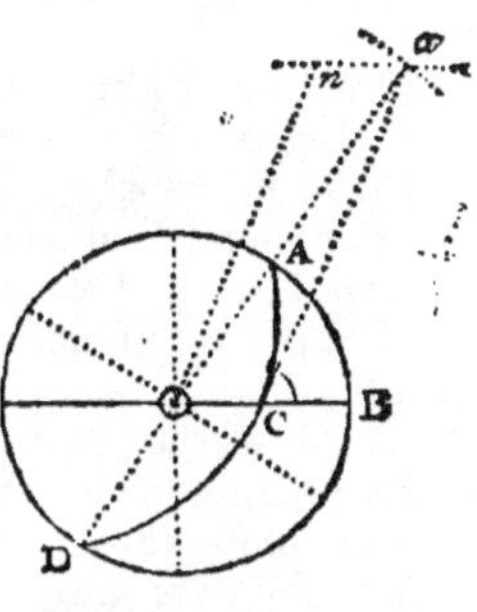

Having deſcribed the primitive circle, and drawn the right circle OB;

Deſcribe (80) an oblique circle ACD, cutting the right circle OB in C, with the given angle 64° 35′, and having the part AC intercepted between the right circle OB and the primitive circle, equal to the given hypothenuſe 64° 40′;

Then ABC is the triangle required.

The ſides required are meaſured by art. 70.

And the required angle by art. 72.

COMPUTATION.

To find the leg opp. the giv. ∠ (130)				*To find the leg adj. the giv.* ∠ (131)			
As Rad.	=90° 00′		10,00000	As Rad.	=90° 00′		10,00000
To ſin. hyp.	=64	40	9,95609	To tan. hyp.	=64	40	10,32476
So ſin. given ∠	=64	35	9,95579	So co-ſ. given ∠	=64	35	9,63266
To ſin. op. leg	=54	43	9,91188	To tan. adj. leg	=42	12	9,95742

Like the given angle.

Acute, as the hypothenuſe and given angle are of like kind.

To find the other angle. (132)

As Rad. ——	=90° 00′	10,00000
To co-ſ. hyp. ——	=64 40	9,63133
So tan. given angle	=64 35	10,32313
To co-t. required angle	=48 00	9,95446

And is acute, as the hypothenuſe and given angle are of like kind.

158. Example III. In the right angled spheric triangle ABC.

Given one leg CB = 42° 12′ } Required the rest.
And its opp. angle CAB = 48 00 }

Constructions.

1st. *To put the required leg on the primitive circle.*

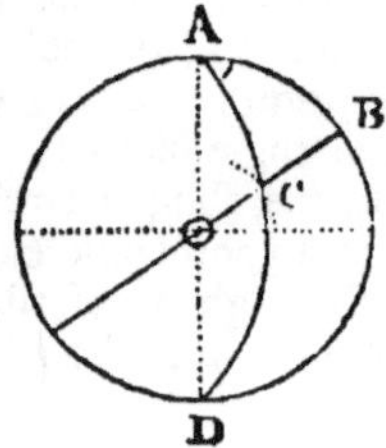

Describe an oblique circle ACD (75), making with the primitive circle the angle CAB, equal to the given angle 48° 00′.

About the center o of the primitive circle describe (67) a small circle at the distance of the complement of the given leg 42° 12′, cutting ACD in C.

Draw the right circle OCB, and ACB is the triangle sought.

2d. *To put the given leg on the primitive circle.*

Draw the right circle OAB, and another OE at right angles.

Make BC equal to the given leg 42° 12′; draw the diameter CD, and another OP at right angles.

About F, the pole of AB, describe a small circle (68), at the distance of the given angle 48° 00′, cutting OP in P.

About P, as a pole (62), describe the oblique circle CAD, cutting AB in A. Then CBA is the triangle required.

The sides are measured by art. 70, and the angles by art. 72.

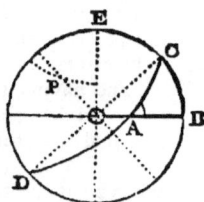

Computation.

To find the hypothenuse.			(133)
As sin. giv. ∠	=48°	00′	0,12893
To sin. giv. leg	=42	12	9,82719
So Rad.	=90	00	10,00000
To sin. hyp.	=64	40½	9,95612

And is either acute or obtuse.

To find the other leg.			(134)
As Rad.	=90°	00′	10,00000
To co-t. giv. ∠	=48	00	9,95444
So tan. giv. leg	=42	12	9,95748
To sin. req. leg	=54	44	9,91192

And is either acute or obtuse.

To find the other angle. (135)

As co-s. given leg ——	= 42°	12′	0,13030
To co-s. given ∠ ——	= 48	00	9,82551
So Rad. ——	= 90	00	10,00000
To sin. required ∠ ——	= 64	35	9,95581

And is either acute or obtuse.

159. Ex-

159. **Example IV.** In the right angled ſpheric triangle ABC.
Given a leg AB=54° 43′ } Required the reſt.
And its adj. angle CAB=48 00 }

Constructions.

1ſt. *To put the given leg on the primitive circle.*

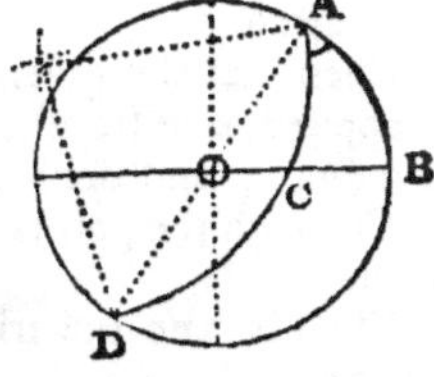

Having deſcribed the primitive, and right circle OB;

Make BA equal to the given leg 54° 43′

Draw the diameter AD.

Through A deſcribe the oblique circle ACD (75) making with the primitive the given angle BAC 48° 00′, cutting OB in C.

Then is ACB the triangle required.

2d. *To put the required leg on the primitive.*

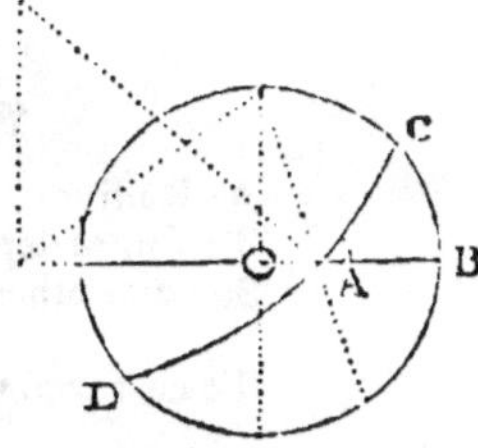

In the right circle OB, take (71) AB, equal to the given leg 54° 43′.

Through the point A, deſcribe (76) the oblique circle CAD, making with AB the angle BAC, equal to the given angle 48° 00′, cutting the primitive circle in C.

Then is ABC the triangle ſought.

The ſides required are meaſured by art. 70.

And the required angle by art. 72.

Computation.

To find the other angle.		(136)	*To find the other leg.*		(137)
As Rad.	=90° 00′	10,00000	As Rad.	=90° 00′	10,00000
To co-ſ. giv. leg	=54 43	9,76164	To ſin. giv. leg	=54 43	9,91185
So ſin. given ∠	=48 00	9,87107	So tan. giv. ∠	=48 00	10,04556
To co-ſ. req. ∠	=64 35	9,63271	To tan. req. leg	=42 12	9,95741

And is like the given angle. | And is like the given leg.

To find the hypothenuſe. (138)

As Rad.	——	= 90° 00′	10,00000
To co-ſ. given ∠	——	= 48 00	9,82551
So co-t. given leg	—	= 54 43	9,84979
To co-t. hypoth.	——	= 64 40	9,67530

And is acute, as the given leg and angle are of a like kind.

160. Ex-

160. EXAMPLE V. In the right angled ſpheric triangle ABC.
Given one leg BA=54° 43′ } Required the reſt.
And the other leg BC=42 12 }

CONSTRUCTION.

To put either leg on the primitive circle.

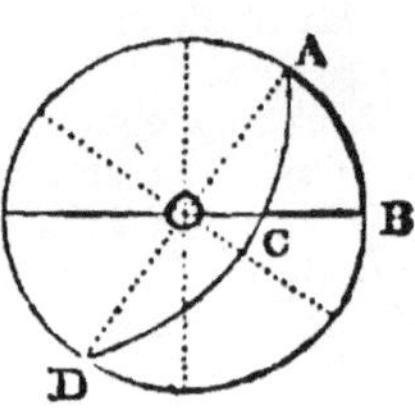

Deſcribe the primitive circle, and draw the right circle OB.

Then, let the given legs 54° 43′, and 42° 12′, be applied, one from B to A, and the other from B to C (74); and draw the diameter AD.

Through the points A, C, D, deſcribe an oblique circle, (II. 72)

Then is ABC the triangle required.

The angles A and C may be meaſured by art. 72.

And the hypothenuſe AC by art. 70.

COMPUTATION.

To find the angle A. (139)

As Radius	——	= 90° 00′	10,00000
To ſin. of leg	AB	= 54 43	9,91185
So co-t. other leg	BC	= 42 12	10,04251
To co-t. op. angle	A	= 48 00	9,95436

And is acute, as the oppoſite leg CB is acute.

To find the angle C. (139)

As Radius	——	= 90° 00′	10,00000
To ſin. of leg	CB	= 42 12	9,82719
So co-t. other leg	AB	= 54 43	9,84979
To co-t. op. angle	C	= 64 35	9,67698

And is acute, becauſe the oppoſite leg AB is acute.

To find the hypothenuſe AC. (140)

As Radius	——	= 90° 00′	10,00000
To co-ſ. either leg	AB	= 54 43	9,76164
So co-ſ. other leg	CB	= 42 12	9,86970
To co-ſ. hypoth.	AC	= 64 40	9,63134

And is acute, as the legs are of the ſame kind.

161. EXAMPLE VI. In the right angled spheric triangle ABC.
Given one angle A=48° 00′ } Required the rest.
And the other angle C=64 35

CONSTRUCTION.

To put either leg, as CB, on the primitive circle.

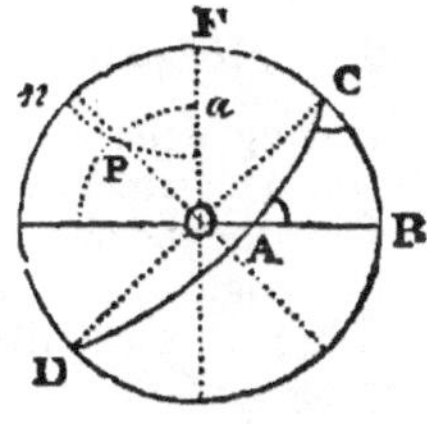

Having described the primitive circle, and drawn the right circle OB;

Then (81) describe the oblique great circle CAD, cutting the primitive circle in the given angle C, and the right circle OB in the given angle A.

The sides are to be measured by art. 70.

COMPUTATION.

To find the leg CB. (141)

As sin. ∠ adj. req. leg	C	= 64°	35	0,04421
To Radius	——	= 90	00	10,00000
So co-s. other angle	A	= 48	00	9,82551
To co-s. of its op. leg	CB	= 42	12	9,86972

And is acute, because the opposite angle is acute.

To find the leg AB. (141)

As sin. ∠ adj. req. leg	A	= 48°	00′	0,12893
To Radius	——	= 90	00	10,00000
So co-s. other angle	C	= 64	35	9.63266
To co-s. of its op. leg	AB	= 54	43	9.76159

And is acute, because the opposite ∠ is acute.

To find the hypothenuse AC. (142)

As Radius	——	= 90°	00′	10,00000
To co-t. either angle as	A	= 48	00	9,95444
So co-t. other angle as	C	= 64	35	9,67687
To co-s. hypoth.	AC	= 64	40	9,63131

And is acute, because the angles are both acute, or like.

162. EXAMPLE VII. In the quadrantal triangle ABC.

Given the quadrantal side AC	= 90° 00′	Required the rest.
an adjacent angle A	= 42 12	
And the opposite angle B	= 64 40	

CONSTRUCTION.

To put the quadrantal side on the primitive circle.

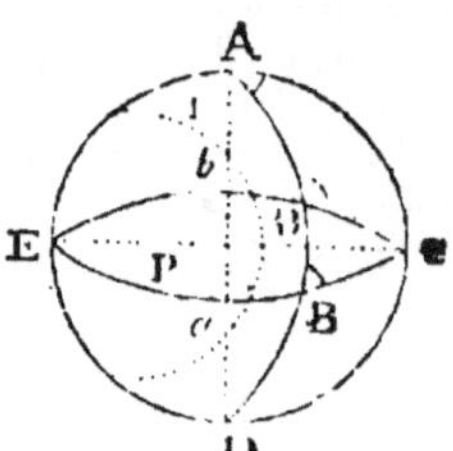

Having described the primitive circle, and drawn the diameters AD, BC, at right angles;

Describe the oblique circle ABD, making with AC an angle of 42° 12′. (75)

Through C describe a great circle CBE, cutting the circle ABD in an ∠ of 64° 40′. (74)

Then is ABC the triangle sought.

The angle C is to be measured by art. 72.

And the sides AB, CB, are measured by art. 70.

COMPUTATION.

Imagine the given triangle ABC to be changed into a right angled triangle, where the supplement of the angle B is to represent the hypothenuse, and the angle A to be one of the legs.

Then will the solution fall under art. 127, 128, 129, in the table; and the numerical computations will be the same as in Example I. Observing that the angles there found are, in this example, the measures of the sides AB, CB; and the side AB in that example stands for the angle C in this.

Now in determining the value of the parts of this triangle, as they arise in the computation, the words like and unlike are to be changed one for the other, where the hypothenuse is concerned in the determination: Thus the leg AB is taken acute, because the supplement of the angle opposite to the quadrantal side, which is here used as the hypothenuse, is unlike the other given angle; and its opposite angle C is to be acute for the same reason: But the kind of the side BC being known by the kind of its opposite angle A, it must be taken acute, as the opposite angle is acute.

In the construction there arises two triangles, either of which will answer the conditions in the example: For the small circle described about P, the pole of the oblique circle ABD, cuts the diameter AD in the points, *a*, *b*; and either of these points may be taken for the pole of the oblique circle wanting to complete the triangle.

Now if *a* be taken for the pole, then in the triangle ABC, the measure of the things sought, will be equal to those arising from the computation: But the angle B is the supplement of what was given.

And if *b* is taken for the pole; then the triangle ABC will arise from the construction; wherein the angles A and B are respectively equal to what is propounded: But then the side AB, and the angle C, will both be obtuse.

SECTION IX.

The Conſtruction and numerical Solution of the caſes of oblique angled ſpheric Triangles.

163. EXAMPLE I. In the oblique angled ſpheric triangle ABC.

Given the ſide	AB = 114° 30′	Required the reſt.
the ſide	BC = 56 40	
And an angle oppoſite to one ſide, BCA	= 125 20	

CONSTRUCTION.

To put the given ſide, adjacent to the known angle, on the primitive circle.

Deſcribe the primitive circle, and draw the diameter BD.

Make BC equal to the ſide adjacent to the given angle = 56° 40′. (70)

Deſcribe the great circle CAE, making the angle BCA equal to the given one, = 125° 20′. (75)

Through B deſcribe a great circle BAD, cutting AE in A, at the diſtance of AB, the other given ſide from B, = 114° 30. (68)

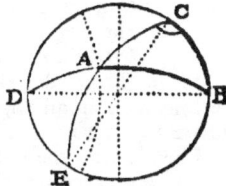

Then ABC is the triangle ſought.

And the parts required are meaſured by art. 70, 72.

COMPUTATION.

To find the angle A, oppoſite to the other given ſide. (144)

As ſin. one ſide	AB = 114° 30′	0,04098	Which may be either acute or obtuſe from the things given: But the conſtruction ſhews it to be acute.
To ſin. op. ∠	C = 125 20	9,91158	
So ſin. oth. ſide	CB = 56 40	9,92194	
To ſin. op. ∠	A = 48 30	9,87450	

To find the angle B between the given ſides. (145)

As Rad.	= 90° 00′	10,00000	As co-t. S. ad. g. ∠ BC	= 56° 40′	0,18197
To tan. giv. ∠ C	= 125 20	10,14941	To co-t. oth. ſide AB	= 114 30	9,65870
So co-ſ. adj ſid. BC	= 56 40	9,73997	So co-ſ. m	= 127 47	9,78723
To co-t. m	= 127 47	9,88938	To co-ſ. n	= 64 53	9,62790

And is obtuſe, as the given angle and its given adjacent ſide are unlike.	Which is acute, being unlike ſide oppoſite given ∠, that ∠ being obtuſe.

Then as the given ſides are unlike, the diff. of m and n, or 62° 54′ = ∠ B.

To find the other ſide AC. (146)

As Rad.	= 90° 00′	10,00000	As co-ſ. S. ad. g. ∠ BC	= 56° 40′	0,26002
To co-ſ. giv. ∠ C	= 125 20	9,76218	To co-ſ. oth. ſide AB	= 114 30	9,61773
So tan. adj. ſid. BC	= 56 40	10,18197	So co-ſ. M	= 138 40	9,87557
To tan. M	= 138 40	9,94415	To co-ſ. N	= 55 29	9,75332

And is obtuſe, as ∠ C and CB are unl.	And is acute, being unl. AB as above.

Then as BC and BA, are unlike the diff. of M and N, or 83° 11′ = AC.

164. Ex-

164. EXAMPLE II. In the oblique angled ſpheric triangle ABC.

Given the angle	BAC= 48° 30′	Required the reſt.
the angle	BCA=125 20	
And the ſide oppoſite to one angle,	AB=114 30	

CONSTRUCTION.

To put the given ſide AB *on the primitive circle.*

Deſcribe the primitive circle; draw the diameter DA; and through A deſcribe the great circle ACD, making the given angle BAC=48° 30′. (75)

Make the arc AB equal to the given ſide= 114° 30′ (70); and draw the diameter BE.

Through B, deſcribe the great circle BCE, cutting ACD in an angle equal to the given angle BCA=125° 20′. (78)

Then is ACB the triangle ſought.

And the parts required are to be meaſured by art. 70, 72.

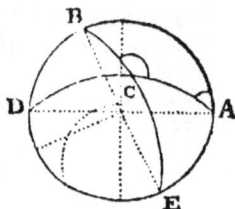

COMPUTATION.

To find the ſide oppoſite the other given angle. (147)

As ſin. one ∠	C=125° 20′	c,08842	Which may either be acute or obtuſe from what is given. But the conſtruction ſhews it to be acute.
To ſin. op. ſide	AB=114 30	9,95902	
So ſin. other ∠	A= 48 30	9,87446	
To ſin. op. ſide	BC= 56 40	9,92190	

To find the ſide AC *between the given angles.* (148)

As Rad.	=90° 00′	10,00000	As co-t. ∠ ad. g. S. A=	48° 30′	0,05319
To co-ſ ∠ ad. g. S. A=	48 30	9,82126	To co-t. other ∠ C=	125 20	9,85059
So tan. gn. S. AB=	114 30	10,34130	So ſine M	=124 31	9,91591
To tan. M	=124 31	10,16256	To ſine N	= 41 19	9,81969

And is obtuſe, being unlike ∠ A, as AB is greater than 90°.	Which may be either acute or obtuſe; either 41° 20′ or 138° 40′.

Then as the given angles are unlike, the difference of M and N, or 83° 12′, is the ſide AC. Or the ſum of 138° 41′, and 124° 31′, leſſened by 180°, leaves 83° 12′.

To find the other angle ABC. (149)

As Rad.	=90° 00′	10,00000	As co-ſ. ∠ ad. g. S. A=	48° 30′	0,17874
To tan. ∠ ad. g. S. A=	48 30	10,05319	To co-ſ. other ∠ C=	125 20	9,76218
So co-ſ. gn. S. AB=	114 30	9,61773	So ſine m	=115 07	9,95686
To co-t. m	=115 07	9,67092	To ſine n	= 52 13	9,89778

And is obtuſe, being unlike ∠ A, as its adj. ſide AB is greater than 90°.	Which may be either acute or obtuſe, viz. 52° 13′, or 127° 47′.

Then as the given angles are unlike, the difference of m and n, or 62° 54′, is the angle B required. Or the ſum of 115° 07′, and 127° 47′, leſſened by 180°, leaves 62° 54′.

165. Example III. In the oblique angled spheric triangle ABC.

Given the side	AB =	114° 30′	Required the rest.
the side	BC =	56 40	
And the contained angle	ABC =	62 54	

Construction.

To put either of the given sides, as BC, *on the primitive circle.*

Describe the primitive circle; draw the diameter BD; and through B describe a great circle BAD, making the given angle ABC=62° 54′. (75)

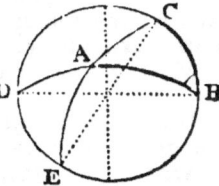

On the circles BCD, BAD, take the arcs BC, BA, respectively equal to the given sides, *viz.* BC=56° 40′, and BA=114° 30′. (70)

Draw the diameter CE, and through C, A, E, describe the great circle CAE; then ABC is the triangle sought.

The required parts of ABC are measured by art. 70, 72.

Computation.

To find the angle C. (150)

As Rad.	= 90° 00′	10,00000	Obtuse, being like side op. req. ∠, the given angle being acute.
To co-s. given ∠ B	= 62 54	9,65853	Take the difference between M and BC, and it is 78° 21′; call it N.
So t. S. op. re. ∠ AB	=114 30	10,34130	
To tan. M	=135 01	9,99983	
As sine N	= 78° 21′	0,00904	And is obtuse, being unlike the given angle, because M is greater than BC, the side adjacent to the required angle.
To sine M	=135 01	9,84936	
So tan. given ∠ B	= 62 54	10,29096	
To tan. req. ∠ C	=125 20	10,14936	

To find the angle A. (150)

As Rad.	=90° 00′	10,00000	Acute, being like side op. req. ∠, the given angle being acute.
To co-s. given ∠ B	=62 54	9,65853	Take the difference between M and BA, and it is 79° 48′; call it N.
So t. S. op. re. ∠ BC	=56 40	10,18197	
To tan. of M	=34 42	9,84050	
As sine N	=79° 48′	0,00692	And is acute, being like the given angle, as M is less than AB, the side adjacent to the required angle.
To sine M	=34 42	9,75533	
So tan. given ∠ B	=62 54	10,29096	
To tan. req. ∠ A	=48 30	10,05321	

To find the other side AC. (151)

As Rad.	= 90° 00′	10,00000	As co-s. M	=135° 01′	0,15039
To co-s. given ∠ B	= 62 54	9,65853	To co-s. N	= 78 21	9,30521
So tan. eith. S. AB	=114 30	10,34130	So co-s. S. used AB	=114 30	9,61773
To tan. M	=135 01	9,99983	To co-s. S. req. AC	= 83 12	9,07333

Obtuse, being like AB, the side used, because the given angle is acute.

The diff. of M and BC, or 78° 21′=N.

And is acute, being like N, because the given angle is acute.

166. Ex-

166. EXAMPLE IV. In the oblique angled spheric triangle ABC.

Given the angle	BCA = 125° 20′	Required the rest.
the angle	BAC = 48 30	
And the included side	AC = 83 12	

CONSTRUCTION.

To put the given side on the primitive circle.

Describe the primitive circle; draw the diameter AD; and through A describe the great circle ABD, making the given ∠BAC=48° 30′. (75)

Make AC equal to the given side=83° 12′. (70)

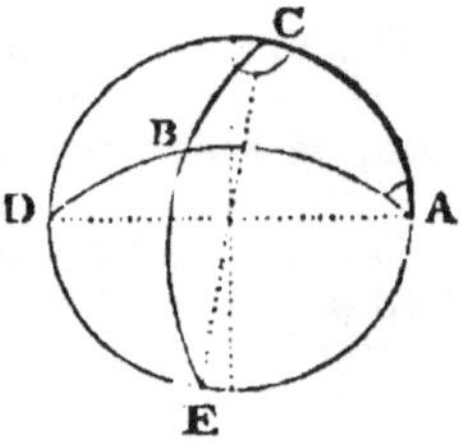

Draw the diameter CE, and through C describe the great circle CBE, making the given angle BCA=125° 20′ (75), cutting ABD in B.

Then is ABC the triangle sought.

And the parts required are measured by art. 70, 72.

COMPUTATION.

To find the side AB. (152)

As Rad.	= 90° 00′	10,00000	Obtuse, being like ∠op. side req. the given side being acute. Take the diff. between m and ∠A, and it is 50° 59′; call it n.
To co-s.gn.side AC	= 83 12	9,07337	
So ta. ∠op. r.S. C	= 125 20	10,14941	
To co-t. M	= 99 29	9,22278	
As co-s. n	= 50° 59′	0,20097	And is obtuse, being unlike n, because the angle opposite to the side required is obtuse.
To co-s. m	= 99 29	9,21615	
So tan.gn. side AC	= 83 12	10,92357	
To tan.req.sid. AB	= 114° 30′	10,34139	

To find the side BC. (152)

As Rad.	= 90° 00′	10,00000	Acute, being like ∠ op. side required, the given side being acute. Take the diff. between m and ∠C, and it is 42° 57′½; call it n.
To co-s.gn.sid. AC	= 83 12	9,07337	
So tan. ∠op.r.S. A	= 48 30	10,05319	
To co-t. of m	= 82 22½	9,12656	
As co-s. n	= 42° 57′½	0,13558	And is acute, being like n, because the angle A opposite to BC, the side required, is acute.
To co-s. m	= 82 22½	9,12283	
So tan. gn. sid. AC	= 83 12	10,92357	
To tan.req.sid. BC	= 56 40	10,18198	

To find the other angle B. (153)

As Rad.	= 90° 00′	10,00000	As sine m	= 99° 29′	0,00598
To co-s.gn.sid. AC	= 83 12	9,07337	To sine n	= 50 59	9,89040
So tan. either ∠C	= 125 20	10,14941	So co-s. ∠ used, C	= 125 20	9,76218
To co-t. m	= 99 29	9,22278	To co-s. req. ∠ B	= 62 54	9,65856

Obtuse, being like ∠ C here used, because the given side is acute.

Take difference of m and ∠A, *viz.* 42° 57′; and call it n.

And is acute, being unlike the angle C here used, as m is greater than the other angle A.

167. Ex-

167. EXAMPLE V. In the oblique angled spheric triangle ABC.

Given the side AB = 114° 30′ }
the side AC = 83 13 } Required the rest.
the side BC = 56 40 }

CONSTRUCTION.

To put either side, as AC, on the primitive circle.

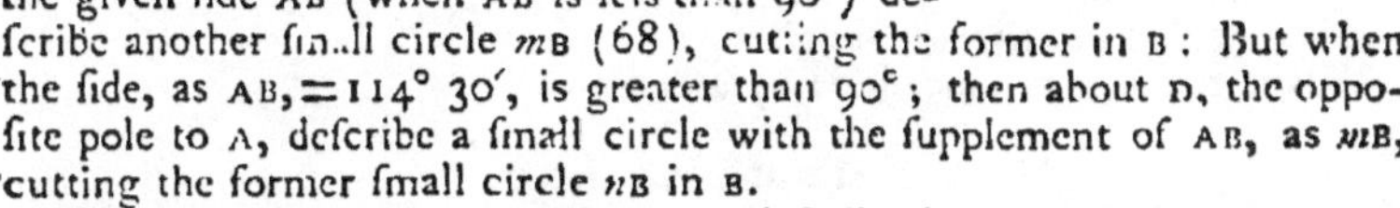

Describe the primitive circle, and from any point in the circumference, as A, set off one of the given sides, as AC, = 83° 13′ (70); and draw the diameters AD, CE.

About C, as a pole, and at a distance equal to the given side BC, = 56° 40′, describe a small circle *n*B. (68)

About A, as a pole, and at a distance equal to the given side AB (when AB is less than 90°) describe another small circle *m*B (68), cutting the former in B: But when the side, as AB, = 114° 30′, is greater than 90°; then about D, the opposite pole to A, describe a small circle with the supplement of AB, as *m*B, cutting the former small circle *n*B in B.

Thro' the points A, B, D, and C, B, E, describe the great circles ABD, CBE. Then is ABC the triangle sought, and the angles are measured by art. 72.

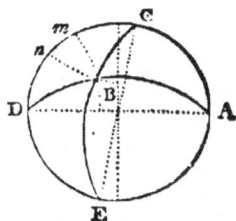

COMPUTATION.

To find the angle C. (154)

Here AC = E = 83° 13′		Ar. Co sine E	= 83° 13′	0,00305
CB = F = 56 40		Ar. Co. sine F	= 56 40	0,07806
		Sine ½ sum	= 70 31½	9,97441
E − F = D = 26 33		Sine ½ diff.	= 43 58½	9,84158
AB = G = 114 30				
		Sum of the four Log. -		19,89710
G + D = 141 03	70° 31′½ = ½ sum			
		½ sum is sin. of 62° 39½′ -		9,94855
G − D = 87 57	43 58½ = ½ diff.			
		Which doubled gives 125° 19′ = ∠C.		

To find the angle A. (154)

Here AB = E = 114° 30′		Ar. Co. sine E	= 114° 30′	0,04098
AC = F = 83 13		Ar. Co. sine F	= 83 13	0,00305
		Sine ½ sum	= 43 58½	9,84158
E − F = D = 31 17		Sine ½ diff.	= 12 41½	9,34184
BC = G = 56 40				
		Sum of four Log. - -		19,22745
G + D = 87 57	43° 58′½ = ½ sum			
		½ sum is sin. of 24° 15′½ -		9,61372
G − D = 25 23	12 41½ = ½ diff.			
		Which doubled gives 48° 31′ = ∠A.		

To find the angle B. (154)

Here AB = E = 114° 30′		Ar. Co. sine E	= 114° 30′	0,04098
BC = F = 56 40		Ar. Co. sine F	= 56 40	0,07806
		Sine ½ sum	= 70 31½	9,97441
E − F = D = 57 50		Sine ½ diff.	= 12 41½	9,34184
AC = G = 83 13				
		Sum of four Log. - -		19,43529
G + D = 141 0	70° 31′½ = ½ sum			
		½ sum is sin. of 31° 28′ -		9,71764
G − D = 25 23	12 41½ = ½ diff.	Which doubled gives 62° 56′ = ∠B.		

168. Ex-

168. Example VI. In the oblique angled spheric triangle ABC.

Given the angle A = 48° 31′ ⎫
the angle B = 62 52 ⎬ Required the rest.
the angle C = 125 20 ⎭

Construction.

To put either two angles, as C and B, at the primitive.

Describe the primitive circle, draw the diameters CD and EF at right angles to one another; and thro' C describe a great circle CAD, making the angle BCA equal to the given angle C=125° 20′. (75)

Describe a great circle BAG, cutting the given great circles CFD, CAD, in the given angles B= 62° 52′, and A=48° 31′. (81)

Then is ABC the triangle sought.

Where the sides are measured by art. 70.

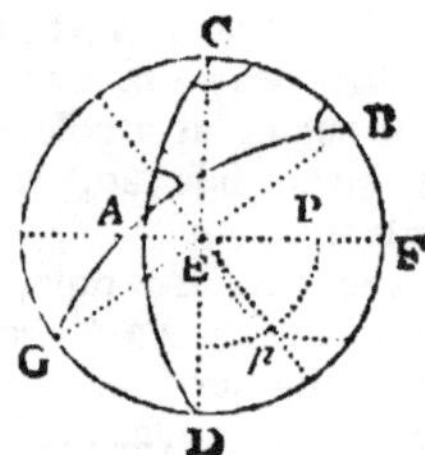

Computation.

To find the side AB. (155)

Here ∠B=E= 62°52′		Ar. Co. sine E = 62°52′	0,05064
∠A=F= 48 31		Ar. Co. sine F = 48 31	0,12543
		Sine ½ sum = 34 30½	9,75322
E—F=D= 14 21		Sine ½ diff. = 20 09½	9,53733
Sup. ∠C=G= 54 40			
		Sum of the four Log.	19,46662
G+D= 69 0	34°30½′=½ sum		
		½ sum is sin. of 32° 45½′	9,73331
G—D= 40 19	20 09½=½ diff.		
		The sup. of its double is 114° 29′=AB.	

To find the side AC. (155)

Here ∠C=E=125°20′		Ar. Co. sine E =125°20′	0,08842
∠A=F= 48 31		Ar. Co. sine F = 48 31	0,12543
		Sine ½ sum = 96 58½	9,99677
E—F=D= 76 49		Sine ½ diff. = 20 09½	9,53733
Sup. ∠B=G=117 08			
		Sum of four Log.	19,74795
G+D=193 57	96°58½′=½ sum		
		½ sum is sin. of 48° 25½′	9,87397
G—D= 40 19	20 09½=½ diff.		
		The sup. of its double is 83° 09′=CA.	

To find the side BC. (155)

Here ∠C=E=125°20′		Ar. Co. sine E =125°20′	0,08842
∠B=F= 62 52		Ar. Co. sine F = 62 52	0,05064
		Sine ½ sum = 96 58½	9,99677
E—F=D= 62 28		Sine ½ diff. = 34 30½	9,75322
Sup. ∠A=G=131 29			
		Sum of four Log.	19,88905
G+D=193 57	96°58½′=½ sum		
		½ sum is the sin. of 61° 39′	9,94452
G—D= 69 01	34 30½=½ diff.		
		The sup. of its double is 56° 42′=BC.	

SECTION X.

169. The principles already delivered have been ſhewn ſufficient for deriving methods for the ſolution of all the caſes in ſpherical Trigonometry: yet as there are many other uſeful and curious particulars which appertain to the ſubject, it was thought proper to add ſome of them for the entertainment of ſpeculative readers. The chief of theſe relations cannot, perhaps, be better inveſtigated, than by imitating the method of the late William Jones, Eſq. who publiſhed in the year 1747, in the Philoſophical Tranſactions, N° 483, ſome properties of Goniometrical lines; which properties are moſtly derived from a general figure which Mr. Jones improved from one communicated to him by the great Dr. Halley. See *Synopſis Palmariorum Matheſeos*, p. 245.

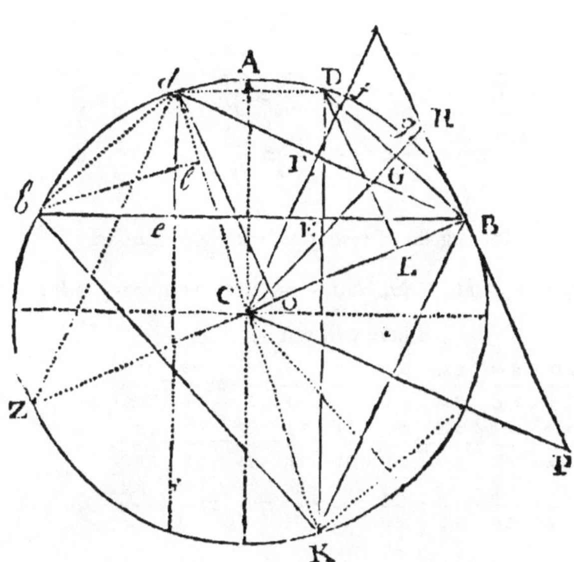

Let AB, AD; or A*b*, A*d*, be any two arcs, each leſs than 90 degrees. B*e* and BE, or *b*E and *be*, be the ſum and difference of their right ſines. KE and DE, the ſum and difference of their co-ſines.

The arcs B*d*, BD; or *b*D, *bd*; expreſs the ſum and difference of the arcs AB, AD. *d*O, DL, are ſines of the arcs B*d*, BD, the ſum and difference of arcs AB, AD: BO, BL, the verſed ſines of that ſum and difference. ZO, ZL = L*d*, the verſed ſines of the ſupplements of their ſum and diff.

Let

Let the arcs B*f*, B*g*, be the half sum, and half diff. of the arcs AB, AD.

BF, BG, the sines
CF, CG, the co-sines
BI, BH, the tangents
CI, CH, the secants
B*d*, BD, twice the sines
KB, K*b*, twice the co-sines
} of the half sum and half diff. of AB and AD.

PB, PC, the co-tangent and the co-secant of the half sum of the arcs AB, AD.

Now the following set of triangles being similar,

viz. CBG, B*de*, KBE, K*bl*, DBL, CHB, BHG, K*db*.

$$\text{Then} \frac{CB}{CG}=\frac{Bd}{Be}=\frac{KB}{KE}=\frac{Kb}{Kl}=\frac{BD}{DL}=\frac{CH}{CB}=\frac{BH}{BG}=\frac{Kd}{Kb}$$

$$\frac{CB}{BG}=\frac{Bd}{de}=\frac{KB}{BE}=\frac{Kb}{bl}=\frac{BD}{BL}=\frac{CH}{BH}=\frac{BH}{HG}=\frac{Kd}{db}$$

$$\frac{CG}{BG}=\frac{Be}{de}=\frac{KE}{BE}=\frac{Kl}{bl}=\frac{DL}{BL}=\frac{CB}{BH}=\frac{BG}{HG}=\frac{Kb}{db}.$$

The following set of triangles being also similar,

viz. CBF, BDE, K*b*E, z*d*O, *d*BO, CIB, BIF, PCB, PIC, K*d*B.

There will result,

$$\frac{CB}{CF}=\frac{BD}{BE}=\frac{Kb}{KE}=\frac{zd}{ZO}=\frac{Bd}{do}=\frac{CI}{CB}=\frac{BI}{BF}=\frac{PC}{PB}=\frac{PI}{PC}=\frac{Kd}{BK}$$

$$\frac{CB}{BF}=\frac{BD}{DE}=\frac{Kb}{Eb}=\frac{zd}{do}=\frac{Bd}{BO}=\frac{CI}{BI}=\frac{BI}{IF}=\frac{CP}{CB}=\frac{PI}{CI}=\frac{dK}{dB}$$

$$\frac{CF}{BF}=\frac{BE}{DE}=\frac{KE}{Eb}=\frac{ZO}{do}=\frac{do}{BO}=\frac{CB}{BI}=\frac{BF}{IF}=\frac{PB}{CB}=\frac{PC}{CI}=\frac{BK}{Bd}.$$

[illegible]. Now the ſeveral values of the radius CB being collected, are placed in [illegible] annexed table; where the letters s, t, ſ, v, ſtand for the ſine, tangent, ſecant, [illegible]ed ſine; and the letters $s^{\backprime}$, $t^{\backprime}$, ${}^{\backprime}\text{ſ}$, the co-ſine, co-tangent, co-ſecant, of the arcs [illegible], a; or of the arcs $\frac{1}{2}\overline{A+a}$, $\frac{1}{2}\overline{A-a}$; and $v^{\backprime}$, the verſed ſine of the ſupplement.

Goniometrical Properties.

(171) $\frac{s^{\backprime},A+s^{\backprime},a}{s,A+s,a}\times t,\frac{1}{2}\overline{A+a}.$	(172) $\frac{s^{\backprime},A+s^{\backprime},a}{s,A-s,a}\times t,\frac{1}{2}\overline{A-a}.$	(173) $\frac{2s^{\backprime},\frac{1}{2}\overline{A-a}}{s,A+s,a}\times s,\frac{1}{2}\overline{A+a}.$	(174) $\frac{2s^{\backprime},\frac{1}{2}\overline{A-a}}{s^{\backprime},A+s^{\backprime},a}\times s^{\backprime},\frac{1}{2}\overline{A+a}.$
(175) $\frac{s,A+s,a}{s^{\backprime},A+s^{\backprime},a}\times t^{\backprime},\frac{1}{2}\overline{A+a}.$	(176) $\frac{s,A-s,a}{s^{\backprime},A+s^{\backprime},a}\times t^{\backprime},\frac{1}{2}\overline{A-a}.$	(177) $\frac{s,A+s,a}{2s^{\backprime},\frac{1}{2}\overline{A-a}}\times \text{ſ},\frac{1}{2}\overline{A+a}.$	(178) $\frac{s^{\backprime},A+s^{\backprime},a}{2s,\frac{1}{2}\overline{A-a}}\times \text{ſ},\frac{1}{2}\overline{A+a}.$
(179) $\frac{s,A-s,a}{s^{\backprime},a-s^{\backprime},A}\times t,\frac{1}{2}\overline{A+a}.$	(180) $\frac{s,A+s,a}{s^{\backprime},a-s^{\backprime},A}\times t,\frac{1}{2}\overline{A-a}.$	(181) $\frac{2s,\frac{1}{2}\overline{A-a}}{s^{\backprime},a-s^{\backprime},A}\times s,\frac{1}{2}\overline{A+a}.$	(182) $\frac{2s,\frac{1}{2}\overline{A-a}}{s,A-s,a}\times s^{\backprime},\frac{1}{2}\overline{A+a}.$
(183) $\frac{s^{\backprime},a-s^{\backprime},A}{s,A-s,a}\times t^{\backprime},\frac{1}{2}\overline{A+a}.$	(184) $\frac{s^{\backprime},a-s^{\backprime},A}{s,a+s,A}\times t^{\backprime},\frac{1}{2}\overline{A-a}.$	(185) $\frac{s^{\backprime},a-s^{\backprime},A}{2s,\frac{1}{2}\overline{A-a}}\times {}^{\backprime}\text{ſ},\frac{1}{2}\overline{A-a}.$	(186) $\frac{s,A-s,a}{2s,\frac{1}{2}\overline{A-a}}\times \text{ſ},\frac{1}{2}\overline{A+a}.$
(187) $\frac{s^{\backprime},\frac{1}{2}\overline{A+a}}{s,\frac{1}{2}\overline{A+a}}\times t,\frac{1}{2}\overline{A+a}.$	(188) $\frac{s^{\backprime},\frac{1}{2}\overline{A-a}}{s,\frac{1}{2}\overline{A-a}}\times t,\frac{1}{2}\overline{A-a}.$	(189) $\frac{2s^{\backprime},\frac{1}{2}\overline{A+a}}{s,\overline{A+a}}\times s,\frac{1}{2}\overline{A+a}.$	(190) $\frac{2s^{\backprime},\frac{1}{2}\overline{A-a}}{s,\overline{A-a}}\times s,\frac{1}{2}\overline{A-a}.$
(191) $\frac{v^{\backprime},\overline{A+a}}{s,\overline{A+a}}\times t,\frac{1}{2}\overline{A+a}.$	(192) $\frac{v^{\backprime},\overline{A-a}}{s,\overline{A-a}}\times t,\frac{1}{2}\overline{A-a}.$	(193) $\frac{2s,\frac{1}{2}\overline{A+a}}{v,\overline{A+a}}\times s,\frac{1}{2}\overline{A+a}.$	(194) $\frac{2s,\frac{1}{2}\overline{A-a}}{v,\overline{A-a}}\times s,\frac{1}{2}\overline{A-a}.$
(195) $\frac{s,\overline{A+a}}{v,\overline{A+a}}\times t,\frac{1}{2}\overline{A+a}.$	(196) $\frac{s,\overline{A-a}}{v,\overline{A-a}}\times t,\frac{1}{2}\overline{A-a}.$	(197) $\frac{2s^{\backprime},\frac{1}{2}\overline{A+a}}{v^{\backprime},\frac{1}{2}\overline{A+a}}\times s^{\backprime},\frac{1}{2}\overline{A+a}.$	(198) $\frac{2s^{\backprime},\frac{1}{2}\overline{A-a}}{v^{\backprime},\overline{A-a}}\times s^{\backprime},\frac{1}{2}\overline{A-a}.$
(199) $\frac{t,\frac{1}{2}\overline{A+a}}{\text{ſ},\frac{1}{2}\overline{A+a}}\times \text{ſ},\frac{1}{2}\overline{A+a}.$	(200) $\frac{s,\frac{1}{2}\overline{A-a}}{t,\frac{1}{2}\overline{A-a}}\times \text{ſ},\frac{1}{2}\overline{A-a}.$	(201) $\frac{s,\frac{1}{2}\overline{A+a}}{t,\frac{1}{2}\overline{A+a}}\times \text{ſ},\frac{1}{2}\overline{A+a}.$	(202) $\frac{s^{\backprime},\frac{1}{2}\overline{A+a}}{t^{\backprime},\frac{1}{2}\overline{A+a}}\times {}^{\backprime}\text{ſ},\frac{1}{2}\overline{A+a}.$
(203) $\frac{t^{\backprime},\frac{1}{2}\overline{A+a}}{r}\times t,\frac{1}{2}\overline{A+a}.$	(204) $\frac{s^{\backprime},\frac{1}{2}\overline{A-a}}{r}\times \text{ſ},\frac{1}{2}\overline{A-a}.$	(205) $\frac{s,\frac{1}{2}\overline{A+a}}{r}\times {}^{\backprime}\text{ſ},\frac{1}{2}\overline{A+a}.$	(206) $\frac{s^{\backprime},\frac{1}{2}\overline{A+a}}{r}\times \text{ſ},\frac{1}{2}\overline{A+a}.$
(207) $\frac{s,\frac{1}{2}\overline{A+a}}{\overline{\text{ſ}-s},\frac{1}{2}\overline{A+a}}\times t,\frac{1}{2}\overline{A+a}.$	(208) $\frac{s,\frac{1}{2}\overline{A-a}}{\overline{\text{ſ}-t^{\backprime}},\frac{1}{2}\overline{A-a}}\times t,\frac{1}{2}\overline{A-a}.$	(209) $\frac{s,\frac{1}{2}\overline{A+a}}{\text{ſ},\frac{1}{2}\overline{A+a}}\times \overline{t+t^{\backprime}},\frac{1}{2}\overline{A+a}$	(210) $\frac{s^{\backprime},\frac{1}{2}\overline{A+a}}{\text{ſ},\frac{1}{2}\overline{A+a}}\times \overline{t+t^{\backprime}},\frac{1}{2}\overline{A+a}.$

 From

From the preceding table a very great number of properties are readily deduced; ſome of which are here annexed, as examples of its uſe; where analogies are, in general, expreſſed by equal ratios.

211. The $\frac{\text{ſum of the ſines of two arcs}}{\text{diff. of the ſines of thoſe arcs}} = \frac{\text{tan. of half the ſum of thoſe arcs}}{\text{tan. of half the diff. of the arcs}}$. (171, 172)

212. The $\frac{\text{ſum of the co-ſin. of two arcs}}{\text{diff. of the co-ſin. of thoſe arcs}} = \frac{\text{co-tan. of half the ſum of the arcs}}{\text{tan. of half the diff. of the arcs}}$. (175, 180)

213. The $\frac{\text{ſine of the ſum of two arcs}}{\text{ſine of the diff. of thoſe arcs}} = \frac{\text{ſum of the tan. of thoſe arcs}}{\text{diff. of the tan. of thoſe arcs}}$.

For $\frac{s,A+s,a}{s,A-s,a} = \frac{t,\frac{1}{2}\overline{A+a}}{t,\frac{1}{2}\overline{A-a}}$ (211.) And $\frac{s,A+s,A+s,A-s,a}{s,A+s,a-s,A+s,A} = \frac{t,\frac{1}{2}\overline{A+a}+t,\frac{1}{2}\overline{A-a}}{t,\frac{1}{2}\overline{A+a}-t,\frac{1}{2}\overline{A-a}}$ by Compoſition.

Then $\frac{t,\frac{1}{2}\overline{A+a}+t,\frac{1}{2}\overline{A-a}}{t,\frac{1}{2}\overline{A+a}-t,\frac{1}{2}\overline{A-a}} = \left(\frac{s,A+s,A}{s,a+s,a}\text{(III. 47, 48)} = \frac{2s,A}{2s,a} = \right)\frac{s,A}{s,a}$.
Here the arcs A, a, are the ſum and diff. of the arcs $\frac{1}{2}\overline{A+a}$, $\frac{1}{2}\overline{A-a}$.

214. The $\frac{\text{coſ. of the ſum of two arcs}}{\text{coſ. of the diff. of the arcs}} = \frac{\text{diff. of tan. of one and cot. of other}}{\text{ſum of tan. of one and cot. of other}}$: taking the tan. of the ſame arc.

For $\frac{t',\frac{1}{2}\overline{A+a}}{t,\frac{1}{2}\overline{A-a}} = \frac{s',A+s',a}{s',a-s',A}$ (212. And $\frac{t',\frac{1}{2}\overline{A+a}-t,\frac{1}{2}\overline{A-a}}{t',\frac{1}{2}\overline{A+a}+t,\frac{1}{2}\overline{A-a}} = \frac{s',A+s',a-s',a+s',A}{s',A+s',a+s',a-s',A}$

Then $\frac{t',\frac{1}{2}\overline{A+a}-t,\frac{1}{2}\overline{A-a}}{t',\frac{1}{2}\overline{A+a}+t,\frac{1}{2}\overline{A-a}} = \left(\frac{2s'A}{2s'a} = \right)\frac{s',A}{s',a}$.

Here the arcs A, a, are the ſum and diff. of the arcs $\frac{1}{2}\overline{A+a}$, $\frac{1}{2}\overline{A-a}$.

215. The ſine of the ſum of two arcs, into radius; is equal to the ſum of the products, of the ſine of the greater by the co-ſine of the leſs, and the ſine of the leſs by the co-ſine of the greater. And,

The ſine of the difference of two arcs, into radius; is equal to the difference of the products, of the ſine of the greater by the co-ſine of the leſs, and the ſine of the leſs by the co-ſine of the greater.

For $\left\{\begin{array}{l} R\times\overline{\tfrac{1}{2}s,A+\tfrac{1}{2}s,a} = s,\tfrac{1}{2}\overline{A+a}\times s',\tfrac{1}{2}\overline{A-a}\ (173). \\ R\times\overline{\tfrac{1}{2}s,A-\tfrac{1}{2}s,a} = s,\tfrac{1}{2}\overline{A-a}\times s',\tfrac{1}{2}\overline{A+a}\ (182). \end{array}\right\}$ Here $\frac{1}{2}\overline{A+a}$ and $\frac{1}{2}\overline{A-a}$ are the arcs.

Hence $\left\{\begin{array}{l} R\times s,A\text{(the ſum)} = s,\tfrac{1}{2}\overline{A+a}\times s',\tfrac{1}{2}\overline{A-a}+s,\tfrac{1}{2}\overline{A-a}\times s',\tfrac{1}{2}\overline{A+a} \\ R\times s,a\text{(the diff.)} = s,\tfrac{1}{2}\overline{A+a}\times s',\tfrac{1}{2}\overline{A-a}-s,\tfrac{1}{2}\overline{A-a}\times s',\tfrac{1}{2}\overline{A+a}. \end{array}\right.$

216. The

216. The co-ſine of the ſum of two arcs, into radius; is equal to the difference, between the product of the co-ſines, and product of the ſines, of thoſe arcs.

The co-ſine of the difference of two arcs, into radius; is equal to the ſum, of the product of the co-ſines, and product of the ſines, of thoſe arcs.

For $\left\{\begin{array}{l} \overline{R \times \tfrac{1}{2}s,A + \tfrac{1}{2}s',a} = s',\tfrac{1}{2}\overline{A+a} \times s',\tfrac{1}{2}\overline{A-a} \ (174). \\ R \times \tfrac{1}{2}\overline{s',a - \tfrac{1}{2}s',A} = s,\tfrac{1}{2}\overline{A+a} \times s,\tfrac{1}{2}\overline{A-a} \ (181). \end{array}\right\}$ $\tfrac{1}{2}\overline{A+a}$ and $\tfrac{1}{2}\overline{A-a}$ being the arcs.

Then $\left\{\begin{array}{l} R \times s',A \text{(the ſum)} = s',\tfrac{1}{2}\overline{A+a} \times s',\tfrac{1}{2}\overline{A-a} - s,\tfrac{1}{2}\overline{A+a} \times s,\tfrac{1}{2}\overline{A-a}. \\ R \times s',a \text{(the diff.)} = s',\tfrac{1}{2}\overline{A+a} \times s',\tfrac{1}{2}\overline{A-a} + s,\tfrac{1}{2}\overline{A+a} \times s,\tfrac{1}{2}\overline{A-a}. \end{array}\right.$

217. $\dfrac{\text{Radius, leſs the co-ſine of an arc}}{\text{Radius, more the co-ſine of an arc}} = \dfrac{\text{Square the tan. of half that arc}}{\text{Square of the Radius}}$

For $\left\{\begin{array}{ll} R - s',\overline{A+a} = (v,\overline{A+a} =) \dfrac{t,\tfrac{1}{2}\overline{A+a}}{R} \times s,\overline{A+a}. & (195) \\ R + s',\overline{A+a} = (v',\overline{A+a} =) \dfrac{R}{t,\tfrac{1}{2}\overline{A+a}} \times s,\overline{A+a}. & (191) \end{array}\right.$

Then $\dfrac{R - s',\overline{A+a}}{R + s',\overline{A+a}} = \dfrac{tt.\tfrac{1}{2}\overline{A+a}.}{RR}$

218. The $\dfrac{\text{ſum of the ſine \& co-ſine of an arc}}{\text{diff. of the ſine \& co-ſine of that arc}} = \dfrac{\text{Radius}}{\text{tan. of diff. of that arc \& }45^\circ}.$

The $\dfrac{\text{ſum of Rad. and tan. of an arc}}{\text{diff. of Rad. and tan. of that arc}} = \dfrac{\text{Radius}}{\text{tan. of diff. of that arc \& }45^\circ}.$

For if $A + a = 90^\circ$; then $\tfrac{1}{2}A = 45^\circ - \tfrac{1}{2}a$; and $\tfrac{1}{2}a = 45^\circ - \tfrac{1}{2}A$.

Alſo $s',a = s,A$: $s,a = s',A$: and $s,A = t,A \times s',A \div R$. (III. 33)

Then $\dfrac{s',A + s',a}{s',a - s',A} = \dfrac{t',\tfrac{1}{2}\overline{A+a}.}{t,\tfrac{1}{2}\overline{A-a}.}$ (212)

Or $\dfrac{s',A + s,A}{s,A - s,A} = \left(\dfrac{t',\overline{45^\circ - \tfrac{1}{2}a + \tfrac{1}{2}a}}{t,\overline{A - 45^\circ + \tfrac{1}{2}A}}\right) = \dfrac{R}{t,\overline{A \backsim 45^\circ}}$*.

Again, $\dfrac{s,A + s',A}{s,A - s',A} = \left((\text{III. }33)\dfrac{t,A \times s',A \div R + s',A}{t,A \times s',A \div R - s',A} = \right)\dfrac{t,A \times s',A + s',A \times R}{t,A \times s',A - s',A \times R}.$

Then $\left(\dfrac{s,A + s',A}{s,A - s',A} = \dfrac{t,\overline{A+R} \times s',A}{t,\overline{A-R} \times s',A} = \right)\dfrac{R + t,A}{R \backsim t,A} = \dfrac{R}{t,\overline{A \backsim 45^\circ}}.$

---

* This mark ∽ ſhews the difference of the values it ſtands between.

219. The difference of the co-fines of two arcs, is equal to the difference of the verfed fines of thofe arcs.

220. The product of the fines of two arcs, is equal to the product of half the radius into the difference of the co-fines, of the fum and difference of thofe arcs.

That is, $s,\frac{1}{2}\overline{A+a} \times s,\frac{1}{2}\overline{A-a} = \frac{1}{2}R \times \overline{s',a - s',A} = s',\overline{\frac{1}{2}\overline{A+a} - \frac{1}{2}\overline{A-a}} - s',\overline{\frac{1}{2}\overline{A+a} + \frac{1}{2}\overline{A-a}}.$ (181)

Or $s,z \times s,x = \frac{1}{2}R \times \overline{s',\overline{z+x} - s',\overline{z-x}}.$ Putting $z = \frac{1}{2}\overline{A+a}$; $x = \frac{1}{2}\overline{A-a}.$

221. The product of the fines of two arcs, is equal to the product of half the Radius into the difference between the verfed fines, of the fum and difference of thofe arcs.

That is, $s,z \times s,x = (\frac{1}{2}R \times \overline{s',\overline{z+x} - s',\overline{z-x}}$ (220) $=) \overline{v,\overline{z+x} - v,\overline{z-x}} \times \frac{1}{2}R.$ (219)

222. Half the Radius $= \frac{\text{fquare of the fine of an arc}}{\text{verfed fine of twice that arc}}.$ (193)

$= \frac{\text{fquare of the co-fine of an arc}}{\text{fup-verfed fine of twice that arc}}.$ (197)

$= \frac{\text{product of the fines of two arcs}}{\text{diff. of ver. fines of the fum and diff. of thofe arcs}}.$ (221)

223. The fq. of Rad. $= \frac{\text{prod. of the fquares, of the fine and cot. of an arc}}{\text{fquare of the co-fine of that arc}}.$

$= \frac{\text{prod. of the fquares of the co-fine \& tan. of an arc}}{\text{fquare of the fine of that arc}}.$

For $R = \frac{s,A \times t',A}{s',A} = \frac{s',A \times t,A}{s,A}$ (187.) Then $RR = \frac{ss,A \times t't',A}{s's',A} = \frac{s's',A \times tt,A}{ss,A}.$

224. The product of Radius, and the co-fine of an arc, is equal to the difference of the fquares, of the fine and co-fine of half that arc.

For $\frac{s's',\frac{1}{2}\overline{A+a}}{ss,\frac{1}{2}\overline{A+a}} = \left(\frac{v',\overline{A+a}}{v,\overline{A+a}}\right.$ (193, 197) $=\left.\right) \frac{R \times s,\overline{A+a}}{R - s',\overline{A+a}}.$ Put $z = \overline{A+a}.$

Then $\frac{R + s',z - R + s',z}{R + s',z + R - s',z} = \frac{s's',\frac{1}{2}z - ss,\frac{1}{2}z}{s's',\frac{1}{2}z + ss,\frac{1}{2}z}.$ By compofition and divifion.

$\frac{2s',z}{2R} = \frac{s's',\frac{1}{2}z - ss,\frac{1}{2}z}{RR}$ (II. 111.) And $R \times s',z = s's',\frac{1}{2}z - ss,\frac{1}{2}z.$

$= \overline{s',\frac{1}{2}z + s,\frac{1}{2}z} \times \overline{s',\frac{1}{2}z - s,\frac{1}{2}z}.$ (II. 119)

In

In any spheric triangle ABC, if in the side CB produced, be taken BE, BD, each equal to BA, and BG be drawn at right angles to CA.

Then CE = BC + BA is the sum } of the legs including the angle at B.
CD = BC − BA is the diff. }

CG and AG are the segments of the base, or side opposite to the angle B. ∠A and ∠C are called base angles. ∠CBG = a, ∠ABG = c are the vertical angles.

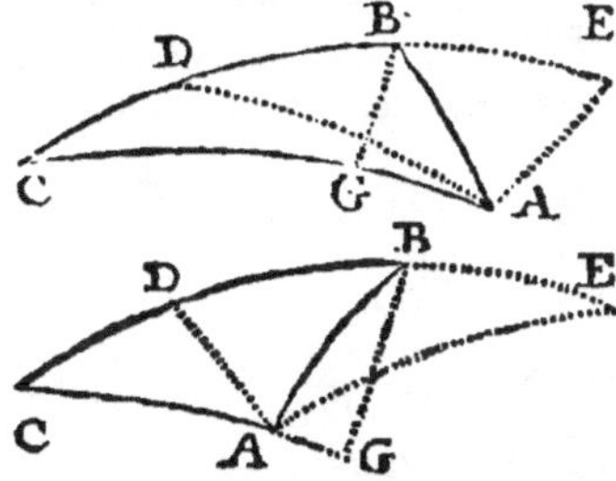

Now a very great number of relations may be formed between the sides and angles; some of which are here enumerated.

225. The sines of the legs, are as the sines of the opposite base angles.

That is, s,BC : s,BA :: s,A : s,C. (110)

$$\text{Hence } \frac{\text{sum of the sines of the legs}}{\text{diff. of the sines of the legs}} = \frac{\text{sum of the sines of the base angles}}{\text{diff. of the sines of the base angles}}$$

by composition.

226. The co-sines of the base angles, are as the sines of the vertical angles.

That is, s',C : s',A :: s,a : s,c. (3d of 122, and 2d of 124)

$$\text{Hence } \frac{\text{sum of co-sines of base angles}}{\text{diff. of co-sines of base angles}} = \frac{\text{sum of the sines of vertical angles}}{\text{diff. of sines of vertical angles}}$$

by composition and division of ratios,

227. The co-sines of the legs, are as the co-sines of the adjacent segments of the base.

That is, s',BC : s',BA :: s',CG : s',AG. (3d of 121, and 2d of 123)

$$\text{Hence } \frac{\text{sum of co-sines of the legs}}{\text{diff. of co-sines of the legs}} = \frac{\text{sum of co-sines of base segments}}{\text{diff. of co-sines of base segments}}$$

by composition and division of ratios.

228. The co-tangents of the legs, are as the co-sines of the adjacent vertical angles.

That is, t',BC : t',BA :: s',a : s',c. (2d of 121, and 2d of 124)

$$\text{Hence } \frac{\text{sum of co-t. of the legs}}{\text{diff. of co-t. of the legs}} = \frac{\text{sum of co-sines of vert. angles}}{\text{diff. of co-sines of vert. angles}}$$

by composition and division of ratios.

229. The tangents of the legs, are as the co-s. of the adjacent vertical angles reciprocally.

$$\text{Hence } \frac{\text{sum of tan. of the legs}}{\text{diff. of tan. of the legs}} = \frac{\text{sum of co-s. of vert. angles}}{\text{diff. of co-s. of vert. angles}}$$

by comp. &c.

230. The

230. The sines of the base segments, are as the tangents of the adjacent base angles reciprocally.

That is, $s,CG : s,AG :: (t',C : t',A ::)\ t,A : t,C$. (2d of 122, and 1st of 123)

Hence $\dfrac{\text{sum of sines of base segments}}{\text{diff. of sines of base segments}} = \dfrac{\text{sum of tan of base angles}}{\text{diff. of tan. of base angles}}$ by composition and division.

231. The tangents of the base segments, are as the tangents of the opposite vertical angles.

That is, $t,CG : t,AG :: t,a : t,c$. (108)

Hence $\dfrac{\text{sum of tan. of base segments}}{\text{diff. of tan. of base segments}} = \dfrac{\text{sum of tan. of vert. angles}}{\text{diff. of tan. of vert, angles}}$ by composition and division of ratios.

232. The $\dfrac{\text{tan. of half the sum of the legs}}{\text{tan. of half the diff. of the legs}} = \dfrac{\text{tan. of half the sum of the base ang.}}{\text{tan. of half the diff. of the base ang.}}$

For $\dfrac{s,BC + s,BA}{s,BC,BA} = \dfrac{s,A + s,C}{s,A - s,C}\ (225) = \dfrac{t,\frac{1}{2}\overline{BC+BA}}{t,\frac{1}{2}\overline{BC-BA}} = \dfrac{t,\frac{1}{2}\overline{A+C}}{t,\frac{1}{2}\overline{A-C}}$. (211)

233. The $\dfrac{\text{tan. of } \frac{1}{2} \text{ sum of base segments}}{\text{tan. of } \frac{1}{2} \text{ sum of the legs}} = \dfrac{\text{tan. of } \frac{1}{2} \text{ diff. of the legs}}{\text{tan. of } \frac{1}{2} \text{ diff. of the base segments}}$.

For $\dfrac{s',BA + s',BC}{s',BA - s',BC} = \dfrac{s',GA + s',GC}{s',GA - s',GC}\ (227) = \dfrac{t',\frac{1}{2}\overline{BC+BA}}{t,\frac{1}{2}\overline{BC-BA}} = \dfrac{t',\frac{1}{2}\overline{CG+GA}}{t,\frac{1}{2}\overline{CG-GA}}$. (212)

Then $\dfrac{t,\frac{1}{2}\overline{BC-BA}}{\overline{G-GA}} = \left(\dfrac{t',\frac{1}{2}\overline{BC+BA}}{t',\frac{1}{2}\overline{CG+GA}}\ (\text{II. } 145) = \right) \dfrac{t,\frac{1}{2}\overline{CG+GA}}{t,\frac{1}{2}\overline{CB+BA}}$. (III. 37)

234. The $\dfrac{\text{sine of sum of legs}}{\text{sine of diff. of legs}} = \dfrac{\text{co-tan. of } \frac{1}{2} \text{ sum of vert. angles}}{\text{tan. of } \frac{1}{2} \text{ diff. of vert. angles}}$

$= \dfrac{\text{co-tan. } \frac{1}{2} \text{ diff. of vert. angles}}{\text{tan. of } \frac{1}{2} \text{ sum of vert. angles}}$.

For $\dfrac{s,\overline{BC+BA}}{s,\overline{BC-BA}} = \left(\dfrac{t,BC + t,BA}{t,BC - t,BA}(213) = \dfrac{s',c + s',a}{s',c - s',a}(226) = \right) \dfrac{t',\frac{1}{2}\overline{a+c}}{t,\frac{1}{2}\overline{a-c}} = \dfrac{t',\frac{1}{2}\overline{a-c}}{t,\frac{1}{2}\overline{a+c}}$.
(212)

235. The $\dfrac{\text{cot. of } \frac{1}{2} \text{ sum of vert. angles}}{\text{tan. of } \frac{1}{2} \text{ sum of the base angles}} = \dfrac{\text{tan. of } \frac{1}{2} \text{ diff. of base angles}}{\text{tan. of } \frac{1}{2} \text{ diff. of vert. angles}}$.

For $\dfrac{t',\frac{1}{2}\overline{A+C}}{t',\frac{1}{2}\overline{A-C}} = \left(\dfrac{s',C + s',A}{s',C - s',A}(212) = \dfrac{s,a + s,c}{s,a - s,c}(226) = \right) \dfrac{t,\frac{1}{2}\overline{a+c}}{t,\frac{1}{2}\overline{a-c}}$ (211)

Hence $\dfrac{t,\frac{1}{2}\overline{A-C}}{t,\frac{1}{2}\overline{a-c}} = \left(\dfrac{t',\frac{1}{2}\overline{A+C}}{t,\frac{1}{2}\overline{a+c}}\ (\text{II. } 145) = \right) \dfrac{t',\frac{1}{2}\overline{a+c}}{t,\frac{1}{2}\overline{A+C}}$. (III. 37)

236. The $\frac{\text{fine of fum of the legs}}{\text{fine of diff. of the legs}}=\frac{\text{fquare of co-t. of } \frac{1}{2} \text{ fum of vert. angles}}{\text{tan. } \frac{1}{2} \text{ fum, into tan. } \frac{1}{2} \text{ diff. of bafe } \angle^{s}}$.

For $\frac{t,\frac{1}{2}\overline{A+C}\times t,\frac{1}{2}\overline{A-C}}{t^{\backprime},\frac{1}{2}\overline{a+c}}=t,\frac{1}{2}\overline{a-c}$. (235)

Then $s,\overline{BC+BA} : s,\overline{BC-BA} :: t^{\backprime},\frac{1}{2}\overline{a+c} : \frac{t,\frac{1}{2}\overline{A+C}\times t,\frac{1}{2}\overline{A-C}}{t,\frac{1}{2}\overline{a+c}}$. (234)

$:: t^{\backprime}t^{\backprime},\frac{1}{2}\overline{a+c} : t,\frac{1}{2}\overline{A+C}\times t,\frac{1}{2}\overline{A-C}$. (II. 151)

237. The $\frac{\text{fine of } \frac{1}{2} \text{ the fum of legs}}{\text{fine of } \frac{1}{2} \text{ the diff. of legs}}=\frac{\text{co-tan. of } \frac{1}{2} \text{ the fum of vert. angles}}{\text{tan. of } \frac{1}{2} \text{ the diff. of the bafe angles}}$.

For $\frac{t^{\backprime}t^{\backprime},\frac{1}{2}\overline{a+c}}{t,\frac{1}{2}\overline{A+C}\times t,\frac{1}{2}\overline{A-C}}=\frac{s,\overline{BC+BA}}{s,\overline{BC-BA}}$ (236). And $\frac{t,\frac{1}{2}\overline{A+C}}{t,\frac{1}{2}\overline{A-C}}=\frac{t,\frac{1}{2}\overline{BC+BA}}{t,\frac{1}{2}\overline{BC-BA}}$. (232)

Then $\frac{t^{\backprime}t^{\backprime},\frac{1}{2}\overline{a+c}\times t,\frac{1}{2}\overline{A+C}}{t,\frac{1}{2}\overline{A+C}\times t,\frac{1}{2}\overline{A-C}\times t,\frac{1}{2}\overline{A-C}}=\frac{s,\overline{BC+BA}\times t,\frac{1}{2}\overline{BC+BA}}{s,\overline{BC-BA}\times t,\frac{1}{2}\overline{BC-BA}}$. (II. 156)

And $\frac{t^{\backprime}t^{\backprime},\frac{1}{2}\overline{a+c}}{tt,\frac{1}{2}\overline{A-C}}=\frac{2ss,\frac{1}{2}\overline{BC+BA}}{2ss,\frac{1}{2}\overline{BC-BA}}$ (195, 193). Then $\frac{s,\frac{1}{2}\overline{BC+BA}}{s,\frac{1}{2}\overline{BC-BA}}=\frac{t^{\backprime},\frac{1}{2}\overline{a+c}}{t,\frac{1}{2}\overline{A-C}}$.

238. The $\frac{\text{cof. of } \frac{1}{2} \text{ fum of the legs}}{\text{cof. of } \frac{1}{2} \text{ diff. of the legs}}=\frac{\text{co-t. of } \frac{1}{2} \text{ the fum of vertical angles}}{\text{tan. of } \frac{1}{2} \text{ the fum of the bafe angles}}$.

For $\frac{t^{\backprime}t^{\backprime},\frac{1}{2}\overline{a+c}}{t,\frac{1}{2}\overline{A+C}\times t,\frac{1}{2}\overline{A-C}}=\frac{s,\overline{BC+BA}}{s,\overline{BC-BA}}$ (236). And $\frac{t,\frac{1}{2}\overline{A-C}}{t,\frac{1}{2}\overline{A+C}}=\frac{t^{\backprime},\frac{1}{2}\overline{BC+BA}}{t^{\backprime},\frac{1}{2}\overline{BC-BA}}$. (232)

Then $\frac{t^{\backprime}t^{\backprime},\frac{1}{2}\overline{a+c}\times t,\frac{1}{2}\overline{A-C}}{t,\frac{1}{2}\overline{A+C}\times t,\frac{1}{2}\overline{A-C}\times t,\frac{1}{2}\overline{A+C}}=\frac{s,\overline{BC+BA}\times t^{\backprime},\frac{1}{2}\overline{BC+BA}}{s,\overline{BC-BA}\times t,\frac{1}{2}\overline{BC-BA}}$. (II. 156)

And $\frac{t^{\backprime}t^{\backprime},\frac{1}{2}\overline{a+c}}{tt,\frac{1}{2}\overline{A+C}}=\frac{2s^{\backprime}s^{\backprime},\frac{1}{2}\overline{BC+BA}}{2s^{\backprime}s^{\backprime},\frac{1}{2}\overline{BC-BA}}$ (191, 197). Then $\frac{s^{\backprime},\frac{1}{2}\overline{BC+BA}}{s^{\backprime},\frac{1}{2}\overline{BC-BA}}=\frac{t^{\backprime},\frac{1}{2}\overline{a+c}}{t,\frac{1}{2}\overline{A+C}}$.

The two laft propofitions folve the problem where two fides, and the included angle, of a fpheric triangle, are given to find the other angles.

Or where two angles and the included fide are given, to find the other fides, ufing the word angles for legs; the given fide for fum of vertical angles; the other fide for bafe angles.

In art. 237, 238, the conclufions were gained from this principle, namely, that *the fides of proportional fquares, are in the fame proportion as thofe fquares.*

239. The

239. The co-sine of an angle, is to Radius;
As the Radius into co-s. of the opposite side, less the product of the co-sines of the including sides,
To the product of the sines of the including sides.

For $\grave{s},CG=(\grave{s},\overline{AC-AG}=)\overline{\grave{s},AC\times\grave{s},AG+s,AC\times s,AG\div R}$. (216)

And $(\grave{s},CG=)\frac{\grave{s},BC\times\grave{s},AG}{\grave{s},AB}(227)=\overline{\grave{s},AC\times\grave{s}AG+s,AC\times s,AG\div R}$.(II.46)

Therefore $\grave{s},BC\times\grave{s},AG=\frac{\grave{s},AB}{R}\times\grave{s},AC\times\grave{s},AG+\frac{\grave{s},AB}{R}\times s,AC\times s,AG$.

Therefore $\frac{R\times\grave{s},BC-\grave{s},AB\times\grave{s},AC}{R}\times\grave{s},AG=\frac{\grave{s},AB\times s,AC}{R}\times s,AG$.

Then $\frac{R\times\grave{s},BC-\grave{s},AB\times\grave{s},AC}{\grave{s},AB\times s,CA}=\left(\frac{s,AG}{\grave{s},AG}(II.\ 163)=\right)\frac{t,AG}{R}$

But $t,AG=\frac{\grave{s},A}{R}\times t,AB$(131). And $\frac{t,AG}{R}=\left(\frac{\grave{s},A}{RR}\times t,AB=\right)\frac{\grave{s},A}{RR}\times\frac{s,AB\times R}{\grave{s},AB}$.
(187)

Then $\frac{\grave{s},A}{R}\times\frac{s,AB}{s,AB}=\frac{R\times\grave{s},BC-\grave{s},AB\times\grave{s},AC}{s,AB\times s,AC}$. And $\frac{\grave{s},A}{R}=\frac{R\times\grave{s},BC-\grave{s},AC\times\grave{s},AB}{s,AC\times s,AB}$.

240. Hence $R\times\grave{s},BC=\frac{\grave{s}A\times s,AC\times s,AB}{R}+\grave{s},AC\times\grave{s},AB$.

241. The versed sine of an angle, is to the square of Radius:
As the diff. of the versed sines of op. side, and diff. of including sides,
To the product of the sines of the sides including that angle.

For (239) $\frac{R\times\grave{s},BC-\grave{s},AC\times\grave{s},AB}{s,AB\times s,AC.}=\left(\frac{\grave{s}A}{R}=\right)\frac{R-v,A}{R}$.

Therefore $RR\times\grave{s},BC-R\times\grave{s},AC\times\grave{s},AB=R\times s,AC\times s,AB-s,AC\times s,AB\times v,A$.

Therefore $RR\times\grave{s},BC+s,AC\times s,AB\times v,A=\overline{\grave{s},AC\times\grave{s},AB+s,AC\times s,AB}\times R$.
$=\grave{s},\overline{AC-AB}\times RR$. (216)

Then $s,AC\times s,AB\times v,A=(RR\times\grave{s},CD-RR\times\grave{s},BC=)\overline{\grave{s},CD-\grave{s},BC}\times RR$.

And $\frac{v,A}{RR}=\left(\frac{\grave{s},CD-\grave{s},BC}{s,AC\times s,AB}=\right)\frac{v,CB-v,CD}{s,AC\times s,AB}$. (219)

242. Hence

242. Hence $\frac{v,A}{2R}=\frac{v,BC-v,CD}{v,CE-v,CD}$. Or $\frac{1}{2}v,A=\frac{v,BC-v,CD}{v,CE-v,CD}$, when $R=1$.

For $(s,AC\times s,AB=)\frac{1}{2}R\times\overline{v,CE-v,CD}\ (222)=\overline{v,CB-v,CD}\times\frac{RR}{v,A}$. (241)

Then $\frac{v,CB-v,CD}{v,CE-v,CD}=\left(\frac{\frac{1}{2}R\times v,A}{RR}=\right)\frac{v,A}{2R}$.

243. The verſed ſine of the ſup. of an angle, is to the ſquare of Radius;
As the diff. of the verſed ſines of the oppoſite ſide, and ſum of the including ſides,
To the product of the ſines of the ſides including that angle.

For (239) $\frac{R\times\grave{s},BC-\grave{s},AC\times\grave{s},AB}{s,AC\times s,AB}=\left(\frac{\grave{s},A}{R}=\right)\frac{v,A-R}{R}$.

Therefore $RR\times\grave{s},BC-R\times\grave{s},AC\times\grave{s},AB=s,AC\times s,AB\times\grave{v},A-R\times s,AC\times s,AB$.

Therefore $RR\times\grave{s},BC-s,AC\times s,AB\times\grave{v},A=R\times\overline{\grave{s},AC\times\grave{s},AB-s,AC\times s,AB}$

$=(RR\times\grave{s},\overline{AC+AB}=)\ RR\times\grave{s},CE$. (216)

Then $RR\times\grave{s},BC-RR\times\grave{s},CE=s,AC\times s,AB\times\grave{v},A$.

And $\frac{\grave{v},A}{RR}=\left(\frac{\grave{s},BC-\grave{s},CE}{s,AC\times s,AB}=\right)\frac{v,CE-v,BC}{s,AC\times s,AB}$.

244. Hence $\frac{\grave{v},A}{2R}=\frac{v,CE-v,CB}{v,CE-v,CD}$. Or $\frac{1}{2}\grave{v},A=\frac{v,CE-v,CB}{v,CE-v,CD}$, when $R=1$.

For $(s,AC\times s,AB=)\frac{1}{2}R\times\overline{v,CE-v,CD}\ (222)=\overline{v,CE-v,CB}\times\frac{RR}{\grave{v},A}$. (243)

Then $\frac{v,CE-v,CB}{v,CE-v,CD}=\left(\frac{\frac{1}{2}R\times\grave{v},A}{RR}=\right)\frac{\grave{v},A}{2R}$.

245. The ſquare of the ſine of half an angle, is to the ſquare of the Radius;
As $\frac{1}{2}$ Radius into the diff. of the verſed ſines of the ſide oppoſite, and diff. of the ſides including that angle,
To the product of the ſines of the ſides including that angle.

For $(v,A=)\frac{ss,\frac{1}{2}A}{\frac{1}{2}R}\ (222)=\frac{v,CB-v,CD}{s,AC\times s,AB}\times RR$. (241)

Then $\frac{ss,\frac{1}{2}A}{RR}=\frac{v,CB-v,CD}{s,AC\times s,AB}\times\frac{1}{2}R=\frac{\grave{s},CD-\grave{s},CB}{s,AC\times s,AB}\times\frac{1}{2}R$. (219)

246. Hence

246. Hence $\frac{ss,\frac{1}{2}A}{RR}=\frac{s,\frac{1}{2}\overline{CB+CD}\times s,\frac{1}{2}\overline{CB-CD}}{s,AC\times s,AB}$ (181)

$$=\frac{s,\frac{1}{2}\overline{CB+AC-AB}\times s,\frac{1}{2}\overline{CB-AC+AB}}{s,AC\times s,AB}\text{; because } CD=AC-AB$$

$$=\frac{s,\overline{H-AC}\times s,\overline{H-AB}}{s,AC\times s,AB}.\text{ Putting } 2H=AC+AB+BC.$$

247. The squ. of the co-sine of half an angle, is to the squ. of Radius;
As $\frac{1}{2}$ Radius into the diff. of versed lines of the side opposite, and sum of the included sides,
To the product of the sines of the sides including that angle.

For $(v',A=)\ \frac{s's',\frac{1}{2}A}{\frac{1}{2}R}\ (222)=\frac{v,CE-v,CB}{s,AC\times s,AB}\times RR.$ (243)

Then $\frac{s's',\frac{1}{2}A}{RR}=\frac{v,CE-v,CB}{s,AC\times s,AB}\times\frac{1}{2}R=\frac{s',CB-s',CE}{s,AC\times s,AB}\times\frac{1}{2}R.$ (219)

248. Hence $\frac{s's',\frac{1}{2}A}{RR}=\frac{s,\frac{1}{2}\overline{CE+CB}\times s,\frac{1}{2}\overline{CE-CB}}{s,AC\times s,AB}.$ (177)

$$=\frac{s,\frac{1}{2}\overline{AC+AB+CB}\times s,\frac{1}{2}\overline{AC+AB-CB}}{s,AC\times s,AB}.\text{ For } CE=AC+AB.$$

$$=\frac{s,H\times s,\overline{H-CB}}{s,AC\times s,AB}.\text{ Putting } 2H=AC+AB+BC.$$

249. The square of the tan. of half an angle, is to the square of Radius;
As the diff. of ver. sines of the side op. and diff. of including sides,
To the diff. of ver. sines of the side op. and sum of including sides.

For $\frac{v,A}{v',A}=\frac{ss,\frac{1}{2}A}{s's',\frac{1}{2}A}\ (222)=\frac{tt,\frac{1}{2}A}{RR}\ (223)=\frac{v,CB-v,CD}{v,CE-v,CB}.$ (241, 243)

250. Hence $\frac{tt,\frac{1}{2}A}{RR}=\frac{s,\frac{1}{2}\overline{CB+CD}\times s,\frac{1}{2}\overline{CB-CD}}{s,\frac{1}{2}\overline{CE+CB}\times s,\frac{1}{2}\overline{CE-CB}}.$ (219, 181)

$$=\frac{s,\frac{1}{2}\overline{CB+AC-AB}\times s,\frac{1}{2}\overline{CB-AC+AB}}{s,\frac{1}{2}\overline{CB+AC+AB}\times s,\frac{1}{2}\overline{AC+AC-CB}}$$

$$=\frac{s,\overline{H-AB}\times s,\overline{H-AC}}{s,H\times s,\overline{H-BC}}.$$

From the articles in the three last pages may be deduced many rules for solving the problem, where the three sides are given to find an angle; and thence, from the three angles given to find a side.

251. When

251. When two ſides and the included angle are given to find the third ſide: Or when the three ſides are given to find an angle; For theſe particular caſes there have been given compendiums by Sir Jonas Moore, in his Mathematics, Vol. II. page 383: Alſo by Nicholas Facio Duillier, in a ſmall tract of his, which is very ſcarce; and by the learned Dr. Pemberton, in the Philoſophical Tranſactions for the year 1760: The principle employed by each of them is the ſame as in Article 245; which will be here illuſtrated on account of its utility in ſome aſtronomical ſubjects.

In the triangle ABC, where CD = AC ∽ AB.

Given AB, AC, ∠A; required BC.

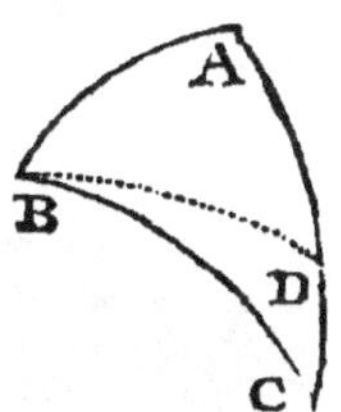

Now $\frac{ss, \frac{1}{2} \angle A}{R^3} = \frac{\frac{1}{2}s`,CB \backsim \frac{1}{2}s`,CD}{s,AC \times s,AB}$. — (245)

And $\frac{ss, \frac{1}{2} \angle A \times s,AC \times s,AB}{R^3} = \frac{1}{2}s`,CB \backsim \frac{1}{2}s`,CD = N$

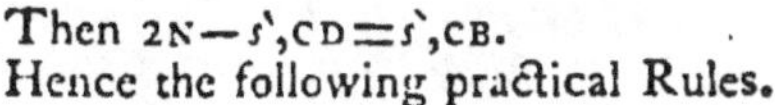

Then $2N - s`,CD = s`,CB$.

Hence the following practical Rules.

252. I. *To twice the log. ſine of half the given angle,*

Add the log. ſines of the two containing ſides;

The ſum, abating three radii in the index, leaves the log. ſine of an arc.

From twice the nat. ſine of that arc; take the nat. co-ſine of the diff. of the given ſides,

Leaves the nat. co-ſine of the third ſide, or of its ſupplement.

253. II. But the ſide required may be found without the uſe of natural ſines. Thus

To twice the log. ſine of half the given angle,

Add the log. ſines of the two containing ſides;

From half the ſum of theſe logs, ſubtract the log. ſine of half the diff. of the ſides.

And the remainder is the log. tangent of an arc;

The log. ſine of which arc, ſubtracted from the ſaid half ſum of logs,

Leaves the log. ſine of half the required ſide.

Take the Example uſed in the ſix caſes of oblique ſpheric triangles.

Where AC = 83° 11′, AB = 56° 40′; ∠A = 125° 20′.

Required BC, which was there found to be 114 30.

Given ∠	=	125°	20′					
its half	=	62	40	—	—		Log. ſine	{ 9,91858 / 9,91858
One ſide	=	83	11	—	—		Log. ſine	9,99692
other ſide	=	56	40	—	—		Log. ſine	9,92194
Arc found	=	40	$53\frac{2}{3}$ its nat. ſine		65467	(256)		9,81602
				its double	130934			
diff. ſides	=	26	30 the nat. co-ſine		89480			
		65	30 the nat. co ſine		41454	(257)		
The ſide required		114	30					

The

The ſaid Example wrought by the ſecond Rule is as follows;

Given ∠ =	125 20				
its half	62 40	log. ſine	{ 9,94858 9,94858		
One ſide =	83 11	log. ſine	9,99692		
Other ſide =	56 40	log. ſine	9,92194		
Sum logs =			39,81602		
half ſum			19,90801	half ſum log.	19,90801
½ diff. ſides =	13 15½		9,36048		
Arc =	74 10	log. tan.	10,54753	Log. ſine 74 10	9,98320
				Log. ſine of 57 15	9,92481
				The required ſide = 114 30	

When the three ſides are given to find an angle;

254. I. *To the nat co-ſ. of the ſide oppoſite the required angle, add the nat. co-ſ. of the diff. of the ſides about that angle; half the ſum is the nat. ſine of an arc. To the log. ſine of that arc, add the arith. comps. of the log. ſines of the ſides about the required angle and alſo the radius.*

The half of this ſum is the log. ſine of half the angle ſought.

Or without uſing the natural ſines.

255. II. *To the log. ſine of half the diff. of the ſides about the angle, add the arith. comp. of the log. ſine of half the baſe; the ſum is the log. ſine of an arc. To the log. co-ſine of this arc, add the log. ſine of half the baſe; reject radius from the ſum, and to the double of what will then remain add the arith. comps. of the log. ſines of the containing ſides.*

Half the ſum is the log. ſine of half the angle.

Exam. Let the three ſides be BC = 114° 30′, AC = 80° 11′, AB = 56° 40′. Required the angle A.

By I. Rule

Baſe BC = 114° 30′					
Its ſupl.	63 30	nat. co-ſine =	41469	(25*)	
Diff. ſides	26 31	nat. co-ſ. =	89480		
Sum			130949	Rad.	10,00000
Half ſum is the nat. ſine. (217)			65474	arc 40° 54′ log. ſine	9,81607
		Ar. co. log. ſine 83 11			0,00308
		Ar. co. log. ſine 56 40			0,07806
					19,89721
		Half the angle ſought 62° 40′ log. ſine			9,94860

By II. Rule.

½ BC = 13° 15½′	Log. ſine	9,36048			
½ BC = 57 15	Ar.Co.L.ſin.	0,07518	log. ſine		9,92482
Log.ſine 15 49½	an arc	9,43566	log. co-ſ. 15° 49½′		9,98322
					9,90804
					2
					19,81608
Ar. Co. Log. ſine AC					0,00308
Ar. Co. Log. ſine AB					0,07806
Sum					19,89722
Half ſum is Log. ſine of 62° 40′					9,94861
Angle ſought is 125 20 = ∠ A.					

As the natural ſines of arcs are not contained in this work, and are on ſome occaſions neceſſary, it will be proper to ſhew how they may be found from the Logarithmic tables contained herein.

256. *Firſt. An arc being given, to find its natural ſine to five places of figures.*

Rule. Take out the Log. ſine of the arc, rejecting the Index;
Seek theſe figures among the logarithms of numbers;
The correſponding number is the natural ſine of the given arc; which is to be reckoned as a decimal fraction of the radius, or unity:
Prefixing the decimal comma (,) if the index of the log. ſine was 9;
But if the index was 8; 7; or 6; prefix ,0; ,00; or ,000; by which means the left hand digit of the natural ſine will ſtand in the place of the firſts, ſeconds, thirds, or fourths. (I. 18)

Ex. I. *Required the natural ſine and co-ſine of* 4° 22′?

Log. ſines	ſine 8,88161	Co-ſine 9,99874
Num. or nat. ſines	0,07614	0,99710

Ex. II. *Required the natural ſine and co-ſine of* 28° 35′?

Log. ſines	ſine 9,67982	Co-ſine 9,94355
Num. or nat. ſines	0,47844	0,87812

If a given log. ſine is found in the table of logs. of numbers, its natural number conſiſting of four places is ſeen at ſight; and its right hand place is 0 when the index of the log. ſine was 9.

But if a given log. ſine is not found to every figure in the tables of log. numbers, its 5th, or right-hand place is thus found.

Take the diff. between the log. num. next greater and leſs, than the given log. ſine; and alſo the diff. between the given log. ſine and its next leſs log. numb.

Then, As 1ſt diff. is to 2d diff. ſo is 10, to the digit for the right hand place.

Thus to 4° 22′, the nat. ſine is 0,07614; and co-ſine is 0,99710.

But to 28° 35′, the log. ſine and co-ſ. does not appear exactly among the log. numb.

And the above-mentioned two differences, for ſine, are 9 and 3; for co-ſ. are 5 and 1.

Then 9 : 3 : : 10 : 3, the 5th place. And 5 : 1 : : 10 : 2, the 5th place.

257. On the contrary. *A natural ſine being given, its correſponding arc may be thus found.*

In the tables of num. and logs. enter with the natural ſine as a num. and take out its log.

Seek this log. in the table of log. ſines, and the correſponding degrees and minutes ſhew the arc required.

Prefixing the index 9, 8, 7, 6; according as the left hand digit ſtood in the place of firſts, ſeconds, thirds, or fourths.

What has been ſaid of the nat. and log. ſines of arcs, is alſo applicable to the nat. and log. tangents of arcs.

END OF BOOK IV.

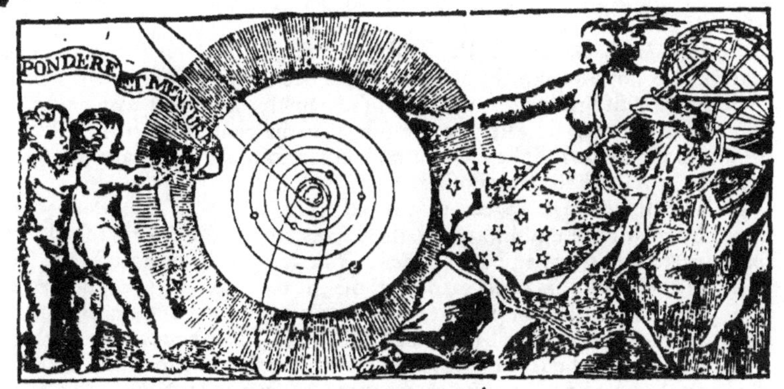

THE ELEMENTS OF NAVIGATION.

BOOK V.

OF ASTRONOMY.

SECTION I.

Of Solar Astronomy.

1. ASTRONOMY is a ſcience which treats of the motions and diſtances of the heavenly bodies, and of the appearances thence ariſing.

There have been great variety of opinions among the philoſophers of preceding ages concerning the ſituation of the great bodies in the univerſe, or of the poſitions of the bodies which appear in the heavens: But the notion now embraced by the moſt judicious Aſtronomers is, that the univerſe is compoſed of an infinite number of ſyſtems, or worlds; in every ſyſtem there are certain bodies moving in free ſpace, and revolving at different diſtances around a SUN, placed in, or near, the center of the ſyſtem; and that theſe *ſuns* and other *bodies* are the ſtars which are ſeen in the heavens.

2. The SOLAR SYSTEM, ſo called by Aſtronomers, is that in which our Earth is placed; and in which the Sun is ſuppoſed to be fixed in or near the center, with ſeveral bodies ſimilar to our Earth revolving round him at different diſtances. This hypotheſis, which is confirmed by all the obſervations hitherto made, is called the COPERNICAN SYSTEM,

from *Nicholas Copernicus*, a Polish Philosopher, who about the year 1500 revived this notion from the oblivion it had been buried in for many ages.

Stars are distinguished into two kinds, namely, *fixed* and *wandering*.

3. The FIXED STARS are the suns, in the centers of their systems, shining by their own light; and are observed to preserve always the same situation in respect to one another.

4. The fixed stars appear of various sizes, which is doubtless occasioned by their different distances; these sizes are usually distinguished into six or seven classes, called Magnitudes: The largest, or brightest, are said to be of the FIRST MAGNITUDE; those in the next class or degree of brightness, are called of the SECOND MAGNITUDE; and so on to the least, or those just discernible to the naked eye. But besides these, there is scattered throughout the heavens a great number of other stars, called TELESCOPIC STARS, because they cannot be seen except through a telescope. And indeed, it is to the assistance of that most admirable instrument, that a great part of the modern Astronomy owes its rise; which will undoubtedly transmit with the greatest honour to the latest posterity the name of GALILEO, among whose many inventions the telescope is ranked.

5. Although the visible fixed stars are probably at very unequal distances from the center of the *solar system*, yet Astronomers, for their ease in computation, consider them as equally distant from our Sun, forming the surface of a sphere which incloses our system, and is called the CELESTIAL SPHERE. This supposition, with regard to the Solar System, may be strictly admitted, considering the immense distance even of the nearest fixed stars from the center of the system.

6. A CONSTELLATION is a number of stars lying in the neighbourhood of one another on the surface of the *celestial sphere*, which Astronomers, for the sake of remembering them with greater ease, suppose to be circumscribed by the outlines of some *animal*, or other *figure*: by this means the motions of the wandering stars are more readily described and compared.

The number of these constellations is 80, each containing several stars of different magnitudes. The number of stars of each magnitude, and also the constellation in which they are ranged, are contained in the following table; where it may be observed, that the constellations are distinguished under three heads; namely, in the *zodiac*, and in the northern, and southern hemispheres.

7. CONSTELLATIONS IN THE ZODIAC.

Names. Northern.	Marks.	Number.	Magnitudes. I	II	III	IV	V	VI	Names. Southern.	Marks.	Number.	Magnitudes. I	II	III	IV	V	VI
Aries.	♈	46	0	1	1	3	5	36	Libra.	♎	33	0	2	1	8	3	19
Taurus.	♉	109	1	1	3	9	24	71	Scorpio.	♏	44	1	3	6	14	5	15
Gemini.	♊	94	1	2	4	8	13	66	Sagittarius.	♐	48	0	1	5	9	11	22
Cancer.	♋	75	0	0	0	6	8	61	Capricornus.	♑	58	0	0	2	5	9	42
Leo.	♌	91	2	2	6	13	11	57	Aquarius.	♒	93	0	0	4	7	28	54
Virgo.	♍	93	1	0	5	11	24	52	Pisces.	♓	110	0	0	1	7	20	74

8. NORTHERN

8. Northern Constellations.

Names.	Numb.	Magnitudes. I	II	III	IV	V	VI	Names.	Numb.	Magnitudes. I	II	III	IV	V.	VI
Little Bear.	12	0	2	1	4	3	2	Camelopardalus.	23	0	0	0	5	7	11
Great Bear.	105	0	5	5	16	30	49	Serpent.	50	0	1	7	6	5	31
Dragon.	49	0	1	7	8	10	23	Serpentarius.	67	0	1	6	12	17	31
Cepheus.	40	0	0	3	7	10	20	Sobieſki's Shield.	8	0	0	0	2	3	3
Greyhounds.	24	0	0	0	1	7	16	Eagle.	29	1	0	5	1	4	18
Bootes.	53	1	0	7	10	12	23	Antinous.	34	0	0	5	2	7	20
Mons Mænalus.	11	0	0	0	1	0	10	Dolphin.	18	0	0	6	0	2	10
Berenice's Hair.	24	0	0	0	6	8	10	Colt.	12	0	0	0	4	1	7
Charles's Heart.	3	0	1	0	0	0	2	Arrow.	13	0	0	0	4	1	8
Northern Crown.	11	0	1	0	6	3	1	Andromeda.	66	0	3	2	10	16	35
Hercules.	92	0	0	12	12	28	40	Perſeus.	67	1	1	5	10	14	36
Cerberus.	9	0	0	0	3	1	5	Pegaſus.	81	0	3	4	9	11	54
Harp.	24	1	0	3	2	8	10	Auriga.	46	1	1	1	9	9	25
Swan.	73	0	1	5	15	20	32	Lynx.	55	0	0	1	8	21	25
Fox.	29	0	0	0	6	11	12	Little Lion.	20	0	0	1	6	5	8
Gooſe.	10	0	0	0	0	2	8	Great Triangle.	10	0	0	0	3	1	6
Lizard.	12	0	0	0	3	5	4	Little Triangle.	5	0	0	0	0	0	5
Caſſiopea.	52	0	0	5	7	7	33	Muſca.	6	0	0	1	2	2	1

9. Southern Constellations.

Names.	Numb.	Magnitudes. I	II	III	IV	V	VI	Names.	Numb.	Magnitudes. I	II	III	IV	V	VI
Whale.	80	0	2	8	13	10	47	Peacock.	14	0	1	3	5	4	1
Eridanus.	72	1	0	10	24	19	18	Southern Crown.	12	0	0	0	1	3	8
Phenix.	13	0	1	5	5	0	2	Crane.	14	0	2	1	2	9	0
American Gooſe.	9	0	0	4	2	3	0	Southern Fiſh.	15	1	0	2	9	2	1
Orion.	93	2	4	3	19	15	50	Hare.	25	0	0	4	9	4	8
Monoceros.	32	0	0	1	10	10	11	Noah's Dove.	10	0	2	0	1	6	0
Little Dog.	14	1	0	1	0	2	10	Charles's Oak.	13	0	1	2	6	4	0
Hydra.	53	0	1	3	14	13	22	Ship Argo.	48	1	6	11	13	14	3
Sextans Uraniæ.	4	0	0	0	0	0	4	Great Dog.	29	1	5	1	4	10	8
Cup.	11	0	0	0	8	2	1	Bee.	4	0	0	0	2	2	0
Crow.	9	0	0	2	2	2	3	Swallow.	11	0	0	0	4	3	4
Centaur.	36	2	6	6	14	8	0	Indus.	12	0	0	0	4	6	2
Wolf.	36	0	0	3	6	18	9	Chamelion.	10	0	0	0	0	9	1
Altar.	9	0	0	1	6	1	1	Flying Fiſh.	7	0	0	0	0	6	1
Southern Triangle.	5	0	1	2	0	2	0	Sword Fiſh.	7	0	0	2	2	1	2

		Stars	I	II	III	IV	V	VI
Conſtellations in the zodiac	12, contain	894	6	12	38	100	169	569
Northern conſtellations	36, contain	243	5	21	92	200	291	634
Southern conſtellations	32, contain	706	9	32	75	185	188	217
Number of ſtars in the 80 conſtellations		2843	20	65	205	485	648	1420

As theſe ſtars are found not to alter their ſituation in reſpect to one another, they ſerve Aſtronomers as fixed points, by which the motions of other

other bodies may be compared; and therefore their relative poſitions have been ſought after with great care for many ages, and catalogues of their places have from time to time been publiſhed by thoſe, who have been at the pains to make the obſervations. Among theſe catalogues, the moſt copious, and, as generally eſteemed, the beſt, is that called the *Hiſtoria Celeſtis* of our countryman FLAMSTEED.

10. The poſitions of the ſtars being obtained, their relative places may be delineated on a ſphere or plane; and thus are the maps or charts of the heavens made, and the conſtellations drawn incloſing their reſpective ſtars. There are two maps, uſually called Celeſtial hemiſpheres, which are prefixed to this book; by the help of which a perſon may readily become acquainted with the poſitions and names of ſome of the principal fixed ſtars, thus:

On a clear night, let theſe prints be laid ſo as to correſpond to the north and ſouth parts of the heavens; then the obſerver looking on the ſtars, and then on the hemiſpheres, will with a little practice know ſome of the ſtars in the heavens, the like poſitions and names of which he has obſerved on the prints.

11. The WANDERING STARS are thoſe bodies within our ſyſtem, or celeſtial ſphere, which revolve round the Sun; they appear luminous or bright, only by reflecting the light they receive from the Sun; and are of three kinds, namely, *primary planets*, *ſecondary planets*, and *comets*.

12. The PRIMARY PLANETS are thoſe bodies, which in revolving round the Sun reſpect him only as the center of their courſes; the motions of which are regularly performed in tracks, or paths, that are found by obſervations to be nearly circular and concentric to one another.

13. A SECONDARY PLANET, commonly called a SATELLITE or MOON, is a body, which, while it is carried round the Sun, does alſo revolve round a primary planet, which it reſpects as its center.

14. COMETS, vulgarly called *blazing ſtars*, are bodies which alſo revolve round the Sun; probably in as regular order as the planets, but in much longer periods of time, from what is hitherto known of them. They are in number many more than all the planets, and their tracks or courſes paſs among the paths of the planets in a great variety of directions.

15. The ORBIT of a planet or comet is that track or path along which it moves.

There are ſix *primary planets*; and reckoned in order from the Sun, their names and marks are, MERCURY ☿, VENUS ♀, the EARTH ♁ or ⊖, MARS ♂, JUPITER ♃, SATURN ♄.

Mars, *Jupiter*, and *Saturn*, are called SUPERIOR PLANETS, as their orbits include that of the *Earth*: but *Venus* and *Mercury*, the orbits of which are contained within the *Earth*'s, are called INFERIOR PLANETS.

16. It has been diſcovered by the help of teleſcopes, that there are ten *ſecondary planets*; the Earth being attended by one, called the Moon, Jupiter by four, and Saturn by five.

Saturn is alſo obſerved to have a kind of circle, called his RING, which ſurrounds the planet at ſome diſtance from his ſurface: and Jupiter has certain appearances, which ſeem like zones or girdles round him; and theſe are called JUPITER's BELTS.

Every primary planet is ſuppoſed to have two motions, namely, *annual* and *diurnal*.

17. The ANNUAL MOTION of a planet is that whereby the planet is carried in its orbit round the Sun; which in every one is found by obſervation to be from weſt to eaſt.

This motion is diſcovered by the planets changing their places in the celeſtial ſphere; upon the ſurface of which they appear to move among the fixed ſtars; and in certain times to return to the ſame ſtars from which they were ſeen to depart; and ſo on continually.

18. The DIURNAL MOTION of a planet is that by which it turns or ſpins about its axis, and is alſo from weſt to eaſt.

This motion is diſcovered by the ſpots that are ſeen by teleſcopes on the ſurfaces of the planets. The ſpots appear firſt on the eaſtern margin, or ſide of the planet, and gradually move from thence acroſs it, till they diſappear on the weſtern ſide, or *limb*; after a certain time they appear again on the eaſtern ſide, and ſo on.

19. Each planet is obſerved always to paſs through the conſtellations *Aries*, *Taurus*, *Gemini*, *Cancer*, *Leo*, *Virgo*, *Libra*, *Scorpio*, *Sagittarius*, *Capricornus*, *Aquarius*, *Piſces*; and it alſo appears, that every one has a track peculiar to itſelf; hence the paths of the ſix planets form among the ſtars a kind of road, which is called the ZODIAC, the middle path of which, called the ECLIPTIC, is the orbit deſcribed by the Earth, with which the orbits of the other planets are compared.

As the ecliptic runs through twelve conſtellations, it is ſuppoſed to be divided into twelve equal parts, of 30 degrees each, called ſigns, having the ſame names with the twelve conſtellations which they run through.

20. The EQUINOCTIAL POINTS are thoſe two points of the Ecliptic, oppoſite to one another, through which the Earth paſſes in its annual motion, when the length of the day and night is equal in all parts on the Earth. One of theſe points, called the VERNAL EQUINOX, anſwers nearly to the 20th of March; and the other, called the AUTUMNAL EQUINOX, nearly to the 22d of September.

21. The *Plane of the Ecliptic* is ſuppoſed to divide the celeſtial ſphere into two equal parts, called the *northern* and *ſouthern celeſtial hemiſpheres*; and any body in either of theſe hemiſpheres is ſaid to have north or ſouth latitude, according to the hemiſphere it is in: So that the LATITUDE of a celeſtial object is its neareſt diſtance from the ecliptic, taken on the ſphere.

The Planes of the other five orbits are obſerved to lie partly in the northern, and partly in the ſouthern hemiſphere; ſo that every one cuts the ecliptic in two oppoſite points, called NODES. One called the ASCENDING NODE, marked thus, ☊, is that through which the planet paſſes when it moves out of the ſouthern into the northern hemiſphere; and the other called the DESCENDING NODE, marked thus, ☋, is that through which the planet muſt paſs in going out of the northern into the ſouthern hemiſphere.

The right line joining the two Nodes of any planet, is called the LINE OF THE NODES.

22. The names of moſt of the conſtellations were given by the ancient Aſtronomers, who reckoned that ſtar in Aries, now marked γ, (according

to *Bayer*'s maps) to be the first point in the ecliptic, this star being next the Sun when he entered the *Vernal Equinox*; and at that time each constellation was in the sign by which it was called. But observations shew, that the point marked in the heavens by the *Vernal Equinox* has been constantly going backward by a small quantity every year, from which cause the stars appear to have advanced forward as much; so that the constellation *Aries* is now removed almost into the sign *Taurus*, the said first star γ having got almost 30 degrees forwards from the equinox; which difference is called the PRECESSION OF THE EQUINOXES, and the yearly alteration is about 50 seconds of a degree, or about a degree in 72 years.

23. It was said in art. 12, that the planets revolved round the Sun in orbits *nearly* circular and concentric; for the several phænomena arising from their motions shew they are not strictly so; and the only curve they can move in, to reconcile all the various appearances, is found to be an Ellipsis:. So that the orbits of the primary planets and comets are Ellipses of different curvatures, having one common focus, in which the Sun is fixed: But every secondary planet respects the primary planet round which it revolves, as the focus of its elliptic motion. For as no other suppositions can solve all the appearances that are observed in the motions of the planets, and as these agree with the strictest physical and mathematical reasoning, therefore they are now received as elementary principles.

24. The line of the nodes of every planet passes through the Sun: For as the motion of every planet is in a plane passing through the Sun, consequently the intersections of these planes, that is, the lines of the nodes, must also pass through the Sun.

25. All the planets, in their revolutions, are sometimes nearer to, sometimes farther from the Sun: This is the consequence of the Sun not being placed in the center of each orbit, and of their being ellipses.

26. The APHELION, or SUPERIOR APSIS, is that point of the orbit where the planet is farthest from the Sun. The PERIHELION, or INFERIOR APSIS, is that point where it is nearest to the Sun: And the transverse diameter of the orbit, or the line joining the two apses, is called the LINE OF THE APSES, or ASPIDES.

27. The planets move faster as they approach the Sun, or come nearer to the perihelion, and slower as they recede from the Sun, or come nearer to the aphelion. This is not only a consequence from the nature of the planets motions about the Sun, but is confirmed by all good observations.

28. If a right line drawn from the Sun through any planet, usually called the *Radius Vector*, is supposed to revolve round the Sun with the planet, then this line will describe or pass through every part of the plane of the orbit; so that the *Radius Vector* may be said to describe the area of the orbit.

29. There are two *chief laws* observed in the Solar System, which regulate the motions of all the planets; namely,

I. *The planets describe equal areas in equal times:* That is, in equal portions of time the *Radius Vector* describes equal areas, or portions of the space contained within the planet's orbit.

II. *The squares of the periodical times of the planets are as the cubes of their mean distances from the Sun:* That is, as the square of the time which a planet A takes to revolve in its orbit, is to the square of the time taken by any other planet B to run through its orbit; so is the cube of the mean distance of A from the Sun, to the cube of the mean distance of B from the Sun.

30. The MEAN DISTANCE of a planet from the Sun is its distance from him, when the planet is at either extremity of the conjugate diameter; and it is equal to half the transverse diameter.

31. The foregoing laws are the two famous laws of KEPLER, a great Astronomer, who flourished in Germany about the beginning of the 17th century, and who deduced them from a multitude of observations: But the first who demonstrated these laws was the incomparable Sir ISAAC NEWTON.

By the second law, the relative distances of the planets from the Sun are known; and were the real distance of any one known, the absolute distances of all the others would be obtained by it.

32. Every thing already said of the planets is found in a great measure to be applicable also to the comets, as well from the observations that have been made of them, as from the physical and mathematical considerations of their motions.

33. Were the motions of the planets to be observed from the Sun, each of them would be ever seen to move the same way, though with different velocities; those nearer to the Sun running their courses through the Zodiac in less time than those at greater distances: And hence it would happen, that some of them overtaking the others would in passing by them appear to be sometimes above, sometimes below, and sometimes as if they touched one another, according to the parts of the orbits in which those planets happened to be with respect to their nodes.

34. When two planets are seen together in the same sign equally advanced, they are said to be in CONJUNCTION: But when they are in direct opposite parts of the Zodiac, they are said to be in OPPOSITION.

35. As the planes of the orbits are inclined to one another, therefore when two planets happen to be in conjunction at the time they come near a node of one of them, they would be seen from the Sun apparently to touch one another; and the farthest of those planets from the Sun would see the nearest moving over the face of the Sun like a black spot, being then directly between the Sun and the remoter planet; so the planet Venus was observed from the Earth in the transits of the years 1761 and 1769. Also, should an opposition of two planets happen near a node of one of them, the Sun, being then directly between them, would hide the light of one from the other. These obscurations, or interceptions of the light of the planets one from the other, are called ECLIPSES.

36. The place that any planet appears to occupy in the celestial sphere, when seen by an observer supposed to be in the Sun, is called its *Heliocentric place:* And indeed all celestial appearances, as seen from the Sun, are called *Heliocentric phænomena.*

37. The

37. The following table exhibits at once some of the most material conclusions that have been deduced from the observations hitherto made, the mean distance of the Earth from the Sun being reckoned at 1000.

Table of the Solar System.

Planets Names.	Marks.	Mean dist. compared to that of the Earth.	Eccentricity.	Inclination of the orbits to the eclipt.	Times of the periodical revolutions.	Diurnal rotations.	True diameter.	N° of moons.
Mercury.	☿	387	81	6° 52′	3 m. or 87^d 23^h	uncertain	0,32	0
Venus.	♀	724	5	3 23	8 m. or 224 17	23^h 0^m 0^s	0,87	0
Earth.	♁	1000	17	0 00	1 y. or 365 6	23 56 4	1,00	1
Mars.	♂	1524	141	1 52	2 y. or 686 23	24 40 0	0,73	0
Jupiter.	♃	5201	250	1 20	12 y. or 4332 12	9 56 0	7,70	4
Saturn.	♄	9538	543	2 20	30 y. or 10759 8	uncertain	4,19	5

38. By all the observations made on the secondary planets, it appears,

1st. That the satellites revolve round their superior planets from west to east, in curve-lined orbits like ellipses, the primary planet being in the focus, and one of the orbit's diameters directed towards the Sun.

2d. That the planes of the orbits of the satellites are inclined to the plane of the orbit of their respective planet.

3d. That, like the primary planets, they describe equal areas in equal times; and the squares of the times of their revolutions are as the cubes of the mean distances from their primary planet.

In every revolution of a moon round its primary planet, there must be two conjunctions betwixt the planet, moon, and Sun: namely, once, when the moon is in that part of its orbit nearest to the Sun; and once, when in that part of its orbit farthest from the Sun: And an eclipse may happen at either conjunction, according as the moon's nodes happen to be posited at those times. For the plane of a moon's orbit is inclined to that of its primary, and so makes two nodes: And whenever the Sun, planet, and moon happen to be at the same time in the line of the nodes, there must be an eclipse; which would occur at every conjunction, but for the inclination of the orbit.

One of the conjunctions, namely, that made by the moon's going beyond the primary, from the Sun, is called the Superior Conjunction; and the other, made by the satellite on the side of the planet next the Sun, is called the Inferior Conjunction.

The following table shews the time taken by each satellite in its revolution, and also its mean distance from the primary in semidiameters of it.

39

	I	II	III	IV	V
	d h m	d h m	d h m	d h m	d h m
Saturn's satell.	1 21 $18\frac{1}{2}$	2 17 $41\frac{1}{3}$	3 12 $25\frac{1}{3}$	15 22 $41\frac{1}{4}$	79 7 48
Dist. from Sat.	$8\frac{7}{8}$ s.diam.	$11\frac{1}{4}$ s.diam.	15 s. diam.	36 s. diam.	108 s.diam.
Jupiter's satell.	1 18 $28\frac{3}{5}$	3 13 $18\frac{5}{6}$	7 3 $59\frac{2}{3}$	16 18 $5\frac{1}{13}$	
Dist. from Jup.	$5\frac{2}{3}$ s.diam.	9 s. diam.	$14\frac{1}{3}$ s.diam.	$25\frac{1}{3}$ s. diam.	
The Moon	29 12 $44\frac{1}{20}$	and is dist. from the Earth $60\frac{1}{5}$ semidiameters.			

40. *Of the figure and light of the Planets.*

That the Sun and planets are spherical bodies is evident from all the observations that have been made of them; and that the Earth is of like figure is not only deduced by analogy, but sufficiently confirmed by observation.*. Now although Astronomers generally say that the planets are spherical, yet they do not mean a Geometrical sphere, but a figure called an oblate spheroid, which is something like the figure that a flexible sphere would be formed into by gently pressing it at its poles. Observations have determined this in Jupiter, and it is known that the Earth is of this figure both from observations and actual mensuration.

That the planets must have this oblate figure, is evident from this consideration; that as they are of matter, and violently whirled on their axes, all the parts would endeavour to fly off, like water from a trundled mop; those in the equator moving swiftest, have the greatest tendency to depart: And although the parts are retained in the sphere by the superior force of gravity, yet the equatorial diameters will be somewhat increased, and the polar lessened.

41. The planets are all opake or dark bodies, and consequently shine only by the light they receive from the Sun: This is known by observing, that those bodies are not visible, when they are in such parts of their orbits as are between the Sun and Earth, or partly so. Now, as all the planets sometimes appear with a strong light, therefore the rays they receive from the Sun must convey to them a degree of warmth proportional in some measure to their distance; which proportion is reciprocally as the squares of the distances; and this must be readily inferred from the heat which the inhabitants of the Earth receive from the Sun.

42. As a planet revolves on its axis, every part of its surface will be turned towards the Sun, and so enjoy its light and heat.

* Observations shew, that in eclipses of the moon the darkened part is bounded by a circular curve; and consequently the body, which casts the shade, or obstructs the light, must be bounded by a like curve: but as these obscurations are caused by different parts of the Earth, consequently its surface must be limited by a circular figure, that is, it must be globular.

SECTION

SECTION II.

Of Terrestrial Astronomy.

43. Terrestrial Astronomy is that which considers the motions of the celestial bodies as seen from the Earth, which is also in motion.

The motions described in the preceding section were such, as would appear to an observer viewing the heavens from the Sun: But were he placed in one of the planets, suppose the Earth, and there observed the motions of the rest, the Sun, and other planets, would appear to him to revolve round the Earth as a center; but the Sun would be the only one that moved uniformly the same way: For the other planets would seem to move sometimes from west to east, and then to stand still; then they would seem to run from east to west; and after standing some time, they would again move from west to east, and so on continually.

44. The place in the celestial sphere that any planet appears in, when seen from the center of the Earth, is called its Geocentric Place.

45. The Direct Motion of a planet is that by which it appears to move from west to east, and this motion is said to be *according to the order of the signs*, or in *consequentia*. When the planet appears to stand still, it is said to be Stationary; and when its motion is apparently from east to west, it is then called Retrograde, or has a motion in *antecedentia*, or contrary to the order of the signs. These different appearances follow partly in consequence of the observer being himself in motion while he is viewing the motions of the planets, and partly because he is not in the center of the motions which he observes.

46. *The Phænomena of the Inferior Planets.* See Fig. 1. Plate IV.

Let ABC represent an arc of the celestial sphere; EOP the Earth's orbit; LNIG the orbit of an inferior planet, as of *Venus*; and S the Sun: Let the Earth at first be supposed to stand still in its orbit at E: Now it is evident that the Sun will appear at the point B, and the planet always within the arc AC. Whilst the planet moves in its orbit from I through Q to N, it will seem to move from B to A in *consequentia:* But passing from N to L, it will seem to an eye at E to return back from A to B, or be *retrograde.* While the planet is at, or near, the point N, and moving as it were in a right line towards the Earth, it will for some time seem to stand still near A, and it is then said to be *stationary.*

47. When the planet is in that part of its orbit N or G, which is contiguous to the tangent EA or EC, it will then appear at A or C, its greatest distance from the Sun, and is said to have then the greatest Elongation: This elongation is measured by the angle SEG. The more distant a planet is from the Sun, the greater will its angle of elonga-tion

tion be; that of Venus is about 48 degrees, and that of Mercury about 28 degrees.

In the ſpace of a revolution, the two inferior planets will, with reſpect to the Earth, undergo two conjunctions; one when it is beyond the Sun at I, the other when it is at L between the Sun and the Earth; the former is called the *ſuperior*, and the latter the *inferior conjunction*.

48. Whilſt Venus goes from her ſuperior conjunction, ſhe appears in the arc BA always to the eaſtward of the Sun, and therefore ſets ſome time after the Sun, and is called the *evening ſtar*. But during the time ſhe is going from her inferior to her ſuperior conjunction, ſhe will be ſeen ſomewhere in the arc BC to the weſtward of the Sun, and ſo will ſet before him in the evening, and riſe before him in the morning; hence ſhe is called the *morning ſtar*.

Hitherto the planet only has been ſuppoſed to move while the Earth ſtood ſtill; but when both move, the foregoing phænomena will be much the ſame, only the planet will be more direct in the fartheſt part of the orbit, and leſs retrograde in the neareſt; the former ariſing from the ſum of their motions, and the latter from the difference.

49. *Of the Phænomena of the Superior Planets.*

The *direct*, *ſtationary*, and *retrograde* appearances of the ſuperior planets are explained much after the ſame manner as thoſe of the inferior ones, but with theſe differences.

1ſt. The retrograde motions of the ſuperior planets happen oftener the ſlower their motions are, as the retrogradations of the inferior planets happen oftener the ſwifter their angular motions are: Becauſe the retrograde motions of the ſuperior planets depend upon the motions of the Earth, but thoſe of the inferior on their own angular motions. A ſuperior planet is retrograde once in each revolution of the Earth; an inferior one, in every one of its own revolutions.

2d. The ſuperior planets do not always accompany the Sun as the inferior do, but are often in oppoſition to him; which neceſſarily follows from the orbit of the Earth being included in the orbits of the ſuperior planets.

50. *Of the apparent Motion of the Sun.*

As a ſpectator in the Sun would ſee the Earth revolve through the ſigns in the ecliptic; ſo to a ſpectator in the Earth the Sun apparently revolves the ſame way, but is always in the oppoſite point of the ecliptic: (For it is well known to every one, eſpecially to thoſe who uſe the ſea, that fixed objects appear to change their place by the motion of the obſerver:) So that the heliocentric place of the Earth, and the geocentric place of the Sun, are always in direct oppoſite points of the ecliptic.

Now although it is the motion of the Earth that really cauſes a great variety in the apparent motions of the other planets, yet as the motion of the Sun being known gives that of the Earth, therefore Aſtronomers ſpeak of of the motion of the Sún; and in their computations uſe the quantities of thoſe motions as if they were real.

51. Beſide the various appearances that ariſe from the annual motion of the Earth, there are many reſulting from its diurnal motion: For that the Earth has a daily motion round its axis muſt neceſſarily be inferred from the moſt ſtrict reaſoning on the motions of the planets: and the notion, that bodies ſo immenſely diſtant as the ſtars are, really revolve round the earth in 24 hours, is now treated as a great abſurdity by every one who has rightly conſidered theſe things: However, as the motions are apparent, and the ſpeaking of them as real is cuſtomary and no way affects the concluſions; therefore Aſtronomers treat of thoſe motions as they appear.

52. Any ſphere revolving as on an axis, muſt have two points on its ſurface at the extremities of its axis, that do not revolve at all; theſe points, with reſpect to the Earth, are called its *poles*.

53. By the Earth's rotation on its axis from weſt to eaſt in a day, the ſurface of the celeſtial ſphere appears to move from eaſt to weſt in the ſame time; and all the celeſtial objects appear to deſcribe circles in the heavens, which are greater or leſs according as they are farther from, or nearer to, the apparent centers of thoſe motions: For there are two points in the heavens which are apparently fixed, and the nearer any ſtars are to theſe points, the ſlower are their motions. Theſe points are called the CELESTIAL POLES; the right line joining them is called the AXIS OF THE SPHERE, and paſſes through the poles of the Earth; the circle in the heavens, equally diſtant from the poles of the celeſtial ſphere, is called the EQUINOCTIAL; the correſponding circle on the Earth is called the EQUATOR, which is equally diſtant from both the poles of the Earth.

54. As the Sun's rays falling on any ſphere enlighten one half of its ſurface; therefore one half of the Earth is always illuminated at once, and conſequently the enlightened part is bounded by a great circle, which may be called the TERMINATOR, from its property of terminating, or bounding, the verges of light and darkneſs. Now, by the rotation of the Earth on its axis once in 24 hours, there will be a conſtant ſucceſſion of light on all parts of its ſurface as they are turned towards the Sun, and of darkneſs in thoſe parts as they move out of his rays; and hence ariſe the viciſſitudes of DAY and NIGHT.

55. If the plane of the equator coincided with the plane of the ecliptic, and the axis of the Earth ſtood perpendicular to it, the terminator would always paſs through the poles of the Earth, and there would be a conſtant equality of day and night in every part of its ſurface, except at the two poles, where there would be conſtant day. But the contrary of this is known to every one, and obſervations ſhew, that the Earth's axis is inclined to the plane of the ecliptic in an angle of about $66\frac{1}{2}$ degrees; therefore the poles of the ecliptic and equator are about $23\frac{1}{2}$ degrees diſtant from one another; conſequently the ecliptic and equinoctial, which in the heavens interſect one another in the oppoſite points of Aries and Libra, make at thoſe interſections angles of about $23\frac{1}{2}$ degrees (IV. 33): This angle is called the OBLIQUITY OF THE ECLIPTIC.

The axis of the Earth being thus inclined to the plane of the ecliptic, and moving parallel to itſelf in all points of the ANNUAL ORBIT, or ecliptic, is the occasion of the inequality of days and nights, and of the different seasons of the year; which two phænomena are explained as follows.

56. It must be observed, that the Sun will appear to be vertical to that part of the Earth, which is cut by a straight line joining the centers of the Sun and Earth.

57. Now when the Earth is at ♑, Fig. 3. Plate IV. the Sun appearing then in ♋ will be vertical to that point of the terrestrial ecliptic, it lying in the right line joining the centers of the Sun and Earth. And this point being in the Earth's northern hemisphere, all those who live there will enjoy summer, or the hottest time of the year, the solar rays falling more copiously, and more perpendicularly, upon their hemisphere at that time.

58. At the same time the inhabitants of the southern hemisphere will have winter, the rays of the sun falling more obliquely, and in less quantity, on them, and consequently affording them less heat.

59. Again, the inhabitants of the northern hemisphere will have their days longer than their nights, in proportion as they are more distant from the equator; while those who live under the equator will have an equal share of day and night all the year round. For in this position the terminator, which is always at right angles to the plane of the ecliptic, will pass $23\frac{1}{2}$ degrees beyond the north pole, and consequently will cut all the circles parallel to the equator which it meets with into two unequal parts: those that are in north latitude will have the greater portions of those parallels in the enlightened hemisphere: but the terminator being a great circle, will cut the equator into two equal parts; therefore half the equator is always illuminated.

60. Hence it necessarily follows, that those who live under the equator will have their days and nights equal: those who live within the limits of $23\frac{1}{2}$ degrees round the north pole, will have no night; and the inhabitants between this limit and the northern neighbourhood of the equator will have their nights shorter than their days. In the mean time those who live in the southern hemisphere will have their nights longer than their days, in proportion as they approach nearer to the south pole; and the regions contained within the limits of $23\frac{1}{2}$ degrees round the south pole will have no day.

61. Suppose the Earth now to move in its orbit from ♑ through the signs ♒, ♓ to ♈, the Sun will seem to run through the signs ♌, ♍ to ♎; and this will be the place of the Sun in autumn.

While the Earth is in ♈, the days and nights will be equal in both hemispheres, and the season is a medium between summer and winter: For at that time the Sun will appear vertical to the equator, because a right line joining the centers of the Sun and Earth will then cut the surface of the Earth in the equator; so that the terminator, the plane of which is always at right angles to the said line, will pass through the poles; consequently, all the Earth will then have an equal share of day and night. And because the rays of the Sun then fall perpendiculary upon the axis of the Earth, it will then follow, that they must fall with an equal obliquity, and with equal number, upon either hemisphere; therefore they must enjoy an equal degree of heat and cold.

Now

Now suppose the Earth to move from ♈ to ♋, the Sun will seem to move from ♎ to ♑, where it will be in its nearest approach to the south pole; and at this time of the year it will be winter in the northern hemisphere. For to this hemisphere the like phænomena will now happen, which did before to the southern, when the Earth was in ♑; and by a parity of reason, when the Earth has got as far as ♎, and the Sun is apparently in ♈, the northern hemisphere will enjoy spring, and the southern will have autumn.

62. The four points of the ecliptic, in which the Earth has been considered in summer, autumn, winter, and spring, are called the four CARDINAL POINTS; ♑ and ♋ are called SOLSTITIAL POINTS; ♎ and ♈, EQUINOCTIAL POINTS.

63. The first point of Cancer is called the SUMMER SOLSTICE; because when the Sun enters it, which is about the 21st of June, he has then got to the greatest extent northwards, and being about to return towards the equator, he seems for a day or two to be at a stand. And for the same reason, the first point of Capricorn, which the Sun enters about the 21st of December, is called the WINTER SOLSTICE, with respect to the northern hemisphere.

64. The first points of Aries and Libra are called the VERNAL and AUTUMNAL EQUINOCTIAL POINTS, from the equality of days and nights all over the surface of the Earth, when the Sun enters those points.

65. *Of the Rising and Setting of the Stars.*

There is only one half of the celestial sphere visible at one time to any observer on the surface of the Earth, the other half being hid by the Earth itself. Now the apparent plane on which the observer stands, seems to be extended to the heavens, and there marks out a circle that divides the visible from the invisible hemisphere; this circle is called the HORIZON, above which all the celestial motions are seen. When this horizon is a great circle of the celestial sphere, it is called the RATIONAL HORIZON: but when by the particular situation of the observer, he sees more or less than half the celestial sphere, then the circle bounding his view is called the SENSIBLE HORIZON.

The horizon is one of the most useful circles in Astronomy; for to this circle, which is the only apparent one, almost all the celestial motions are referred. It is the common termination of day and night; it marks out the times of the rising and setting of the Sun and stars, and many other particulars, of which hereafter.

66. *Of Parallaxes.*

The PARALLAX of any object is the difference between the places that object is referred to in the celestial sphere, when seen at the same time from two different places within that sphere: Or, it is the angle under which any two places in the inferior orbits are seen from a superior planet, or even from the fixed stars: But the parallaxes which are most used by Astronomers are those which arise from seeing the object from the centers

ters of the Earth and Sun; from the Surface and center of the Earth; and from all three compounded.

67. The difference between the heliocentric and geocentric place of a planet, is called the *parallax of the annual orbit* (namely, that of the Earth); that is, the angle at any planet, subtended by the distance between the Sun and Earth, is called the parallax of the Earth's, or annual orbit.

68. The difference in the two longitudes is called the parallax of longitude; and that of the two latitudes is called the parallax of latitude.

69. In the SYZIGIES, that is, in the *oppositions* or *conjunctions*, the Sun and planet being equally advanced in the same sign, or in like places in opposite signs, the parallax of latitude is then greatest.

70. And when the planet is in its QUADRATURES, that is, when it is 90 degrees distant from the Sun, the parallax of longitude is then the greatest.

71. To explain the parallaxes which respect the Earth only. Fig. 2. Plate IV.

Let HSW represent the Earth, where T is the center; OR part of the Moon's orbit, P*rg* part of a planet's orbit, and Z*a*A part of a great circle in the celestial sphere. Now to a spectator at S upon the surface of the Earth, let the Moon appear in G, that is in the sensible horizon of S, and it will be referred to A; but if viewed from the center T, it will be referred to the point D, which is its true place.

The arc AD will be the Moon's parallax; the angle SGT the parallactic angle: Or the parallax is expressed by the angle under which the semidiameter TS of the Earth is seen from the Moon.

If the parallax is considered with respect to different planets, it will be greater or less as those objects are more or less distant from the Earth. Thus the parallax AD of G is greater than the parallax A*d* of *g*. If it is considered with respect to the same planet, it is evident that the horizontal parallax (or the parallax when the object is in the horizon) is greatest of all; and diminishes gradually as the body rises above the horizon, until it comes to the zenith, where the parallax vanishes, or becomes equal to nothing. Thus AD and A*d*, the horizontal parallaxes of G and *g*, are greater than *a*B and *ab*, the parallaxes of R and *r*; and the objects O or P, seen from S or T, appear in the same place Z, or the zenith.

72. By knowing the parallax of any celestial object, its distance from the center of the Earth may be easily obtained by Trigonometry. Thus, if the distance of G from T is sought; in the triangle STG, the side ST being known, and the angle SGT determined by observation, the side TG is thence known.

The parallax of the Moon may be determined by two persons observing her from different stations at the same time, she being vertical to the one, and horizontal to the other: and it is generally concluded to be about 57 minutes of a degree; consequently her mean distance TG is about 60 semidiameters of the Earth, or 60 times TS.

But the parallax most wanted is that of the Sun, by which his absolute distance from the Earth would be known; and thence the absolute diſtances of all the other planets would be obtained from their relative diſtances found by the ſecond *Keplerian Law*.

Before the year 1761 ſome Aſtronomers reckoned the Sun's parallax at 12½ ſeconds, others at 10; theſe different parallaxes gave very different diſtance between the Sun and the Earth; the former making the diſtances near 8270 diameters of the Earth, and the latter 10313 diameters.

But in the years 1761 and 1769 the planet Venus paſſed between the Earth and the Sun, and was ſeen like a black ſpot moving over the face of the Sun. Theſe phenomena (which had not happened in more than 100 years before) were obſerved by many Aſtronomers from different parts of the Earth, and the reſult of their obſervations make the Sun's mean parallax about 8⅔ ſeconds, and hence the mean diſtance between the Sun and Earth comes very nearly to 11900 diameters of the Earth: And from what was ſhewn many years ago by the excellent Dr. Halley, if theſe obſervations were made with the accuracy he ſuppoſed, the diſtance between the Sun and the Earth might be obtained to leſs than a 500th part of the whole diſtance.

73. *Of the Meaſure of the Earth.*

The relative diſtances of the planets are diſcovered by the 2d *Keplerian Law*, and their relative magnitudes are gathered from the angles which they appear under (when viewed with very accurate inſtruments) compounded with their diſtances. Now as theſe diſtances and magnitudes can by means of the parallaxes be compared with the diameter of the Earth, conſequently this diameter being accurately known would ſerve as a meaſure with which the magnitudes and diſtances of all the other planets might be compared.

To find the meaſure of the Earth is a problem of ſuch importance in Aſtronomy, that it has been attempted by ſome of the moſt conſiderable men in almoſt all the preceding ages. But its ſolution was not brought to any degree of accuracy till the year 1635, when it was very nearly aſcertained by our countryman Richard Norwood, an eminent mathematician at that time. The principle he proceeded upon was this, that as 360 degrees were contained in every great circle, both of the celeſtial ſphere and of the Earth, and as theſe circles are conſidered as concentric to the center of the Earth; therefore, were the meaſure of a degree known on a great circle of the Earth, correſponding to a degree of a great circle of the heavens, then, by analogy, the whole circumference of a great circle of the Earth would be known in that meaſure, and conſequently its diameter would be obtained. (II. 197)

Norwood ſolved this problem in the following manner: He choſe two diſtant places which were know to lie nearly north and ſouth one of the other, as London and York; and by a method like that of Traverſe ſailing (explained in Book VII.) he found their difference of latitude, or, the diſtance between the parallels of latitude paſſing through thoſe places; or, which is the ſame thing, the length of that arc of the terreſtrial meridian. He alſo with a good inſtrument found the diſtance between

between the zeniths of thoſe places, and conſequently he thence knew the quantity of the celeſtial arc anſwering to the meaſured terreſtrial one. Then ſaying, As that celeſtial arc is to a great circle of the celeſtial ſphere, or 360 degrees; ſo is the arc of the terreſtial great circle meaſured in feet, to the circumference of a great circle of the Earth in feet meaſure.

And thus he found that about $69\frac{1}{2}$ Engliſh miles anſwered to one degree; hence the circumference of the Earth appears to be 25020 miles, and its diameter about 8000 miles.

By the ſame kind of reaſoning, the diſtances found in art. 72. from the parallaxes, were obtained.

For $12\frac{1}{2}''$: 360° : : 1 ſemi-diam. : 103680	the	Circumference of the Earth's orbit in ſemi-diameters of the Earth.
10 : 360 : : 1 ſemi-diam. : 129600		
$8\frac{2}{3}$: 360 : : 1 ſemi-diam. : 149538		

And 6,283185 : 103680 : : 1 : 16539,5	the	Mean diſt. of the Earth from the Sun, in ſemi-d. of the Earth. (II. 197)
6,283185 : 129600 : : 1 : 20626,4		
6,283185 : 149538 : : 1 : 23799,8		

Then 16539,5 × 4000 = 66158000	the	Mean diſtance of the Earth from the Sun, in miles.
20626,4 × 4000 = 82505600		
23799,8 × 4000 = 95199200		

71. *Of the Moon.*

The Moon revolves in her orbit from weſt to eaſt round the Earth, and is carried perpetually with it through the annual orbit round the Sun, making in the ſpace of one year 13 *periodical*, and 12 *ſynodical revolutions.*

75. A PERIODICAL MONTH, or REVOLUTION, is the time the Moon takes up in revolving from one point of her orbit to the ſame point again, and conſiſts of 27 d. 7 h. 43 m.

76. A SYNODICAL MONTH, or REVOLUTION, is the time the Moon ſpends in paſſing from one conjunction with the Sun to another, which is 29 d. 12 h. 44 m.; being 2 d. 5 h. 1 m. longer than the *Periodical Month.* For whilſt the Moon is paſſing from her former conjunction with the Sun round to it again; the Earth has proceeded forwards in its annual courſe, as it were leaving the Moon behind it; ſo that, in order to complete her next conjunction with the Sun, ſhe muſt not only come round to her former point again, but alſo go beyond it.

77. Beſides this monthly motion of the Moon round the Earth, ſhe has alſo a motion round her axis, which is performed exactly in the ſame time with her periodical revolution: Hence it comes to paſs, that the ſame face of the Moon is always turned towards the Earth, her diurnal motion turning juſt as much of her face to us, as her periodical motion turns it from us.

78. Though the ſame ſide of the Moon is ever turned towards us, yet it is not always viſible, but ſeems daily to put on different appearances,

 called

called PHASES: For the Moon being an opake body like the rest of the planets, borrows its light from the Sun, having always one hemisphere enlightened by the solar rays.

When the enlightened hemisphere is wholly turned from the Earth, as at her change or time of new-moon, the planet then being betwixt us and the Sun, the Moon's whole enlightened face, or *disk*, must needs be invisible to the Earth. When she passes from this state, and turns some little portion of the illuminated half to us, she must appear horned, the CUSPS or points being turned from the Sun towards the east. When the Moon is in her quadratures, or at 90 degrees from the Sun, then half the illuminated face becomes visible: She afterwards continues to shew more than half the enlightened disk, until she comes in opposition to the Sun or time of full-moon, when the whole of the illuminated orb is presented to us; from whence receding, she must put on the like phases as before, but in an inverse order, the cusps being now turned towards the west.

79. *Of Solar and lunar Eclipses.*

Eclipses of the Sun and Moon can only happen about the times of the conjunctions and oppositions: those of the Sun fall out at the conjunctions, when the Moon intercepts the light of the Sun from the Earth; and those of the ~~Sun~~ occur in the oppositions, when the Earth getting between the Sun and Moon, the latter loses her light during the time of that interposition.

The cause why there is not an eclipse in every syzigie is the inclination of the plane of the Moon's orbit to that of the ecliptic, which is about $5^{\circ}\ 18'$: for it is certain, that unless the Sun, Earth, and Moon, are all in the plane of the ecliptic, or nearly so, the shadows of the Earth and Moon can never fall on one another, but must be directed either above or below. Now they can never be in the same plane, and in one right line, except when the Moon is in her nodes, the nodes and Sun's center being in the same right line.

80. The solar and lunar eclipses do not happen every year in the same places of the zodiac, but in succeeding years they fall in places gradually removed backwards, or towards the antecedent signs: For since the nodes are found to go continually backwards, the eclipses must also observe the same order.

81. Eclipses of the Moon are either *total* or *partial*: the total happen when the node falls in or near the center of the shadow: and the partial, when the node happens to be on either side the center, within or without the shadow. Now the longer the duration of a partial eclipse is, so much the greater is that part of the Moon which enters into the shadow of the Earth.

82. Hence it is usual to conceive the Moon's diameter as divided into 12 parts, called DIGITS, by which the greatness of partial eclipses is measured, they being said to be of so many digits as they are parts covered by the Earth's shadow: Thus if 5 of the 12 parts are covered, it is called an eclipse of 5 digits.

83. As the planet Mars is never eclipsed by the Earth, it is plain the shadow of the latter does not reach so far as the orbit of the former, but

but tapers to a point at a lefs diftance; and confequently the Earth's fhadow muft be a cone, the vertex of which is extended beyond the orbit of the Moon. It naturally follows from hence, that the Sun is a much larger body than the Earth; it is indeed, in diameter, above 100 times that of the Earth.

84. If a perfon was placed juft at the vertex, or point of this fhadow, he would fee nothing of the Sun but a fmall rim of light round his difk; and the farther the obferver was removed from the vertex, the larger would the rim of light appear, and confequently the fewer rays would be intercepted by the opake body, till at laft it would appear only as a fpot in the Sun; in like manner as the planets Venus and Mercury appear when they are feen to pafs over the Sun's difk.

85. What has hitherto been faid of the fhadow of the Earth includes that of the atmofphere furrounding the Earth: for in lunar eclipfes the fhadow of the atmofphere is to be confidered. And hence it is that the Moon is vifible in eclipfes, the fhadow caft by the atmofphere being not near fo dark as that caft by the Earth.

86. The Moon always enters the weftern fide of the fhadow with her eaftern limb, and quits it with her weftern limb; and in her approach to and recefs from the fhadow, fhe muft pafs through a PENUMBRA, or imperfect fhade, which is caufed by the Earth itfelf.

87. In the fame manner, in which it has been fhewn that the Moon muft come into the fhadow of the atmofphere, when fhe is at full and at or near a node, it may alfo be fhewn, that her fhadow muft fall upon the Earth at the time of new Moon, provided fhe is in or near a node: But the penumbra of the Moon's fhadow is much more fenfible in folar eclipfes, than that accompanying the fhadow of the Earth in lunar ones.

88. It is obferved, that to determinate parts of the Earth folar eclipfes are not feen fo oft as lunar ones; which is owing to the fhadow of the Moon being lefs than that of the Earth: For the Earth's fhadow often covers all the Moon; but that of the Moon cannot cover all the Earth; and as it fometimes falls on one part, fometimes on another, it caufes folar eclipfes, in general, to be more frequent than lunar ones; yet to any determinate place on the Earth there are more eclipfes of the Moon vifible than of the Sun.

What has hitherto been faid, may fuffice to give beginners a general idea of the motions of the bodies in the folar fyftem, and of fome of the phenomena thence arifing; thofe who defire to be farther acquainted with particulars, may find them fully treated of in M. de la Caille's Elements of Aftronomy, publifhed in Englifh a few years fince *; and alfo in the works of Gregory, Keil, and others.

* Tranflated by the Author of thefe Elements.

SECTION III.

The Aſtronomy of the Sphere.

DEFINITIONS and PRINCIPLES.

89. By the Aſtronomy of the ſphere is meant the finding, from proper things given, the meaſure of certain arcs and angles formed on the ſurfaces of the celeſtial and terreſtrial ſpheres, by the apparent motions of the bodies which are ſeen in the heavens.

The ſurfaces of thoſe ſpheres are ſuppoſed to be concentric to the center of the Earth, and to have correſpondent circles deſcribed on both ſpheres.

90. GREAT CIRCLES are thoſe which divide either ſphere into two equal parts.

LESSER CIRCLES, thoſe which divide the ſphere into unequal parts.

The POLES of a circle are the points on the ſphere equally diſtant from that circle.

An AXIS is a right line ſuppoſed to connect the poles.

The CELESTIAL AXIS is that right line about which the heavens ſeem to revolve.

The NORTH and SOUTH POLES of the world are thoſe two points where the axis cuts the celeſtial ſphere.

91. The EQUINOCTIAL or EQUATOR, is the great circle of the ſphere equally diſtant from the poles of the world.

92. MERIDIANS, or HOUR CIRCLES, or CIRCLES of RIGHT ASCENSION, or CIRCLES OF TERRESTRIAL LONGITUDE, are great circles perpendicular to the equator, and paſſing through the poles of the world.

93. The ECLIPTIC is a great circle inclined to the equator in an angle of about 23½°, and cutting it in two points diametrically oppoſite.

The ecliptic is ſuppoſed to be divided into 12 equal parts, called SIGNS, beginning from one of its interſections with the equator; each ſign containing 30 degrees, named and noted thus:

Aries	*Taurus*	*Gemini*	*Cancer*	*Leo*	*Virgo*
♈	♉	♊	♋	♌	♍
Libra	*Scorpio*	*Sagittarius*	*Capricornus*	*Aquarius*	*Piſces*
♎	♏	♐	♑	♒	♓

The firſt ſix are called *northern*, and the latter ſix *ſouthern* ſigns.

94. The CARDINAL POINTS of the ecliptic are the four firſt points of the ſigns ♈, ♋, ♎, ♑; thoſe of ♈ and ♎ are called EQUINOCTIAL POINTS, and thoſe of ♋ and ♑ are called SOLSTITIAL POINTS.

95. The EQUINOCTIAL COLURE is a meridian paſſing through the *equinoctial points*; and the SOLSTITIAL COLURE is another meridian paſſing through the *ſolſtitial points*. The colours cut one another at right angles in the poles of the world.

96. CIR

96. Circles of Celestial Longitude are great circles perpendicular to the ecliptic.

97. The Latitude of any point in the heavens is an arc of a circle of longitude intercepted between that point and the ecliptic, and is called north or south latitude, as the point is on the north or south side of the ecliptic.

98. Parallels of Celestial Latitude are small circles parallel to the ecliptic.

99. The Longitude of any object in the heavens is an arc of the ecliptic intercepted between the first point of Aries and a circle of longitude passing through that point.

100. The Right Ascension of any object is an arc of the equator, contained between the first point of Aries and a meridian passing through that point: Or, it is the angle formed by the equinoctial colure, and the meridian passing over that point.

101. The Declination of any object is an arc of a meridian contained between that point and the equinoctial: If the point is on the north side of the equinoctial, it is called *north declination*; but if on the south side, it is called *south declination*.

102. The Obliquity of the Ecliptic is the angle made by the intersection of the equator and ecliptic, and is measured by the Sun's greatest declination; which, according to modern observations, is about 23° 28′.

103. Parallels of Declination are small circles parallel to the equinoctial. The Tropic of Cancer is a parallel of declination at 23° 28′ distant from the equinoctial in the northern hemisphere; and the Tropic of Capricorn is the parallel of declination as far distant in the southern hemisphere.

104. The Arctic Polar Circle is a parallel of declination at 23° 28′ distant from the north pole; and the Antarctic Polar Circle is the parallel of declination as far distant from the south pole.

105. The Zenith is the point of the heavens directly over a place; and the Nadir is the point directly underneath.

106. The Horizon is that great circle of the sphere which is equally distant from the *zenith* and *nadir* of any place, and divides the sphere into the upper and lower hemispheres.

107. The Rising of a celestial object is when its center appears in the eastern part of the horizon; and its Setting is when its center disappears in the western quarter of the horizon.

108. Azimuth, or Vertical Circles, are great circles perpendicular to the horizon, passing through its poles, which are the *zenith* and *nadir*.

109. The Prime Vertical is that vertical circle which passes through the east and west points of the horizon, and is at right angles to the *meridian of the place*, which is a vertical circle passing through the north and south points of the horizon.

110. As the meridian of a place is called the *twelve o'clock hour circle*, so the hour circle at right angles to the meridian is called the *six o'clock hour circle*.

111. The Azimuth of any celestial object is an angle at the zenith formed by the meridian of any place, and a vertical circle passing through

that object when it is above or below the horizon: And it is meaſured by the arc of the horizon intercepted between thoſe vertical circles.

112. The AMPLITUDE of any object in the heavens is uſually taken as an arc of the horizon contained between the eaſtern point of it, and the center of the object at its riſing, or between the weſtern point of it and the center of the object at its ſetting; or it may be taken as an angle at the zenith, included between the meridian of a place and a vertical circle paſſing through the object at its riſing or ſetting.

113. The ALTITUDE of any object in the heavens is an arc of a vertical circle intercepted between the center of that object and the horizon.

114. The ZENITH DISTANCE of any object is an arc of a vertical circle contained between the center of that object and the zenith.

The altitude and zenith diſtance are complements one of the other.

115. The MERIDIAN ALTITUDE, or MERIDIAN ZENITH DISTANCE, is the altitude or zenith diſtance when the object is on the meridian of the place.

116. The CULMINATING of any celeſtial object, is the time it *tranſits*, or comes to the Meridian. And the MEDIUM COELI, or MID-HEAVEN, to any place, is that degree of the ecliptic, or part of the heavens, over the meridian of that place, at any time. Or the MID-HEAVEN is the diſtance of the meridian from the firſt point of Aries, reckoned on the equinoctial.

117. The Nonageſimal degree is the 90th degree of the Ecliptic, reckoned from its interſection with the eaſtern point of the horizon, at any given time.

Conſequently the altitude or height of the nonageſimal degree above the horizon is equal to the diſtance of the poles of the Ecliptic and Horizon; and is the meaſure of the angle which the ecliptic makes with the horizon.

118. ALMICANTHERS, or PARALLELS OF ALTITUDE, are ſmall circles parallel to the horizon.

119. A PARALLEL SPHERE is that poſition of the ſphere in which the circles, apparently deſcribed by the diurnal rotation, are parallel to the horizon; which can happen only at the poles.

120. A RIGHT SPHERE is that in which the diurnal motions are at right angles to the horizon: Thus it appears in all places under the equator.

121. An OBLIQUE SPHERE has all the diurnal motions oblique to the horizon: And thus the motions appear to all parts of the Earth, except under the poles and equator.

122. DIURNAL ARCS are thoſe parts of the parallels of declination of celeſtial objects which are apparently deſcribed between the times of the riſing and ſetting of thoſe objects: And NOCTURNAL ARCS are the parts of thoſe parallels apparently deſcribed from the time of ſetting to the time of riſing.

123. SEMI-DIURNAL and SEMI-NOCTURNAL ARCS, or the halves of diurnal and nocturnal arcs, are the parts of the parallels intercepted between the meridian and the horizon. The correſponding part of the equator anſwering to the ſemi-diurnal arc, gives the times between noon and the riſing or ſetting; and the equatorial part anſwering to the ſemi-nocturnal

nocturnal arc, ſhews the time between midnight and the time of ſetting or riſing.

124. The OBLIQUE ASCENSION of any object in the heavens, is an arc of the equinoctial intercepted between the firſt point of Aries and the eaſtern part of the horizon when that object is riſing; and the OBLIQUE DESCENSION is an arc of the equinoctial intercepted between the firſt point of Aries and the weſtern part of the horizon at its ſetting.

125. The ASCENSIONAL DIFFERENCE belonging to any celeſtial object is an arc of the equinoctial intercepted between the horizon and the hour-circle which the object is on when it riſes or ſets; or it is the difference between the right and oblique aſcenſion of that object. In the Sun, it is the time that he riſes or ſets before or after the hour of ſix.

126. The LATITUDE of any place on the Earth is an arc of a terreſtrial meridian contained between that place and the equator; or it is an arc of a celeſtial meridian intercepted between the zenith of the place and the equinoctial; being north or ſouth, according to the ſide of the equator it is on.

127. The LONGITUDE of any place on the Earth is an arc of the equator contained between the meridian of that place and the meridian which is choſen for the firſt, where the reckoning of longitude begins: Or, it is the angle at the pole formed by the firſt meridian and that of the place.

128. REFRACTION, in an aſtronomical ſenſe, is the difference between the true and apparent altitudes of celeſtial objects; they appearing more elevated above the horizon than they really are, on account of the denſity of the Earth's atmoſphere, or air and vapours ſurrounding it.

129. The TWILIGHT is that medium between light and darkneſs, which happens in the morning before ſun-riſe, and in the evening after ſun-ſet.

This is occaſioned by the atmoſphere's refracting the ſolar rays upon any place, although the Sun is below the horizon of that place, and by obſervation it is found to begin and end when the Sun is about 18° below the horizon.

130. The CREPUSCULUM is a ſmall circle parallel to the horizon at 18° below it, where the twilight begins and ends.

131. The LATITUDE OF A PLACE is expreſſed by an arc of the meridian, ſhewing the diſtance between the zenith of that place and the equinoctial; or, by an arc of the meridian, ſhewing the height of the pole above the horizon.

For under the pole, or in the latitude of 90 degrees, the pole is in the zenith, or is 90 degrees above the horizon; ſo that, in this caſe, the horizon coincides with the equinoctial.

And as many degrees as the obſerver goes from the pole towards the equator, ſo many degrees does his horizon go below the equator on one ſide, and approach the pole on the other ſide.

Therefore the pole approaches the horizon juſt as much as the zenith approaches the equator; that is, the height of the pole above the horizon, is equal to the diſtance of the zenith from the equinoctial, which is equivalent to the diſtance of the obſerver from the equator, or is equal to the latitude.

132. ASTRONOMICAL TABLES in general contain numbers ſhewing either the meaſure of the diſtances of the heavenly bodies from certain limits which are uſed to repreſent remarkable *times* and *places*; or, the times when thoſe bodies had, or will have, given poſitions relative to thoſe limits.

Some of the chief aſtronomical tables are,
Solar and lunar tables for finding the places of thoſe luminaries at given times.
Tables for finding the places of the other planets.
Stellar tables for finding the places of the ſtars.
Tables ſhewing the Sun's place, declination, and right aſcenſion for given times.
Tables of refractions for correcting obſervations on altitudes.
Tables of the equation of time; or the difference between the times ſhewn by a ſun-dial and a well-regulated clock.
&c.

The aſtronomical tables chiefly wanted in this work are placed at the end of this book; and are preceded by an account of their conſtruction and uſe.

133. As the Earth makes one revolution on its axis in a common day of 24 hours; therefore every point of the equator will deſcribe the circle of 360 degrees in 24 hours; and conſequently, if 360 degrees give 24 hours, any other number of degrees will give its proportional hours: And if 24 hours give 360 degrees, any other number of hours will give its proportional number of degrees.

And hence are derived methods for converting arcs of circles into meaſures of time, and meaſures of time into arcs of circles.

To reduce degrees, minutes, &c. to time.

Multiply by 24, and divide by 360; or multiply by 4, and divide by 60: *Or*, Divide the given degrees by 15 for hours; multiply the remainder by 4 for minutes, adding to the product 1 minute for every 15′ of a degree; the overplus minutes of a degree, multiplied by 4, give ſeconds of time, *&c.*

Or thus: Let the quotient of the given degrees by 60 ſtand for the firſt name; the remaining degrees for the ſecond name; and the other given names in order following: Then this number multiplied by 4, will give the hours, minutes, ſeconds, &c. in order.

To reduce time into degrees.

Multiply the given hours by 15 gives degrees, to which add 1° for every 4 minutes of time; for every overplus minute reckon 15′ of a degree; and for every ſecond of time take 15″ of a degree.

Or thus: Divide the time by 4, carrying by ſixties, the quotient will be in order, ſixties of degrees, degrees, minutes, ſeconds, &c.: Then ſixties of degrees and degrees being reduced, will give the degrees, &c. required.

Exam. I. *Reduce* 69° 20′, 45″, *to its corresponding time.*

$15)\ 69^{\circ}\ 20'\ 45''\ (4^{h}\ 37^{m}\ 23^{s}$

$9\times4+1=37$

$5\times4+3=23$

Exam. II. *Reduce* 4^{h}, 37^{m}, 23^{s}, *to its corresponding degrees.*

4^{h}	37^{m}	23^{s}	
15			
60°	0′	0″	for 4 hours.
9	15	0	for 37 minutes.
	5	45	for 23 seconds.
69°	20′	45″	

Exam. III. *Reduce* 237°, 44′, 37″, *to its equivalent time.*

$60)\ 237^{\circ}$

3 57 44 37

4

Answer $15^{h}\ 50^{m}\ 58^{s}\ 28^{t}$

Exam. IV. *Reduce* 15^{h}, 50^{m}, 58^{s}, 28^{t}, *to its equivalent degrees.*

$4)\ 15^{h}\ 50^{m}\ 58^{s}\ 28^{t}$

$3^{s}\ 57^{\circ}\ 44'\ 37''$

Or $237^{\circ}\ 44'\ 37''$ Answer.

As the Sun is constantly changing his place, the tables of his right ascension shew for every day at noon (when he comes to the meridian of the place for which the tables are made) what part of the equator is intercepted between that meridian and the equinoctial point ♈. The tables for the stars shew the equatorial arcs contained between the point ♈ and the section of circles of right ascension, passing through those stars: The measures of the arcs of right ascension are reduced to time.

There are few days when one or more stars do not come to the meridian with the Sun, and then they have the same right ascension with him: Also, at some time of the year, the Sun must have the same right ascension which any proposed star has; though at other times he may have a less, and so precedes, or comes to the meridian before that star; or a greater, and so follows the star, and comes to the meridian later. And hence is derived the following method.

Of Finding the Culminating of the Stars.

134. *To find the time when any star in the table will be on the meridian.*

Rule. Subtract the sun's right ascension for the proposed day from the right ascension of the given star; the difference will be the time of the star's culminating nearly. Say as 24^{h} is to the daily change of the sun's right ascension, so is the time of culminating, nearly, to a fourth number; which being subtracted from the time of culminating nearly, will give the true time of the star's culminating. If this time be less than 12^{h} it happens in the afternoon; but if more than twelve hours, the excess above 12^{h} will shew the time next morning.

N. B. 24^{h} must be added to the star's right ascension, if the sun's right ascension be greatest.

Exam.

EXAM. I. *At what time will the ſtar Arcturus come to the meridian of London on the 1ſt of September, 1780?*

Right aſcen. of Arcturus	14^h	5′	42″
Sun's right aſcenſion	10	44	34
Time of culmin. nearly	3	21	8
And $3^h\ 21\frac{1}{4}^m$ give			30
True time of ſtar's culm.	3	20	38

Ex. II. *On the 26th of Feb. 1780, at what hour will the ſtar Virgin's Spike be on the meridian of London?*

Virg. Spike's right aſc.	13^h	13′	38″
Sun's right aſcenſion	22	37	10
Time of culm. nearly	14	36	28
And 14^h, $36\frac{5}{8}^m$ give		2	18
True time of ſtar's culm.	14	34	10

If the time of the ſtar's culminating be wanted for any other meridian than that of Greenwich, or London, add the longitude in time to the time of culminating nearly, if the longitude be weſt, or take their difference if it be eaſt, and uſe that ſum or difference inſtead of the time of culminating nearly: obſerving, only, in the latter caſe, that if the longitude in time be greater than the time of culminating nearly, that the min. and ſec. reſulting from the proportion, muſt be added to the time of culminating nearly, inſtead of being ſubtracted from it.

EXAM. *On the 26th of February, 1784, what time will Syrius be on the meridian of a place which is in longitude 166° 30′ E. of London?*

Rt. aſcen. Syrius, 1780	6^h	35′	28″
Preceſſion for 4 years	+		11
Time of culm. nearly	7	58	36
Long. in time	11	6	00
Difference	3	7	24

} Rt. aſc. of Syrius, 1784	6^h	35′	39″
Sun's right aſcen.	22	37	10
Time of culm. nearly	7	58	29
And $3^h\ 7^m$, 4 give +			29
True time of ſtar's culm.	7	58	58

To find if any ſtar in the table will be on, or near the meridian at a given time, reckoned from the preceding noon.

RULE. To the given time add the Sun's right aſcenſion for that time; the ſum (rejecting 24 hours, if above) is the right aſcenſion of the mid-heaven; which being ſought among thoſe of the ſtars, will ſhew what ſtar will be on, or near the meridian at the time propoſed.

EXAM. I. *What ſtar will be on the meridian of London about 10 o'clock at night on the 25th January, 1784?*

Given time 10 hours P. M.	10^h	0^m
Sun's right aſcenſion at noon	20	31
And for 10 hours more		2
Sum (abating 24 hours) anſwers to Syrius.	6	33

Ex. II. *On the 10th May, 1784, what ſtar will be on the merid. of Lond. about 30 min. after 4 in the morning?*

Given time	16^h	30′
Sun's right aſcenſion at noon	3	12
And for 16 hours more		3
Right aſcenſion mid-heaven anſwers nearly to Altair.	19	45

SECTION

SECTION IV.

Of the Projection of the Sphere.

135. PROBLEM I.

To project the ſphere upon the plane of the ſolſtitial colure, or upon the plane of the meridian of any place, thoſe planes being ſuppoſed to coincide.

For this projection, the eye is ſuppoſed to be in the firſt point of Aries, or the common interſection of the equator, ecliptic, and equinoctial colure; that being the pole of the plane of projection, or primitive circle. Pl. IV. Fig. 4.

1ſt. With the chord of 60 degrees deſcribe a circle PESQ to repreſent the ſolſtitial colure, the center of which ♈ is its pole. (IV. 62)

2d. A diameter EQ will be the equator, and another PS at right angles to it will ſhew the equinoctial colure (IV. 60), or the axis of the world, the extremities of which P, S, will be the north and ſouth poles.

3d. *For the parallels of declination.* On the primitive circle, beginning at E and Q, apply the chords of the given degrees of declination, ſuppoſe every 10 degrees, and alſo the diſtances of the *tropics* and *polar circles* from the equator, namely, $23\frac{1}{2}^\circ$ and $66\frac{1}{2}^\circ$. Then from the center ♈ in the axis PS produced, apply the reſpective ſecants of the complements of the degrees laid on the primitive (IV. 58), and theſe will give the centers of the correſponding parallels of declination; from which centers, with the extents to the ſeveral diviſions in the circumference, deſcribe the ſmall circles 10, 10; 20, 20; *&c.* and theſe will be the parallels of declination required: Among which *a* ♋, *b* ♑, are the tropics of Cancer and Capricorn; and *cc*, *dd*, the arctic and antarctic polar circles.

4th. *For the circles of right aſcenſion, or hour circles.* In the diameter EQ produced lay off from the center ♈ both ways the tangents of 15°, 30°, 45°, 60°, 75°, reſpectively, and they will give the centers of circles to be deſcribed through P and S, and cutting the equator in the points repreſenting the 24 hours; the ſolſtitial colure being the 12 o'clock, and the equinoctial colure, PS, the ſix o'clock hour circles. And in like manner may any other of this kind of circles be drawn. (IV. 75)

5th. *The ecliptic* ♋ ♑ is drawn, making with the equator an angle of $23\frac{1}{2}^\circ$; the poles of which *c*, *d*, are the interſections of the polar circles with the ſolſtitial colure.

6th. *Parallels of celeſtial latitude* are drawn parallel to the ecliptic, in the ſame manner as the circles of declination are drawn parallel to the equator.

7th. *Circles of celeſtial longitude* are deſcribed through *c*, *d*, the poles of the ecliptic, in the ſame manner as the circles of right aſcenſion were deſcribed through P, S, the poles of the equator; and thus were the diviſions of the ecliptic found that are marked with the ſigns.

8th. *The horizon* is repreſented by drawing a diameter HR, making an angle with the axis PS, equal to the latitude of the place; and the poles of the horizon Z, N, the zenith and nadir, are at 90° diſt. from the circle HR.

9th. *Azimuth*, or *vertical circles*, making any angle with the meridian, are deſcribed like circles of right aſcenſion: Thus ZN is the prime vertical, and ZAN is another azimuth, 45° from the ſouth.

10th, *Almi-*

10th. *Almicanthers, or parallels of altitude*, are in this projection drawn parallel to the horizon, in like manner as the circles of declination were drawn parallel to the equator.

136. ## PROBLEM II.

To project the sphere upon the plane of the horizon.

In this projection, the eye is supposed in the nadir, one of the poles of the horizon, or plane of projection. Plate IV. Fig. 5.

1st. *The horizon* is represented by the primitive circle, where the upper XII is the north, the lower XII the south, E the west, and Q the east points.

2d. *The azimuth circles* are represented by diameters drawn through Z, the center or pole of the horizon: Thus the diameter XII, XII is for the meridian, and EZQ for the prime vertical; and other azimuth circles, forming any angle with the meridian, are readily drawn by laying off their distances in the primitive from the north or south points.

3d. *Parallels of altitude* are concentric to the primitive, and are described about the pole Z with the half tangent of their distance from it: Thus the small circle, the diameter of which is *ab*, is a parallel of altitude 10° above the horizon, or at 80° distant form its pole Z.

4th. The distance of the *equinoctial* from the zenith is equal to the latitude of the place, and therefore this circle makes with the horizon an angle, which is measured by the complement of the latitude; then setting off from the center Z in Z XII continued, the tangent of 50° (the latitude in this example being 40°), it will give the center of the circle EAQ, representing the equinoctial; and the half tangent of 50°, set the same way from Z, will give P, the pole of the world.

5th. *The six o'clock hour circle* passes through the poles of the world, making with the horizon an angle equal to the measure of the latitude; therefore taking in the meridian, from Z towards A, the tangent of the latitude 40°, it gives G, the center of the six o'clock hour circle EPQ.

6th. *The hour circles* pass through the poles of the world, and make with one another angles of 15 degrees: Therefore (IV. 55) in a line DF, drawn through G, at right angles to the meridian, set off on both sides of G the tangents 15°, 30°, 45°, 60°, 75°, to the radius PG, and they will give the centers of the several hour circles passing through P, cutting the horizon and equinoctial in the hour points.

7th. *The polar circles, tropics, and other circles of declination*, are described parallel to the equinoctial, about its pole P, at given distances from it, either by finding the centers of such parallels, as shewn in B. IV. 66; or by setting off on each side of Z the half tangents of their greatest and least distances from Z; then the middles of those intervals are the centers sought. Thus; the arctic circle is distant from P $23\frac{1}{2}$°; then to, and from ZP=50°, add and take $23\frac{1}{2}$°; there remain $73\frac{1}{2}$° and $26\frac{1}{2}$°; the half tangents of these set off from Z give *p* and *q*; then a circle described on the diameter *pq* is the arctic circle.

In like manner will the centers of the tropic of Cancer *c* ♋ *c*, and of Capricorn *d* ♑ *d*, be obtained.

8th. *The northern portion of the ecliptic* ♈ ♋ ♎ is described from a center distant from Z towards P, the tangent of $73\frac{1}{2}$°, = ∠ the ecliptic makes with the horizon.

9th. *Cir-*

9th. *Circles of longitude* ♈ *p* ♎, *p* ♉, *p* ♊, *p* ♌, *p* ♍, are described thro' *p*, the pole of the ecliptic, from centers in the line BFC; in like manner as the hour circles were described through P, the pole of the equator.

10th. *Circles of celestial latitude*, VIII *q* IX, are described about *p*, as the circles of declination were described about P, the pole of the equinoctial.

137. PROBLEM III.

To project the sphere upon the plane of the equator.

In this projection the eye is supposed to be in one of the poles of the equator, suppose in the south pole, and projecting the north hemisphere. Plate IV. Fig. 6.

1st. *The equator* is represented by the primitive circle, the center and pole of which is P.

2d. *The hour circles* are expressed by diameters making angles of 15° with one another; of which XII P XII is the meridian, or solstitial colure, and VI P VI the 6 o'clock circle, or equinoctial colure.

3d. *Circles of declination* are circles parallel and concentric to the equator, described from its center with radii equal to the half tangents of their several distances from the pole P, or half co-tangents of their degrees of declination: Thus *pq* the arctic circle, and *a* ♋ the tropic of Cancer, are described with the half tangents of 23½° and 66½° respectively; and so of the others.

4th. *The ecliptic* making an angle of 23½° with the equator; the tangent of these degrees laid from P towards *a* will give the center for describing the ecliptic ♈ ♋ ♎, the pole of which *p* is in the polar circle.

5th. *Circles of longitude* are described through *p*, the pole of the ecliptic, in like manner as the hour circles were described through P, the pole of the equator in the last problem; and thus were the divisions ♉, ♊, ♌, ♍, obtained.

6th. *Circles of celestial latitude* are projected in the same manner as the circles of declination in the last problem.

7th. *The horizon of any place*, suppose of London, being inclined to the equator in an angle equal to the co-latitude, 38° 28′; the tangent of this laid from P towards ♋, and the half tangent laid from P to Z, will give the center, and Z the pole, of the horizon HOR.

8th. *The prime vertical* HZR making an angle with the equator equal to 51° 32′, the latitude of the place, its center is found by laying the tangent of 51° 32′ from P towards O.

9th. *Azimuth circles*, making given angles with the meridian ZO, are thus described: In a line drawn through the center of the prime vertical, at right angles to the meridian, take distances from that center, equal to the tangents of the proposed azimuth angles, the semidiameter of the prime vertical being the radius, those distances give the centers sought; and thus was the azimuth circle ZA described.

10th. *Parallels of altitude* are described about Z, the pole of the horizon, at the distances of the co-altitudes, in the same manner as the circles of declination were described about P, the pole of the equator in the last problem; and thus was the small circle V *b* VII described at 10° distance from the horizon, or 80° distant from its pole Z.

138. PROBLEM IV.

To project the ſphere upon the plane of the ecliptic.

The eye is here ſuppoſed to be in one of the poles of the ecliptic, and thence viewing the northern hemiſphere. Plate IV. Fig. 7.

1ſt. *The ecliptic* is here repreſented by the primitive circle, the center of which *p* is its pole.

2d. *Circles of longitude* are here repreſented by diameters; thoſe that make angles of 30° with one another, being drawn through the diviſions marked with the ſigns of the zodiac.

3d. *Parallels of celeſtial latitude* are circles deſcribed about *p*, concentric to the ecliptic; ſuch is the ſmall circle, the diameter of which is *ab*, repreſenting the parallel of 10° of latitude.

4th. *The equator* making an angle with the ecliptic of $23\frac{1}{2}$°; therefore the tangent of this inclination laid from *p* towards ♋ will give the center of the equator ♈ XII ♎; and the half tangent of $23\frac{1}{2}$° laid from *p* the ſame way, gives P for the pole of the equator.

5th. *The equinoctial colure*, which here makes the *ſix o'clock circle*, makes an angle with the ecliptic of $66\frac{1}{2}$°; therefore the tangent of $66\frac{1}{2}$° laid from *p* towards ♑, gives the center of the 6 o'clock circle ♈ P ♎.

6th. *Hour circles* paſſing through P, and making angles of 15° with one another, are deſcribed from centers, found in a right line paſſing through the center of ♈ P ♎, and drawn at right angles to the ſolſtitial colure ♈ *p* ♑; by laying off in that line the tangents of 15°, 30°, 45°, 60°, 75°, reckoned from the center of ♈ P ♎, on both ſides, the ſemi-diameter of this circle being the radius. Theſe hour circles cut the equator in the hour points.

7th. *Parallels of declination*, ſuch as the tropic of Cancer, and the arctic circle, the diameters of which are 12, 12, and *pq*, are deſcribed by laying off from *p* the half tangents of their greateſt and leaſt diſtances: Thus *q* being diſtant from *p* 47°, makes $pq=\frac{1}{2}$ tangent of 47°, the middle of *pq* will be the center of the polar circle.

8th. *The horizon* HOR is to make an angle with the ecliptic equal to the difference between the co-latitude and the obliquity of the ecliptic, when P is projected to the north of *p*; otherwiſe that angle is equal to the ſum of thoſe quantities. And for London, where the ſaid difference =(38° 28′—23° 28′=) 15° 00′, the tangent of 15° 00′, gives the center of HOR, and the half tangent gives Z the zenith.

9th. *The prime vertical* HZR is deſcribed by laying from *p*, towards O, the co-tangent of *p*Z for a center.

10th. *Azimuth circles* are deſcribed through Z, making given angles with the meridian ZO, by finding their centers in a line drawn through the center of HZR, in the manner deſcribed for the hour circles, Prob. II.

11th. *Parallels of altitude* are repreſented by deſcribing ſmall circles parallel to the horizon HOR, at given diſtances from it; or, which comes to the ſame, deſcribing ſmall circles about the pole Z, at diſtances equal to the complements of the given altitudes: And thus the circle *cde* was deſcribed for a parallel of 33° of altitude.

SECTION

SECTION V.

Problems of the Sphere.

139. PROBLEM V. Pl. V.

Given the Sun's longitude, and the obliquity of the ecliptic;
Required the Sun's right aſcenſion and declination.

EXAM. *Let the obliquity of the ecliptic, or the Sun's greateſt declination, be 23° 28′, and the Sun's place 13° 16′ in Taurus: Required the reſt.*

CONSTRUCTION.

In the primitive circle PESQ, repreſenting the ſolſtitial colure, the center of which is ♈, draw a diameter EQ for the equator, and at right angles to EQ draw a diameter PS for the equinoctial colure: Make E ♋ = 23° 28′, and draw a diameter ♋ ♑ for the ecliptic, in which (IV. 71.) take ♈ ☉ = 43° 16′ for the Sun's diſtance from the point ♈: Through P ☉ S deſcribe a circle of right aſcenſion.

COMPUTATION. See Book IV. art. 130, 131.

In the right angled ſpheric triangle ♈ ☉ B.

Given Sun's longitude	♈ ☉ = 43° 16′	Req. right aſcen.	♈ B.
Obliquity of the Eclip.	∠ ☉ ♈ B = 23 28	declin.	B ☉.

To find the declination.			*To find the right aſcenſion.*		
As Radius	= R	10,00000	As Radius	= R	10,00000
To ſ. Sun's lon.	= 43° 16′	9,83594	To t. Sun's lon.	= 43° 16′	9,97371
So ſ. ob. eclip.	= 23 28	9,60012	So co-ſ. obl. ecl.	= 23 28	9,96251
To ſ. Sun's decl.	= 15 50	9,43606	To t. rt. aſcen.	= 40 48	9,93622

140. While the Sun is moving from ♈ to ♋, or is in the firſt quadrant of the ecliptic, the given longitude is the hypothenuſe in the triangle ♈ ☉ B, the declination B ☉ is north, and ♈ B is the right aſcenſion.

When the Sun has paſt the ſolſtice ♋, and is deſcending towards ♎, he is then ſaid to be in the ſecond quadrant, and his longitude or diſtance from ♈ being taken from 180°, the remainder ♎ ☉ becomes the hypothenuſe, and the declination is ſtill north; but the arc B ♎ found for the right aſcenſion is only the ſupplement, and muſt therefore be taken from 180°.

The Sun having paſt the point ♎, and deſcending towards ♑ has got into the third quadrant; the longitude then, reckoned from ♈, will be greater than 180°: In this caſe the exceſs above 180°, or the diſtance the Sun is removed from ♎, will be the hypothenuſe ♎ ☉; the declination will be ſouth; and the arc ♎ A, found for the right aſcenſion, muſt be added to 180°, to give the right aſcenſion eſtimated from ♈.

When the Sun has paſt the ſolſtice ♑, and is aſcending towards ♈, he is then in the fourth quadrant; therefore the longitude is greater than 270°, and muſt be taken from 360°, to give the hypothenuſe ♎ ☉. Here the declination is ſouth, and the right aſcenſion ♎ A, found by the proportion, muſt be taken from 360°, to give the right aſcenſion from ♈.

At equal diſtances from the equinoctial points ♈ or ♎, the Sun will have equal quantities of declination; but will be of different names, according as it is on the north or ſouth ſide of the equinoctial.

141. PROBLEM VI. Pl. V.

Given the obliquity of the ecliptic, and the Sun's declination; Required the Sun's longitude and right ascension.

EXAM. *The obliquity of the ecliptic, being 23° 28′, what is the Sun's longitude and right ascension when he has 20° 43′ of north declination?*

CONSTRUCTION.

Having described the solstitial colure, and drawn the equator EQ, the axis PS, and the ecliptic ♋ ♑, as before; make En, Qn, equal to the given declination, and (3d 133) describe the parallel of declination *nn*, its intersection with the ecliptic gives ☉ the Sun's place; through P, ☉, S, describe the circle of right ascension P ☉ S.

COMPUTATION.

In the right-angled spheric triangle ♈ ☉ B.

Given the ob. eclip. ∠ ☉ ♈ B = 23° 28′ } Required Sun's long. ♈ ☉.
the Sun's decl. ☉ B = 20 43 } rt. ascen. ♈ B.

To find the Sun's longitude.			*To find the Sun's right ascension.*		
As s. obliq. eclip.	= 23° 28′	0,39988	As Radius	= R	10,00000
To sin Sun's decl.	= 20 43	9.54869	To co-t. obl. eclip.	= 23° 28′	10,36239
So radius	= R	10,00000	So tan. Sun's dec.	= 20 43	9,57772
To sin. ☉ longit.	= 62 40	9,94857	To sin. rt. ascen.	= 60 36	9,94011

Therefore the Sun is in ♊ 2° 40′, or in ♋ 27° 20′, according as the time of the year is before or after the summer solstice.

142. PROBLEM VII. Pl. V.

Given the obliquity of the ecliptic, and the Sun's right ascension; Required the Sun's longitude and declination.

EXAM. *When the Sun's right ascension is 60° 31′, what is the longitude and present declination, the obliq. of the eclip. being 23° 28′?*

CONSTRUCTION.

The solstitial colure, equator, axis, and ecliptic being described as before, make ♈ B = given right ascension (4th 133), and describe the circle PBS, cutting the ecliptic in ☉ the Sun's place.

COMPUTATION.

In the right-angled spheric triangle ♈ ☉ B; the leg ♈ B and ∠ ☉ ♈ B being known, the hypoth. ♈ ☉, and other leg ☉ B, are found as in art. 137, 138. Book IV.

As Rad. . co-s. ob. eclip. : : co-t. rt. [as. : co-t. ☉ long.	As Rad. : tan. obl. eclip. : : sin. rt. [as. : tan. decl.
As Rad. : co-s. 23° 28′ : : co-t. 60° 31′ [: co-t. 62° 35′	As Rad. : tan. 23° 28′ : : sin. 60° 31′ [: tan. 20° 42′

Three other problems may be formed out of the four things concerned, or obliquity of the ecliptic, declination, longitude, and right ascension: But these being of little more importance than as an exercise for right-angled spheric triangles, they are therefore omitted.

143. PRO-

143. PROBLEM VIII. Pl. V.

Given the latitude of the place, and the Sun's declination;
Required the Sun's altitude and azimuth at 6 o'clock.

EXAM. *At London, in lat. 51° 32′ N., on the longest day, when the Sun's declination is 23° 28′: Required the Sun's altitude and azimuth at 6 o'clock in the morning or evening.*

CONSTRUCTION.

Describe the meridian, draw the horizon HR, and prime vertical ZN; make RP=latitude 51° 32′ N.; draw the 6 o'clock hour circle PS, the equator EQ, the 23° 28′ N. parallel of declination *n m*, cutting the 6 o'clock hour circle PS in ⊙; and through Z, ⊙, N, describe the azimuth circle Z ⊙ N, cutting the horizon in A; then the things given and required fall in either of the triangles Z ⊙ P or ♈ ⊙ A, they being supplemental triangles one to the other.

COMPUTATION.

In the spheric triangle Z ⊙ P, right-angled at P.

Given the co-latit. ZP=38° 28′ } Required the co-altitude Z ⊙.
the co-decl. ⊙P=66 32 } the azimuth ∠ ⊙ ZP.

Or in the spheric triangle ♈ A ⊙, right-angled at A.

Given the latit. A ♈ ⊙=51° 32′ } Required the altitude A⊙.
the decl. ♈ ⊙=23 28 } the co-azimuth ♈A.

To find the altitude A⊙.

As Radius	= R		10,00000
To sin. decl.	= 23° 28′		9,60012
So sin. lat.	= 51 32		9,89375
To sin. alt.	= 18 10		9,49387

To find the azimuth AR.

As Radius	= R		10,00000
To co-s. lat.	= 51° 32′		9,79383
So tan. decl.	= 23 28		9,63761
To co-t. azim.	= 74 53		9,43144

For the arc AR measures the ∠RZA, the azimuth. (IV. 9)

144. On the shortest day at London, the parallel of S. declination cuts the 6 o'clock hour circle below the horizon; and as the triangles ♈A⊙, ♈a⊙, are congruous, the depression below the horizon, on the shortest day at 6 o'clock, will be equal to the altitude at the same hour on the longest day; and the azimuth will also be equal, if estimated from the south.

So that on the 21st of June, at London, the Sun will bear N. 74° 53′ E. at 6 o'clock in the morning, and N. 74° 53′ W. at 6 in the evening; but on the 21st of December, at the same hours, it will bear S. 74° 53′ E., and S. 74° 53′ W.

From a due consideration of this Problem it is evident, that as the declination increases, the altitude increases and the azimuth lessens; and the contrary happens while the declination is diminishing: So that on the days of the equinoxes, on which the Sun has no declination, the altitude at 6 o'clock will be nothing, or the Sun will be in the horizon; and the azimuth being then 90 degrees, the Sun will be due east in the morning, and west in the evening; that is, on the days of the equinoxes the Sun rises and sets at six, in the east and west points of the horizon.

Given the latitude of the place, and the Sun's declination;
Required the altitude and hour when the Sun is due east or west.

EXAM. *At London, in latitude 51° 32′ N., what is the Sun's altitude, and the hour when he is due east or west, on the longest day, or when the declination is 23° 28′ N.?*

CONSTRUCTION.

Describe the primitive circle to represent the meridian of London, draw the horizon HR, and the prime vertical ZN; make RP = 51° 32′, the given latitude, draw the 6 o'clock hour circle PS, the equator EQ, the parallel of declination *mn* (3d 135), cutting the prime vertical in ☉, and through P☉S describe (II. 72) the hour circle P☉S, cutting the equator in A.

Here the things concerned in the Problem fall in either of the triangles PZ☉ or ♈A☉.

COMPUTATION.

In the spheric triangle PZ☉, right-angled at Z.

Given the co-latit. PZ = 38° 28′ } Required the co-altitude Z☉
the co-decl. P☉ = 66 32 } the hour fr. noon ∠ZP☉.

Or in the spherical triangle ♈A☉, right angled at A.

Given the latit. ∠A♈☉ = 51° 32′ } Required the altitude ♈☉.
the decl. A☉ = 23 28 } the hour after 6 ♈A.

To find the altitude ♈☉.		*To find the hour after* 6.	
As s. lat. ∠A♈☉ = 51° 32′	0,10625	As Radius = R	10,00000
To sin. decl. A☉ = 23 28	9,60012	To co-t. lat. A♈☉ = 51° 32′	9,90009
So Radius = R	10,00000	So tan. decl. A☉ = 23 28	9,63761
To sin. alt. ♈☉ = 30 34	9,70637	To s. h. fr. 6. A♈ = 20 11	9,53770

Which 20° 11′ converted into time (132), gives 1 h. 20 m. 44 s. for the time after 6 in the morning, and before 6 in the evening, when the Sun will appear due east or west; which will be at 7 h. 20 m. 44 s. in the morning, and 4 h. 39 m. 16 s. in the afternoon.

Or, the compl. of 20° 11′, *viz.* 69° 49′ put into time, which gives 4 h. 39 m. 16 s., shews the time before and after noon, when the Sun will be due east or west.

146. This Problem worked for the shortest day, namely in the △♈*a*☉, which is congruous to ♈A☉, would give the Sun's depression at the time when he was east or west, which would be before 6 in the morning, and after 6 in the evening, by as much as was found above, *viz.* 1 h. 20 m. 44 s.

By this Problem it appears, that when the latitude of the place, and the Sun's declination, have the same name, then, the greater the declination and latitude, the greater the altitude and time from 6: and having contrary names, the same things happen; but with this difference, that in the former case the days lengthen on account of the increase of the latitude and declination; whereas in the latter case the days shorten on that account.

147. PRO-

Given the latitude of a place and the Sun's declination;
Required his amplitude and afcenfional difference.

EXAM. *At London, lat. 51° 32′ N. on the 21ft of June, being the longeft day, when the Sun's declination is 23° 28′ N. How far from the north does the Sun rife and fet, at what time, and what is the length of the day and night?*

CONSTRUCTION.

Let the primitive circle reprefent the meridian of the place, and the diameter HR the horizon; from R, the north point, take RP = 51° 32′ for the latitude, draw the axis, or 6 o'clock hour circle PS, and at right angles to it draw the equator EQ; make E*n*, Q*m* = 23° 28′, the declination, and (3d 135) defcribe the parallel of declination *n m*, cutting the horizon in ☉, the place of the Sun at its rifing and fetting; through which defcribe (II. 72) the hour-circle P ☉ S.

COMPUTATION.

Now as the arc QR = co-latitude, meafures the ∠ Q ♈ R.

In the fpheric triangle ♈ ☉ A, right-angled at A.

Given Sun's decl.	A ☉ = 23° 28′	Required the amplitude	♈ ☉
co-latit.	∠ A ♈ ☉ = 38 28	the afcen. diff.	♈ A.

To find the amplitude ♈ ☉.

As fin. A ♈ ☉, co-l.	= 38° 28′	0,20617
To fin. decl. A ☉	= 23 28	9,60012
So Radius	= R	10,00000
To fin. amp. ♈ ☉	= 39 48	9,80629

This 39° 48′ is the amplitude reckoned from the eaft or weft points of the horizon: But its complement 50° 12′ fhews how far from the north the Sun rifes or fets on the longeft day at London.

To find the afcenfional difference ♈ A.

As Radius	= R	10,00000
To t. lat. ∠ P ♈ ☉	= 51° 32′	10,09991
So tan. decl. A ☉	= 23 28	9,63761
To f. af. diff. ♈ A	= 33 07	9,73752

Which 33° 07′ converted into time (132) gives 2 h. 12 m. 28 s. for the time which the Sun rifes before, and fets after, the hour of fix on the longeft day.

Suppofe *rs* to be a parallel of declination as far fouth, as *m n* is north; then the hour circle P ☉ S, paffing through ☉ the place of the fun at its rifing or fetting, will form a triangle ♈ ☉ B = A ♈ ☉ A, where the amplitude is to the fouthward of the eaft and weft points.

148. Hence it is evident, *that when the latitude and declination have the fame name, the Sun rifes before, and fets after 6: But when they are of contrary names, the Sun rifes after, and fets before 6.*

149. And

149. And as the Sun defcribes the parallel of declination $n\ m$ in 24 hours, being at n when it is noon, and at m when it is midnight; therefore the time in paffing from m to ☉, or the time of rifing being doubled, gives the length of the night; and the time of fetting being doubled, muft give the length of the day.

Then to, and from	6h	0m	0s
Add and fubtract the afcen. diff.	2	12	28
Sum, gives ☉ fetting	8	12	28
Diff. gives ☉ rifing	3	47	32
Length of day is	16	24	56
Length of night is	7	35	04

But when it is the fhorteft day at London, which is, when the Sun has 23° 28′ fouth declination; then the lengths of the day and night change places; the day being 7 h. 35 m. 04 s. long, and the night 16 h. 24 m. 56 s.

150. When the latitude and declination have the fame name, the difference between the right afcenfion and the afcenfional difference, is the oblique afcenfion; and their fum is the oblique defcenfion..

But when they are of contrary names, their fum is the oblique afcenfion, and their difference is the oblique defcenfion.

151. When the declination is equal to the co-latitude of any place (which can only happen to places within the polar circles), than the parallel of declination will not cut the horizon, and confequently the Sun will not fet in thofe places during the time his declination exceeds the co-latitude: And the fame may be faid of all thofe ftars, the polar diftance of which is lefs than the latitude of the place; or, which is the fame thing, that have declinations lefs than the co-latitude, for thofe ftars will never defcend below the horizon of that place. But this is to be underftood only when the Sun or ftars are in the fame hemifphere with the given place; for when the Sun or ftars are in a contrary hemifphere to any place, the co-latitude of which does not exceed the declination of thofe celeftial objects, then they will never rife above the horizon of that place, and confequently are never vifible there.

152. PROBLEM XI. Pl. V.

Given the latitude of a place, the Sun's declination and altitude; Required the hour from noon, and the Sun's azimuth.

EXAM. *In the latitude of 51° 32′ N. the Sun's altitude was obſerved to be 46° 20′, when his declination was 23° 28′ N. What was the Sun's azimuth, and the hour when the obſervation was made?*

CONSTRUCTION.

Let the primitive circle ZRNH repreſent the meridian of London, HR the horizon, ZN the prime vertical; make RP = 51° 32′ the height of the pole at London; draw the axis PS, and the equator EQ; lay off the declination E*n*, Q*m*, 23° 28′ N. the altitude H*r*, R*s*, 46° 20′; and (IV. 68) deſcribe the parallel of declination *n m*, and the parallel of altitude *rs*, cutting one another in ☉, the place of the Sun at that time; through Z, ☉, N, deſcribe an azimuth circle Z☉N, and through P, ☉, S, deſcribe an hour circle P☉S: Then the angles ☉ZP, ☉PZ, being meaſured (IV. 72), will give the azimuth and hour from noon required.

COMPUTATION.

In the oblique-angled ſpheric triangle P☉Z.

Given the co-latitude - ZP = 38° 28′
the co-alt. or zen. diſt. Z☉ = 43 40
the co-dec. or pol. diſt. ☉P = 66 32

} Required the azim. ∠ ☉ZP and the h. fr. noon ∠ ☉PZ. See art. 167. Book IV.

To find the azimuth ∠ ☉ZP.

Here Z☉ = 43° 40′
ZP = 38 28
Z☉ − ZP = 5 12 = D
P☉ = 66 32
71 44 | 35° 52′
2)
61 20 | 30 40

Then Co-ar. ſin. co-lat.	= 38° 28′	0,20617
Co-ar. ſin. co-alt.	= 43 40	0.16086
Sin. ½ ſum co-decl. & D	= 35 52	9,76782
Sin. ½ diff. co-decl. & D	= 30 40	9,70761
The ſum of the four logs.		19,84246
The ½ ſum gives 56° 31½′		9,92123

Which doubled, gives 113° 03′ for the azimuth ſought, reckoning from the north.

To find the hour from noon, ∠ ☉PZ.

Here P☉ = 66° 32′
PZ = 38 28
P☉ − PZ = 28 4 = D
☉Z = 43 40
71 44 | 35° 52′
2)
15 36 | 7 48

Then Co-ar. ſin. co-decl.	= 66° 32′	0,03749
Co-ar. ſin. co-lat.	= 38 28	0,20617
Sin. ½ ſum co-alt. & D	= 35 52	9,76782
Sin. ½ diff. co-alt. & D	= 7 48	9,13263
The ſum of the four logs.		19,14411
The ½ ſum gives 21° 55′		9,57206

This doubled, gives 43° 50′ for the meaſure of the hour from noon, which is 2 h. 55 m. 20 s.

Hence it appears, that the obſervation was made either at 9 h. 4 m. 40 s. in the morning, or at 2 h. 55 m. 20 s. in the afternoon.

The azimuth being firſt found, the hour from noon might have been found by the proportion between oppoſite ſides and angles.

Had the declination and latitude been of contrary names, the ſame kind of operation would have been uſed to find the things required, only the ſide ☉ P would have been obtuſe; by adding the declinat. to 90°, inſtead of ſubtracting it, as in the caſe of the lat. and decl. having like names.

153. PROBLEM XII. Pl. V.

Given the latitude of the place, and the Sun's declination;
Required the time when the twilight begins and ends.

EXAM. *At what time does the twilight begin and end at London, when the Sun's declination is 15° 12′ N. the latitude of the place being 51° 32′ N.*

CONSTRUCTION.

Let the circle ZRNH repreſent the meridian of the place, HR the horizon, ZN the prime vertical, and *ts* the Crepuſculum, or ſmall circle parallel to the horizon deſcribed at 18 degrees below it (IV. 68); lay off the latitude RP, draw the axis PS, the equator EQ, and deſcribe the parallel of declination *n m*, and where *n m* cuts *t s* in ☉, is the Sun's place at the time of the beginning or end of the twilight; through ☉ deſcribe (II. 72) the vertical circle Z☉N, and the hour circle P☉S; then the ∠ ZP☉ being meaſured (IV. 72) will give the time before or after noon as required.

COMPUTATION.

In the oblique-angled ſpheric triangle Z☉P.

Given the co-lat. ZP = 38° 28′ } Req. the hour from noon = ∠ ZP☉
the polar diſt. P☉ = 74 48 } The manner of ſolution is the
the zenith diſt. Z☉ = 108 00 } ſame as in laſt Problem.

Here P☉ = 74° 48′
PZ = 38 28

P☉ − PZ = 36 20 = D
☉Z = 108 00

144 20 | 72° 10′
2) ——
71 40 | 35 50

Then Co-ar. ſin. polar diſt.	= 74° 45′		0,01547
Co-ar. ſin. co-latit.	= 38	28	0,20617
Sine ½ ſum. of zen. d. & D	= 72	10	9,97861
Sine ½ diff. of zen. d. & D	= 35	50	9,76747
The ſum of theſe four logs.			19,96772
The half ſum gives 74° 28½′			9,98386

Which doubled, gives 148° 57′ for ∠ ZP☉.

And 148° 57′ reduced to time gives 9 h. 55 m. 48 s. either before or after noon; that is, the twilight begins at 2 h. 04 m. 12 s. in the morning, and ends at 9 h. 55 m. 48 s. in the evening on the given day, at London.

154. When the declination becomes greater than the difference between the co-latitude and 18 degrees, then the parallel of declination *n m* will not cut the parallel *t s* 18 degrees below the horizon, and conſequently at that time there will be no night at that place, but the twilight will continue from Sun-ſetting to Sun-riſing; and on this account it is, that from the 22d of May to the 21ſt of July nearly, there is no total darkneſs at London, the Sun's declination during that interval being greater than 20° 28′, which is the difference between 18° and 38° 28′, the complement of the latitude.

155. PRO-

Given the time of the year, the latitude of a place, and the altitude of a known fixed ſtar;
Required the hour of the night when the obſervation was made.

EXAM. *Some time in the night, on the 1ſt of September 1780, ſuppoſe the ſtar Arcturus, the declination of which is 20° 30′ N. ſhould be obſerved at London to be 27° 12′ above the horizon: At what hour would the obſervation be made?*

CONSTRUCTION.

Deſcribe the meridian of the place, draw the horizon HR, the zenith and nadir of which are Z and N, and deſcribe the parallel of altitude *rs* at 27° 12′ above the horizon; take P the north pole 51° 32′ above the horizon for the latitude of the place, and S the ſouth pole as much below the horizon; draw the equator EQ, and deſcribe (3d 135) the ſtar's parallel of declination *n m*; and where this parallel *n m* cuts the former *r s* in ✱, is the poſition of the ſtar at the time of obſervation; deſcribe (II. 72) the vertical circle Z ✱ N, and the hour circle P ✱ S, and the angle ZP ✱ being meaſured (IV. 72) gives the hour from, or to, the time of the ſtar's culminating.

COMPUTATION.

In the oblique-angled ſpheric triangle P ✱ Z.

Given the co-latitude PZ	= 38°	28′	Required ∠ ZP ✱, or the hour from culminating.
the co-altitude Z ✱	= 62	48	
the polar diſt. ✱ P	= 69	30	

Here P ✱ = 69° 30′
PZ = 38 28

P ✱ − PZ = 31 2 = D
Z ✱ = 62 48

93 50 | 46° 55
2)
31 46 | 15 53

Then Co. ar. ſin. co-lat.	= 38°	28′	0,20617
Co. ar. ſin. pol. diſt.	= 69	30	0,02841
Sin. ½ ſum zen. diſt. & D	= 46	55	9,86354
Sin. ½ diff. zen. diſt. & D	= 15	53	9,43724
The ſum of the four logs.			19,53536
The ½ ſum gives 35° 51′			9,76768

Which doubled, gives 71° 42′ = ∠ ZP ✱.

This 71° 42′ turned into time (132) gives 4 h. 46 m. 48 s. for the time which has elapſed ſince the ſtar was on the meridian.

Now, at the time of obſervation, September 1ſt, 1780. (133)

The right aſcenſion of Arcturus was	14h	5′	42″	
The right aſcenſion of the ſun at noon †	10	44	34	
Time of culminating nearly	3	21	08	
And 24h is to 3′ 37″ as 3h 21′¼ is to			30	
The ſtar ſouths, or culminates at	3	20	38	
The time that the ſtar has paſſed the meridian	4	46	48	
The ſum is the hour of the night	8	07	26	P. M.

† Aſtronomical tables at the end of Book V.

And

And whether to ſubtract or add will always be known by the ſtar's being in the eaſtern part of the horizon, or aſcending; or by being in the weſtern part of the horizon, or deſcending.

156. PROBLEM XIV. Pl. V.

Given the obliquity of the ecliptic, and a ſtar's right aſcenſion and declination;

Required its latitude and longitude.

EXAM. *What is the latitude and longitude of a ſtar, its right aſcenſion being 16 h. 14 m., its declination 25° 51′ N., and the obliquity of the ecliptic 23° 28′?*

CONSTRUCTION.

Let the primitive circle repreſent the ſolſtitial colure, in which draw the equator EQ, mark its poles P, S, and deſcribe (3d 135) the parallel of the ſtar's declination *n m*.

The right aſcenſion 16 h. 14 m. = 243° 30′, which being 63° 30′ above 180°, falls in the third quadrant; therefore make (IV. 75.) ♈ *a* = 63° 30′, deſcribe (4th 135) the circle of right aſcenſion, cutting the parallel *n m* in ✱, the point of the heavens repreſenting the ſtar.

Make E♋ = 23° 28′, the obliquity of the ecliptic, draw the ecliptic ♋ ♑, find its poles *p*, *q*, and through *p*, ✱, *q* deſcribe a circle of longitude; then the arc *p* ✱ meaſured (IV. 70) will give the co-latitude, and the ∠ P*p* ✱ will ſhew the longitude.

COMPUTATION.

In the oblique-angled ſpheric triangle *p* P ✱.

Given the obliq. ecliptic *p*P = 23° 28′ } Required the co-lat. *p* ✱.
the co-declination P✱ = 64 09 } and the longit. ∠ P*p* ✱.
the right aſcen. ∠ *p*P✱ = 243 30 } See art. 150, 151. B. IV.

To find the latitude.

As Radius = R	10,00000	As co-ſ. 4th arc = 61° 34′	0,32227
To co-ſ. rt. aſc. = 26° 30′	9,95179	To co-ſ. 5th arc = 38 06	9,89594
So tan. co-decl. = 64 09	10,31471	So ſine decl. = 25 51	9,63950
To tan. 4th arc = 61 34	10,26650	To ſin. lat. = 46 06½	9,85771
Obl. eclipt. = 23 28			
Fifth arc = 38 06			

Here the ſtar's latitude is 46° 06½′ N. becauſe the declinat. is N., and greater than the obliquity of the ecliptic.

To find the longitude.

As ſine 5th arc = 38° 06′	0 20969
To ſine 4th arc = 61 34	9,94417
So tan. rt. aſc. = 26 30	9,69774
To tan. longit. = 234 36	9,85160

Here the longitude 144° 36′ being added to 90°, gives 234° 36′ for the ſtar's longitude, reckoning from the firſt point of Aries.

For the right aſcenſion being in the third quadrant, the ſtar is there alſo. Now in 234° 36′, are 7 ſigns 24° 36′; that is the ſtar's place, or longitude is 24° 36′ in the 8th ſign, or 24° 36′ in ♏.

By the preceſſion of the equinoxes, the fixed ſtars, although they always keep the ſame latitudes, yet are continually altering their longitude, right

right aſcenſion, and declination; the alteration in longitude is uniformly 50 ſeconds and 3-10ths yearly (22), but that of the right aſcenſion and declination is conſtantly varying: So that many ſtars, which once had north declination, come to have ſouth; while others change from S. to N. declination.

157. PROBLEM XV. Pl. V.

Given the right aſcenſions and declinations of two fixed ſtars; Required their diſtance.

EXAM. *What is the diſtance between the fixed ſtars, Betelgueſe in the eaſt ſhoulder of Orion, and Aldebaran in Taurus; the former having 7° 21′ N. declinat. with 5 h. 43 m. 16 s. right aſcenſion; and the other 16° 03′ N. declinat. with 4 h. 23 m. 20 s. of right aſcenſion.*

CONSTRUCTION.

As Aldebaran precedes Betelgueſe in right aſcenſion, let the primitive circle repreſent the circle of right aſcenſion paſſing through Betelgueſe; deſcribe the circle of right aſcenſion PAS, making with PBS an angle of 19° 59′, (IV. 75) equal to the difference between the given right aſcenſions.

Deſcribe the parallels of declination B*m*, *rs*, at the given diſtances 16° 03′ N. and 7° 21′ N. (3d 133); and the interſections A, of Aldebaran's declination, and B, of Betelgueſe's, with their reſpective circles of right aſcenſion, will be the poſitions of thoſe ſtars from one another: Then draw a great circle BAC, through B and A, and the intercepted arc BA (meaſured by art. 70. Book IV.) ſhews the diſtance of thoſe two ſtars.

COMPUTATION. (IV. 151)

In the oblique-angled ſpheric triangle PAB.

Given the co-decl. of Ald. PB=73° 57′ }
the co-dec. of Betelgueſe PA=82 39 } Required their diſt. AB.
diff. of right aſcen. ∠APB=19 39 }

Radius	=R	10,00000	Co-ſ. 4th arc	82° 11′	0,86645
To co-ſ. diff rt. aſ.	19° 59	9,97303	To co-ſ. 5th arc	8 14	9,99550
As co-t. Betelg. dec.	7 21	10,88944	As ſin. Betelg. dec.	7 21	9,10697
To tang. 4th arc	82 11	10,86247	To co-ſ. diſt.	21 25	9,96892
Aldeb. co-dec.	73 57				
Remains 5th arc.	8 14				

The ſame reſult would have come out, had the declination of Aldebaran been uſed in the proportions.

158. PROBLEM XVI. Pl. V.

Given the latitudes and longitudes of two known fixed ſtars; Required their diſtance.

EXAM. *Aliath, in the Great Bear,* *Lon.* ♍ 5° 49′ *Lat.* 54° 18′ *N.*
Arcturus, in Bootes, *Lon.* ♎ 21 10 *Lat.* 30 54 *N.*

The conſtruction of this Problem is like that of the laſt; only inſtead of circles of right aſcenſion read circles of longitude, and uſe parallels of latitude inſtead of parallels of declination.

The

The computation is also like that of the last, there being given two co-latitudes and the included angle, which is the difference between the given longitudes: Thus Arcturus's long. is 6s 21° 10′, and Aliath's is 5s 5° 49′; their difference is 1s 15° 21′, or 45° 21′.

Hence the distance will be found to be 39° 45′.

159. PROBLEM XVII. Pl. V.

Given the latitude and longitude of a fixed star, and also the obliquity of the ecliptic;

Required the right ascension and declination of that star.

EXAM. *Suppose the latitude of a star is 7° 09′ N. its longitude ♈ 29° 01′: What is the right ascension and declination of that star, the obliquity of the ecliptic being 23° 28′?*

The construction of this Problem is much like that of Prob. XIV.; only here the intersection of a parallel of latitude *cb* with a circle of longitude *p*A*q*, will give the place of the star.

The computation is also as in Prob. XIV; for here are given P*p* = 23° 28′, *p*A = 82° 51′, and the ∠ P*p*A = 60° 59′, the longitude from the first point of ♋, to find PA the co-declination, and ∠*p*PA the right ascension.

The declination of the star will be found to be 17° 49′ N. (IV. 151)

And the right ascension will be 24° 19′. (IV. 150)

160. PROBLEM XVIII. Pl. V.

Given the meridional altitude of any celestial object, suppose a comet, its distance from a known star, and the latitude of the place;

Required the declination and right ascension of that comet.

EXAM. *Suppose a comet was observed on the meridian at London, when its altitude was 51° 55′, and its distance from the star Arcturus was 59° 47′: What was the declination and right ascension of the comet at that time?*

CONSTRUCTION.

In the primitive circle, representing the meridian of the place, draw the horizon HR and prime vertical ZN; lay off the given latitude RP = 51° 32′, draw the axis PS, the equator EQ, and (3d 135) *n m* Arcturus's parallel of declination = 20° 21′. From the south point of the horizon lay off the given altitude of the comet = 51° 55′ from H to O: About the point O as a pole, at the given distance between the comet and Arcturus, describe (IV. 68) a small circle *a a* cutting the parallel *n m* in ✳, the position of Arcturus at that time: Describe the circle of right ascension P ✳ S, and a great circle through O and ✳.

COMPUTATION.

Since HE = 38° 28′, the co-lat. and the alt. HO = 51° 55′, then EO = (HO − HE =) 13° 27′, is the decl. sought; which is north, as the altitude exceeds the co-lat.; consequently the polar distance OP = 76° 33′.

Then in the triangle P✱O are given the three ſides to find the ∠OP✱, the difference between the right aſcenſions of the comet and Arcturus. And (IV. 154) the ∠OP✱ will be found $=62° 24' =$ 4h. 9 m. 36 s. which is the difference of their right aſcenſions: Now if Arcturus had paſſed the meridian, the right aſcenſion of the comet was 18 h. 15 m. 16 s. but if Arcturus had not paſſed the meridian, the right aſcenſion of the comet was 9 h. 56 m. 4 s.; it being, in the former caſe, equal to the ſum, and in the latter to the diff. of Arcturus's right aſcen. and the ∠OP✱.

161. PROBLEM XIX. Pl. V.

Given the latitude of a place, the Sun's declination and Azimuth; Required his altitude and the time of the obſervation.

EXAM. *In the latitude of* 13° 30′ *N. and when the Sun has* 23° 28′ *N. declination: What is the Sun's altitude and time of the day, when he is ſeen on the ENE azimuth circle?*

CONSTRUCTION.

Let the primitive circle repreſent the meridian of the place, in which HR repreſents the horizon, and ZN the prime vertical; make RP equal to the latitude, draw the 6 o'clock hour circle PS, the equator EQ, and (3d 153) the parallel of 23° 28′ of declination *n m*: The tangent of 67° 30′ being laid from the center *a* towards H, gives the center of the vertical circle ZDN, which cuts the parallel *n m* in the points A and B; and ſhews that at two diſtant times in the forenoon the Sun will have the azimuth propoſed: Through the point A and B deſcribe the hour circles PAS, PBS (II. 72); the angles ZPA, ZPB, ſhewing the times from noon, may be meaſured by art. 72. Book IV.; and the altitudes DA, DB, by art. 70. Book IV.

COMPUTATION. See art. 146. Book IV.

In the ſpheric triangle PZA, or PZB, there are known,

The co-lat. PZ $=76° 30'$; the co-decl. PA, or PB $=66° 32'$; the azim. ∠PZD $=67° 30'$.

To find ZA, or ZB, and the ∠ZPA, or ∠ZPB.

As Radius : co-ſ. azimuth :: co-t. lat. : to tan. of a 4th arc $M=57° 54'$.

And as ſin. lat. : ſin. decl. :: co-ſ. M to co-ſ. of a 5th arc $N=24° 56'$.

Then M + N, or $57° 54' + 24° 56' = 82° 50' =$ ZA, is the comp. of leaſt alt.

And M − N, or $57° 54' - 24° 56' = 32° 58' =$ ZB, is the comp. of the gr. alt.

Therefore, when the Sun has 7° 10′, or 57° 02′, of alt. he is on the given azimuth.

Again, As co-ſ. dec. : ſin. azim. :: co-ſ. leaſt alt. : ſin. hour fr. noon 87° 55′.

And as co-ſ dec. : ſin. azim. :: co-ſ. greater alt. : ſin. h. fr. noon 33° 14′.

But $87° 55' = 5^h\ 51^m\ 40^s$; and $33° 14' = 2^h\ 12^m\ 56^s$, the reſpect. times fr. noon.

Conſequently the Sun will be ſeen on the ENE azimuth at 6 h. 08 m. 20 s. and again at 9 h. 47 m. 4 s. both in the morning: Alſo, in the afternoon he will be on the WNW azimuth at 2 h. 12 m. 56 s. and at 5 h. 51 m. 40 s.

162. Now to find at what time, and at what altitude, the greateſt azimuth will happen at that place on the ſaid day;

As the azimuth circle in this caſe is to touch the parallel *n m*, therefore the greateſt diſtance of the azimuth from the equator will be 23° 28′; and as their poles muſt be at the ſame diſtance (IV. 33) therefore a ſmall circle *r* deſcribed about the poles, at the diſtance of 23° 28′ (IV. 66),

its

its interſection p with the horizon, is the pole of the circle ZCN; then deſcribe an hour circle PCS through p.

In the ſpheric triangle ZPC right angled at C. (IV. 34)

Given the co-lat. PZ=76° 30′, and the co-decl. PC=66° 32′.

Required the greateſt azim. ∠PZC=70° 37′, the diſt. ZC=54° 08′, and the hour from noon =56° 26′=3 h. 45 m. 44 s.

So that the azimuth is altered only 3° 7′ in 2 h. 6 m.; and conſequently the variation of the compaſs may be obſerved with more certainty in the torrid zone than elſewhere.

163. PROBLEM XX. Pl. XIV. Fig. 1.

In the latitude of 20° 00′ N. ſtands a horizontal dial, the gnomon of which is perpendicular to the plane of the horizon: It is required to know at what hour in the afternoon on the longeſt day, the ſhadow of that gnomon ſhall ſtand ſtill; and how many degrees ſhall the ſhadow run back.

Construction. Let the circle ZRNH be the meridian of the place, HR the horizon, the poles of which are Z, N; RP=20°, the latitude P and S the north and ſouth poles: About P deſcribe the tropic of Cancer *aa*, cutting the horizon in L; about S, a ſmall circle being deſcribed at the diſt. of 23° 28′, the complement of the diſt. of *aa* from P, its interſection p with the horizon, is the pole of the azimuth circle which will touch the parallel *aa* in ☉, the place of the Sun when he has the greateſt azimuth that day: Through Z, ☉, N, deſcribe a vertical circle cutting the horizon in K; and through ☉ and L deſcribe the hour circles P☉S, PLS.

Then will the ∠ZP☉ be equivalent to the hour when the ſhadow will ſtand ſtill; and KL, the difference between the meaſures of the azimuth and amplitude, will ſhew how much the ſhadow will run back.

Computation. In the right-angled ſpheric triangle PRL.			In rt. angl. ſpheric triangle P☉Z.		
Given	∠R	= 90° 00′	Given	∠☉	= 90° 00′
lat.	= RP	= 20 00	co-lat.	= ZP	= 70 00
co-decl.	= PL	= 66 32	co-dec.	= P☉	= 66 32
Requir. ampl.	= RL	= 64 56	Required hour	= ∠ZP☉	= 33 06
			azim.	= ∠☉ZP	= 77 28

Then 33° 02=2 h. 12 m. 08 s.: And 77° 28′—64° 56′=12° 32′.

So that the ſhadow will ſtand ſtill at 2 h. 12 m. 08 s. and will run back 12° 32′.

164. PROBLEM XXI. Pl. XIV. Fig. 2.

A comet, the declination of which was 47° 00′ N. was obſerved to be diſtant from a ſtar, to the eaſtward of it, 49° 00′; the ſtar's declination was 36° 00′ N. and its right aſcenſion 45° 00′: What was the latitude and longitude of that comet?

Construction.

On the plane of the ſolſtitial colure, where P and E are the poles of the equator and ecliptic, put the ſtar at A by its right aſcenſion and declination: About P and A deſcribe ſmall circles, at the diſtances of the comet from thoſe points, their interſection ☉ gives the place of the comet; deſcribe great circles through A☉, P☉, E☉, then E☉ will be the co-latitude, and ∠PE☉ the co-longitude; and their meaſures may be obtained from articles 70 and 72 of Book IV.

Compu-

COMPUTATION. In the triangle AP☉.

Given the ✱'s co-dec. PA = 54° 00′
comet's co-dec. P☉ = 43 00
their diſtance A☉ = 49 00

Req. com. rt. aſ. fr. ✱ ∠ AP☉ = 65 48
Then 65° 48′ — 45° 00 = 20° 48′.
And 90° 00′ — 20° 48′ = 69° 12′ = ☉PE

In the triangle EP☉.

Given comet's co-decl. P☉ = 43° 00′
obliq. of ecliptic PE = 23 28
comet's rt. aſ. ∠ EP☉ = 69 12

Req. comet's co-lat. E☉ = 39 54
and co-longit. ∠ PE☉ = 83 42
Which being taken from 90°, leaves ♈ 6° 18′ for the long. required.

165. PROBLEM XXII. Pl. XIV. Fig. 3.

At London, on the 10th of December 1780, at what time of the night will the ſtars Aldevaran and Rigel be on the ſame azimuth circle?

Aldeb. decl. = 16° 03′ N.; right aſc. = 4 h. 23 m. 19 s. Rigel's decl. = 8° 28′ S.; right aſc. = 5 h. 03 m. 58 s.

Their difference of right aſcenſions is 40 m. 39 s. or 10° 10′.

CONSTRUCTION. On the plane of the equinoctial put Aldebaran at A, and Rigel at B, by their right aſcenſions and declinations, then a great circle through B and A will be the azimuth they are on at the time ſought; and the parallel of London's lat. deſcribed about P, will cut the azimuth circle BA in zz the zenith, through which draw the meridians PZ, PZ.

Here the neareſt interſection to the ſtars is taken for the zenith, for as the ſtars are both above the horizon, the greateſt zenith diſtance is leſs than 90 degrees.

COMPUTATION. In the △ APB.

Given B's co-decl. PB = 98° 28′
A's co-decl. PA = 73 57
diff. rt. aſc. ∠ APB = 10 10

Required the ∠ BAP = 156 58

In the triangle APZ.

Given A's co-decl. PA = 73° 57′
the co-lat. PZ = 38 28
the ſuppl. of BAP or ∠ PAZ = 23 02

Req. ∠ APZ = 142° 35′, or = 24 01

Now the ſtar Aldebaran comes to the meridian at 11 h. 8 m. 27 s. in the evening; which leſſened by 1 h. 36 m. 4 s. (24° 01′) gives 9 h. 32 m. 23 s. for the time in the evening when thoſe ſtars will be on the ſame azimuth.

166. PROBLEM XXIII. Pl. XIV. Fig. 4.

At what time in the evening will the ſtars Betelgueſe and Pollux have one common altitude above the horizon of London, on the 10th of December 1780?

Betelgueſe right aſcen. = 5 h. 43 m. 16 s.; decl. = 7° 21′ N. Pollux right aſcen. = 7 h. 31 m. 51 s.; decl. = 28° 32′ N.

Their difference of right aſcenſion is 1 h. 48 m. 35 s. = 27° 09′.

CONSTRUCTION. On a primitive circle, where any point P repreſents the pole of the equinoctial, put the ſtar Pollux at B, and Betelgueſe at A, by their declination and difference of right aſcenſions; through A, B, deſcribe a great circle; through C, the middle of AB, deſcribe a great circle at right angles to AB, and cutting PA in D; then a ſmall circle deſcribed about P, at the diſtance of 38° 28′, the co-lat. will cut the circle CD in Z the zenith.

For the ſtars A and B having a common altitude, are equally diſtant from Z.

COMPUTATION. In the triangle APB.

Given A's co-decl.	PA = 82° 39′	Required the	∠BAP =	47° 01′
B's co-decl.	PB = 61 28		AB =	33 14
diff. rt. asc.	∠ APB = 27 09	Its half	AC =	16 37

In the triangle ACD.

Given the	∠C = 90° 00′	Required the	∠D =	45° 30′
	∠A = 47 01		AD =	23 38
	AC = 16 37	Theref. PA—AD = PD	=	59 01

In the triangle PDZ.

Given the co-lat.	PZ = 38° 28′	Required	∠ZPD =	48° 56
	PD = 59 01	Or it is	=	75° 46
	∠PDZ = 45 30			

Now the ſtar Betelgueſe comes to the meridian at 12h. 28m. 8s. that is between twelve and one o'clock in the morning (133); from which take 3 h. 15 m. 44 s. as the ſtars are to the eaſt of the meridian, and it leaves 9 h. 12 m. 24 s. in the evening, for the time when thoſe ſtars have the ſame altitude.

167. PROBLEM XXIV. Pl. XIV. Fig. 5.

Wanting to know the latitude and longitude of a comet C, *its diſtance from two known ſtars* A *and* B *were obſerved, and are as follows:*

A's *lat.* = 49° 12′ *N. Lon.* = 16° 39′ ♓; *diſtance from* C = 49° 05′.
B's *lat.* = 30 05 *N. Lon.* = 2 48 ♊; *diſtance from* C = 45 57.
Hence the place of the comet C *is required.*

CONSTRUCTION. On the plane of the ſolſtitial coloure, where E is the pole of the ecliptic, put the ſtars A and B by their latitudes and longitudes, and deſcribe a great circle through A and B; then ſmall circles deſcribed about A and B as poles, at the reſpective diſtances of the comet, their interſection C will give its place; deſcribe great circles through A, C; B, C; E, C; and E C will be the co-latitude, and from ∠ AEC will be obtained the longitude.

COMPUTATION. In the △ ABE.

Given A's co-lat.	AE = 40° 48′
B's co-lat.	BE = 59 55
diff. longit.	∠ AEB = 76 09
Required	AB = 59 01
and	∠ EAB = 78 31

In the triangle ABC.

Given the diſtance	AB = 59° 01′
diſtance	AC = 49 05
diſtance	BC = 45 57
Required the	∠ BAC = 56 27
Then ∠ EAB + ∠ BAC = ∠ EAC =	134° 58

In the triangle CEA.

Given A's co-lat.	AE = 40° 48′	Required the co-lat. EC = 81° 33′
diſtance	AC = 49 05	diff. long. AEC = 32 43
and the	∠ EAC = 134 58	Hence lat. is 8° 27′ N. lon. 19° 22′ in ♈

168. PROBLEM XXV. Pl. XIV. Fig. 6.

The diſtance of the ſtar C *being obſerved from two ſtars* A *and* B, *the latitude and diſtance of which are known, and alſo the longitude of one of them; thence to find the lat. and long. of* C.

Suppoſe A's lat. to be 5° 30′ N.; its diſt. from C = 39° 40′: B's lat. 9° 57′ N. its long. Taurus, 18° 16′, and diſt. from C 10° 7½′: And the diſtance of AB 44° 43′: Required the long. and lat. of C.

CON-

CONSTRUCTION. On a circle of longitude, where E is the pole of the ecliptic, put the ſtar B by its lat.; about the points B and E deſcribe circles at the diſtances of A from thoſe points, their interſection gives the place of A: alſo circles deſcribed from A and B, at the diſtances of C reſpectively from them, their interſection is the place of C: Then deſcribe the great circles EA, EC; AC, AB; BC; and EC will be the co-lat. and ∠BEC the longitude, of C from B.

COMPUTATION. In the Δ AEB
Given A's co-lat. AE = 84° 30′
B's co-lat. BE = 80 03
the diſtance AB = 44 43
Required the ∠ABE = 92 14

In the triangle ABC.
Given the diſtance AB = 44° 43′
diſtance AC = 39 40
diſtance BC = 10 07½
Required the ∠ABC = 55 22

In the triangle BEC.
Given B's co-lat. BE = 80° 03′
the diſtance BC = 10 07½
(∠ABE — ∠ABC =) ∠CBE = 36 52

Required C's co-lat. CE = 72° 01′
C's lon. fr. B, ∠BEC = 6 22
And its abſolute long. ♉ 11 54

169. PROBLEM XXVI. Pl. XIV. Fig. 7.

From the altitudes of two known fixed ſtars, and the altitude of a planet when in the ſame azimuth with one of theſe ſtars; to find the place of the planet.

EXAMPLE. Obſerved the Moon and Cor Leonis in the ſame azimuth, when the Moon's zenith diſtance was 36° 37′.

Cor Leonis's zen. diſt. = 45° 00′; decl. 13° 02′ N.; rt. aſ. $9^h\ 56^m\ 39^s$.
Cor Hydra's zen. diſt. = 49 16; decl. 7 43 S.; rt. aſ. $9^h\ 16^m\ 47^s$.

CONSTRUCTION. On the plane of the equinoctial, the pole of which is P, draw the colures, and in the ſolſtitial, take E for the pole of the ecliptic; put the given ſtars at B and A by their declinations and right aſcenſions: About B and A as poles, with their reſpective zenith diſtances, deſcribe circles cutting in Z the zenith; through Z and B deſcribe an azimuth circle, and making Z☽ equal to the ☽'s zenith diſtance, it gives her place: Then deſcribe the great circles ZA, AB, E☽; and the arc E☽ will be the co-latitude, and ∠PE☽ the longitude from the firſt point of ♋.

COMPUTATION. In the Δ ABP.
Given A's co-decl. PA = 97° 43′
B's co decl. PB = 76 58
diff. rt. aſ. ∠BPA = 9 58
Required the ∠ABP = 153 57½
the ſide AB = 22 59½

In the triangle AZB.
Given A's zen. diſt. ZA = 49° 16′
B's zen. diſt. ZB = 45 00
the ſide AB = 22 59½
Required the ∠ABZ = 89 38½
Then ∠ ABP — ABZ = ∠ ZBP = 64° 19′ = ∠ ☽BP.

In the triangle B☽P.
Given B's co-decl. BP = 76° 58′
(BZ — Z☽ =) ſide B☽ = 8 23
∠PB☽ = 64 19
Requ. ☽'s co-decl. P☽ = 73 26½
☽'s rt. aſ. fr B, ∠BP☽ = 7 53
Then 90° + ∠ ♈PB + ∠ BP☽ = ∠EP☽ = 128° 43′.

In the triangle P☽E.
Given obl. of eclip. PE = 23° 28′
☽'s co-decl. P☽ = 73 26½
☽'s co-rt. aſ. ∠EP☽ = 128 43
Requir. ☽'s co-lat. ☽E = 88 41
☽'s lon. fr. ♋, ∠PE☽ = 48 25
And its abſolute long. is ♌ 18 25

SECTION VI.

Of various methods to find the Latitude.

The ufual way at fea to find the latitude is from the Sun's meridional altitude and declination; the manner of doing this will be particularly fhewn in Book IX. But as it frequently happens at fea, that the meridian altitude cannot be taken, therefore the mariner fhould be furnifhed with other means to come at the knowledge of this moft ufeful article. To help him in this point, and as a farther exercife in the Aftronomy of the Sphere, the following problems are collected together.

170. PROBLEM XXVII. Pl. V.

Given the Sun's declination and his amplitude;
Required the latitude of the place.

EXAM. *Being in a place where the compafs had no variation, on a day when the Sun's declination was* 15° 12′ *N., I obferved him to rife* 62° 30′ *from the north towards the eaft: Required the latitude of that place.*

CONSTRUCTION.

Having defcribed the primitive circle, drawn the horizon HR, and (IV. 71) taken RO=62° 30′; then about O as a pole defcribe (IV. 66) a fmall circle, at the diftance of 74° 48′=co-decl., cutting the primitive in P, the place of the north pole: Draw the axis PS, the equator EQ, and the circle POS, cutting the equator in A.

COMPUTATION.

In the fpheric triangle ♈OA right angled at A.

Given the co-amp. ♈O=27° 30′	Then f.♈O : rad. :: f. AO : f.∠A♈O.
the declin. AO=15 12	Hence the latitude will be 55°
Required the co-latitude A♈O.	24′ N.

171. PROBLEM XXVIII. Pl. V.

Given the Sun's declination, and his afcenfional difference;
Required the latitude of the place.

EXAM. *When the Sun had* 20° 01′ *of declination S., he was obferved to fet at* 4 *h.* 30 *m.: Required the latitude of the place.*

As the afcenfional difference is the time that the Sun rifes or fets before or after 6 o'clock; therefore 6 h.—4 h. 30 m.=1 h. 30 m.=22° 30′= afcenfional difference.

CONSTRUCTION. In the primitive circle reprefenting the meridian of the place, draw the equator EQ, the axis PS, the parallel of declination *ro*, 20° 01′ S.: Make ♈B=22° 30′, the afcenfional difference; defcribe the circle of right afcenfion PBS, cutting *ro* in O; then a diameter HR through O will be the horizon, and RP the lat. fought.

COMPUTATION. In the fpheric triangle ♈BO, right angled at B.

Given the afc. diff. ♈B=22° 30′	Then rad.:cot.OB::f.♈B:cot.∠O♈B.
the declin. OB=20 01	Or rad.:cot.dec.::fin.af.diff.:tan.lat.
Required the co-lat. ∠O♈B.	Hence the lat. will be 46° 25′ N.,

being contrary to the decl. when the afc. diff. falls between noon and fix.

172. PRO-

Given the Sun's declination, and altitude at six o'clock;
Required the latitude of the place.

EXAM. *Being at sea, on a day when the Sun's declination was 20° 04′ N. his altitude at six o'clock in the evening was 18° 45′: What was the latitude of the place of observation?*

CONSTRUCTION. Having described the meridian, drawn the horizon HR, the prime vertical ZN, and the parallel *st* of 18° 45′ of altitude; from the center ♈, with the half tangent of the declination = 20° 04′, cut the parallel *st* in O: Through O draw the axis PS, and the azimuth circle ZON (II. 72), and the measure of RP will give the latitude sought.

COMPUTATION. In the spheric triangle ♈AO, right-angled at A.

Given the decl. ♈O = 20° 04′ N. | Then sin. ♈O : rad. :: s. AO : s. ∠O♈A:
the altit. AO = 18 45 | Or sin. decl. : rad. : : sin. alt. : sin. lat.
Required the lat. = ∠O♈A | Which is 69° 32′ N., as the decl. is N.

173. PROBLEM XXX. Pl. V.

Given the Sun's declination, and his altitude when due east or west;
Required the latitude of the place.

EXAM. *In a place where the compass had no variation, the Sun was observed to be due east when his declination was 16° 38′ N., and his altitude 20° 12′: What is the latitude of that place?*

CONSTRUCTION. In the meridian HZRN, draw the horizon HR, the prime vertical ZN, and make ♈O = the half tan. of the alt. 20° 12′: About O as a pole, at the distance of 73° 22′, the co-decl., describe (IV. 66) a small circle, cutting the meridian in P the elevated pole; draw the axis PS, equator EQ, and through P, O, S, describe an hour circle POS; then the measure of PR shews the latitude.

COMPUTATION. In the spheric triangle ♈AO, right-angled at A.

Given the alt. ♈O = 20° 12′ | Then sin. ♈O : rad. : : sin. AO : sin. ∠A♈O.
the decl. AO = 16 38 N. | Or sin. alt. : rad. : : sin. decl. : sin. lat.
Required the latit. = ∠A♈O. | Which is 56° 00′ N., as the decl. is N.

But had the declination been S., the other intersection of the parallel circle and meridian must have been taken for the elevated pole, and the latitude would be south.

174. PROBLEM XXXI. Pl. V.

Given the Sun's altitude and the hour of the day on either equinox;
Required the latitude of the place.

EXAM. *On the day the Sun entered the vernal equinox, his alt. was found 22° 56′ at 9 o'clock in the morning. In what lat. was that observation made?*

CONSTRUCTION. Describe the meridian, draw the horizon, the prime vertical, and (IV. 68) the parallel *st* of 22° 56′ of altitude; from the center ♈, with the half tan. of 45° = 3 h., the time from 6 o'clock, cut *st* in O, and describe the vertical circle ZON, cutting the horizon in B.

COMPUTATION. In the spheric triangle ♈BO, right-angled at B.

Given the time after 6, ♈O = 45° 00′ | As s. ♈O : rad. : : s. BO : s. ∠B♈O.
the altitude BO = 22 56 | Or s. time : rad. : : s. alt. : co-s. l.
Required the co-latitude B♈O. | Which is 56° 34′.

175. PROBLEM XXXII. Pl. V.

Given the Sun's altitude, declination and azimuth;
Required the latitude of the place.

EXAM. *Being at ſea in a place where the compaſs had no variation, in the afternoon when the Sun was 42° 30′ high, his bearing was S. 57° 45′ W. and his declination 22° 30′ N.: What is the latitude of that place?*

CONSTRUCTION. Draw the meridian, the horizon HR, the prime vertical ZN, and the parallel *s t* at 42° 30′ above the horizon (IV. 68): The tangent of 57° 45′ ſet from A towards R gives the center of the azimuth circle ZON, cutting the parallel of altitude *s t* in O: About O as a pole (IV. 66), at the diſtance of 67° 30′, equal to the co-declination, deſcribe a ſmall circle, cutting the meridian in P, the place of the pole; then the meaſure of RP gives the latitude ſought.

COMPUTATION. In the oblique-angled ſpheric triangle ZOP.

Given the zenith diſt. ZO = 47° 30′
the polar diſt. PO = 67 30
the azimuth ∠PZO = 122 15
} Required the co-latitude PZ.

As rad.	= R		10,00000	As ſin. alt.	= 42°	30′	0,17032
To co-ſ. azim.	= 122°	15′	9,72723	To ſin. decl.	= 22	30	9,58284
So co-t. alt.	= 42	30	10,03795	So co-ſ. 4th.	= 30	13	9,93658
To tan. 4th.	= 30	13	9,76518	To co-ſ. 5th.	= 60	42	9,68974

Then the difference between the 5th and 4th arcs, that is 30° 13′ taken from 60° 42′, the remainder 30° 29′ is the co-lat. Therefore 59° 31′ N. is the latitude ſought.

176. PROBLEM XXXIII. Pl. V.

Given the Sun's declination, his altitude and the hour of the day;
Required the latitude of the place.

EXAM. *Being at ſea, the Sun's altitude was obſerved to be 37° 20′ at 9 h. 45 m. in the morning, his declination at that time being 22° 30′ N.: What is the latitude of the place of obſervation?*

CONSTRUCTION. In the meridian PESQ, draw the equator EQ, axis PS, and parallel of declin. *n m*, 22° 30′ diſt. from the equator (3d 135). Set off from the center A towards Q the tang. of 33° 45′ = 2 h. 15 m., the diſtance between the time of obſervation and noon, which gives the center of the hour circle POS, cutting the parallel *n m* in O: about the point O as a pole, deſcribe (IV. 66) at the diſt. of 52° 40′, the zen. diſt., a ſmall circle, cutting the meridian in Z the zenith; through Z O deſcribe an azimuth circle ZON; then the meaſure of ZE will give the lat. ſought.

COMPUTATION. In the oblique-angled triangle ZOP.

Given the zenith diſtance ZO = 52° 40′
the polar diſtance PO = 67 30
the hour from noon ∠ZPO = 33 45
} Required the co-lat. ZP.

As rad. : co-ſ. hour A. M. : : co-t. decl. : tan. 4th arc = 63° 31′.
As ſin. decl. : ſin. alt. : : co-ſ. 4th arc : co-ſ. 5th arc = 45 02.
Their difference is the co-latitude 18° 29′. Therefore the lat. is 71° 31′ N.

177. PROBLEM XXXIV. Pl. V.

Given the altitude of one of two known fixed ſtars, when they have the ſame azimuth;
Required the latitude of the place.

Exam. *Being at ſea in an unknown latitude, I obſerved the ſtar Schedar in Caſſiopeia, and Almaach in Andromeda, to have the ſame azimuth, when the altitude of Schedar was 37° 15′: What is the latitude of that place?*

Construction. Let the primitive circle repreſent the equator, the pole of which is P, and any point ♈ the place where the right aſcenſion begins, from whence lay off ♈a=27° 37′ for Almaach's right aſcenſion, and ♈b=7° 2′ for Schedar's; draw the circles of right aſcenſion Pa, Pb: Deſcribe (3d 137) Almaach's and Schedar's parallels of declination, cutting Pa, Pb, in A, B; A being Almaach, and B Schedar. A great circle paſſing through A and B (IV. 61) will be the azimuth they are on. About B at the diſtance of 52° 45′, Schedar's zenith diſtance, deſcribe (IV. 66) a ſmall circle, cutting the ſaid azimuth circle in Z, the zenith of the place; draw PZ, which meaſured on the half tangents gives the co-latitude of the place of obſervation.

Computation.

1ſt. In the oblique-angled ſpheric triangle ABP.

Given		
Given Almaach's co-dec.	PA =	48° 44′
Schedar's co-dec.	PB =	34 40
their diff. of r. aſc. ∠ APB		20 33

Required the angle of poſition ABP. For the ſolution, ſee IV. 165.

As rad.	90° 00′	10,00000
To co-ſ. ∠ APB	20 35	9,97135
So is tan. AP	48 44	10,05676
To tan. 4th arc	46 51	10,02811
The ſide BP	34 40	
The 5th arc	12 11	

As ſin. 5th arc	12° 11′	0,67563
To ſin. 4th arc	46 51	9,86306
So is tan. ∠ APB	20 35	9,57466
To tan. ∠ B	52 23	10,11335

2d. In the oblique ſpheric triangle PBZ.

Given		
Given Schedar's co-dec.	PB =	34° 40′
Schedar's co-alt.	BZ =	52 45
angle of poſition	PBZ =	52 23

Required the co-lat. PZ. For the ſolution, ſee IV. 165. Here ∠ PBZ = ſup. ∠ PBA.

As rad.	= R	10,00000
To co-ſ. ∠ poſit.	= 52° 23′	9,78550
So co-t. Sch. decl.	= 55 20	9,83984
To tan. 4th arc	= 22 53	9,62541
Which taken from	52 45 = BZ	
Leaves 5th arc	29 52	

As co-ſ. 4th arc	= 22° 53′	0,03560
To co-ſ. 5th arc	= 29 52	9,93811
So ſin. Sch. dec.	= 55 20	9,91512
To ſin. latit.	= 50 44	9,88883

178. PROBLEM XXXV. Pl. V.

Given the difference of time between the rising of two known ſtars; Required the latitude of the place.

EXAM. *Being at ſea in an unknown place, the ſtar Aldebaran was obſerved to riſe 3 h. 15 m. later than the bright ſtar in Aries: Required the latitude of that place.*

Bright ſtar in ♈ decl. 22° 25′ N.; right aſcen. 1 h. 54 m. 49 s. Aldebaran's decl. 16° 03′ N.; right aſcenſion 4 h. 23 m. 19 s.

CONSTRUCTION.

Let the primitive circle repreſent the equator, deſcribe (3d 137) the parallels of declination of the two ſtars, that of Aries being 22° 25′ N. and of Aldebaran 16° 03′ N.: Draw P*a* for the circle of right aſcenſion paſſing through the ſtar in ♈, which ſuppoſe in A: From *a* lay off *ab*, =37° 7½′=diff. of right aſcenſions; and *ac*=48° 45′=3 h. 15 m., the diff. of time between their riſing; draw *b*P, *c*P, cutting the parallels of declination in B, C: Through the points B, C, deſcribe (IV. 61) the great circle HOR; draw PO at right-angles to HR; then the meaſure of PO will give the latitude ſought.

COMPUTATION.

In the oblique-angled ſpheric triangle PBC.

Given B's co-decl. PB=73° 57′	Rad.:co-ſ.∠BPC::t.PB:t.M=73° 38′.
A's co-decl. PC=67 35	From M take PC, leaves N = 6 03′.
∠APC—∠APB=∠BPC=11 37½	As ſin.N : ſ. M : : tan. ∠CPB : t.∠C=
Required the angle PCB.	Hence ∠ PCO=61° 54′. [118° 06′.

In the ſpheric triangle PCO, right-angled at O.

Given C's co-decl. PC=67° 35′	As rad. : ſin. PC : : ſin. ∠ PCO : ſin.
and the ∠ PCO=61 54	[PO=54° 38′.
Required the latitude PO.	Therefore the latitude is 54° 38′.

179. PROBLEM XXXVI. Pl. V.

Two known fixed ſtars being obſerved to have the ſame altitude; Required the latitude of the place of obſervation.

EXAM. *In the evening, the ſtars Capella and Procyon were obſerved at the ſame time to have each 38° 00′ of altitude: Required the latitude of the place where that obſervation was taken.*

Capella's decl.=45° 45′ N. right aſcen. 5 h. 0 m. 28 s. Procyon's decl. =5° 47′ N. right aſcen.=7 h. 27 m. 48 s.

CONSTRUCTION.

On the plane of the equator, repreſented by the primitive circle, deſcribe (3d 137) the parallels of the given declinations; take *ab*=36° 50′. the diff. of the given right aſcenſions; draw P*a*, P*b*, then A repreſents Procyon, and B Capella.

About A and B as poles, deſcribe (IV. 66) arcs of ſmall circles, at the diſtance of 52°, the co-altitude, and their interſection gives Z the zenith of the place: Through the points A, B; Z, A; Z, B; deſcribe great circles (IV. 61) and draw ZP, the meaſure of which will give the co-latitude of the place of obſervation.

COMPU-

COMPUTATION.

In the oblique angled spheric triangle APB.

Given A's co-decl.	AP=84° 13′	Rad. : cos. ∠P : : t. BP : t. M=37° 57
B's co-decl.	BP=44 15	And M tak. fr. PA leaves N=46 16
diff. rt. asc.	∠APB=36 50	Sin. N : sin. M : : tan. ∠P : tan. ∠BAP [=32° 31
Required the stars distance AB.		
And the angle BAP.		Cos. M : cos. N : : cos. BP : cos. BA=51 06

In the oblique angled spheric triangle AZB.

Given A's co-alt.	ZA=52° 00′	The angle BAZ will be found= 68° 04′.
B's co-alt.	ZB=52 00	
stars distance	AB=51 06	Then ∠BAZ—∠BAP=∠PAZ= 35° 33′.
Required the angle ZAB.		

In the spheric triangle AZP.

Given A's co-alt.	ZA=52° 00′	Rad. : cos. ∠A : : t. ZA : t. M=47° 29′
A's co-declin.	AP=84 13	M taken from PA leaves N=36 44
the angle	ZAP=35 30	Cos. M : cos. N : : cos. ZA : cos. PZ=43 06
Required the co-lat. ZP.		Therefore the latitude is 46° 54′ N.

180. PROBLEM XXXVII. Pl. V.

Given the altitudes of two known stars;
Required the latitude of the place.

EXAM. *The altitude of the Hydra's heart was observed to be* 40° 44′, *and of the Lion's heart* 45° 00′: *What is the latitude of the place of observation?*

Hydra's heart, decl = 7° 43′ S.; right ascen. = 9 h. 16 m. 47 s.
Lion's heart, decl. = 13° 02′ N.; right ascen. 9 h. 56 m. 39s.

CONSTRUCTION.

If this problem is constructed on the plane of the equator, it will be in every respect like the last; only the small circles, described about A and B, are to be unequally distant from their respective poles A, B.

COMPUTATION.

Here, as in the last, there will be three spheric triangles to work in; namely, the triangles APB, ZAB, and ZPB.

In the triangle APB, where AP=97° 43′, BP=76° 58′, ∠APB=9° 58′.

As rad. : cos. ∠APB : : tan. BP : tan. M=76° 46′½. Then AP—M=N =20° 57′½.

As sin. N : sin. M : : tan. ∠APB : tan. ∠BAP=25° 34′.

And as cos. M : cos. N : : cos. BP : cos. BA=22 59.

In the triangle BAZ, where AZ=49° 16′, BZ=45° 00′, AB=22° 59′.

The angle BAZ will be found equal to 68° 56′.

Then ∠BAZ—∠BAP=∠PAZ=43° 22′.

In the triangle APZ, where AP=97° 43, AZ=49° 16′, ∠PAZ=43° 22′.

As rad. : cos. ∠PAZ : : tan. AZ : tan. M=40° 10′. Then AP—M= N=57° 33′.

And as cos. M : cos. N : : cos. AZ : cos. PZ=62° 59′.

Hence the latitude sought is 27° 10 N.

181. PROBLEM XXXVIII. Pl. V.

Given the Sun's declination, two altitudes, and the time between the obſervations;
Required the latitude of the place.

EXAM. *On a day when the Sun's declination was 20° 00′ N., in the forenoon the Sun's altitude was obſerved to be 18° 30′, and 3 hours after, his altitude was 44° 00′: What was the latitude of the place?*

CONSTRUCTION.

Let the primitive circle repreſent that hour circle on which the Sun was at the firſt obſervation, EQ being the equator, then A*a*, the parallel of 20° of declination, gives A the Sun's place at firſt; and as CQ is the tangent of 45°, Q will be the center of the hour circle PBS three hours diſtant from the former, its interſection B with the parallel of declination, is the Sun's place at the ſecond obſervation: About A as a pole, at the diſtance of 71° 30′, the firſt zenith diſtance, deſcribe (IV. 66) a ſmall circle; about B, as a pole, at the diſtance of 46° 00′, the ſecond zenith diſtance, deſcribe (IV. 66) another ſmall circle, cutting the former in Z the zenith: Through Z, A; Z, B; A, B; P, Z; deſcribe (IV. 61) great circles; then PZ is the co-latitude required.

COMPUTATION.

Here are three triangles to work in; namely, ABP, ABZ, BPZ.

In the iſoſceles ſpheric triangle APB.

Given AP = 70° 00′	Suppoſe the perpendicular P*b* is drawn.
BP = 70 00	Rad. : tan. BP*b* : : coſ. PB : co-t. ∠PBA = 81° 56′.
∠APB = 45 00	Rad. : ſin. PB : : ſin. ∠BP*b* : ſin. B*b* = 21° 04½′.
Req. ∠ABP and AB.	Then B*b* double gives AB = 42° 09′.

In the oblique angled ſpheric triangle ABZ.

Given AZ = 71° 30′	Then working with the three ſides, the angle ABZ
BZ = 46 00	will be found = 114° 11′.
AB = 42 09	And ∠ABZ — ∠PBA = PBZ = 32° 15′.
Required ∠ABZ.	

In the oblique angled ſpheric triangle PBZ.

Given PB = 70° 00′	As rad. : coſ. ∠PBZ : : tan. BZ : tan. M = 41° 13′.
BZ = 46 00	And PB — M = N = 28° 47′.
∠PBZ = 32 15	As coſ. M : coſ. N : : coſ. BZ : coſ. PZ = 30° 59′.
Req. the co-lat. PZ.	Therefore the latitude is 54° 01′ N.

182. If the Sun's altitude can be taken both before and after noon, when he has equal heights, then the time between theſe two obſervations being biſected, will give the time when the Sun was on the meridian: Now the co-declination, the co-altitude, and the time from noon at either obſervation being known, the latitude may be readily computed in one oblique angled triangle, in which are known two ſides, and an angle oppoſite to one of them to find the other ſide, which is the co-latitude; for which ſee the problem, art. 176.

Given the Sun's declination, two altitudes, and the difference of the magnetic azimuths;
Required the latitude of the place.

EXAM. *On the 21st of May, the Sun's declination being 20° 16′ N., in the morning when the Sun was on the ESE. point of the compass, his altitude was 43° 30′; and when he bore S. 20° 30′ E. his altitude was 58° 30′: What is the latitude of the place of observation?*

CONSTRUCTION.

Let the primitive circle represent the azimuth circle which the Sun was on at the greater altitude, 58° 30′, A being the Sun's place at that time, HR the horizon, and Z the zenith; draw *aa* a parallel of 43° 30′ of altitude, and (IV. 75) describe a vertical circle, making an angle with AZ, of 47° 00′, the difference of the observed azimuths; the place where this cuts the parallel of altitude *aa*, gives B the Sun's place at the first observation: Then small circles being described about A and B, as poles at the distances of 69° 44′, the co-declination (IV. 66), their intersection will give P the place of the pole: Through A, B; P, A; P, B; and Z, P, describe great circles (IV. 61); then PZ is the co-latitude sought.

COMPUTATION.

1st. In the spheric triangle AZB:	Given AZ =	A's co-alt.	= 31° 30′
	BZ =	B's co-alt.	= 46 30
	AZB =	diff. of az.	= 47 00
	Required ∠ ABZ		= 45 41
	AB		= 32 17
2d. In the isosceles spheric △APB:	Given AP =	A's co-decl.	= 69 44
	BP =	B's co-decl.	= 69 44
	AB =	distance	= 32 17
	Required ∠ ABP		= 83 52
3d. In the spheric triangle ZBP:	Given BZ =	B's co-alt.	= 46 30
	PB =	B's co-decl.	= 69 44
	∠ZBP		= 38 11
	Requir. ZP =	co-lat.	= 39 21

Therefore the latitude of the place is 50° 39′ N.

184. PROBLEM XL. Pl. V.

Two known ſtars being obſerved on the ſame azimuth, and two other known ſtars being obſerved on another azimuth, and the time between the obſervation being known; to find the latitude of the place.

EXAM. *The ſtars Aldebaran in Taurus, and Rigel in Orion, were obſerved on the ſame azimuth; and 2 h. 35 min. after, the ſtars Caſtor in Gemini and the Hydra's heart were alſo obſerved on another azimuth: What was the latitude of the place of obſervation?*

CONSTRUCTION.

On the plane of the equator put the ſtars Aldebaran and Rigel at A, B, alſo the ſtars Caſtor and Hydra at *c*, *d*, by means of their right aſcenſions and declinations (2d and 3d of 137): Let the ſtars *c*, *d*, be removed forwards $2^h\ 35^m$, or 38° 45′ to C, D; through A, B, and D, C, deſcribe (IV. 61) great circles interſecting in Z, the zenith of the place; draw the great circles AC and PZ; then the meaſure of PZ gives the co-latitude required.

COMPUTATION.

Aldebaran's declin.	= 16° 03′ N.	right aſcen.	= $4^h\ 23^m\ 19^s$	= 65° 50′.
Rigel's	= 8 28 S.		= 5 03 58	= 75 59½.
Caſtor's	= 32 21 N.		= 7 20 33	= 110 08.
Hydra's heart	= 7 43 S.		= 9 16 47	= 139 12.

1ſt. In the triangle PAB, where PB = 98° 28′, PA = 73° 57′, ∠APB = 10° 09½′.
Then the ∠PAB will be 156° 59′, and the ∠PAZ, the ſuppl. = 23° 01′.

2d. In the triangle PCD, where PD = 97° 43′, PC = 57° 39′, ∠CPD = 29° 04′.
Then the ∠PCD will be 140° 09′, and the ∠PCZ, the ſuppl. = 39° 51′.

3d. In the triangle APC, where AP = 73° 57′, CP = 57° 39′, ∠APC = 5° 33½′, which is the difference between 2 h. 35 m. and the difference of the right aſcenſions of A and C.
Then the ∠PAC will be 16° 12′, ∠PCA = 161° 30′, and AC = 17° 03′.
Now ∠PAC + ∠PAZ = ∠CAZ = 39° 13′; and ∠PCA − ∠PCZ = ∠ACZ = 121° 39′.

4th. In the triangle ACZ, where AC = 17° 03′; ∠CAZ = 39° 13′; ∠ACZ = 121° 39′.
Then CZ will be found equal to 28° 26′.

5th. In the triangle CPZ, where CZ = 28° 26′, CP = 57° 39′, ∠PCZ 39° 51′.
Then PZ will be found equal to 38° 49′.
And the latitude of the place of obſervation is 51° 11′. N.

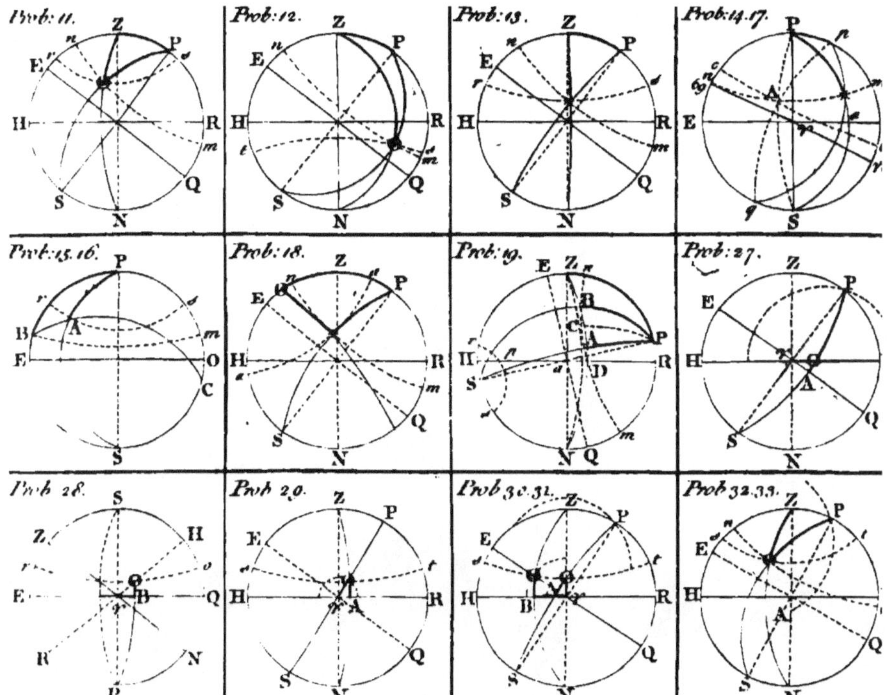
Prob:11.
Z P E H R Q S N
Prob:12.
Z P E H R Q S N
Prob:13.
Z P E H R Q S N
Prob:14.17.
P A E S
Prob:15.16.
P B A E O C S
Prob:18.
Z P E H R Q S N
Prob:19.
E Z B C A P D R S N Q
Prob:27.
Z P E H A Q S N
Prob 28.
S H E B Q R N P
Prob 29.
Z P E H R A Q S N
Prob 30.31.
Z P E H B R Q S N
Prob 32.33.
Z P E H A Q S N

There might be given a great variety of other problems to find the latitude from various circumſtances; but the trouble of ſolving them, as well as ſome of the foregoing ones, is too great to render them of general uſe: And indeed ſome of them were only inſerted as trigonometrical exerciſes for young ſtudents; it being generally allowed that the ſciences are moſt readily learned by working many examples: And on this account it was judged, that the few following queſtions might not only be entertaining to thoſe who have a love for theſe matters; but on ſome occaſions might be uſefully applied at ſea.

185. PROBLEM XLI.

Given the Sun's meridian, or mid-day altitude $=62° \; 00'$.
And its mid-night depreſſion, below the horizon, $=22 \; 00$.
Required the latitude of the place, and the Sun's declination.

SOLUTION. Let the circle HZR be the meridian;
arc H*m*, the meridian alt.; its ſine F*m*;
arc R*n*, the mid-night depreſſion; its ſine *nf*;
mn, the parallel of declination;
Q*q*, parallel to *mn* the equator;
PS, at right angles to Q*q*, the axis, or 6 o'clock circle.

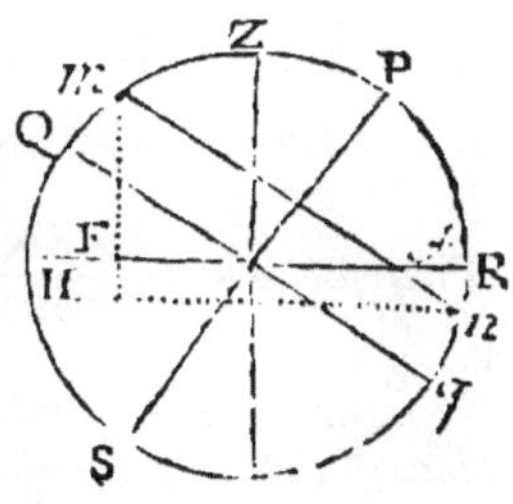

Now $HQ+Qm=Hm$ } For $HQ=Rq$; and $Qm=qn$.
And $HQ-Qm=Rn$ }

Then $HQ = \dfrac{Hm+Rn}{2} =$ co-latitude $=42° \; 00'$.

And $Qm = \dfrac{Hm-Rn}{2} =$ declination $=20° \; 00'$.

In the following problems, as it was the method of computation which was chiefly intended for the information of beginners, the conſtruction is ſuppoſed to be done: And the lines and letters, as here deſcribed, are to be underſtood to repreſent the ſame things in each figure.

186. **PROBLEM XLII.**

Some time in the month of May, 1780, at a place in the western ocean, the Sun's meridian altitude was observed to be 62° 00′; and $1^h\ 48^m\ 14^s$ after, the altitude was found to be 54° 30′: Required the latitude of that place, and the Sun's declination.

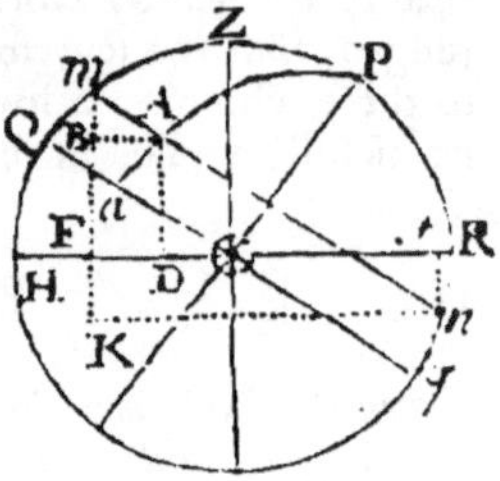

Let *m* and A be the Sun's places at the given times.

*m*F, AD, the sines of the observed altitudes.

*m*B the difference of those right sines.

∠QP*a*, the given interval of time,

and Q*a*, the versed sine of that interval.

Now Q*a* : Q*q* : : *m*A : *mn* (II. 182). And *m*A : *mn* : : *m*B : MK. (II. 167)
Therefore Q*a* : Q*q* : : *m*B : *m*K = *m*F + *nf*.

$$\text{And } mK = \frac{Qq \times mB}{Qa} = \frac{2 \times \text{radius} \times \text{diff. of sines of alts.}}{\text{versed sine of hour from noon}}.$$

But versed sine of an arc = twice square of the sine of half that arc. (IV. 193)

$$\text{Therefore } mK = \frac{2 \times R \times \text{diff. sines of alts.}}{2ss, \tfrac{1}{2} \text{ hour à noon *}} = \frac{\text{diff. of sines of alt.}}{ss, \tfrac{1}{2} \text{ hour à noon}}.\ \text{Radius}$$

being 1.

Or L, diff. sines of alts.—2L*s*, ½ hour *à* noon = L, sum sines, *m*F + *nf*.

Here $1^h\ 48^m\ 14^s$ = 27° 3′ 30″, (131) | Alt. 62° 00′ nat. sine = 0,88295 (IV. 256)
| Alt. 54 30 nat. sine = 0,81412

And ½ hour *à* noon = 13° 31′ 45″. | Diff. of sines of alts. = 0,06883

Now diff. sines alts. = 0,06883; its log. 8,83778 †

½ hour *à* noon = 13° 31′ 45″; twice its log. sine 8,73822 ‡

*m*K = 1,2574 the number to log. 10,09946 ‖

*m*F = 0,8829 the nat. sine of 62° 00′ the meridian altitude.

nf = 0,3745 the nat. sine 21° 59′ 36″ the mid-night depr.

Sum 83 59 36, its ½ 41° 59′ 48″ = co-lat.

Diff. 40 00 24 its ½ 20 00 12 = dec.

Latitude 48° 0′ 12″ N. observations made on the 19th of May.

---

* The mark *à* is used for the word *from*.

† Here 8, is the index; because 6, the left-hand digit of 0,06881, is in the place of 2ds.

‡ The log. sin. of 13° 31′ is 9,36871; and of 13° 32′ is 9,36924; their diff. is 53; then 60″ : 53 : : 45″ : 40; and 9,36871+40=9,36911; its double is 8,73822, rejecting 10 in the doubled index.

In subtracting 8,73822 from 8,83765; the index of the minuend is to be increased by 10 for a radius; or augment 0, the index of the remainder, by 10.

‖ The log. 10,09946, having 10 for its index, shews that the left-hand place of its corresponding number stands in the place of units.

To find the degrees, minutes, and seconds to a given natural right sine.

Now *nf* = 0,3745 its log. is ,57345; which sought among the log. sines, falls between those of 21° 59′ and 22° 00′; the difference of their logs. is 31; and the difference between the given log. and that of 21° 59′ is 19; then 31 : 19 : : 60″ : 36″; so that *nf* answers to 21° 59′ 36″. (iv. 257.)

187. PRO-

187. PROBLEM XLIII.

Being at sea, some time in July, in North lat. the Sun was observed to rise at 4 h. 24 m. 36 s. A. M.; and in the same place, his altitude at noon was 62° 00′: Required the latitude of that place, and day of the month.

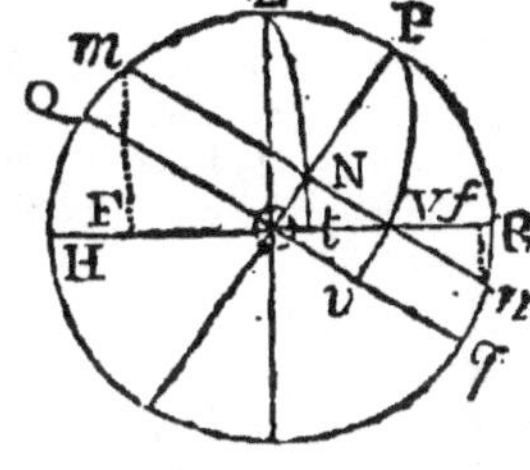

Let *m*, v, *n*, be places of the Sun, at noon, at rising, and at midnight.

*m*F, *nf*, sines of mer. alt. and midnight depr.

ov the sine of the ascensional difference.

vq the versed sine of the time of setting from midnight.

Q*v*=radius+sine of the ascensional difference.

Now Q*v* : *vq* : : (*m*v : v*n* : :) *m*F : *nf*.

Then $nf = \frac{vq \times mF}{Qv}$; or Ls, *nf*=L`, Q*v*+Ls, *m*F+L*v*, ∠VPR.

Or, L`, Q*v*+Ls, merid. alt.+2Ls, ½ time *à* midnight+L, 2=Ls, midnight depression.

Here *ov*=(*s*, 1 h. 35 m. 24 s.=*s*, 23° 51′=)0,40435; and Q*v*=1,4043.
Time from midnight=4 h. 24 m. 36 s.=66° 09′; its half=33° 4½′.

Q*v*=1,4043	its L`	9,85254
*m*F=*s*, 62°	its Ls,	9,94593
vq={ *ss*, 33° 4½′	2Ls,	9,47397
{ 2	its L	0,30103
nf=21° 59′ 40″	its Ls,	9,57347

Merid. alt.	=62° 0′ 0″
Midnt. depr.	=21 59 40
Sum	=83 59 40; its ½=41° 59′ 50″
Diff.	=40 0 20; its ½=20 0 10
Latitude	=48° 0′ 10″ N.
Declination	=20° 0′ 10″ N. on July 23d.

(185.)

At a place in the northern hemisphere, some time in the month of May, the Sun was observed to have 14° 43½′ altitude at 6 h. P. M. and to set at 7 h. 35 m. 24 s.: Required the latitude of that place, and day of the month.

Let *m*, N, V, *n*, be places of the Sun, at noon, 6 o'clock, setting, and midnight. See the fig. to Problem 43.

*m*F, N*t*, sines of the altitudes at *m* and N.

O*v*, *vq*, and Q*v*, the same as in the last problem.

Now O*v* : *vq* : : (N*v* : V*n* : :) N*t* : *nf*. Then L, *nf* = L`, O*v* + L, N*t* + L, *vq*.
Also O*v* : Q*v* : : (NV : V*m* : :) N*t* : *m*F. And L, *m*F = L` O*v* + L, N*t* + L, Q*v*.
Here O*v* = *s*, 23° 51′ = 0,40434; and Q*v* = 1,4043.
qv = *v*, 66° 09′ = 2*ss*, 33° 4½′.

Then O*v* = *s*, 23° 51′	its L`*s*,	0,39325	
N*t* = *s*, 14° 43½′	L*s*,	9,40514	
qv = { *ss*, 33° 4½′	2L*s*,	9,47397	
{ 2		0,30103	
nf s, 22° 0′		9,57339	

And O*v* = *s*, 23° 51′	its L`*s*,	0,39325
N*t* = *s*, 14 43½	its L*s*,	9,40514
Q*v* = 1,40 43	its L,	10,14746
*m*F = *s*, 62 0	L*s*,	9,94585

Then $\frac{62° + 22°}{2} = 42°$ the co-latitude.

And $\frac{62 - 22}{2} = 20°$ the declination answering to May 19th. (185.)

189. PROBLEM XLV.

At a place in the western ocean, some time in July, the Sun's altitude was observed to be 36° at 3 h. 51 m. 49 s. P. M.; and was seen to set at 7 h. 35 m. 24 s. P. M.: Required the latitude of the place, and day of the month.

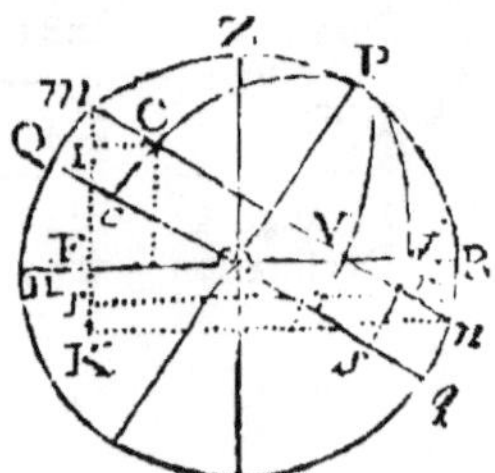

Let *m*, C, V, *n*, be the Sun's places, at noon, at 3 h. 51 m. 49 s. at setting, and at midnight.

mf, IF, the sines of the altitudes at *m*, C;

nf the sine of the midnight depression.

O*c*, O*v*, the sines of the times from 6 *h*, and *cv*, their sum.

Now

Now *cv* : QV : :(CV : V*m* : :) IF : *m*F. Or Ls,*m*F = L`,*cv* + Ls,IF + L,QV.
And *cv* : *qv* : :(CV : V*n* : :) IF : *nf*. Or Ls,*nf* = L`,*cv* + Ls,IF + LV,*q*PV
Here O*c* = *s*, 2h. 8m. 11s. = *s*, 32° 2′ 45″ = 0,53059 }
O*v* = *s*, 1h. 35 m. 24s. = *s*, 23 51 00 = 0,40434 } *cv* = 0,93493;
QV = 1,4043; *qv* = *v*, 66°9′ = 2*ss*, 33°4′30″; or L,*qv* = 2L*s*, 33°4½′ + L2.

Then L`, *cv* = 0,93493	0,02922.	And L`,*cv* = 0,93493	0,02922
L*s*, IF = 36° 00′	9,76922	L*s*,IF = 36° 00′	9,76922
L,QV = 1,4043	10,14746	L,*qv* { *ss*, 33° 4½′	9,47397
		2	0,30103
L, *m*F = 62° 00′	9,94590		
		L*s*,*nf* 22° 00′	9,57344

Then $\frac{62° + 22°}{2}$ = 42 the co-latitude.

And $\frac{62 - 22}{2}$ = 20 the declination, anſwering to July 23. (185.)

190. PROBLEM XLVI.

Some time in the month of May, at a place in the weſtern ocean, the day broke at 1 *h.* 45 *m.* 36 *s. A. M.; and at* 8 *h.* 8 *m.* 11 *s. A. M. the Sun's altitude was obſerved to be* 36°: *Required the latitude and day of the month.*

Let *m*, C, *r*, *n*, be the Sun's places, at noon, at 8 h. 8 m. 11 s., at the beginning of twilight, and at midnight.
*m*F, IF, the ſines of the altitudes at *m*C.
FT, FK, the ſines of the depreſſions at *r*, *n*.
O*c*, O*s*, the ſines of the times from 6 h., and *c s* their ſum.

Now *cs* : Q*s* : : (C*r* : *mr* : :) IT : *m*T. And *m*T — FT = *m*F.
Alſo *cs* : *qc* : : (C*r* : C*n* : :) IT : IK. And IK — IF = *nf*.
Here IF = *s*, 36° 00′ = 0,58778 }
FT = *s*, 18 00 = 0,30902 } IT = 0,89680
O*c* = *s*, 2h. 8m. 11s. = *s*, 32° 2′ 45″ = 0,53059; and *qc* = 1,5306
O*s* = *s*, 4h. 14m. 24s. = *s*, 63 36 00 = 0,89571; and Q*s* = 1,8957

Then *cs*	9,84579	*cs*	9,84579	*m*T — FT = *m*F = 0,8829 the *s*, 62° 00′
IT	9,95269	IT	9,95269	IK — IF = *nf* = 0,37458 the *s*, 22 00
Q*s*	10,27777	*qc*	10,18486	Hence the lat. 48° N.
*m*T	10,07625	IK	9,98334	Decl. 22° 00′ N., anſwering to May 19th.
*m*T = 1,1919		IK = 0,96237		

191. PROBLEM XLVII.

In the month of May, at some place in the western ocean, the Sun's altitude at 6h A. M. was 14° 43½′; and at 8h. 8 m. 11s. its altitude was 36°: Required the latitude of the place and day of the month.

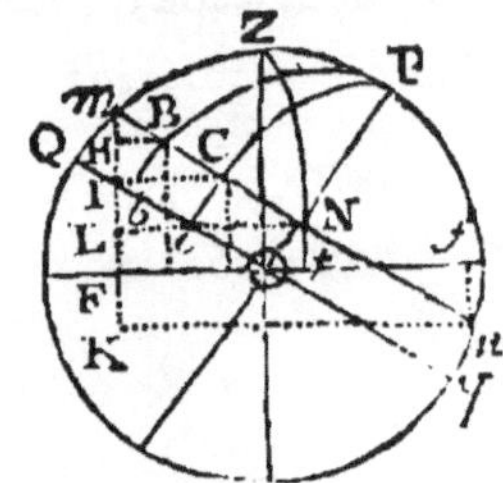

Let *m*, C, N, *n*, be the Sun's places at noon, at 8 h. 8 m. 11s., at 6 h., and at midnight.
*m*F, IF, LF, the sines of the alts. at *m*, C, N.
nf the sine of the midnight depression.
oc the sine of 2 h. 8 m. 11s.

Now *oc* : OQ : : (NC : N*m* : :) IL : *m*L. Then *m*L + LF = *m*F.
And *oc* : *cq* : : (NC : C*n* : :) IL : IK. Then IK — IF = *nf*.

Hence L,*m*L = L`,*oc* + rad. + L,IL. And L,IK = L`,*oc* + L*cq* + L,IL.

Here *oc* = *s*, 2 h. 8 m. 11s. = *s* 30° 2′ 45″ = 0,53059; and *cq* = 1,5306.
IF = *s*, 36° 0′ = 0,58778; and LF = *s*, 14° 43½′ = 0,25418; so IL = 0,3336

oc = 32° 2′ 45″	its L`*s*,	0,27524	*oc* = 32° 2′ 45″	its L`*s*,	0,27524
IL = 0,3336	its L.	9,52323	II = 0,3336	its L.	9,52323
Rad.		10,00000	*cq* = 1,5306	its L.	10,18486
*m*I = 0,62874		9,79847	IK = 0,96234		9,98333

Then *m*F = 0,88292 the sine of 62° 00′ the meridian altitude.
And *nf* = 0,37456 the sine of 22 00 the midnight depression.
Hence the latitude is 48° N. decl. 20° N. on May 19th. (185).

192. PROBLEM XLVIII.

At a place in the western ocean, in the month of July, the Sun's altitude was found to be 46° at 2h 49m 9s P. M.; and to be 36° high at 3h 51m 49s P. M.: Required the latitude of the place and day of the month.

Let *m*, B, C, *n*, be the Sun's places at noon, at 2 h. 49 m. 9 s., at 3 h. 51 m. 49 s., and at midnight; and *m*F, HF, IF, the sines of the alts. at *m*, B, C. *ob*, *oc*, the co-sines of the time from noon; or the sines of the time to 6 o'clock.

Now *bc* : Q*c* : : (BC : *m*C : :) HI : *m*I. Then *m*I + IF = *m*F.
And *bc* : *bq* : : (BC : B*n* : :) HI : HK. Then HK — HF = FK = *nf*.

Here *ob* = *s*, 3 h. 10 m. 51s. = *s*, 47° 42′ 45″ = 0,73978 }
oc = *s*, 2 h. 8 m. 11s. = *s*, 32 2 45 = 0,53059 } Hence *bc* = 0,20919
HF = *s*, 46° = 0,71934; IF = *s*, 36° = 0,58778; HI = 0,13156; *bq* = 1,7398.
Also Q*c* = (ver. sine of 57° 57′ 15″ =) 2*ss*, ½ 57° 57′ 15″ = 2*ss*, 28° 58′ 37″.

Then

Then $bc=$	0,20919	0,67947	And	$bc=0,20919$	0,67947
$HI=$	0,13156	9,11912		$HI=0,13156$	9,11912
$QC=$	{ ss, 28° 58′ 37″	9,37050		$bq=1,7398$	10,24050
	{ 2	0,30103			
				$HK=1,0942$	10,03909
$mI=,29520$		9,47012			

Then $mF=0,88298$ the fine of 62° the mer. alt. } Hence lat. $=$ 48° N. decl.
And $nf=0,37486$ the fine of 22 the mid. depr. } 20° on July 23.

193. PROBLEM XLIX.

Being at fea in the weftern ocean, the Sun was obferved to have 27° 24′ of altitude when due W.; and to have 14° 43½′ alt. at 6 h. P. M.: Required the latitude of that place, and the Sun's declination.

Let C, N, be the Sun's places at W., and at 6 h.
OC, Nt, the fines of their altitudes.
Cc $=$ ON, the arcs of declination.
∠ COc $=$ ∠ NOt $=$ latitude.

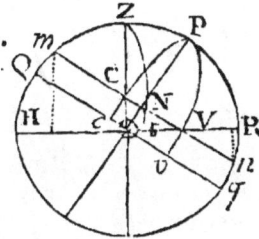

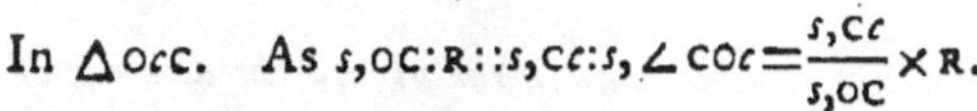

In △OcC. As s,OC : R :: s,Cc : s, ∠ COc $= \frac{s,Cc}{s,OC} \times R$.

In △OtN. As s,ON : R :: s,Nt : s, ∠ NOt $= \frac{s,Nt}{s,ON} \times R$.

Then $\frac{s,Cc}{s,OC} = \left(\frac{s,Nt}{s,ON} = \right) \frac{s,Nt}{s,Cc}$. And ss,Cc $= s$,OC $\times s$,Nt.

Or s, alt. W. $\times s$, alt. at 6 $= ss$,decl. Or $\frac{Ls,\text{ alt. W.} + Ls,\text{ alt. at } 6}{2} = Ls$,decl.

And L′s,alt. W. + Ls,decl. $=$ Ls,lat.

OC $= s$, 27° 24′	its L,s		9,66295
Nt $=$ 14 43½	its L,s		9,40514
		Sum	19,06809
Cc $=$ 20° 00′			9,53404
Oc $=$ 27 24	its L′		0,33705
∠ QOZ $=$ 48 00			9,87109

194. PROBLEM L.

At a place in the weftern ocean, the Sun at rifing was obferved to be 59° 15′ 40″ from the true north point of the horizon; and at 6 h. A. M., the altitude was obferved 14° 43½′: Required the latitude and declination.

Let V, and N, be the places of the Sun at rifing and at 6 h. A. M.
Nt, the fine of the alt. at 6. ON, Vv are arcs of declination.
Ov, the afcenfional diff. ∠ NOt $=$ lat.; ∠ VOv $=$ co-latitude.
OV, $=$ co-amplitude.

S Now

Now in $\triangle$ OVv. As R : s,OV : : s,VOv : s,Vv $= \frac{s,\text{OV} \times s,\text{VO}v}{\text{R}}$.

in $\triangle$ NOt. As s,NOt : R : : s,Nt : s,ON $= \frac{\text{R} \times s,\text{N}t}{s,\text{NO}t}$.

Then $\frac{s,\text{OV} \times s\text{VO}v}{\text{R}} = \frac{s,\text{N}t \times \text{R}}{s,\text{NO}t}$; and s,VO$v \times s$,NOt $= \frac{s,\text{N}t}{s,\text{OV}} \times$ RR.

That is, $\frac{s,\text{N}t}{s,\text{OV}} = s,\text{NO}t \times s',\text{NO}t$; hence $\frac{2s,\text{N}t}{s,\text{OV}} = (2s,\text{NO}t \times s',\text{NO}t =)\, s,2\text{NO}t$.

(IV. 189)

Therefore L$'s'$, ampl. + Ls, alt. at 6 + L,2 = Ls, double the latitude. If the latitude is less than 45°; otherwise it is double the co-latitude.

L$'s$, ampl.	59° 15′ 40″	0,29147	Rad.	R		10,00000
Ls, alt. 6	14 43 30	9,40514	s', ampl.	59° 15′ 40″		9,70853
L, 2		0,30103	s', lat.	47 59		9,82565
Ls,	84° 02′	9,99764	s, decl.	20 00		9,53418
Co-lat. is	42 01					

195. PROBLEM LI.

Being at sea in the western ocean, some time in the night, the distance of two stars when both were on the meridian, was observed to be 20°; and 1^h 49^m after, the difference of their altitudes was 14° 35½′, and the difference of their azimuths 30° 9½′: Required the latitude of the place.

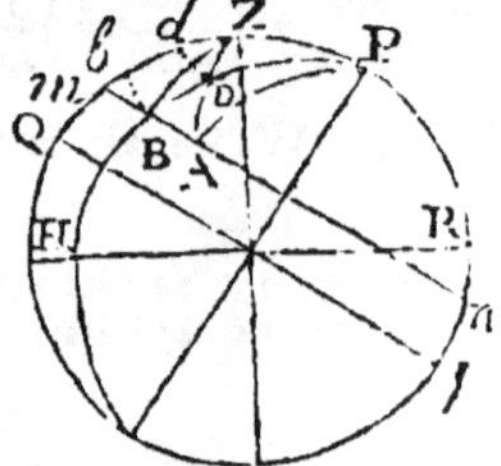

As the stars were on the meridian when first observed; their distance, difference of declination, and difference of altitudes, at that time, are equal: If they are first at d, b, and in the difference of time revolve to D, B; then is known ∠P, ∠DZB, DB, and ZB—ZD. Let ZB—ZD = N; and find ZB + ZD = M.

Now (IV. 239) $s,\text{ZB} \times s,\text{ZD} \times s',\text{DZB} + s',\text{ZD} \times s'\text{ZB} = s',\text{DB}$.
Or (IV. 181, 174) $\overline{\tfrac{1}{2}s',\text{N} - \tfrac{1}{2}s',\text{M}} \times s',\text{DZB} + \tfrac{1}{2}s',\text{N} + \tfrac{1}{2}s',\text{M} = s',\text{DB}$.
Or $\overline{s',\text{DZB} \times \tfrac{1}{2}s',\text{N}} - \overline{s',\text{DZB} \times \tfrac{1}{2}s'\text{M}} + \tfrac{1}{2}s'\text{N} + \tfrac{1}{2}s'\text{M} = s',\text{DB}$.
Or $\overline{s',\text{DZB} + 1} \times \tfrac{1}{2}s',\text{N} + \overline{1 - s',\text{DZB}} \times \tfrac{1}{2}s',\text{M} = s',\text{DB}$.

Then $s',\text{M} = \left(\frac{2s',\text{DB} - \overline{1 + s'\text{DZB}} \times s',\text{N}}{1 - s'\,\text{DZB}} = \right) \frac{2s',\text{DB} - v',\text{DZB} \times s',\text{N}}{v,\text{DZB}}$.

Or $s',\text{M} = \left(\frac{2s',\text{DB}}{v,\text{DZB}} - \frac{v',\text{DZB} \times s'\text{N}}{v,\text{DZB}} = \right) \frac{2s',\text{DB}}{2ss,\tfrac{1}{2}\text{DZB}} - \frac{2s's',\tfrac{1}{2}\text{DZB} \times s',\text{N}}{2ss,\tfrac{1}{2}\text{DZB}}$.

(IV. 193, 197)

Let 2L$'s$,½DZB + Ls',DB = L,A; and 2L$'s$,½DZB + 2L$'s$,½DZB + Ls',N = L,B.

Then s'M = A — B.		2L$'s$.½DZB	1,16952	2L$'s$,½DZB	1,16952
Here DB = 20° 00′		Ls',DB	9,97200	2Ls',½ZB	9,96960
∠DZB = 30	9½	A = 13,884	1,14251	Ls',N	9,98576
½∠DZB = 15	4¾	B = 13,331		B = 13,331	1,12488

ZB—ZD = N = 14 35½ s',M = 0,553; and ZB + ZD = 56° 25½′.

Then

Then $\frac{1}{2}$ ſum $+ \frac{1}{2}$ diff. $=$ ZB $= 35° \; 30\frac{1}{2}'$; and $\frac{1}{2}$ ſum $- \frac{1}{2}$ diff. $=$ ZD $= 20° \; 55'$.
Now s,DB : s,DZB : : s,ZB : s,PDZ ; and s,ZPD : s,PDZ : : s,ZD : s,ZP $42° \; 1'$.
Hence the latitude is $47° \; 59'$ N.

196. PROBLEM LII.

By obſervations made at a place in the weſtern ocean, it was found that the Sun's altitude was 36° S., when his azimuth was N. 100° 5′ E. and his alt. was 46° S., when his azimuth was N. 114° 28′ E. What was the latitude of the place and the Sun's declination?

Let A, B, be the Sun's places when obſerved.
In the triangles PAZ, PBZ, where PA $=$ PB.

By IV. 239. $\begin{cases} \grave{s},ZP \times \grave{s}ZA - \grave{s},PZA \times s,ZP \times s,ZA = \grave{s},PA. \\ \grave{s},ZP \times \grave{s},ZB - \grave{s},PZB \times s,ZP \times s,ZB = \grave{s},PA. \end{cases}$

Then $\grave{s},PZB \times s,ZB \times s,ZP - \grave{s},PZA \times s,ZA \times s,ZP = \grave{s},ZB \times \grave{s},ZP - \grave{s},ZA \times \grave{s},ZP$.

Or $\overline{\grave{s},PZB \times s,ZB - \grave{s},PZA \times s,ZA} \times s,ZP = \overline{\grave{s},ZB - \grave{s},ZA} \times \grave{s},ZP$.

Then $\frac{\grave{s},PZB \times s,ZB \backsim \grave{s},PZA \times s,ZA}{\grave{s},ZB - \grave{s},ZA} = \left(\frac{\grave{s},ZP}{s,ZP} = (\text{III. } 33) \; t,ZP = \right) \grave{s}$, RP the latitude.

Let $L\grave{s}$, PZB $+ Ls$, ZB $=$ L,A : And $L\grave{s}$,PZA $+ Ls$,ZA $=$ L, B. Then $\frac{A \backsim B}{\grave{s}ZB - \grave{s},ZA} = \grave{t},RP$.

Here A $= 0,14164$; B $= 0,28770$; $\grave{s}$,ZB $= 0,71933$; $\grave{s}$,ZA $= 0,58779$.
Then $\frac{0,13154}{0,14606} = ,9005 = t,42°$. Hence lat. is 48° N. decl. 20° N.

197. PROBLEM LIII.

Given two altitudes of the Sun and the time from noon when thoſe altitudes were taken; thence to find the latitude and declination.

EXAM. *At* 8 *h*. 8 *m*. 11 *s*. *A. M.*, *the alt. was* 36° ; *and at* 9 *h*. 10 *m*. 51 *s*. *the alt. was* 46° ; *at a place in the weſtern ocean, ſome time in May*, 1763.

Let B, A, be the Sun's places obſerved;
m, n, thoſe of noon and midnight;
Fe, Fd, Fm, FK, repreſent the ſines of the diſtances of thoſe places from the horizon HR, to the diameter Qq; and $d = $ Fd $-$ Fe.

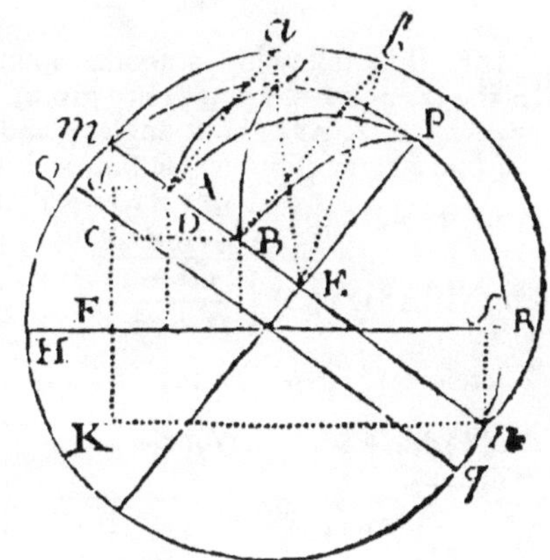

On mn deſcribe the ſemicircle mbn, repreſenting half the parallel of declination, and let Aa, Bb, be at right angles to mn: Then will the angles mEb, mEa, repreſent the times from noon, at the obſervations B, A; and mB, mA, are as the verſed ſines of thoſe times.

And mB $-$ mA $=$ AB.
Then AB : de : : mB : me ; and me + Fe $=$ Fm, the ſine of Hm.

Alſo AB : de : : mn : mK ; and Km — Fm = FK, the ſine of Rn.
Hence the latitude and declination are found. (185)

Here AB $= (\grave{s},ma - \grave{s},mb =) s,\frac{mb+ma}{2} \times 2s,\frac{mb-ma}{2} =) s,\text{M} \times 2s,\text{N}.$ (IV. 181)

And $de = (s,\text{2d alt.} - s,\text{1ſt alt.} =) \grave{s},\frac{\text{2d}+\text{1ſt}}{2} \times 2s,\frac{\text{2d}-\text{1ſt}}{2} = \grave{s},\text{W} \times 2s,\text{V}.$ (IV. 182)

Now $\text{L},\frac{de}{\text{AB}} \times mn = \text{L},m\text{K} = \text{L}\grave{s},\text{M} + \text{L}\grave{s},\text{N} + \text{L}s,\text{W} + \text{L},s\text{V},\text{L},2.$

And $\text{L},\frac{de}{\text{AB}} \times m\text{B} = \text{L},me = \text{L},m\text{K} + 2\text{L}s,\tfrac{1}{2}\angle m\text{E}b.$

In this example, the $\angle m\text{E}b$ = 3 h. 51 49 = 57° 57¼′; its ½ = 28° 58⅝′.
$\angle m\text{E}a$ = 2 h. 49 9 = 42 17¼.

57° 57¼′		46		L$\grave{s}$,M	50° 7¼′		0,11498
42 17¼		36		L$\grave{s}$,N	7 50		0,86553
				L$\grave{s}$,W	41 0		9,87778
100 14½	50° 7¼′ = M	82	41° 0′ = W.	Ls,V	5 0		8,94030
				L,2			0,30103
15 40	7 50 = N	10	5 0 = V.				
s,36° = Fe = 0,58778				L,Km	1,25783		10,09962
me = 0,29521				2Ls,½mb	28° 58⅝′		9.37050
Fm = 0,88299 = 62° 0′ 19″				L,me	0,29521		9,47012
Km = 1,25810							
FK = 0,37511 = 22 1 51				42 0′ 55″ the co-latitude.			
84 2 10				19 59 14 the decl. on May 20th.			
39 58 28							

198. The following is another ſolution, on different principles.
In the triangles BPZ, APZ, are given, (ſee the foregoing figure.)
BZ, AZ ; BPZ, APZ, hour angles ; and PB = PA ;
To find PB, PZ ; for whoſe ſum and diff. put M and N.

Now (IV. 239) $\begin{cases} s,\text{PB} \times s,\text{PZ} \times \grave{s},\text{BPZ} + \grave{s},\text{PB} \times \grave{s},\text{PZ} = \grave{s},\text{BZ}. \\ s,\text{PA} \times s,\text{PZ} \times \grave{s},\text{APZ} + \grave{s},\text{PA} \times \grave{s},\text{PZ} = \grave{s},\text{AZ}. \end{cases}$

Or (IV. 181. 174) $\begin{cases} \overline{\tfrac{1}{2}\grave{s},\text{N} - \tfrac{1}{2}\grave{s},\text{M}} \times \grave{s},\text{BPZ} + \overline{\tfrac{1}{2}\grave{s},\text{N} + \tfrac{1}{2}\grave{s},\text{M}} = \grave{s},\text{BZ}. \\ \overline{\tfrac{1}{2}\grave{s},\text{N} - \tfrac{1}{2}\grave{s},\text{M}} \times \grave{s},\text{APZ} + \overline{\tfrac{1}{2}\grave{s},\text{N} + \tfrac{1}{2}\grave{s},\text{M}} = \grave{s},\text{AZ}. \end{cases}$

Therefore $(\tfrac{1}{2}\grave{s},\text{N} - \tfrac{1}{2}\grave{s},\text{M} =) \frac{\grave{s},\text{BZ} - \overline{\tfrac{1}{2}\grave{s},\text{N} + \tfrac{1}{2}\grave{s},\text{M}}}{\grave{s},\text{CPZ}} = \frac{\grave{s},\text{AZ} - \overline{\tfrac{1}{2}\grave{s},\text{N} + \tfrac{1}{2}\grave{s},\text{M}}}{\grave{s},\text{APZ}}.$

And $(\tfrac{1}{2}\grave{s},\text{N} + \tfrac{1}{2}\grave{s},\text{M} =) \grave{s},\text{BZ} - \overline{\tfrac{1}{2}\grave{s},\text{N} - \tfrac{1}{2}\grave{s},\text{M}} \times \grave{s},\text{BPZ} = \grave{s},\text{AZ} - \overline{\tfrac{1}{2}\grave{s},\text{N} - \tfrac{1}{2}\grave{s},\text{M}} \times \grave{s},\text{APZ}.$

Hence $\grave{s},\text{BZ} \times \grave{s},\text{APZ} - \overline{\tfrac{1}{2}\grave{s},\text{N} + \tfrac{1}{2}\grave{s},\text{M}} \times \grave{s},\text{APZ} = \grave{s},\text{AZ} \times \grave{s},\text{BPZ} - \overline{\tfrac{1}{2}\grave{s},\text{N} + \tfrac{1}{2}\grave{s},\text{M}} \times \grave{s},\text{BPZ}.$

Therefore

Therefore $s',BZ\times s',APZ - s',AZ\times s',BPZ = \overline{s',APZ - s',BPZ}\times\overline{\tfrac{1}{2}s',N + \tfrac{1}{2}s',M}$.
Again $s',AZ - s',BZ = \overline{s',APZ - s',BPZ}\times\overline{\tfrac{1}{2}s',N - \tfrac{1}{2}s',M}$.

Therefore $\tfrac{1}{2}s',N + \tfrac{1}{2}s',M = \dfrac{s',BPZ\times s',AZ - s',APZ\times s',BZ}{s',APZ - s'BPZ.}$ } Hence IV. 216.

And $\tfrac{1}{2}s',N - \tfrac{1}{2}s',M = \dfrac{s',AZ - s',BZ}{s',APZ - s',BPZ}$

$$s',M = \left(\frac{s',AZ + s',BPZ\times s',AZ - s',BZ - s',APZ\times s',BZ}{s',APZ - s',BPZ} = \right)$$
$$\frac{\overline{1 + s',BPZ}\times s',AZ - \overline{1 + s',APZ}\times s',BZ}{s',APZ - s'BPZ}.$$

$$s',N = \left(\frac{s',BPZ\times s',AZ - s',AZ - s',APZ\times s',BZ + s',BZ}{s',APZ - s',BPZ} = \right)$$
$$\frac{\overline{1 - s',BPZ}\times s',AZ - \overline{1 - s',APZ}\times s',BZ}{s',APZ - s',BPZ}.$$

$$\text{Or, } sM = \left(\frac{v',BPZ\times s',AZ - v',APZ\times s',BZ}{s',APZ - s',BPZ} = \right)$$
$$\frac{2s's',\tfrac{1}{2}BPZ\times s',AZ - 2s's',\tfrac{1}{2}APZ\times s',BZ}{s',APZ - s',BPZ}.$$

$$\text{And } s',N = \left(\frac{v,BPZ\times s',AZ - v,ABZ\times s',BZ}{s',APZ - s',BPZ} = \right)$$
$$\frac{2ss,\tfrac{1}{2}BPZ\times s',AZ - 2ss,\tfrac{1}{2}APZ\times s',BZ}{s',APZ - s',BPZ}.$$

Here BPZ $=57^\circ\ 57\tfrac{1}{4}'$, its $\tfrac{1}{2} = 28^\circ\ 58\tfrac{5}{8}'$; APZ $= 42^\circ\ 17\tfrac{1}{4}'$, its $\tfrac{1}{2} = 21^\circ\ 8\tfrac{5}{8}'$. BZ $= 54^\circ$; AZ $= 44^\circ$; $s',BPZ = 0,53060$; $s',APZ = 0,73978$, their difference $= 0,20918$.

2Ls's',	28° 58⅝′	{ 0,30103 9,88384	2Lss,	28° 58⅝′	{ 0,30103 9,37050
Ls',	44	9,85693	Ls',	44	9,85693
L,A	1,10104	10,04180	L,a	0,33764	9,52846
2Ls's',	21° 8⅝′	{ 0,30103 9,93946	2Lss,	21° 8⅝′	{ 0,30103 9,11438
Ls',	54	9,76922	Ls',	54	9,76922
L,B	1,02260	10,00971	L,b	0,15298	9,18463
L,A—B	0,07844	8,89454	L,a—b	0,18466	9,26637
Ls',APZ—s',BPZ	0,20918	9,32052	Ls',APZ—s,BPZ	0,20918	9,32052
Ls',M	112° 1½′	9,57402	Ls',N	28° 0′	9,94585

Hence the latitude is 48° 00′ N.; declination 19° 59′, which anſwers to the 20th of May.

199. And hence is readily derived the investigation of that method, published in the year 1759, and then used by some for finding the true latitude at sea, by knowing the latitude by account (or dead reckoning), the Sun's declination, two altitudes of the Sun, and the time between the observations. Thus. See the last figure.

Let M and N represent the half sum and half diff. of the times from noon; W and V, the half sum and half diff. of the two altitudes.
AB the diff. of the co-sines of the times from noon, to the radius E*m*.
AD the diff. of the sines of the altitudes.
∠EAD represents the latitude; E*m* the co-s. of the declination.

Now (197) $s,M \times 2s,N = AB$ reduced to the rad. $\frac{1}{2}$ Q*q*; and $s',W \times 2s,V = AD$. But in the triangle ABD.

$$s',\text{lat.} : R :: AD : AB = \frac{1}{s',\text{lat.}} \times AD, \text{ to rad. } Em.$$

$$\text{And } s',\text{decl.} : R :: AB : AB \times \frac{1}{s'\,\text{decl.}} = \frac{1}{s',\text{decl.}} \times \frac{1}{s',\text{lat.}} \times AD = AB \text{ reduced}$$

to the radius $\frac{1}{2}$ Q*q*.

$$\text{Then } s,M \times 2s,N = \frac{1}{s',\text{decl.}} \times \frac{1}{s',\text{lat.}} \times s',W \times 2s,V.$$

$$\text{And } s,M = \frac{1}{s',\text{decl.}} \times \frac{1}{s',\text{lat.}} \times \frac{1}{s,N} \times s',W \times s,V.$$

Then M+N = ∠*m*E*b*, the time from noon at the least altitude.
And M−N = ∠*m*E*a*, the time from noon at the greatest altitude.
Hence the versed sines of the arcs *mb* or *ma*, are known to rad. $\frac{1}{2}$ Q*q*.
Now R : E*m* :: *v,ma* : *m*A = E*m* × *v,ma*; or *m*B = E*m* × *v,mb*.
And R : *s,m*A*d* :: *m*A : *md* (:: *m*B : *me*.)
Then F*m* = F*d* + *dm*, or to F*e* + *em*, is the sine of the mer. alt.

Hence the two operations.
1st. L*s'*, decl. + L*s'*, lat. + L*s'*,N + L*s'*,W + L*s*,V = L*s*,M.
Hence the times are known; viz. arcs *ma*, *mb*.
2d. L*s'*, decl. + L*s'*, lat. + L,2 + 2L*s*,$\frac{1}{2}$*ma* = L,*md*.

Then by the merid. alt. and declination the latitude may be found. If this latitude and that assumed are the same, then the latitude by account, or dead reckoning, may be taken as the true latitude.

But if they differ, it is plain that the ∠*m*A*d*, the co-latitude, is less or greater than was assumed.

200. PROBLEM LIV.

Given three descending (or ascending) altitudes of the Sun, taken on the same day at unequal known intervals of time; thence to find those times, the latitude of the place of observation, and the Sun's declination. Thus, suppose in July, 1763, the altitudes were 54° 30′, 46°, and 36°; and the intervals of time 60 m. 55 s. and 62 m. 40 s.; required the rest.

Let

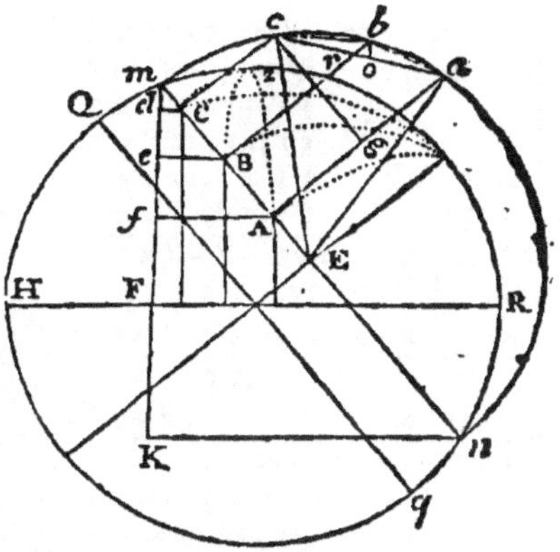

Let *m a n* be the parallel of declination described on *m n*, and *a*, *b*, *c*, the places of the Sun when observed; *a* A, *b* B, and *c* C the sines of the times from noon to the radius E*m*; *m*, *n*, the places at noon and midnight; and let *f* F, *e* F, *d* F, *m* F, F K, represent the sines of the distances of those places from the horizon HR. Draw *c g* parallel to A C; then if the ∠ *gc*E, which is equal to the ∠ *m*E*c*, the time from noon when the greatest altitude was taken, could be found, the times from noon when the other two were taken would be known also. Now *c b* being one interval, and *b a* the other, *b c* and *b a*, the chords of these arcs, will be known, as also *c a*, which is the chord of their sum. Draw *b o* perpendicular to *a c*. Now in the right angled △ *c b o*, the ∠ *b c o* = $\frac{1}{2}$ the arc *b a* (II. 120), and the side *c b* = twice the sine of $\frac{1}{2}$ the arc *b c*, consequently R : *s*,*b c o* (= *s* $\frac{1}{2}$ arc *b a*) : : *b c* (= 2 *s*, $\frac{1}{2}$ arc *b c*) : *b o*; and R : *s*, *c b o* (*s*`, $\frac{1}{2}$ arc *b a*) : : *b c* (2 *s*, $\frac{1}{2}$ arc *b c*) : *c o*. Now *d f*, *d e*, the diff. of the sines of the altitudes, are known; and the lines *f d*, AC, *a c*, are cut proportionally in *e*, B and *r*; consequently, *d f* : *d e* : : (CA : CB : :) *e a* : *c r*, and *c o* — *c r* = *r o* : In the triangle *b o r*, (III. 46) *r o* : *b o* : : R : *t*`, ∠ *r b o* = ∠ *r cg*. Now ∠ *a c* E (= compt. of $\frac{1}{2}$ whole interval *a c*) — ∠ *r c g* = ∠ *g c* E = ∠ *c* E *m* = time from noon when greatest altitude was observed; therefore the time is known, as well as *cm* the versed sine of that time from noon.

Again R : *s*`,*a c g* : : *ac* : *c g* = AC.
And AC : *mc* : : *f d* : *dm*. Then F*d* + *dm* = F*m*, the sine of H*m*.
And AC : *mn* : : *f d* : *m*K. Then K*m* — F*m* = FK, the sine of R*n*.

This Problem has, at times, for near a century past, exercised the talents of many ingenious persons, as well in Russia, Germany, Holland, and France, as in England; perhaps, on account of its apparent use at sea: And among the different solutions there seems none shorter or more intelligible, particularly to beginners, than that above; however, for the sake of the more inquisitive, another solution, which has been commonly given, is here subjoined.

201. In the last figure, the three triangles CPZ, BPZ, APZ, are those concerned; in which the same two sides are common in each.

$$\left.\begin{array}{l} s`,CPZ \times s,PC \times s,PZ + s`,PC \times s`,PZ = s`,ZC \\ s`,BPZ \times s,PC \times s,PZ + s`,PC \times s`,PZ = s`,ZB \\ s`,APZ \times s,PZ \times s,PC + s`,PC \times s`,PZ = s`,ZA \end{array}\right\} \text{by IV. 239.}$$

Then $\overline{s`,CPZ - s`,BPZ} \times s,PC \times s,PZ = (\overline{s`,ZC - s`,ZB} =)\ d.$ (II. 48.)
And $\overline{s`,CPZ - s`,APZ} \times s,PC \times s,PZ = (\overline{s`,ZC - s`,ZA} =)\ D.$
Hence $D \times \overline{s`,CPZ - s`,BPZ} = d \times \overline{s`,CPZ - s`,APZ}.$ (II. 147)
Then $D \times s`,CPZ - d \times s`,CPZ = D \times s`,BPZ - d \times s`,APZ.$

 Or,

Or, $D \times s',CPZ - d \times s',CPZ$ $(= \overline{D-d} \times s',CPZ) = D \times s',BPZ - d \times s',APZ$.
But, $BPZ = CPZ + BPC$, and $APZ = CPZ + APC$.

Consequently, $\left\{ \begin{array}{l} s',BPZ = s',CPZ \times s',BPC - s,CPZ \times s,BPC. \\ s',APZ = s',CPZ \times s',APC - s,CPZ \times s,APC. \end{array} \right\}$ (IV. 216.)

Hence $\overline{D-d} \times s'$. CPZ $=$. $\left\{ \begin{array}{l} D \times s',CPZ \times s',BPC - D \times s,CPZ \times s,BPC - \\ d \times s',CPZ \times s',APC + d \times s,CPZ \times s,APC. \end{array} \right\}$ by substitu.

Or, $\overline{D - D \times s',BPC - d + d \times s',APC} \times s',CPZ = \overline{d \times s,APC - D \times s,BPC} \times s,CPZ$. Wherefore,

$$\frac{D - D \times s',BPC \backsim d - d \times s',APC}{d \times s,APC \backsim D \times s,BPC.} \left(= \frac{\overline{1 - s',BPC} \times D \backsim \overline{1 - s',APC} \times d}{d \times s,APC \backsim D \times s,BPC} \right)$$

$$= \frac{v.BPC \times D \backsim v.APC \times d}{s,APC \times d \backsim s,BPC \times D} = \frac{s,CPZ}{s',CPZ} = t,CPZ,$$ the measure of the time from noon when the greatest altitude was observed.

Here $Fd = s,54° 30' = 0,81412$; $Fe = s,46° 00 = 0,71934$; $Ff = s,36° 00 = 0,58779$. Then $df = 0,22633$; $de = 0,09478$.

The arc cb, or $\angle CPB$, $=$ 1 h. 0 m. 55 s. $= 15° 13\frac{3}{4}'$; its $\frac{1}{2} = 7° 36\frac{7}{8}$.
arc ab, or $\angle BPA$, $=$ 1 h. 2 m. 40 s. $= 15\ 40$; its $\frac{1}{2} = 7\ 50$.
arc ca, or $\angle CPA$, $=$ 2 h. 3 m. 35 s. $= 30\ 53\frac{3}{4}$; its $\frac{1}{2} = 15\ 26\frac{7}{8}$.

To find the hour by the 1st method.

Radius	90° 00'	10,00000
Is to s, $\frac{1}{2}$ ba	7 50	9,13447
As s, $\frac{1}{2}$ bc	7 $36\frac{7}{8}$	9.12224
To $\frac{1}{2}$ ob	,01806	8,25671
Radius	90° 00'	10,00000
Is to s, $\frac{1}{2}$ bc	7 $36\frac{7}{8}$	9,12224
As s' $\frac{1}{2}$ ba	7 50	9.99593
To $\frac{1}{2}$ co	,13127	9.11817
As fd	22633 A.C.	0,64526
Is to de	,09478	8,97672
So is $\frac{1}{2}$ ac (s, $\frac{1}{2}$ cEa)	15° $26\frac{7}{8}'$	9.42547
To $\frac{1}{2}$ cr	,11154	9,04745
$\frac{1}{2}$ co	,13127	
As $\frac{1}{2}$ ro	,01973	1,70480
Is to $\frac{1}{2}$ bo	,01806	8,25671
So is Rad.	90 00	10,00000
To t', $\angle rbo$	47 $32\frac{1}{8}$	0,06151
$\angle acE$	74 $33\frac{1}{8}$	h m s
$\angle gcE = \angle mEc = 27$	1 $=$	1 48 4
Time of 2d observation		2 48 59
Time of 3d observation		3 51 39

To find the hour by the 2d method.

D ($= fd$)	,22633	9,35474
s, $\angle BPC$	15° $13\frac{3}{4}'$	9,41943
D $\times s$,BPC	,05945	8,77417
d ($= de$)	,09478	8,97672
s, $\angle APC$	30° $53\frac{3}{4}'$	9,71052
$d \times s$,APC	,04867	8,68724
D ($= fd$)	,22633	9,35474
v, $\angle BPC$	15° $13\frac{3}{4}'$	8,54552
D $\times v$,BPC	,00795	7,90026
d ($= de$)	,09478	8,97672
v,APC	30° $53\frac{3}{4}'$	9,15198
$d \times v$,APC	,01345	8,12870
D $\times v$,BPC	,00795	
$d \times v$,APC $-$ D $\times v$,BPC	,00550	17,74036
D $\times s$,BPC $- d \times s$,APC	,01078	8,03262
tang.	27° $1\frac{3}{4}'$	9,70774
Hence the h. fr. n. of 1st ob. is		$1^h\ 48'\ 7''$
Of the second observation		2 49 2
Of the third observation		3 51 42

Consequently from any two of these, with their corresponding altitudes the latitude and declination may be found by Problem 53.

Here the altitudes are supposed to be descending ones, or in the afternoon.

202. If

202. If the altitudes were taken at equal intervals of time; the two first proportions are useless: For $a\,b$ and $b\,c$ being equal, the point o falls in the middle of the chord $c\,a$; and $b\,o$, the versed sine, is known.
Then $df : de :: (\text{CA} : \text{CB} ::)\, ca : cr$; and $co - cr = ro$.
And $bo : ro ::$ Rad. : $t, rbo, = acg$; and $ac\text{E} - acg = gc\text{E} = c\text{E}m$.
Hence the times from noon are known; and also mc, the versed sine of $c\text{E}m$.
Again, in $\triangle\, acg$. R : $s', acg :: ac : cg = \text{AC}$.
And AC : $mc :: fd : dm$. Then $\text{F}d + dm = \text{F}m$.
Also AC : $mn :: fd : m\text{K}$. Then $\text{K}m - \text{F}m = \text{FK}$.

Here $d\text{F} = 0{,}81412$, $c\text{F} = 0{,}71934$; $f\text{F} = 0{,}58779$; $df = 022633$; $de = 0{,}09478$.
Also, arc $cb = 1$ h. 1 m. $47\frac{1}{2}$ s. $= 15°\ 26\frac{7}{8}'$; $co = 0{,}26636$; $bo = 0{,}03613$.
Then $df : de :: ca : cr = 0{,}22309$: and $co - cr = 0{,}04327$.
And $bo : ro ::$ Rad. : $t, rbo = 50°\ 8\frac{3}{8}'$ —; then $74°\ 33'\frac{1}{8} - 50°\ 8'\frac{1}{8} = 24°\ 24\frac{3}{4}'$.

	h	m	s	
Then $24°\ 24\frac{3}{4}' =$	1	37	39	from noon at first alt.
And $24°\ 24\frac{3}{4}' + 15°\ 26\frac{7}{8} = 39°\ 51\frac{5}{8} =$	2	39	$26\frac{1}{2}$	from noon at 2d alt.
Also $39\ 51\frac{5}{8} + 15\ 26\frac{7}{8} = 55\ 18\frac{1}{2} =$	3	41	14	from noon at 3d alt.

Here the altitudes are supposed to be ascending ones, or in the forenoon.
Again, rad. : $s, cag :: ac : \text{AC} = 0{,}34142$.
And AC : $mc :: fd : dm = 0{,}05927$; then $m\text{F} = 0{,}87338 = s$, $60°\ 51'$.
Also AC : $mn :: fd : m\text{K} = 1{,}32581$; then $\text{FK} = 0{,}45243 = s$, $26°\ 54'$.
Hence the latitude is $46°\ 7\frac{1}{2}$ N. and the declin. $16°\ 58\frac{1}{2}'$; or on May 7th.

203. But the operation in this case may be much contracted. Thus, since $(df : de :: ca :)\ cr = \frac{de \times ca}{df}$; thence $ro = \left(co - \frac{de \times 2co}{df} =\right) \frac{df - 2de \times co}{df}$.

And $(bo : ro :: \text{R} :)\ t, rbo = \left(\frac{ro}{bo} = \frac{\text{D} \times co}{df \times 2ss, \frac{1}{2}cb} =\right) \frac{\text{D} \times \frac{1}{2}co}{df \times ss, \frac{1}{2}cb}$;
where $\text{D} = df - 2de$.
But $\text{R} \times v, cb = ss, \frac{1}{2}cb = \frac{1}{2}s, cb \times t, \frac{1}{2}cb$. (IV. 193, 195)
Then $t, rbo = \frac{\text{D}}{df \times t, \frac{1}{2}cb}$; or $\text{L}t, rbo = \text{L}'t, \frac{1}{2}cb + \text{L}', df + \text{L}, \text{D}$.
Also $(\text{R} : s', acg :: ac :)\ \text{AC} = (s', acg \times ac =)\ s', acg \times 2s, cb$.
And $(\text{AC} : mn :: fd :)\ m\text{K} = \left(\frac{mn \times fd}{\text{AC}} = \frac{2 \times fd}{s, acg \times 2s, cb} =\right) \frac{fd}{s, acg \times s, cb}$.
And $(\text{AC} : mc :: fd :)\ md = \left(\frac{mc \times fd}{\text{AC}} = \frac{fd \times 2ss, \frac{1}{2}m\text{E}c}{s', acg \times 2s, cb} =\right) \frac{fd}{s', acg \times s, cb} \times ss \frac{1}{2} m\text{E}c$.
Hence $\text{L}'s', acg + \text{L}'s, cb + \text{L}, fd = \text{L}, m\text{K}$.
And $\text{L}'s', acg + \text{L}'s, cb + \text{L}, fd + 2\text{L}s, \frac{1}{2}m\text{E}c = \text{L}, md$.

Here $df = 0{,}22633$; $2de = 0{,}18955$; and $\text{D} = (df - 2de =)\ 0{,}03678$.
Also $\frac{1}{2}cb = 7°\ 43'\ 26''$; and $ac\text{E} = 74°\ 33\frac{1}{8}'$.

L, t\`, 7° 43′ 26″	0,86764	L\`s\`, acg = 50° 09′	0,19329
L\`, ds = 0,22633	0,64526	L\`s, bc = 15 26⅞	0,57452
L, D = 0,03678	8,56561	L, sd = 22633	9,3547
L, t, rbc = 50° 09′	10,07851	L, mK, = 1,32602	10,12255
acB = 74 33⅛		2Ls, ½mEc = 12° 12$\frac{1}{16}$′	8,64998
mEc 24 24⅛; half is 12° 12$\frac{1}{16}$′		L, m d = 0,05923	8,77253

PROBLEM LV.

204. Given the obliquity of the ecliptic, the latitude of a place, and the apparent time at that place. To find the longitude of the nonagesimal degree.

CONSTRUCTION.

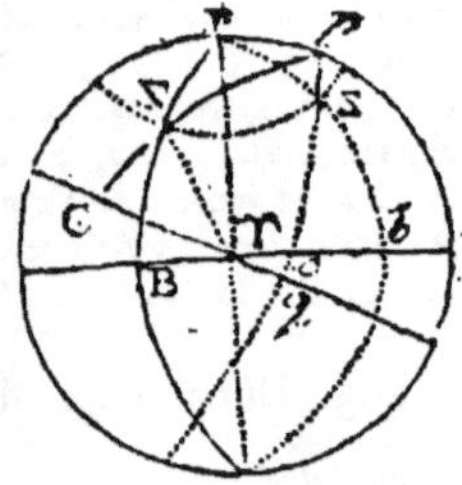

The given time applied to the sun's right ascension, gives the right ascension of the mid-heaven.

Then let the primitive circle represent the solstitial colure, where P, p, represent the poles of the equator ♈ B, and ecliptic ♈ C, the center ♈ being their intersection. In the equator apply the right ascension of the mid-heaven from ♈ to B, and the circle PZB, being described, is that meridian, the intersection of which by a parallel of latitude described about P, gives Z, the place of the zenith; through Z describe a circle of longitude pZC, and the point C is the nonagesimal degree, and ♈C its longitude.

COMPUTATION.

In the triangle P p Z. Given P p the obliquity of the ecliptic,
PZ the co-latitude.
∠ZPp the right as. of the mid-heaven.

Required Zp —— { IV. 237, 238, and 144. }
∠PpZ

DETERMINATION.

When the right ascension of the mid-heaven falls in the first quadrant, its quantity in degrees, increased by 90, gives the angle Z P p, and the acute angle P p Z is the complement of the longitude of the nonagesimal degree.

When in the second quadrant, the said right ascension in degrees taken from 270, leaves the angle Z P p; and the acute angle P p Z, increased by 90 degrees, is the longitude of the nonagesimal degree.

When the said right ascension falls in the third quadrant, its degrees, taken from 270, leaves the angle Z P p, and the angle P p Z, increased by 90 degrees, is the longitude sought.

When in the fourth quadrant, the ſaid right aſcenſion in degrees, leſſened by 270, leaves the angle z P *p*; and the ſupplement of the angle, P *p* z, ſo long as it continues to be obtuſe, being added to three right angles, or 270 degrees, gives the longitude of the nonageſimal degree; but after it becomes acute, its complement is the longitude required.

Note. In theſe determinations the latitude of the place is ſuppoſed to be north, and leſs than the diſtance of the tropic from the neareſt pole.

EXAMPLE. *At Greenwich, in latitude 51° 28⅔′ N. the obliquity of the ecliptic being 23° 28′: What is the longitude of the nonageſimal degree on the 14th of May* 1780, *at* 1 *h.* 24*m.* 24*s. P. M. at* 3 *h.* 40 *m.* 2 *s. P. M. at* 13 *h.* 22 *m.* 26 *s. P. M. and at* 15 *h.* 38 *m.* 4 *s. P. M.?*

The ſeveral right aſcenſions of the mid-heaven are thus found:

	h m s	h m s	h m s	h m s
1780. May 14th, at	1 24 24	3 40 2	13 22 26	15 38 4
The Sun's right aſcen.	3 27 36	3 27 58	3 29 34	3 29 56
Right aſc. mid. hea. in time	4 52 0	7 8 0	16 52 0	19 8 0
Right aſc. mid hea. in degrees	73° 00′	107° 00′	253° 00′	287° 00′
	90 00	270 00	270 00	270 00
The angle z P *p*, or z P *p*	163 00	163 00	17 00	17 00

The two following operations are wrought by IV. 237. and 238.

P z	38° 31⅓′			
P *p*	23 28			
Sum	61 59⅓, half is	30° 59⅔′	Ar. co. *s.* 0,28823	Ar. co. *s.* 0,06691
Diff.	15 3⅓, half is	7 31⅔	*s.* 9,11729	*s.* 9,99624
∠ z P *p*	163 00, half is	81 30	*t.* 9,17450	*t.* 9,17450
Half diff. ∠'s z and *p*		2 10⅔	*t.* 8,58002	
Half ſum		9 4[illegible]	— —	— *t.* 9,23765
The angle *p*		11 59		
		90 00		
The difference		78 01	is the long. nonag. in 1ſt quad.	
The ſum		101 59	is the long. nonag. in 2d quad.	

Sum	61° 59⅓′, half	30° 59⅔′	Ar. co. *s.* 0,28823	Ar. co. *s.* 0,06691
Diff.	15 3⅓, half	7 31⅔	*s.* 9,11729	*s.* 9,99624
∠ z P *p*	17 00, half	8 30	*t.* 10,82550	*t.* 10,82550
Half diff. ∠'s z and *p*		59 34	*t.* 10,23102	
Half ſum		82 38	— —	— *t.* 10,88865
The angle at *p*		142 12,	its ſupplement is	37° 48′
		90 00		270 00
Long. nonag. in 3d qd.		232 12	Long. nonag. in 4th qd.	307 48

*** The altitude of the nonageſimal being equal to z *p*, the diſtance of the zenith from the pole of the ecliptic, it is found by the ſines of oppoſite ſides and angles in the ſpheric triangle z P *p*: that is, ſin. long. nonag. : co-ſ. lat. : : ſin. ∠ z P *p* : ſin. alt. nonageſimal.

SECTION

SECTION VII.

Of Practical Astronomy.

205. DESCRIPTION and USE of ASTRONOMICAL INSTRUMENTS.

By PRACTICAL ASTRONOMY is meant the knowledge of observing the celestial bodies with respect to their position, and time of the year; and of deducing from those observations, certain conclusions useful in calculating the time, when any proposed position of those bodies shall happen.

For this purpose the Astronomer, or Observer, should have an observatory properly furnished.

An OBSERVATORY is a room, or place, conveniently situated, contrived, and furnished with proper astronomical instruments for observing the motions of the heavenly bodies: it should have an uninterrupted view, from the zenith, down to (or even below) the horizon, at least towards its cardinal points; and for this purpose that part of the roof which lies in the direction of the meridian, in particular, should have moveable covers, which may be easily removed and put on again: by which means an instrument may be directed to any point of the heavens between the horizon and zenith, as well to the northward as southward.

The furniture should consist of some, if not all, of the following instruments.

1st. A PENDULUM CLOCK for shewing equal time.

2d. An Achromatic REFRACTING TELESCOPE, or a REFLECTING ONE, of two feet at least in length, for observing particular phænomena.

3d. A MICROMETER for measuring small angular distances.

4th. An ASTRONOMICAL QUADRANT for observing meridian altitudes of the celestial bodies.

5th. A TRANSIT INSTRUMENT for observing objects as they pass over the meridian.

6th. An EQUATORIAL SECTOR to observe angular distances of several degrees, and the differences of right ascension and declination.

7th. An EQUAL ALTITUDE INSTRUMENT for finding when an object has the same altitude on both sides of the meridian.

It is not intended to give in this work any other than a general account of these instruments, most of which have met with considerable improvements (if they were not contrived) by the late Mr. George Graham, F. R. S. one of the most eminent artists in mechanical contrivances that this, or any other nation has produced: those readers who are curious to see a minute description of such, and other, instruments, together with their use fully exemplified, may consult the second volume of Dr. Smith's complete Treatise of Optics, Stone's Treatise of Mathematical Instruments, the Philosophical Transactions, and the works of many writers who have treated on such subjects.

206. Of

206. *Of the Pendulum Clock.*

A clock which ſhews time in hours, minutes, and ſeconds, ſhould be choſen; with which the obſerver, by hearing the beats of the pendulum, may count them by his ear, while his eye is employed on the motion of the celeſtial object he is obſerving.

Juſt before the object arrives at the poſition deſired, the Obſerver ſhould look on the clock and remark the time; ſuppoſe it $9^h\ 15^m\ 25^s$; then ſaying 25, 26, 27, 28, &c. reſponſive to the beats of the pendulum, till he ſees through the inſtrument the object arrived at the poſition expected, which ſuppoſe to happen when he ſays 38; he then writes down $9^h\ 15^m\ 38^s$ for the time of obſervation, annexing the year and day of the month.

If two perſons are concerned in making the obſervation, one may read the time audibly, while the other obſerves through the inſtrument, the Obſerver repeating the laſt ſecond read, when the deſired poſition happens.

207. *Of the Teleſcope.*

The REFRACTING TELESCOPE is an inſtrument with which almoſt every perſon is acquainted, eſpecially the marine gentlemen; it will therefore be ſufficient to remark here, that an *aſtronomical teleſcope* has only two convex glaſſes; viz. the eye-glaſs, or that which is uſed next to the eye; and one at the other end, uſually called the object-glaſs, which has much the longer focal diſtance: ſuch an inſtrument, although it inverts all objects, is yet as uſeful for viewing thoſe in the heavens, as if it ſhewed them erect; the Obſerver knowing that the motions are in an oppoſite direction to thoſe he ſees through this teleſcope: But the Achromatic Refracting Teleſcope, which has been lately invented by Mr. Dolland, has its object-glaſs compounded of three glaſſes, and combined with two eye-glaſſes placed near each other. This inſtrument, which ſhews objects in their true poſition, need not exceed three feet and a half in length.

The REFLECTING TELESCOPE, as is generally well known, ſhews objects in their true poſitions; and as it is much ſhorter than the old refracter, it is therefore in much greater eſteem by ſome.

A *teleſcope*, uſed in aſtronomical obſervations, ſhould have a metal frame fixed in the focus of its object-glaſs, carrying fine ſilver wires ſtretched at right angles to one another; one of them is to be vertical, and the other horizontal; the interſection of thoſe wires ought to be exactly in the middle of the focus of the object-glaſs; a line paſſing through this interſection and the center of the object-glaſs, is called the line of ſight, or line of *collimation*.

208. *Of the Micrometer.*

A MICROMETER is an inſtrument uſed to meaſure ſmall angular diſtances by being placed in the focus of a teleſcope. This is effected by turning a ſcrew, which moves a fine wire in a poſition parallel to itſelf, and alſo parallel to a fixed wire; both being in a plane at right angles to the line of collimation: the diſtance of theſe parallel wires is meaſured by the number of turns the ſcrew has taken to cauſe their receſs; which number of turns is ſhewn on a graduated circular plate (like that of a clock) by an

index,

index, or hand, which revolves by the turning of the ſcrew: now the diviſions on the plate, anſwering to a known angle or arc intercepted between the parallel wires, being known by experiment, any other diſtance, to which the wires can recede, may be known by proportion; and ſo a table of angles anſwering to every diviſion on the circular plate may be formed, by which the obſerved angles will be readily known.

Thus in obſerving the diameter of a planet; when the wires are removed ſo far aſunder, as to become parallel tangents at the ſame time to oppoſite points of the planet, the meaſure of the receſs of the wires will ſhew the diameter of the planet in minutes and ſeconds.

There is another micrometer publiſhed by the late very ingenious Mr. Dollond *, an account of which was given to the Royal Society by Mr. James Short, F. R. S. and publiſhed in the Philoſophical Tranſactions for the year 1753, which is thus.

Let a good circular object-glaſs be neatly cut into two ſemicircles; and each ſemicircle fitted in a metal frame, ſo that their diameters ſliding on one another (by the means of a ſcrew) may have their centers ſo brought together as to appear like one glaſs, and ſo form one image; or by their centers receding may form two images of the ſame object: it being a property of ſuch glaſſes, for any ſegment, to exhibit a perfect image of an object, although not ſo bright as the whole glaſs would give it.

Now proper ſcales being fitted to this inſtrument, to ſhew how far the centers recede, relative to the focal length of the glaſs, will alſo ſhew how far the two parts of the ſame object are aſunder relative to its diſtance from the object-glaſs; and conſequently give the angle under which the diſtance of the parts of that object are ſeen.

209. *Of the Aſtronomical Qudrant.*

An Astronomical Quadrant is an inſtrument in the form of a quarter of a circle, contained under two radii at right angles to one another, and an arch equal to one fourth part of the circumference of the circle, and conſiſts of the following parts.

1ſt. *Its frame.* This is uſually compoſed of iron or braſs bars, ſet at right angles to one another in as ſtrong and neat a manner as a workman can contrive, to preſerve the face of the inſtrument in the ſame plane, and be as little affected by heat and cold as is poſſible.

2d. *Its center.* This center, which is a very fine point, ſhould be contained in a ſeparate piece of work ſcrewed to the bars; and ſo contrived, that if the index, or teleſcope, by frequent motion in a length of time, ſhould become irregular in its rotation, by the parts wearing, a new collar and ſocket may be fitted to the firſt center, and the inſtrument reſtored to its original accuracy.

* The firſt notion of ſuch a micrometer was given by *Roemer*, a Dane, in the year 1675; Mr. *Savery*, an Engliſhman, alſo thought of ſuch a contrivance, which he communicated to the Royal Society in the year 1743; Mr. *Bouguer*, a Frenchman, alſo propoſed it in the year 1748; and Mr. *Dollond*, an Engliſhman, publiſhed it in the year 1753: but the public are obliged to Mr. *Short* for putting the theory into execution, otherwiſe it might ſtill have continued only as an ingenious thought.

3d. *Its*

3d. *Its limb.* This is a braſs arch of about two inches broad, well fixed to the ſaid frame-work, and generally continued a little farther at each end than the extent of 90 degrees; the two perpendicular radii may be alſo covered with plates of braſs ſcrewed to them; and the whole face of the inſtrument is to be worked ſmooth, and brought into the ſame plane with the greateſt care.

4th. *Its diviſions.* The arcs of 60, 30, and 90 degrees, and alſo the intermediate degrees, together with ſuch ſubdiviſions as the ſize of the degrees will conveniently contain, are laid down by accurate methods well known to good workmen.

5th. *Its index or teleſcope.* This, which is uſually a braſs tube containing the proper glaſſes and croſs wires, is fixed near the object end to a braſs plate, a little above a circular hole, or ſocket, in the plate: this ſocket goes round a collar concentric to the center, and fixed to the center-piece: ſo that, although the axis of the teleſcope does not, as a radius, paſs through the center, yet it always keeps at the ſame diſtance from it in every poſition: to the eye-end of the tube is ſcrewed a flat plate, which ſlides along the limb with the teleſcope; this plate, called the VERNIER, contains certain diviſions, which, uſed with thoſe on the limb, give the angle to minutes or ſeconds of a degree, according to the ſize of the inſtrument: the beginning of the diviſions called the index, on the *Vernier*, is as far diſtant from the axis, or line of collimation, as the center is; and therefore the poſition of an object is given as truly, as if the line of collimation coincided with a radius.

6th. *Its pedeſtal.* This part, which ſhould, by its conſtruction, be very ſteady, may be either moveable or fixed: the moveable pedeſtal is commonly a ſtrong pillar ſtanding on a tripod, or three-footed ſtand; with holes through each foot, either to ſcrew them to a floor, or to pin them to the ground: the fixed pedeſtal may be either a ſtrong timber frame, or the wall of the obſervatory, or a ſtone ſhaft built from the ground through the middle of the floor of the obſervatory. On the top of the pillar, of either ſort of pedeſtal, may be fixed a piece of machinery called the *arm*, which is attached by ſcrews to the middle of the plane of the quadrant, on the under ſide. The arm is contrived to give to the inſtrument, either an horizontal, vertical, or oblique motion; which motions ſhould be ſteady, and free from jerks, or ſhakes: but when a wall, or ſtone ſhaft, is uſed as the ſupporter, the quadrant is then fixed to the wall, or ſhaft (without its arm attached) and is called a MURAL ARCH; its plane is adjuſted to that of the meridian, and this is the beſt method of fixing the quadrant for taking the meridian altitude of the ſtars, or planets.

7th. *Its plummet.* This is a ſufficient ball, or weight, hanging to one end of a very fine ſilver wire, the upper end being fixed in the radius continued above the center. Now when the face of the quadrant is ſet in the plane of an azimuth circle, one of its radii is brought into a vertical poſition by the help of the plummet, the wire being made to biſect the center-point and the diviſion of 90° on the arch; and to diſtinguiſh theſe biſections with accuracy, they are to be examined with a ſmall proſpect, or magnifying-glaſs: the ball ſhould hang freely in a veſſel of water to check its vibrations.

210. *Of the transit Instrument.*

This instrument consists of a telescope fixed at right angles to an horizontal axis, which axis must be so supported, that the line of collimation of the telescope may move in the plane of the meridian.

The axis, to the middle of which the telescope is fixed, should gradually taper towards its ends, and terminate in cylinders well turned and smoothed: and a proper balance is to be put on the tube, so that it may stand at any elevation when its axis rests on the supporters.

Two upright posts of wood or stone, firmly fixed at a proper distance, are to sustain the supporters of this instrument: these supporters are two thick brass plates, having well smoothed angular notches in their upper ends to receive the cylindrical arms of the axis: each of the notched plates are contrived to be moveable by a screw, which slides them upon the surfaces of two other plates immoveably fixed to the two upright posts; one plate moving in a vertical, and the other in an horizontal, direction, to adjust the telescope to the planes of the horizon and meridian: to the plane of the horizon, by a spirit level hung in a parallel position to the axis, and to the plane of the meridian in the following manner.

Observe the times by the clock when a circumpolar star, seen through this instrument, transits both above and below the pole: and if the times of describing the eastern and western parts of its circuit are equal, the telescope is then in the plane of the meridian; otherwise, the notched plates must be gently moved till the time of the star's revolution is bisected by both the upper and lower transits, taking care at the same time that the axis remains perfectly horizontal.

When the telescope is thus adjusted, a mark must be set at a considerable distance (the greater the better) in the horizontal direction of the intersection of the cross-wires, and in a place where it can be illuminated in the night-time by a lanthorn hanging near it; which mark being on a fixed object, will serve at all times afterwards to examine the position of the telescope by, the axis of the instrument being first adjusted by means of the level.

211. *To adjust the Clock by the Sun's Transit over the Meridian.*

Note the times by the clock, when the preceding and following edges of the sun's limb touch the cross wires: the difference between the middle time and 12 hours, shews how much the mean, or time by the clock, is faster or slower than the apparent, or solar time for that day; to which the equation of time being applied, will shew the time of mean noon for that day, by which the clock may be adjusted.

212. *Of the Equatorial Sector.*

This is an instrument contrived for finding the difference in right ascension and declination between two objects, the distance of which is too great

great to be obſerved by means of a micrometer. It conſiſts of the following particulars.

1ſt. A braſs plate called a ſector, formed like a T, having the ſhank (as a radius) of about $2\frac{1}{2}$ feet long, and 2 inches broad, and the croſs piece (as an arch) of about 6 inches long, and $1\frac{1}{2}$ inch broad; upon which, with a radius of 30 inches, is deſcribed an arch of 10 degrees, each being ſubdivided into as ſmall parts as are convenient.

2d. Round a ſmall cylinder, containing the center of this arch, and fixed in the ſhank, moves a plate of braſs, to which is fixed a teleſcope, having its line of collimation parallel to the plane of the ſector, and paſſing through the center of the arch and the index of a *Vernier*'s dividing plate, which ſlides on the arch, and is fixed to the eye end of the teleſcope. This plate, with the teleſcope and Vernier, are moved on the cylinder, by means of a long ſcrew which is at the back of the arch, and communicates with the Vernier through a ſlit cut in the braſs work, parallel to the divided arch.

3d. A circular braſs plate, of 5 inches diameter, round the center of which there moves a braſs croſs, which has the oppoſite ends of one bar turned up perpendicularly about 3 inches. Theſe ſerve as ſupporters to the ſector, and are ſcrewed to the back of its radius, ſo that the plane of the ſector is parallel to the plane of the circular plate, and revolves round the center of that plate in this parallel poſition.

4th. A flat axis of 18 inches long is ſcrewed to the back of the circular plate, along one of its diameters; ſo that the axis is parallel to the plane of the ſector: the whole inſtrument is ſupported on a proper pedeſtal, in ſuch a manner that the ſaid axis is parallel to the axis of the earth; and proper contrivances are annexed for fixing it in that poſition.

Now the inſtrument, thus ſupported, can revolve round its axis, parallel to the earth's axis, with a motion like that of the ſtars; the plane of the ſector being always parallel to the plane of ſome hour circle, and conſequently every point of the teleſcope deſcribes a parallel of declination: and if the ſector be turned round the joint of the circular plate, its graduated arch may be brought parallel to an hour circle; and conſequently any two ſtars, between which the difference of declination is not greater than the number of degrees in that arch, may be obſerved by the inſtrument.

213. *To obſerve their paſſage.* Direct the teleſcope to the preceding ſtar, and fix the plane of the ſector a little to the weſtward of it; move the teleſcope by the ſcrew, and obſerve the time ſhewn by the clock at the tranſit of each ſtar over the croſs wires, and alſo the diviſion ſhewn by the index; then is the difference of the arches the difference of declination; and that of the times ſhews the difference of right aſcenſion of theſe ſtars.

214. *Of the Equal-Altitude Inſtrument.*

An EQUAL-ALTITUDE INSTRUMENT is that uſed to obſerve a celeſtial object, when it has the ſame altitude on both the eaſt and weſt ſides of the meridian, or in the morning and afternoon; and conſiſts of a teleſcope of about 30 inches long (with 2 vertical, and 3 or 5 horizontal, wires in its focus) ſupported on the end of an iron bar, or axis, of 30 inches long, and about an inch in diameter. The axis is ſuſtained in a vertical poſition by paſſing through a hole in the upper end of a braſs box, whilſt its lower end ſupports the lower point of the axis. The box, which is about 21 inches long, with ends about 4 inches ſquare, has only two ſides, which are fixed at right angles to each other. To one of theſe ſides are fixed four flat arms, with a hole in each, by which the box is fixed in a vertical poſition to an upright poſt with ſcrews. On the lower end of the box lies a braſs plate, which ſlides in grooves, and can be moved gently backwards or forwards by means of a ſcrew. In this plate a fine hole is punched to receive the ſmooth conical point, which the lower end of the axis is formed into. On the upper end of the box are two plates, which ſlide alſo in grooves; and, by the means of ſcrews, can be moved gently ſideways, till their angular notches embrace the axis; which, in this part, is made perfectly cylindrical, and very ſmooth.

To the upper part of the axis is fixed, by its radius, a braſs ſextant (or arch of 60°, to a radius of ſeven or eight inches) with the arch downwards, ſo that the center is juſt above the top of the axis: alſo a ſpirit level is fixed at right angles acroſs the axis, juſt under the arch, ſo as to be clear of the upper end of the box.

To the under part of the teleſcope is fixed a braſs ſemicircle, of the ſame radius with the ſextant, both arches having a common center-pin. In the ſemicircle is a groove cut through the plate parallel to its limb, to receive two ſcrew-pins, which go into the ſextantal arch near its ends; by theſe ſcrew-pins the two arches may be preſſed cloſe, and the teleſcope fixed in any deſired elevation; which might be nearly aſcertained, by graduating the ſemicircle, and putting a Vernier's ſcale on the ſextant.

To uſe the Inſtrument. Fix the box to the poſt, put the axis into the box, letting the conical point drop into the punched hole, ſcrew on the level, and annex the teleſcope, obſerving to inſert the center and arch pins; then, by the help of the ſcrew-plates at the bottom and top ends of the box, correct the vertical poſition of the axis, ſo that the ſame end of the air-bubble in the level may ſtand at the ſame point throughout the whole revolution of the axis, which will thereby be known to be then truely vertical, ſo that the teleſcope will deſcribe a parallel of altitude: direct the tube to the ſun, or ſtar, and fix it at the deſired elevation by preſſing the two arches together with the two ſcrew pins.

Some inſtruments have been contrived to anſwer both kinds of obſervation; viz. either a tranſit, or equal altitudes.

215. *To adjuſt the Clock by equal altitudes of the Sun.*

Having rectified the inſtrument by the level, and being provided with a piece of tranſparently coloured or ſmoked glaſs to preſerve the eye; then at any convenient time from about 6 to 3 hours before noon, direct the teleſcope to the ſun, and fix it by the arch, ſo that the whole body of the ſun ſhall be above the upper wire (the aſcent of the ſun appearing through the teleſcope as a deſcent): mark the times ſhewn by the clock, when the preceding edge of the ſun touches each of the wires; and alſo when the

the following edge touches those wires, writing down those times; the instrument being turned horizontally on its axis to follow the Sun, and keep his center in the middle of the telescope between the vertical wires. About the same time after noon (taking care to be early enough) turn the instrument on its vertical axis, the telescope remaining fixed at the same elevation as in the morning, and rectifying its horizontal situation by the level, observe the Sun in its descent, which through the telescope apparently ascends, and write down the times, when the preceding edge touches each wire, and also when they are touched by the following edge, keeping the Sun in the middle of the telescope; and the sets of observations are made.

There are as many sets of observations, as there are horizontal wires: for the fore and afternoon contacts of the same edge of the Sun with the same wire, make one set; and the same edge which precedes in the forenoon, follows in the afternoon; and that which follows in the forenoon, precedes in the afternoon; therefore the

<table>
<tr><td>1st,
2d,
3d, &c.</td><td>A. M. preceding, and the</td><td>last,
last but one,
last but 2, &c.</td><td>P. M. following,</td></tr>
</table>

make a set.

<table>
<tr><td>1st,
2d,
3d, &c.</td><td>A. M. following, and the</td><td>last,
last but one,
last but 2, &c.</td><td>P. M. preceding,</td></tr>
</table>

make a set.

Then to each set, or pair of observations, find the middle time, which added to the time of the morning observation, gives the time shewn by the clock when the Sun was on the meridian, if the observations were made within two or three days of the solstice, when the Sun's declination would not sensibly alter between the fore and afternoon observations: but on other days, this time must be corrected, by applying an equation to it, shewing the alteration in time, arising from the alteration in declination between the fore and afternoon observations.

The time, by the clock, of the solar or apparent noon being thus obtained, the time of the mean noon may be had by applying the proper equation of time.

When the time of noon is sought from two or more pairs of observations, if they give different times, it is best to take the medium between them, which is found by dividing the sum of all the times by their number.

216. PROBLEM LV.

Given the latitude, the declination of the Sun, and interval of time between the Sun's having equal altitudes before and after noon, to find the distance from noon of the middle point of time between the observations.

1st. Find the change made in the Sun's declination during the interval between the observations; which will nearly bear the same proportion to the change made between the noon of the day, on which the observations are made, and the noon of the day immediately preceeding or following, as the interval of time between the observations to 24 hours.

2dly. Add the co-tangent of the latitude to the co-sine of half the interval of time reduced to degrees and minutes of the equator; the sum, rejecting the radius, is the tangent of an arc to be taken less than a quadrant, when the interval of time is less than twelve hours, and greater than a quadrant, should the interval of time exceed twelve hours.

3dly. Add together the arithmetical complements of the sine of this arc, and of the sine of the Sun's distance from the pole at noon, the logarithmic sine of the difference of these arcs, the logarithmic co-tangent of half the interval of time in degrees, and the logarithm of half the change in the Sun's declination during the interval between the observations; the sum, rejecting twice the radius, is the logarithm of an arc, which, divided by 15, gives the distance of the middle point between the observations from noon, in seconds of time.

4thly. When the Sun's distance from the elevated pole increases, this middle point of time precedes noon, otherwise it falls beyond.

DEMONSTRATION.

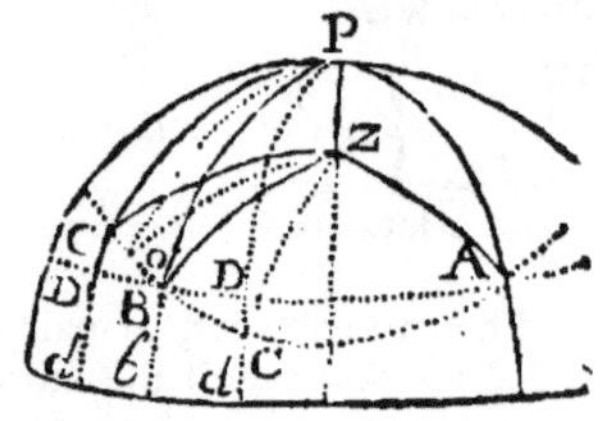

Let P be the pole of the equator *bd*, Z the zenith, A the morning place, C the afternoon place, ABD a parallel of declination, ABC a parallel of altitude.

Then the afternoon hour angle, ZPC, differs from the morning hour angle, ZPA, by the hour angle BPC, the points A and B having the same declination and distance from the zenith; and the arc P*o* bisecting the ∠BPC, the ∠ZP*o* will be half the interval of time, which being increased or diminished by half the ∠BPC, will give the position of the meridian to A or C; also P*o* will be the Sun's distance from the pole at noon.

Now here the difference between PB, P*o*, PC being but small, the ∠BP*o* will be to the difference between P*o* and PB, or PC, that is, half PB ∽ PC, nearly as $\grave{t}$, P*o*Z to *s*, P*o* *.

Again, in the triangle *o*PZ, an arc M being taken, that as rad. : $\grave{t}$, ZP*o* :: *t*, PZ : *t*, M the arc M to be less than a quadrant, when the ∠ZP*o* is acute, but greater, should the ∠ZP*o* be obtuse; then (IV. 123)

$s,\overline{Po \backsim M} : s,M :: \grave{t},PoZ : \grave{t},ZPo$, and consequently

$s,\overline{Po \backsim M} \times \grave{t},ZPo = s,M \times \grave{t},PoZ$.

But $\angle BPo : \frac{PB \backsim PC}{2} :: \grave{t},PoZ : s,Po :: s,M \times \grave{t},PoZ : s,M \times s,Po$;

therefore $\angle BPo : \frac{PB \backsim PC}{2} :: s,\overline{Po \backsim M} \times \grave{t},ZPo : s,M \times s,Po$, conformably to the rule above laid down.

---

* See *Cotes. Æstimat. Error. in Mixt. Math. Theorem* 23.

217. **EXAMPLE.**

In the latitude 50° N. on the 27th of October, 1780, the Sun was obferved to have equal altitudes at 9 h. 11 m. 50 s. A. M. and at 2 h. 22 m. 22 s. P. M. by a clock adjufted nearly to the true meafure of time, to find what correction may be wanted to fet this clock to the true hour of the day, the Sun's diftance from the pole on the 27th day at noon being 103° 6′ 34″, and on the 28th 103° 26′ 38″.

Here the interval of time is 5 h. 10 m. 32 s. its half is 2 h. 35 m. 16 s. in degrees and minutes of the equator 38° 49′, and the difference in declination in one day is 20′ 4″.

Then 24 h. : 5 h. 10 m. 32 s. : : 20′ 4″ : 4′ 20″ = 260″, the alteration in declination, the half of which is 2′ 10″ = 130″.

Then

Latitude	50°	log. t′, 9,92381	33° 10′ 32″	L. s,	0,26185
½ time =	38° 49′	log. s′, 9,89162	103 06 34	L. s,	0,01147
			69 56 02	log. s,	9,97280
	33° 10′ 32″	log. t, 9,81543	38 49 0	log. t′,	10,09447
			130″	log.	2,11394
			corr. = 285″	log.	2,45453
			or 19 fec. of time.		

Hence, for fetting the clock to the true hour of the day, add the half interval of time 2 h. 35 m. 16 s. to 9 h. 11 m. 50 s.; the fum 11 h. 47 m. 6 s. is the middle time between the obfervations, as noted by the clock.

And 11 h. 47 m. 6 s. + 19 s. = 11 h. 47 m. 25 s. will be the time pointed out by the clock, when the Sun paffes the meridian, and fhews the clock to be 12 m. 35 s. behind the Sun.

Though the clock fhould not keep time with perfect exactnefs, yet if the deviation is but fmall, the correction computed will not differ much from the truth; and the clock being examined again within a few days, will fhew whether it keeps time truly, or moves too faft or too flow, and its rate of going may be corrected accordingly.

218. The method here directed fuppofes the fhip to be ftationary: But the Abbé de la Caille propofes a method of correcting a watch at fea, even while the fhip is in motion, by taking two equal altitudes of the Sun with a quadrant, one before and the other after noon.

His method is this. With the common altitude obferved, together with the latitudes at the time of each obfervation, and the Sun's correct declination to thofe times, the times from noon are to be computed at both obfervations, which times being applied to the two times of obfervation, give the refpective times of noon: then the mean of the two noons being taken, will give the time fhewn by the watch when it was the true midday.

Or. Half the difference of the computed noons being applied to either of them, will alfo give the true time of noon.

And although the latitudes ufed in the computations be fomething erroneous, yet the altitudes being equal, the error in each of the computed diftances from noon will be nearly the fame, if the change in latitude and longitude between the obfervations be duly attended to.

219. *Of the Vernier's dividing plate.*

When the relative unit of any line is to be divided into many ſmall equal parts, thoſe parts may be too many to be conveniently introduced, or if introduced, they may be too cloſe to one another to be readily eſtimated; and on theſe accounts there has been a variety of methods contrived for eſtimating the aliquot parts of the ſmall diviſions, into which the relative unit of a line may be commodiouſly divided; among thoſe methods that is moſt juſtly preferred which was publiſhed by PETER VERNIER (a gentleman of Franche Comté) at Bruſſels, in the year 1631; and which, by ſome ſtrange fatality, is moſt unjuſtly, although commonly, called by the name of NONIUS: for *Nonius*'s method is not only very different from that of *Vernier*'s, but much leſs convenient.

Vernier's method is derived from the following principle.

If two equal right lines, or circular arcs A, B, are ſo divided, that the number of equal diviſions in B is one leſs than the number of equal diviſions of A; then will the exceſs of one diviſion of B above one diviſion of A be compounded of the ratios of one of A to A, and one of B to B.

For let A contain 11 parts; then one of A to A, is as 1 to 11; or $\frac{1}{11}$.

Let B contain 10 parts; then one of B to B, is as 1 to 10; or $\frac{1}{10}$.

Now $\frac{1}{10}-\frac{1}{11}=\left(\frac{1\times 11}{10\times 11}-\frac{1\times 11}{11\times 10}\right.$ (II. 148) $\left.=\frac{11-10}{10\times 11}=\frac{1}{10\times 11}=\right)$ $\frac{1}{10}\times\frac{1}{11}$.

Or. If B contains n parts, and A is of $n+1$ parts;

Then $\frac{1}{n}$ is one part of B, and $\frac{1}{n+1}$ is one part of A.

And $\frac{1}{n}-\frac{1}{n+1}=\left(\frac{1\times\overline{n+1}}{n\times\overline{n+1}}-\frac{1\times n}{\overline{n+1}\times n}\right.$ (II. 148) $=\frac{n+1-n}{n\times\overline{n+1}}=$ $\left.\frac{1}{n\times\overline{n+1}}=\right)\frac{1}{n}\times\frac{1}{n+1}$.

Or thus. Let A and B be unequal right lines, or circular arcs; and let any part of A, conſidered as the relative unit, be divided into n parts; and a part of B, equal to $m+1$ parts of A, be divided into m parts: then will $\frac{1}{m}$th of B $=\frac{1}{n}$th of A $=\frac{1}{m}$th of B $\times\frac{1}{n}$th of A.

But n parts of A : 1 unit of A : : $m+1$ parts of A : $\frac{m+1}{n}$ units of A.

But m parts of B $=$ ($m+1$ parts of A $=$) $\frac{m+1}{n}$ units of A.

Then m parts of B : $\frac{m+1}{n}$ units of A : : 1 part of B : $\frac{m+1}{m\times n}$ units of A.

Therefore $\frac{m+1}{m\times n} - \frac{1}{n} = \left(\frac{m+1}{m\times n} - \frac{m\times 1}{n\times m} = \frac{m+1-m}{m\times n} = \frac{1}{n\times m} =\right)$ $\frac{1}{m}\times\frac{1}{n}$.

The moſt commodious diviſions, and their aliquot parts, into which the degrees on the circular limb of an inſtrument may be ſuppoſed to be divided, depend on the radius of that inſtrument.

Let R be the radius of a circle in inches; and a degree to be divided in n parts, each degree being $\frac{1}{p}$th of an inch.

Now the circumference of a circle in parts of its diameter, 2R inches, is $3,1415926\times 2R$ inches. (II. 197)

Then $360^\circ : 3,1415926\times 2R :: 1^\circ : \frac{3,1415926}{360}\times 2R$ inches.

Or, $0,01745379\times R$ is the length of one degree, in inches.
Or, $0,01745379\times R\times p$ is the length of 1°, in pth parts of an inch.
But as every degree contains n times ſuch parts,
Therefore $n=0,01745379\times R\times p$.

The moſt commodious perceptible diviſion is $\frac{1}{8}$ or $\frac{1}{10}$ of an inch.

EXAM. *Suppoſe an inſtrument of 30 inches radius: into how many convenient parts may each degree be divided? how many of thoſe parts are to go to the breadth of the Vernier, and to what parts of a degree may an obſervation be made by that inſtrument?*

Now $0,01745\times R=0,5236$ inches, the length of each degree.

And if p be ſuppoſed about $\frac{1}{8}$ of an inch for one diviſion.

Then $0,5236\times p=4,188$, ſhews the number of ſuch parts in a degree.
But as this number muſt be an integer, let it be 4, each being 15′.
And let the breadth of the *Vernier* contain 31 of thoſe parts, or $7\frac{3}{4}$°, and be divided into 30 parts.

Here $n=\frac{1}{4}$; $m=\frac{1}{30}$; then $\frac{1}{4}\times\frac{1}{30}=\frac{1}{120}$ of a degree, or 30″,
Which is the leaſt part of a degree that inſtrument can ſhew.

If $n=\frac{1}{5}$, and $m=\frac{1}{36}$; then $\frac{1}{5}\times\frac{1}{36}=\frac{60}{5\times 36}$ of a minute, or 20″.

220. The following table, taken as examples in the inſtruments commonly made from 3 inches to 8 feet radius, ſhews the diviſions of the limb to neareſt tenths of inches, ſo as to be an aliquot of 60′s, and what parts of a degree may be eſtimated by the Vernier, it being divided into ſuch equal parts, and containing ſuch degrees, as their columns ſhew.

Rad. inches	Parts in a deg.	Parts in Vernier.	Breadth of Ver.	Parts observed.	Rad. inches	Parts in a deg.	Parts in Vernier.	Breadth of Ver.	Parts observed.
3	1	15	$15\frac{1}{4}^\circ$	4′ 0″	30	5	30	$7\frac{1}{2}^\circ$	0′ 20″
6	1	20	$10\frac{1}{4}$	3 0	36	6	30	$5\frac{1}{4}$	0 20
9	2	20	$10\frac{1}{4}$	1 30	42	8	30	$3\frac{7}{8}$	0 15
12	2	24	$12\frac{3}{4}$	1 15	48	9	40	$4\frac{5}{9}$	0 10
15	3	20	$6\frac{1}{4}$	1 0	60	10	36	$3\frac{7}{10}$	0 10
18	3	30	$10\frac{1}{4}$	0 40	72	12	30	$2\frac{7}{12}$	0 10
21	4	30	$7\frac{1}{4}$	0 30	84	15	40	$2\frac{2}{3}$	0 6
24	4	36	$9\frac{1}{4}$	0 25	96	15	60	4	0 4

By altering the number of divisions, either in the degrees or in the Vernier, or in both, an angle can be observed to a different degree of accuracy. Thus to a radius of 30 inches, if a degree be divided into 12 parts, each being five minutes, and the breadth of the Vernier be 21 such parts, or $1\frac{3}{4}^\circ$, and divided into 20 parts, then $\frac{1}{12} \times \frac{1}{20} = \frac{1^\circ}{240} = 15''$: or taking the breadth of the Vernier of $2\frac{1}{12}^\circ$, and divided into 30 parts; then $\frac{1}{12} \times \frac{1}{30} = \frac{1^\circ}{360}$, or $10''$: Or $\frac{1}{12} \times \frac{1}{50} = \frac{1^\circ}{600} = 6''$; where the breadth of the Vernier is $4\frac{1}{4}^\circ$.

SECTION VIII.

Practical Astronomy.

The Elements of the Earth's Motion.

221. By the theory of the Sun, or Earth, is meant the knowledge of all the requisites, or elements, necessary for determining its place in the ecliptic at any proposed time.

222. Mean Motion, or Mean Angular Velocity, is a motion made uniformly in the circumference of a circle, the center of motion being the center of that circle.

The mean motion of a planet is the degree and parts shewing its distance from the first point of Aries, reckoned in the order of the signs.

223. Anomaly, or True Anomaly, is an angle made by two lines drawn from the center of motion, one to the Aphelion, or Apogee, and the other to the place of the revolving body, or planet: Or, Anomaly is the angular distance of a planet from its Aphelion, the angular point being the center of motion.

224. Mean Anomaly is that made by an uniform circular motion about the center, and is the same as mean motion, beginning at the Aphelion.

225. Ex-

225. Eccentric Anomaly is an angular distance from the aphelion, determined in a circle on the transverse axis by a normal to that axis, passing through the planet's place in its elliptical orbit.

226. The Equation of the Center, sometimes called the *prosthaphæresis*, is the distance between the mean and true anomalies.

227. The *motion of the equinoxes* is the same as the *precession of the equinoxes*, which is backwards, or contrary to the order of the signs; by which the stars appear to have advanced forwards from the equinoctial point Aries: this motion is about 50 seconds of a degree in a year.

228. *The motion of the apsides* is a slow motion of the Earth's orbit around the Sun in the order of the signs; discovered by the apogeon changing its place among the fixed stars: this motion is found, by comparing distant observations together, to be about 16 seconds of a degree in a year, in respect to the fixed stars; and about 66 seconds ($=50''+16''$) with respect to the equinoxes.

229. A Tropical or Solar Year is the time elapsed between two successive passages of the Sun through the same Equinoctial or Solstitial points of the ecliptic.

230. A Siderial Year is the time the Sun takes between his departure from any fixed star to his next return to that star.

231. An Anomalastic Year is the interval of time between two succeeding passages of the Sun through the same apsis.

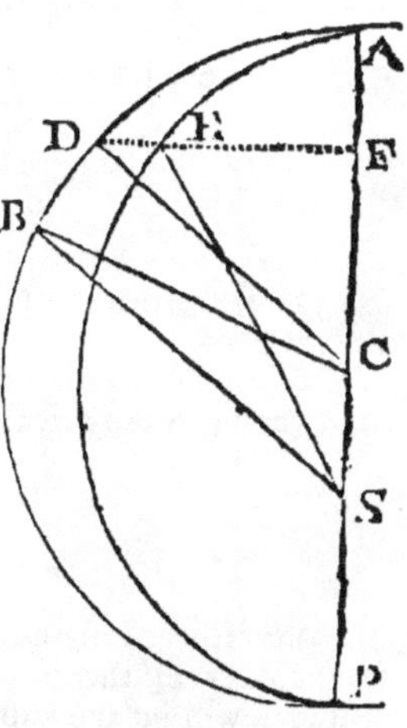

232. By the annexed figure the foregoing articles may be easily comprehended.

On the line of the apsides AP describe a circle ADP, called the excentric; and an ellipsis AEP for the Earth's orbit, having the excentricity CS.

Let S be the place of the Sun, C the center of the orbit, A the aphelion, P the perihelion; SA the aphelion, or apogeon distance; SP the perigeon distance.

Let E be a true place of the earth in its orbit; D a corresponding place in the excentric, in FE continued, normal to AP.

Let the ∠ ACB represent the mean anomaly; the ∠ ACD is the eccentric anomaly; and the ∠ ASE is the true anomaly; the difference between ∠ ACB and ∠ ASE is the equation of the center.

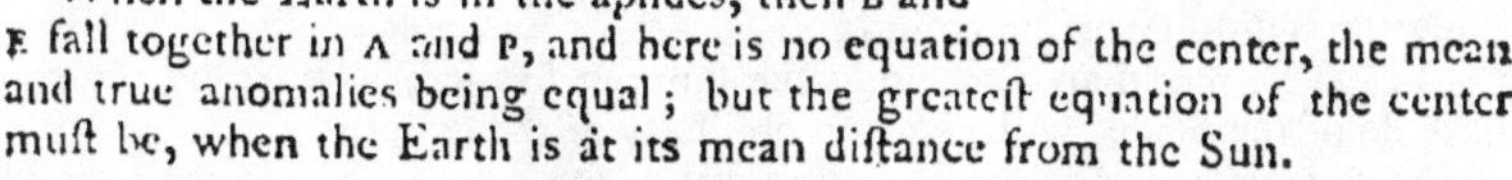
When the Earth is in the apsides, then B and E fall together in A and P, and here is no equation of the center, the mean and true anomalies being equal; but the greatest equation of the center must be, when the Earth is at its mean distance from the Sun.

233. Observations shew, that in this age the Earth passes the apogee on the 30th of June, when its daily motion is $57'\ 12''$; and passes the perigee on the 30th of December, when the daily motion is $61'\ 12''$: and is at the mean distance about the 28th of March and 30th of September, when its daily motion is $59'\ 8''$.

234. PRO-

234. PROBLEM LVI.

To find the Latitude of a Place.

Solution. Select a ſtar, the diſtance of which from the pole ſtar does not exceed 8 or 10 degrees; and obſerve with a quadrant the greateſt and leaſt meridional altitudes; then

If both obſervations are on the ſame ſide of the zenith;
Half the ſum of the *alts.* is the latitude, on the ſame ſide of the zenith.

If the obſervations are on different ſides of the zenith;
Half the difference of the altitudes is the co-latitude, on the ſame ſide of the zenith, with the leſſer altitude.

For let HZR be the meridian, HR the horizon, Z the zenith, RB, RA, two altitudes on the ſame ſide of the zenith; H*b*, R*a*, two altitudes on contrary ſides of the zenith.

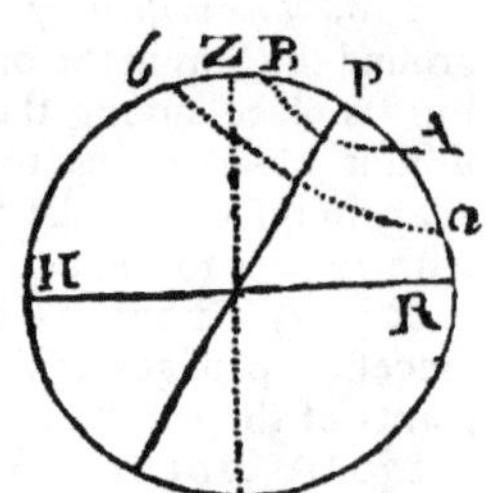

Then, the arc AB, or *ab*, being biſected, will give P the poſition of the elevated pole.
For a ſtar is equally diſtant from P in its revolution.
Therefore PA=PB; or P*a*=P*b*; and RP equal to the latitude.

$$\text{Hence RP} = \left(\text{RA} + \text{PA} = \frac{2\text{RA}}{2} + \frac{2\text{PA}}{2} = \frac{\text{RA} + \text{RA} + \text{AB}}{2} = \right) \frac{\text{RA} + \text{RB}}{2}$$

$$\text{And RP} = \left(\text{R}a + \text{P}a = \frac{2\text{R}a}{2} + \frac{2\text{P}b}{2} = \frac{\text{R}a + \text{R}a + ab}{2} = \frac{\text{RP}b + \text{R}a}{2}\right.$$

$$\left. = \frac{180^\circ - \text{H}b \backsim \text{RA}}{2} = \right) 90^\circ - \frac{\text{H}b \backsim \text{R}a}{2}.$$

235. Remarks. 1. There will be about 12 hours between the two obſervations.

2. This method is ſubject to a ſmall error, on account of the leſſer altitude being more affected by refraction, than the greater.

236. PROBLEM LVII.

To find the Obliquity of the Ecliptic.

Solution. Let the meridian altitude of the Sun's center be obſerved on the days of the ſummer and winter ſolſtice; the difference of thoſe altitudes will be the diſtance of the tropics; and half that diſtance will ſhew the obliquity of the ecliptic.

Or. The meridian altitude at the ſummer ſolſtice, leſſened by the co-latitude of the place, will give the obliquity of the ecliptic.

From good obſervations the obliquity of the ecliptic, about the time of the vernal equinox 1772, was found to be 23° 28′.

Diſtant obſervations compared together, ſhew that the obliquity is decreaſing at the rate of about one minute in 120 years.

237. Remark,

237. Remark. By the ſecond method the declinations of the fixed ſtars, or of any other celeſtial phenomenon, may be found; obſerving that their declination is of the ſame name, viz. north or ſouth, with the latitude of the place, when its complement is leſs than the altitude; otherwiſe, of a contrary name with the latitude.

238. PROBLEM LVIII.

To find the Time of an Equinox.

Solution. In a place the latitude of which is known, let the Sun's meridian altitude be taken on the day of the equinox, and on the day preceding, and that following it. Then the difference between thoſe altitudes and the co-latitude will be the Sun's declinations at the times of obſervations. (236)

If either of the altitudes is equal to the co-latitude, that obſervation was made at the time of the equinox.

But if the co-latitude is unequal to either of the altitudes, proceed thus. Let DG repreſent the equator; AC the ecliptic, E the equinoctial point; the points A, B, C, the places of the Sun at the times of obſervation; the arcs AD, BF, CG, the correſponding declinations.

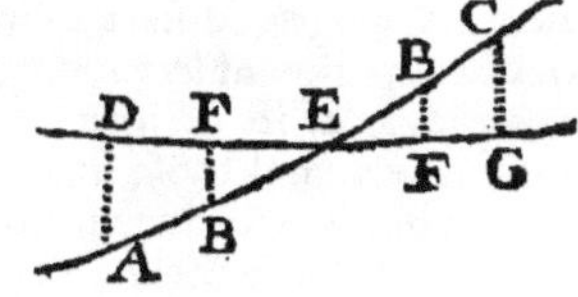

Now uſing either the two firſt, or two laſt obſervations, ſuppoſe the latter, in the right-angled ſpherical triangles CEG, BEF, in which there are known the obliquity of the ecliptic, and the declinations; find EC, EB: then BC, the ſum or difference of EC, EB, is the ecliptic arc deſcribed in 24 hours. Then ſay,

As BC to BF, ſo 24 hours for BC, to the time correſponding to BE.

And this time ſhews the diſtance of the equinox from the time of the middle obſervation.

239. PROBLEM LIX.

To find the length of the tropical, periodical, and anomaliſtical revolutions of the earth.

Solution. Let two obſervations be choſen, among the moſt authentic of thoſe on record, of the time when the Sun had like poſitions, viz.

1ſt. In regard to his longitude, or place in the ecliptic.

2d. In regard to the right aſcenſion of ſome noted ſtar.

3d. In reſpect to the line of the apſides.

The greater the interval (ſuppoſe 80 or 100 years) between each two obſervations, the more accurate will be the reſult: then that interval being divided by the number of revolutions made during that time, will give the time of one periodical revolution.

According to Mayer's tables the numbers are theſe,

A tropical year	is made in	365^d	5^h	48^m	42^s.
A periodical, or ſiderial revolution		365	6	9	7.
An anomaliſtic revolution		365	6	15	29.

240. Remarks,

240. REMARKS. 1. The tropical year being ſhorter than the ſiderial by 20 m. 25 s., ſhews that the Sun has returned to the ſame point of the ecliptic, before he has made one complete revolution with regard to the ſtars; and conſequently every point of the ecliptic muſt have moved in *antecedentia* during that tropical period, and ſo have produced what is called the preceſſion of the equinoxes.

Now 365 d. 6 h. 9 m. 7 s. : 360° : : 20 m. 25 s. : 50″,3, or nearly 50″, for the preceſſion in one year.

If there was no preceſſion, the tropical and ſiderial years would be equal.

241. 2. A ſiderial revolution being performed ſooner by 6 m. 22 s. than the anomaliſtic, ſhews that the line of the apſides has a motion in *conſequentia*: now 365 d. 15 h. 29 m. : 360° : : 6 m. 22 s. : 15″,7, the yearly quantity by which the Sun's apogee is advanced in reſpect to the ſtars: and as the equinoxes move in *antecedentia*, and the apſides in *conſequentia*, their ſum 66″ (=50,3+15,7) ſhews the motion of the apſides from the equinoxes.

242. 3d. From the compariſon of many obſervations it appears, that the length of the ſolar year, deduced from two very diſtant obſervations made at the time when the Sun was in the ſame point of the ecliptic near its apogee, differs by many ſeconds from the length of the year deduced by like obſervations, when the Sun was in another part of the ecliptic, near its perigee; thoſe made near the apogee giving the revolutions leſs, and thoſe made near the perigee making them greater, than the revolutions deduced from obſervations taken at the Sun's mean diſtance; this alſo ſhews, that the line of the apſides has a motion in *conſequentia*; and that the length of a tropical revolution ſhould be determined from very diſtant obſervations, made at the times when the Sun is at its mean diſtance from the Earth; or that the mean revolution ſhould be taken between thoſe deduced from obſervations made on the Sun's place, when he is in both the apogee and perigee.

243. PROBLEM LX.

To find the right aſcenſion of ſome noted fixed ſtar.

Having a good clock well regulated to mean or equal time, a large aſtronomical quadrant fixed in the plane of the meridian, and an equal altitude or tranſit inſtrument: then, on ſome day a little before or after the vernal equinox, when the daily alteration of the Sun's declination is about 18 or 20 minutes, obſerve the Sun's meridian altitude; and by equal altitudes find the times when both Sun and ſtar come to the meridian; the difference of theſe times is their difference of right aſcenſion.

Again. At ſome time a little after or before the autumnal equinox, before the Sun has paſſed the ſaid declination, obſerve his meridian altitude; and by equal altitudes find the times of the Sun and ſame ſtar's coming to the meridian, the difference of thoſe times is alſo the difference of their right aſcenſions.

If the vernal and autumnal meridian altitudes are the ſame, then thoſe obſervations were made, when the Sun was on the ſame parallel of declination: now the ſum, or diff. of the two obſerved differences of right aſcenſion, ſhews the equatorial arc deſcribed by the Sun between thoſe times; which arc, being biſected, ſhews the diſtance of the neareſt ſolſtice from the Sun, at the time when the obſervations have equal altitudes; and that diſtance corrected and taken from 90°, ſhews the Sun's right aſcenſion at the vernal obſervation, or its complement to 360 degrees.

From hence, and the firſt difference of right aſcenſion between the Sun and ſtar, the ſtar's right aſcenſion will be obtained.

244. If the two meridian altitudes of the Sun are not the ſame, their difference ſhews the difference of the mid-day declinations, when thoſe obſervations were taken: now from ſome tables of right aſcenſion and declination take the Sun's daily alteration in declination and right aſcenſion on the day the leſſer altitude was taken; then ſay, *As the daily change of decl. is to that of right aſcen.; ſo is the diff. of the altitudes, to the correction in right aſcenſion.*

This correction being added to the vernal, or ſubtracted from the autumnal difference of right aſcenſion, as either is leaſt, reduces that difference of right aſcenſion to what it would be when the declination is the ſame with the other; and then the difference between thoſe two differences of right aſcenſion, ſo reduced, gives the equatorial arc, as before recited.

245. At the Royal Obſervatory at Greenwich, in the year 1770, obſervations were made on the Sun and the ſtar α Aquilæ.

March 15, Sun's mer. zen. diſt. cleared of refraction and parallax, was 53° 28′ 29″; and their diff. of rt. aſc. was 60° 30′ 7,8″.

Sep. 28th. Sun's mer. zen. diſt. cleared of refraction and parallax, was 53° 36′ 26″; and their diff. of rt. aſc. was 109° 59′ 22,8″.

Then 7′ 57″ is the diff. of zen. diſts. or the alteration in declination.

Alſo 23′ 40″ and (3^m 39^s or) 54′ 45″ are the diffs. of decl. and rt. aſc. between the 15th and 16th days of March 1770.

Now 23′ 40″ : 7′ 57″ : : 54′ 45″ : 18′ 23,5″ the increaſe of the difference of right aſcenſion after the noon of the 15th of March.

Then 60° 30′ 07,8″ − 18′ 23,5″ = 60° 11′ 44,3″ which is the firſt diff. rt. aſc. when the Sun had the ſame decl. as at the ſecond obſervation.

Here, the times of the two obſervations fall neareſt the winter ſolſtice.

Then 60° 11′ 44,3″ + 109° 59′ 22,8″ = 170° 11′ 7″; its half 85° 5′ 33,5″ is the diſtance of the winter ſolſtice from the Sun.

Hence 270° + 85° 5′ 33,5″ + 18′ 23,5″ = 355° 23′ 57″ is the Sun's rt. aſc. on March 15th.

Alſo 355° 23′ 57″ − 60° 30′ 7,8″ = 294° 53′ 49,2″ is the rt. aſc. of α Aquilæ.

246. The right aſcenſion of one ſtar being known, the right aſcenſions of all the reſt are found by noting the times ſhewn by the clock, when thoſe ſtars come to the meridian: for the differences of thoſe times, from the tranſit of the choſen ſtar, are the differences of right aſcenſion; by which the right aſcenſion of all the obſerved ſtars will be known; taking care to augment or diminiſh the right aſcenſion of the choſen ſtar by thoſe differences, according as the choſen ſtar is preceded, or followed by the other obſerved ſtars.

247. PROBLEM LXI.

To find the Sun's Place.

SOLUTION. Let the time be obſerved both when the Sun, and a ſtar (the right aſcenſion of which is known) paſſed the meridian, and hence the Sun's right aſcenſion is known.

With that right aſcenſion, and the obliquity of the ecliptic, compute (142) the longitude, and thus his place in the ecliptic will be known.

248. PROBLEM LXII.

To find the greateſt Equation of the Center.

SOLUTION. At the times when the Sun is near his mean diſtance, let his longitude be found; their difference will ſhew the true motion for that interval of time.

Find alſo the Sun's mean motion for that interval of time.

Then half the difference between the true and mean motions will ſhew the greateſt equation of the center.

Obſervation made at the Royal Obſervatory at Greenwich, ſhews that
1769 October 1ſt. at $23^h\ 49^m\ 12^s$ mean time, ☉ long. was $6^s\ 9^\circ\ 32'\ 0{,}6''$
1770 March 29th. at 0 4 50 mean time, ☉ long. was 0 8 50 27,5

The diff. of time 178d. 0 15 38; True diff. long. 5 29 18 27
The tropical year = 365 d. 5 h. 48 m. 42 s. = 365,2421527
The obſerved interval = 178 0 15 38 = 178,01085648.
Then 365,2421527 : 178,01085648 :: 360° : 175,455948 mean motion.
So $175^\circ\ 27'\ 21''$ of mean motion, anſwers to $179^\circ\ 18'\ 27''$ true motion.
Their diff. = $3^\circ\ 51'\ 6''$; its half $1^\circ\ 55'\ 33''$ is the greateſt equation of the center according to theſe obſervations.

249. PROBLEM LXIII.

To find the eccentricity of the Earth's orbit.

SOLUTION. Say, As the diameter of a circle in degrees,
To the diameter in equal parts;
So the greateſt equation of the center in degrees,
To the eccentricity in equal parts.

The greateſt equation of the center $1^\circ\ 55'\ 33'' = 1^\circ{,}9258333$, &c.
The diam. of a circle being 1, its circumf. is 3,1415926. (II. 197)
Then 3,1415926 : 1 :: 360° : 114°,5915609 equal to the diameter.
And 114,5916c9 : 1,00&c. :: 1,9258333 : 0,0168061 the eccentricity.
Hence 1,016806 (= 1,000000 + 0,016806) = aphelion diſtance.
And 0,983194 (= 1,000000 — 0,016806) = perihelion diſtance.

PROBLEM LXIV.

To find the time and place of the Sun's Apogee.

Solution. On each day of two ſucceſſive apſides let the Sun's place and the time be obſerved.

Then if the interval of thoſe times and places is equal to the halves of 365 d. 6 h. 15 m. 29 s. and 360° 1′ 6″; thoſe obſervations were made when the Sun was in the apſides.

For ſuch intervals of time and place belong to no other points of the Earth's orbit.

But if thoſe obſerved intervals of time and place differ from the ſaid halves, take the difference between the interval of place and 180° 0′ 33″.

Then to the daily motion of the Sun's apogee (233), the ſaid diff. and 24 h. find the proportional time; which proportional time and difference, being applied to the time, and places, of the apogeon obſervation, gives a time and place when it is 180° 0′ 33″ diſtant from the obſerved perigeon place: now if the interval of theſe times is equal to 182 d. 15 h. 7 m. 44½ s. the times and places of the apſides are known.

But if the interval of time differs from 182 d. 15 h. 7 m. 44½ s., ſay, *As the diff. between the perigeon and the apogeon daily motions, is to the daily motion of the apogee; ſo is the diff. of the interval of time, to a ſecond correction of the time of the apogee.*

This correction applied to the apogeon time, corrected as above, will give the true time of the Sun's apogee.

Alſo, to the laſt correction of time find the proportional motion of the Sun's apogee; and apply it to the laſt corrected place of the apogee, and the true place of the apogee will be obtained.

By obſervations made at the Royal obſervatory at Greenwich in the year 1769.

July 1ſt.	at 0h	3m	20s	mean time ☉ long. =	3s	9°	46m	38,5″
December 29th. at	0	2	49	mean time ☉ long. =	9	8	10	58,1
Interval 180 d.	23	59	29.	Interval of place =	5	28	24	19,6
The Sun's motion in half an anomaliſtic year					6	0	0	33
The Sun's place at firſt obſervation is too forward by						1	36	13,4

Then 57′ 12″ : 1° 36′ 13,4″ : : 24 h. : 40 h. 22 m. 24 s. to be taken from the time of July 1ſt, to make the diſtance of the times anſwer to the half of 360° 1′ 6″; and it leaves June 29 d. 7 h. 40 m. 56 s.; at which time, the ſun was in 3s 8° 10′, 25,1″, which is diſtant from the December obſervation by 180° 0′ 33″: But here the interval of time is 182 d. 16 h. 21 m. 53 s.; which is greater than 182 d. 15 h. 7 m. 44½ s. the half anomaliſtic revolution, by 1 h. 14 m. 8½ s.; therefore the Sun has ſome time to run before he comes to the apogee.

Now 4′ 0″ : 57′ 12″ : : 1 h. 14 m. 8½ s. : 17 h. 13 m. 14 s. correction of time.

And 24 h. : 17 h. 13 m. 14 s. : : 57′ 12″ : 42′ 6,8″. correction of place.

Then June 29 d. 7 h. 4 m. 56 s. + 17 h. 13 m. 14 s. gives

June 30 d. 0 h. 21 m. 10 s. for the time of the apogee.

And 3s 8° 20′ : 25,1″ + 42′ 6,8″ gives 3s 8° 52′ 33″ for the place of the apogee.

251. PROBLEM LXV.

At any given time to find the Sun's mean anomaly.

Solution. Let an epocha of the Sun's passage through its aphelion be accurately determined. Then say,
As the time of a tropical revolution, or solar year,
To the interval between the aphelion and given time;
So is 360 degrees,
To the degrees shewing the mean anomaly.
Or. From the tables of mean motions find the Sun's mean motion for the given time, and this will be the mean anomaly.

252. If the Sun's motion in the ecliptic was uniform, his true place for any time could be found by the tables of his mean motion; but the Sun's longitude found by those tables, called his mean longitude, must be corrected on account of his irregular motion.

As the Earth revolves in an elliptical orbit about the Sun, placed in one of its foci, its angular motion round the Sun will differ from the angular motion it would have, were the Sun in the center of the ellipsis.

Now the table of mean motions gives the angular motions from the center of the ellipsis in a circle described on the line of the apsides, and reckoned from the first point of Aries; this motion, lessened by that of the apogee, gives the Sun's mean longitude, or mean anomaly, from the aphelion point.

But the motion of the Earth being in an elliptic orbit, its true anomaly will differ from its mean; this difference, called the equation of the center, is the correction wanted to reduce the mean motions to the true ones.

253. To find the equation of the center, or to solve (what is called) the Keplerian problem, is the most difficult operation, particularly in orbits the eccentricity of which bears a considerable proportion to the mean distance: how to do this has been shewn by Newton, Gregory, Keil, La Caille, and many others, by methods little differing from one another: it consists chiefly in finding an intermediate angle, called the eccentric anomaly, as shewn in the following problem.

254. PROBLEM LXVI.

The Sun's mean anomaly being known, and the dimensions of its orbit, to find the eccentric anomaly.

SOLUTION. Say,
As the aphelion distance,
To the perihelion distance;
So is the tan. $\frac{1}{2}$ the mean anomaly,
To the tan. of an arc.
Which arc added to half the mean anomaly gives the excentric anomaly.

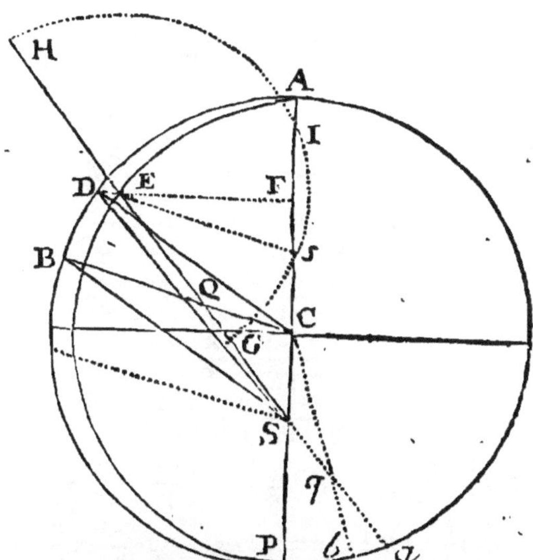

For let ADPB be the excentric.
AEP the Earth's orbit, C the center, S the Sun A the aphelion, P the perihelion, E the true place, D the corresponding place in the excentric, and B the mean place.

Now it is evident, that the less the eccentricity is, the nearer will the elliptic orbit approach the excentric circle; the nearer will the true and mean places, E and B, approach one another; and the less will be the difference between the mean, the excentric, and the true anomalies; also the nearer will the lines CD, SB, approach to parallelism, or coincidence: so that in orbits of small eccentricities CD and SB may be taken as parallel lines, particularly in the Earth's orbit, where CS is only about $\frac{1}{60}$ of CP.

Therefore $\angle$ ASB = $\angle$ ACD the excentric anomaly.

Then in the triangle BCS, where the sum of the sides BC + CS = SA; the diff. of the sides BC — CS = SP, and $\angle$ BCS (= supplement of ACB) are known; the $\angle$ CSB may be found. (III. 48)

Thus SA : SP : : tan. $\frac{1}{2}$ (sum $\angle s$, CSB + B =) $\angle$ ACB : tan. of an arc.

Then $\frac{1}{2}$ $\angle$ ACB + that arc = $\angle$ CSB (III 47.) the excentric anomaly.

255. PROBLEM LXVII.

The Sun's excentric anomaly, and the dimensions of its orbit being known, to find the true anomaly.

SOLUTION. Say, As the square root of the aphelion distance,
To the square root of the perihelion distance,
So tangent of half the excentric anomaly,
To tangent of half the true anomaly.

For let a semicircle be described from E through the other focus s, cutting AP in s, I, and SE, produced, in G, H.

Then (II. 172) SH : SI : : Ss : SG = $\left(\frac{SI \times Ss}{SH} = \frac{\overline{Ss + sI} \times Ss}{SE + Es} =\right) \frac{2CF \times 2CS}{2CA}$.

Or $CF \times CS = (\frac{1}{2}SG =) \frac{1}{2}SE - \frac{1}{2}Es$; $CA (= \frac{1}{2}SE + \frac{1}{2}Es)$ being radius, and $= 1$.
Therefore $SE = (1 + CS \times CF$ (III. 47) $=) 1 + CS \times s\text{'},ACD$. (III. 9)

Again. In Δ SFE. As $SE : R :: SF : s\text{'}, ASE = \left(\frac{SF}{SE} = \right) \frac{SC + s\text{'},ACD}{1 + SC \times s\text{'},ACD}$.

Then $1 + s\text{'},ASE : 1 - s\text{'},ASE :: 1 + \frac{SC + s\text{'},ACD}{1 + SC \times s\text{'},ACD} : 1 - \frac{SC + s\text{'},ACD}{1 + SC \times s\text{'},ACD}$.

$$\text{Or } \frac{1 - s\text{'},ASE}{1 + s\text{'},ASE} = \left(\frac{1 + SC \times s\text{'},ACD - SC - s\text{'},ACD}{1 + SC \times s\text{'},ACD + SC + s\text{'},ACD}\right.$$

$$= \frac{1 - SC + SC \times s\text{'},ACD - s\text{'},ACD}{1 + SC + SC \times s\text{'},ACD + s\text{'},ACD}$$

$$= \frac{SP + \overline{CS - 1} \times s\text{'},ACD}{SA + \overline{CS + 1} \times s\text{'},ACD} = \left.\frac{SP - s\text{'},ACD \times SP}{SA + s\text{'},ACD \times SA}\right)$$

$$= \frac{1 - s\text{'},ACD}{1 + s\text{'},ACD} \times \frac{SP}{SA}.$$

But $\frac{1 - s\text{'},ASE}{1 + s\text{'},ASE} = tt,\frac{1}{2}ASE$; and $\frac{1 - s\text{'},ACD}{1 + s\text{'},ACD} \times \frac{SP}{SA} = tt,\frac{1}{2}ACD \times \frac{SP}{SA}$. (IV. 217)

Then $\frac{SP}{SA} \times tt,\frac{1}{2}ACD = tt,\frac{1}{2}ASE$. Or $\frac{SP}{SA} = \frac{tt,\frac{1}{2}ASE}{tt,\frac{1}{2}ACD}$.

Therefore $\left(\frac{\sqrt{SP}}{\sqrt{SA}} = \frac{t,\frac{1}{2}ASE}{t,\frac{1}{2}ACD}\right.$. Or$\left.\right) \sqrt{SA} : \sqrt{SP} :: t,\frac{1}{2}ACD : t,\frac{1}{2}ASE$.

256. REMARK. *The* $\angle CQS = \angle ACB \backsim \angle ASE$ (II. 95), *is the equation of the center, to be applied to the mean anomaly; and is ſubtractive from the aphelion to the perihelion, or in the firſt ſix ſigns of anomaly; and additive from the perihelion to the aphelion, or in the laſt ſix ſigns of anomaly.*

For the lines CB, SE; C*b*, SE, which coincide in SA, SP, will in every other poſition croſs one another; in Q while revolving from A to P, and in *q* while revolving from P to A: in the firſt half revolution, the mean anomaly, or the external $\angle$ ACB, exceeds the $\angle$ ASE, the true anomaly, by the $\angle$ CQS (II. 96): in the latter half, the true anomaly, or external $\angle$ PS*a*, exceeds the mean anomaly, or $\angle$ PC*b*, by the $\angle$ S*q*C.

SECTION IX.

Practical Astronomy.

Of the EQUATION of TIME.

257. Time, which of itfelf flows uniformly, has its parts meafured by the motion of fome vifible object; and the Sun being the moft confpicuous moving object in the heavens, its motion has been chofen as the moft proper meafure of the parts of time, as well for the day, as for the year.

258. The aftronomical day, at any place, begins when the Sun's center is on the meridian of that place; and is divided into 24 hours, reckoned in a numeral fucceffion from 1 to 24: the firft 12 are fometimes diftinguifhed by the mark P. M., fignifying *poft meridiem*, or afternoon; and the latter 12 are marked A. M., fignifying *ante meridiem*, or before noon: but aftronomers generally reckon through the 24 hours, from noon to noon; and what is by the civil, or common way of reckoning, called morning hours, is by Aftronomers reckoned in the fucceffion from 12, or midnight, to 24 hours.

Thus 5 o'clock in the morning of April the 10th, is by aftronomers called April the 9th, at 17 h.

259. *The Sun's daily motion in longitude* is the arc of the ecliptic run through in that day; and his *daily motion in right afcenfion* is the correfponding arc of the equator; and the mean daily motion in either circle is meafured by 59′ 8″ nearly. For 365 d. : 1 d. : : 360° : 59′ 8″.

260. An ASTRONOMICAL or SOLAR DAY is the interval of time between two fucceffive tranfits of the Sun's center over the fame meridian; and is meafured by the fum of the whole equator, and an arc of it equal to the daily motion in right afcenfion.

For at the end of a diurnal rotation, which by obfervations is known to be uniform, the meridian has returned to the fame ftar, or point of the ecliptic, which it was againft at the preceding noon; but the Sun, during this rotation, has removed from that ftar to another, which has a greater right afcenfion: therefore, before the meridian can be again oppofite to the Sun, fo much of another rotation muft be defcribed, as is equal to the daily motion in right afcenfion.

261. A SIDERIAL DAY is the interval between two fucceffive returns of the fame meridian to the fame fixed ftar, is lefs than the folar day, and is meafured by 360°.

262. A MEAN or EQUATORIAL DAY is the time elapfed between two fucceffive tranfits of the Sun over the meridian, and is meafured by 360° 59′ 8″ nearly.

263. MEAN or EQUAL TIME is that fhewn by a *clock*, whofe 24 hours meafure the time which the Sun takes to defcribe an equatorial arc equal to 360° 59′ 8″ nearly.

264. The difference between the meafures of a mean folar day and a fiderial day, viz. 59′ 8″, reduced to time (132), gives 3 m. 56 s.; which fhews, that a ftar which was on the meridian with the Sun on

one noon, will return to that meridian 3 m. 56 s. before the next noon; therefore a clock, which meafures mean or equal days by 24 hours, will give 23 h. 56 m. 4 s. for the length of a fiderial day.

265. Apparent, or True Time, is that fhewn by a *fun-dial*; where 24 hours, or a day, is meafured by the fum of 360°, and that day's motion in right afcenfion.

266. The folar days are unequal to one another, for obfervations fhew that the fun's daily motion in right afcenfion is continually varying.

The true and mean folar days are never equal, but when the Sun's daily motion in right afcenfion is 59′ 8″; which happens about February 11th, May 14th, July 26th, and November 1ft: at all other times the lengths of the *true* and *mean* days differ. The accumulation of thefe differences produces the equation of time; and fometimes the apparent noon will precede the time of the mean noon, and fometimes fall after it; their difference amounting to above 16 minutes at the beginning of November.

267. The Equation of Time is the difference between the times fhewn by a *clock* and a *fun-dial*; or between the *mean* and true noons; or between the Sun's right afcenfion and his mean longitude when turned into time at the rate of 15° to an hour.

This difference arifes on two accounts. Firft, becaufe of the obliquity of the ecliptic the daily motions in longitude and right afcenfion are unequal. Secondly, becaufe of the unequal motion of the Earth in an elliptic orbit.

In the firft and third quadrants, or between the figns ♈♋, ♎♑, the right afcenfion being lefs than the longitude (140), or the mean motion taken in the equator; the point of right afcenfion is to the weft, and therefore the apparent noon precedes, or comes in *confequentia* to the meridian before the mean noon: but in the 2d and 4th quadrants, or between the figns ♋♎, ♑♈, the right afcenfion being greater than the longitude or mean motion, taken in the equator, the mean noon is weftward, and therefore precedes, or comes in *confequentia* to the meridian before the apparent noon.

From the aphelion to the perihelion, or in the firft fix figns of anomaly, the mean noon precedes the apparent; and in the laft fix figns of anomaly the apparent noon precedes the true; their difference in either cafe is the equation of the center, which convert into time.

Now becaufe the points of Aries, and of the Sun's apogee, the places where the two parts of the equation of time commence, do conftantly recede from one another; therefore the whole equation of time made up of thofe two parts will ferve only for a few years, and requires to be corrected from time to time.

268. *To calculate the equation, or difference between the mean and apparent noons, for any propofed day.*

Find the mean and true anomalies for that time (255); their difference, or the equation of the center, is one part.

The true anomaly gives the Sun's longitude; with which, and the obliquity of the ecliptic, compute the right afcenfion (139); the difference between the longitude and right afcenfion gives the other part.

The fum, or diff. of the two parts, turned into time, gives the equation fought.

SECTION

SECTION X.

Practical Astronomy.

To make SOLAR TABLES.

269. I. *Tables of the mean motions of the Sun.* (301, 302, 303, 304.)

Divide 360 degrees by a ſolar revolution, the quotient ſhews the mean motion for one day 0° 59′ 08″ &c.

Take the multiples of one day's motion from 1 to 365 for every day in the year; and theſe properly diſpoſed, according to the month days, will give the mean motions for every day of each month. (304)

The 24th part of one day's motion will give that for one hour, and its multiples to 24 times will ſhew the mean motions anſwering to each hour: from hence, thoſe for the minutes of an hour, the ſeconds of a minute, &c. are eaſily obtained. (303)

The mean motion of a year of 365 days (viz. for the laſt of December) being doubled, tripled, and quadrupled, thoſe for 1, 2, 3, and 4 years will be obtained, adding one day's mean motion to the 4th year, it being leap-year, and containing 366 days: the motion for leap-year being increaſed by thoſe of 1, 2, 3, and leap-years, give thoſe for 5, 6, 7, and 8 years: the mean motion for 8 years being increaſed by thoſe for 1, 2, 3, and 4 years, give thoſe for 9, 10, 11, and 12 years: and thus increaſing the mean motion for the laſt leap year by thoſe of 1, 2, 3, and 4 years, the mean motions may be continued for any number of abſolute years. (301)

270. In the following tables the numbers uſed were,

Length of the year	365d.	5h.	48m.	54¾s.
Yearly motion of the apogee,		0°	1′	5″.
Place of the apogee, beginning the year 1760,	3s	8	47	25.
Greateſt equation of the Earth's orbit.		1	55	39.

271. Now 365 d. 5 h. 48 m. 54¾ ſ. = 365,2423003472 days.

Then 365,2423003472 d. : 360° : : 1 d. : 0,9856470613 degrees.

Hence the mean motion for 1 day =	0s	0°	59′	8″	19‴	45iv	54v	50vi
January 5th	5 days =	0	4	55	41	38	49	34	10
January 30th	30 days =	0	29	34	9	52	57	25	0
March 31ſt	90 days =	2	28	42	29	38	52	15	0
June 29th	180 days =	5	27	24	59	17	44	30	0
December 26th	360 days =	11	24	49	58	35	29	0	0
December 31ſt	365 days =	11	29	45	40	14	18	34	10

Now 1 year's mean motion	=11ſ.	29°	45′	40″	14‴	18^{iv}	34^{v}	10^{vi}.
2 years	=11	29	31	20	28	37	8	20.
3 years	=11	29	17	0	42	55	42	30.
4, or leap year	= 0	0	1	49	17	0	11	30=3y.+1y.+1d.
5 years	=11	29	47	29	31	18	45	40=4y.+1y.
6 years	=11	29	33	9	45	37	19	50=4y.+2y.
7 years	=11	29	18	49	59	55	54	0=4y.+3y.
8 years B	= 0	0	3	38	34	0	23	0=4y.×2.
20 years B	= 0	0	9	6	25	0	57	30=4y.×5.
100 years B	= 0	0	45	32	5	4	47	30=20y.×5.
1000 years B	= 0	7	35	20	50	47	55	0=100y.×10.

Where B ſtands for biſſextile, or leap-year.

272. But to find the mean motions for the years related to any particular epocha, the mean motion for ſome particular time in that epocha muſt be known. Thus,

Let the mean motion of the Sun be determined by obſervation (or otherwiſe) when the Sun is in ſome noted point of the ecliptic, ſuppoſe near Aries: or let the time of its entrance into the ſign Aries be well aſcertained. Take the difference between the time of that ingreſs and the 31ſt of December at noon, in days, hours, minutes, and ſeconds (reckoning the end of the 31ſt of December to be the beginning of January at noon,) and find the mean motions for thoſe days, hours, minutes, and ſeconds, and it will ſhew the motion from Aries, for the 31ſt of December, or the mean motion at the beginning of the year propoſed; or the radix for that year with relation to the propoſed epocha.

The relative mean motions for one year being known, thoſe for any number of ſucceeding years belonging to that epocha, may be had, by adding ſuch of the before found abſolute years to the firſt relative year, as will make the number wanted: and the mean motions for any paſt year of that epocha will be found by leſſening the radical years by ſuch a number of the abſolute years, as will produce the relative years required. (302)

And in this manner are tables conſtructed, by which the mean motions of the Sun for any time, paſt, or to come, may be computed.

273. Suppoſe in the year 1760, the Sun entered Aries on the 20th of March, at 13 h. 42 m. 3¼ s. P. M.: required the Sun's mean motion for the beginning of the year 1760.

Now 1760 being leap-year, February has 29 days, and from the equinox to the commencement of the year is 80 d. 13 h. 42 m. 3¼ s.

Then 1 d. : 0,9856470613 deg. :: 80 d. 13 h. 42 m. 3¼ s. : 79,41444 &c. degrees.

Therefore at the beginning of the year 1760, the Sun's mean longitude was 2ˢ 19° 24′ 52″ ſhort of Aries; or his mean longitude was 9ˢ 10° 35′ 8″, which is the radical mean place for the year 1760.

274. II. *Of the mean motions of the Sun's apogees.* (301, 302)

The yearly motion of the apogee being determined (241); the motion for any number of abſolute years will be that multiple of one year's year's motion, and ſo for any part of a year: the monthly motions will be 5 ſeconds for ſome months, and 6 for others, to make 65 in the 12 months.

Let the time of the Sun's paſſage through the aphelion be accurately determined by obſervation (250), and alſo its place in the ecliptic; then the diſtance of the place of the apogee from Aries will be known at that time: let this diſtance be leſſened by the apogee's motion from the laſt day of the year preceding the propoſed epocha to the time of the apogeon paſſage, and the mean motion of the apogee will be known for the beginning of that year, taken as a radix.

Then that radical mean motion, increaſed by the multiples of the yearly motion, will give thoſe for ſucceeding years: but being diminiſhed by thoſe multiples will give them for paſt years.

The Sun's mean motion for any time, leſſened by that of the apogee for that time, gives the Sun's mean anomaly.

275. III. *Of the equation of the Sun's center.* (305)

To every degree of the firſt ſix ſigns of mean anomaly aſſumed, find the true anomaly (253, 254): the difference between the mean and true anomalies will be the equations of the center to thoſe degrees of mean anomaly; which ſerve alſo for the degrees of the laſt ſix ſines; as equal anomalies are at equal diſtances on both ſides of either apſide.

Set the equations of the center orderly to their ſigns and degrees of anomaly, the firſt ſix being reckoned from the top of the table downwards, and ſigned at top with the title *ſubtract*; the laſt ſix, for which the ſame equations ſerve, but taken in a contrary order, viz. from the bottom of the table reckoned upwards, are ſigned at bottom with the title *add*; and let the difference between every adjacent two equations, called tabular differences, be ſet in another column.

From theſe equations of the center, augmented or diminiſhed by the proportional parts of their reſpective tabular differences for any given minutes and ſeconds, are deduced equations of the center to any given mean anomaly.

276. Aſtronomical tables are uſually computed to anſwer to two given denominations only; as to ſigns and degrees: degrees and minutes; months and days; &c.: for if made to more names, ſuch tables would ſwell into a bulk ſo great, as to be tedious to compute, expenſive to print, and of no great advantage in the uſe; but it generally happens in calculations, that numbers are wanted from tables to anſwer to given numbers of three, or more denominations as to ſigns, degrees, minutes, and ſeconds; months, days, hours, minutes, and ſeconds; &c.: and to obtain from the tables numbers anſwering to all the given names, the tabular numbers are to be increaſed or diminiſhed by a proportional part of their difference.

Thus. *To find the equation of the center to* 4ˢ 21° 44′ 36″?

Now the equation to this number will fall between thoſe belonging 4ˢ 21° and 4ˢ 22°; which equations are 1° 13′ 59″ and 1° 12′ 24″ (205) Their diff. is 1′ 35″=95″; the pro. pt. of which is to be taken for 44′ 36″.

And as the diff. 1° or 60′ : diff. 95″ : : 44′,6 : 70″,6 = 1′ 11″ the proportional part.

Now to 4ˢ 21° 0′ 0″,	1° 13′ 59″	is the equation of the center.
And to 0 0 44 36 ,	1 11	is the prop. part to be subtracted
Then to 4 21 44 36 ,	1 12 48	is the equation of the center.

When the tabular numbers are increasing, the proportional part is to be added; but when decreasing, the proportional part is to be subtracted.

277. IV. *Tables of the Sun's true place.* (308)

The Sun's true place at any proposed time is thus found.

Collect together the mean motions of the Sun, and also those of the apogee, for the given year, month, day, (hour, minute, and second, if given); and their sum will be the mean motions of the Sun and its apogee.

The Sun's mean motion, lessened by that of the apogee, gives the mean anomaly; to which find the proper equation of the center by proportioning for the minutes and seconds.

Then the Sun's mean motion, augmented or diminished by the equation of the center, as the title of its table directs, gives the Sun's true longitude, or place, for that given time.

The Sun's place thus found to every day for four successive years, viz. for leap-year, and 1, 2, 3 years after; and those places ranged under their proper years, according to their respective months and days, constitute the tables of the Sun's place.

These tables find the Sun's place at noon only; but the place for any intermediate time is found by applying to the noon-place the proportional part of the daily difference at that time.

278. *To find the Sun's longitude, suppose on May 4, 1788, at the time of apparent noon?*

In the table of the Sun's longitude (308) for 1788, against May 4th, stands 1ˢ 14° 36′ 02″, which shews that the Sun's longitude, reckoned from Aries, is 44° 36′ 02″; or that his place is in ♉ 14° 36′ 02″.

But to find the Sun's place at any other hour, suppose on May 4th, at 7 h. 24 m. 36 s. apparent time, proceed thus,

The difference between the noon places of the 4th and 5th of May is 57′ 59″ = 3479″, answering to 24 hours in time. (308)

Then 24 h. : 7 h. 24 m. 36 s. : : 3479″ : 1074″ = 17′ 54″, the proportional part.

And 1ˢ 14° 36′ 02″ + 17′ 54″ = 1ˢ 14° 53′ 56″, the Sun's longitude at that time.

279. Or, the Sun's place may be found by the tables of mean motions.

From

From the apparent time $7^h\ 24'\ 36''$ take the equation of time (316) equal to $3'\ 35''$ and the remainder, $7^h\ 21'\ 1''$, is the mean time.

3. ⊙'s m. mot.	(302)	$9^s\ 10°\ 47'\ 53''$
d 4	(305)	4 2 13 13
ours	(303)	17 15
inutes	(303)	52
cond	(303)	0
's mean longitude		1 13 19 13
Equat. center +		1 34 44
Sun's true longitude		1 14 53 57

Mot. ap.	3 9 17 45		(302)
	22		(307)
	3 9 18 07	m. apogee.	
Diff.	10 4 1 06	m. anom.	

Now to $10^s\ 4°$ the equation of the center is $1°\ 34'\ 45''$ (305) And the diff. is $70''$ decreasing. $60' : 70'' :: 1'\ 06'' : 1''$ the proportional part. And $1°\ 34'\ 45'' - 1'' = 1\ 34\ 44$ equation of the center.

280. *To find the Sun's longitude at any given time and place.*

Seek, in the table of the longitudes of places, at the end of Book VI. for the difference of longitude between London and the proposed place; and convert the diff. of longitude into time.

If the proposed place is to the eastward of London, take the diff. between the proposed time and diff. of longitude, and this will shew the corresponding time at London; after noon, if the proposed time is greater than the diff. of longitude; but before noon, if the proposed time is least.

If the proposed place is to the westward of London, the sum of the proposed time and diff. of longitude will be the corresponding time at London.

The Sun's place found to the corresponding time at London, will be the Sun's longitude sought for the proposed time and place.

Thus. In a place 6 h. to the east of London, when it is 8 h. P. M. at that place, it is 2 h. P. M. at London; and when it is 4 h. P. M. at that place, it is 2 h. before noon at London.

For when it is noon at London, it is 6 h. P. M. at the other place.

Also, in a place 6 h. to the west of London; when it is 8 h. P. M. at that place, it is 14 h. P. M. at London.

For when it is noon at the proposed place, it is 6 h. P. M. at London.

281. V. *Tables of the Sun's declination.* (309)

With each of the Sun's longitudes, already found, and the obliquity of the ecliptic, find the declination to each day of the four years. (139)

Or thus. To each degree of the three first signs of the ecliptic, taken as longitudes, find the declination (139): and of these declinations, regularly ranged to their sign and degree, take the difference of each adjacent two, which set against them in another column; and this auxiliary table is prepared, answering to each sign and degree of longitude (306): for to equal longitudes, taken on both sides of each equinox, belong equal declinations.

Now these auxiliary declinations augmented, or diminished (according as they are increasing or decreasing, by the proportional part of their difference,

difference, for the minute and seconds in any given longitude, will give the declination for that longitude.

And this being done for every day in the four years, using the longitudes already computed, will give the declinations sought: which are to be ranged according to their year, month, and day. (309)

282. To find the Sun's declination. Suppose on May 4, 1788, at noon. In the table of the Sun's declination (309) for 1788, against May 4, stands 16° 14′ 13″ for the Sun's declination, which is N. as being between the vernal and autumnal equinoxes.

283. But if the declination was wanted on May 4, 1788, at 7 h. 24 m. 36 s. P. M. proceed thus.

The difference between the noons of May 4 and 5, is 16′ 59″, which answers to 24 h. Then 24 h. : 17′ 0″ : : 7 h. 24 m. 36 s. : 5′ 15″, the proportional part.

And as the declination is increasing; then 16° 14′ 13″ + 5′ 15″ gives 16° 19′ 28″ for the Sun's decl. at the proposed time.

284. But art. 311 is a table for finding the proportional part at sight, for fitting the noon declination to any other time. Thus.

Seek in the left-hand column for a daily difference, nearest to the given one; against which, in a column marked at top with hours, nearest to those given, stands the proportional part sought.

Thus against 17′ 0″ of daily diff. and to 7 h. 24 m. time, stand 5′ 15″, the proportional part sought.

Although this table goes no farther than 8 h., yet it may be applied quite to 12 h. or 180 degrees.

285. Exam. *What will be the Sun's declination at London, on the 25th of August, 1788, at 10 h. 35 m. P. M.?*

In 1788, the daily diff. between the noons of the 25th and the 26th of August is 20′ 58″ decreasing. (309)

Now 10 h. 35 m. is equal to 2 h. 35 m. + 8 h. 0 m.

To the diff. 20′ 58″, and to 2 h. 35 m., answers 2′ 16″. (311)

To the diff. 20′ 58″, and to 8 h. 0 m., answers 6′ 59″.

The sum 9′ 15″ is the proportional part, by which the decl. 10° 28′ 29″ to August 25th, is to be diminished; so 10° 19′ 14″ is the decl. sought.

Here 20′ 58″, is taken as if it was 21′ 0″.

And 2 h. 35 m. is ¾, the interval between 2 h. 20 m. and 2 h. 40 m.

Now 21′ gives 2′ 2″ for 2^h 20′, and 2′ 20″ for 2^h 40′; the diff. is 18″, three fourths of which is 14″: and this being added to 2′ 2″ gives 2′ 16″ for 21′ with 2^h 35′. Moreover 21′ with 8 h. gives 7′ 00″; but I take one second less because the daily diff. in declination is 2″ less than 21′ 00″.

286. From the table of declination, fitted to the meridian of London, or Greenwich, the declination may be found at any time, under any other meridian, at a given difference of longitude from London. Thus.

Required

Required the Sun's declination at noon under a meridian 110° to the west of London, on the 24th of February, 1788.

(311) Now at 110° to the weſt of London, it is noon 7 h. 20 m. after it is noon at London; that is, when it is 7 h. 20 m. P. M. at London, it will be noon at the propoſed place; ſo the declination found to that time at London (285) will be the declination ſought.

In 1788, the diff. between the declinations of the 24th and 25th of February, is 22′ 13″ decreaſing (309): and againſt 22′ 20″ of daily diff., and under 110°, or 7 h. 20 m., is 6′ 49″ in table, art. 311, which taken from 9° 27′ 33″, leaves 9° 20′ 44″, the declination ſought.

EXAM. II. *What is the Sun's declination on September 2d, 1788, at 20 h. 30 m., under a meridian 100° to the eaſtward of London?*

Now under a meridian 100° to the eaſtward of London, it is noon 6 h. 40 m. before it is noon at London (311); or when it is noon at London, it is 6 h. 40 m. after noon at the propoſed place; and when 20 h. 30 m. after noon at that place, it is 13 h. 50 m. after noon at London; ſo the declination found at that time (285), will be the declination ſought.

In 1788, the daily diff. at September 2d, is 22′ 6″ (309), againſt which (in tab. art. 311), and under 8 h. and 5 h. 50 m., ſtand 7′ 21″ and 5′ 21″, their ſum 12′ 42″ taken from the decl. to September 2, viz. 7° 36′ 30″, leaves 7° 23′ 48″, the declination ſought.

Here 5 h. 50 m. fall in the middle between 5 h. 40 m. and 6 h. 0 m. ſo 5′ 21″, the middle between 5′ 12″ and 5′ 30″, is taken.

287. VI. *Tables of the Sun's right aſcenſion.* (310)

To the obliquity of the ecliptic, and each degree in the three firſt ſigns of longitude, find the right aſcenſions (139), and of each take the ſupplement.

Range the right aſcenſions according to their ſign and degree for the three firſt ſigns; and for the three next ſigns, range the ſupplements, ſo that the 4th ſign begins with the leaſt ſupplement, and the 6th ſign ends with the greateſt: becauſe the right aſcenſions in the 2d and 4th quadrants are the ſupplements of thoſe in the firſt and third.

Let the differences of theſe right aſcenſions, viz. each adjacent two, through the ſix ſigns be taken, and ſet in other columns. (307)

Then this auxiliary table, uſed like that of declination, will give the right aſcenſion to each day in the four years.

288. *To find the Sun's right aſcenſion, ſuppoſe on June 12 at noon, in the year 1788, at London.*

In the table of the Sun's right aſcenſion (310) for 1788, againſt June 12, ſtands 5 h. 25 m. 19 ſ., which is the right aſcenſion ſought, and ſhews how much later the Sun paſſed the meridian of London than the equinoctial point Aries.

EXAM.

EXAM. II. *Required the Sun's right ascension at London on the 2d of November, 1788, at 9 h. 30 m. P. M.?*

Between the 2d and 3d of November, 1788, the daily diff. is 3 m. 58 s. which answers to 24 h. Then 24 h.: 3 m. 58 s. : : 9 h. 30 m. : 1 m. 34 s., the proportional part.

Then the right ascension on the 2d at noon, 14 h. 33 m. 20 s. + 1 m. 34 s. gives 14 h. 34 m. 54 s. for the right ascension at the time required.

By this table the right ascension may also be found at any time in places that are to the eastward, or westward, of London, the difference of longitude of those places being known; by finding the time at London corresponding to the given time at the proposed place, and seeking the right ascension to that corresponding time at London.

The table at art. 311, pages 222, 223, may be applied to the tables of the Sun's longitude and right ascension, as well as to those of the declination, for finding the proportional parts of the difference between the noon of adjoining days, which shall answer to any intermediate hours.

Thus in the Ex. page 296. To find the pro. pts. of 58′ to 7 h. 24 m. 36 s.
Now ¼th of 58′ is 14′ 30″; which falls between 14′ 20″ and 14′ 40″.
And the time 7 h. 24 m. 36 s. falls between 7 h. 20 m. and 7 h. 40 m.
The mean of the equations under 7 h. 20 m. and 7 h. 40 m. and against 14′ 20″ and 14′ 40″, are 4′ 26″ and 4′ 38″, their diff. is 12″.
And 20 : 12 : : 4,6 : 2½ : and 4′ 26″ + 2½ = 4′ 28½ the pro. pts. to ¼ of 58″.
Then the proportional parts to 58′, are 17′ 54″.
Again. In the Exam. above. To find the parts proportional to 3 m. 57 s. as 9 h. 30 m. is to 24 h.
Here 3 m. 57 s. being taken as 4 m.; and 4 h. 40 m. as the half of 9 h. 30 m.
The equation is 47″; which doubled gives 1′ 34″ for the proportional parts required.

289. VII. *Of the right ascensions and declinations of the fixed Stars.* (312)

This table, which contains 120 of the principal fixed stars, viz. 60 having north declination, and 60 with south declination, are fitted to the year 1780; and are selected partly from the catalogue which is given in the Nautical Almanac for 1773, as deduced from Dr. Bradley's Observations; and partly from that given by M. de La Caille, which, he says, "are all derived from his own observations made, during ten years attention to this business, either at Paris, or at the Cape of Good Hope; "that the positions are ascertained with all the accuracy that could be derived from the modern Astronomy; and that he had all proper helps, "with regard to instruments, assistants, and convenience, and neither "care or pains were wanting to perfect the work.

"The right ascensions were determined by a multitude of corresponding altitudes of each, taken with a quadrant of three feet radius, to have "their passage over the meridian with the greatest exactness. Almost all "the stars in the northern hemisphere have been compared with the "bright star in the Harp; and those in the southern hemisphere, with "Syrius; that is to say, on each day that the time of the star's passing "the meridian had been found by equal altitudes, that of α Lyræ and "Syrius were found in like manner; the right ascensions of these two "stars

" ſtars having been ſettled by a great many obſervations taken when " they were in the propereſt ſituation for this purpoſe.

" The declinations have been deduced from a ſufficient number of " obſervations of their zenith diſtances, taken with an inſtrument of ſix " feet radius, made with great care for this purpoſe."

The table conſiſts of nine columns; that on the left hand contains the name of the conſtellation; the next ſhews in what part of the conſtellation the ſtar is; in the 3d are the names by which certain ſtars are diſtinguiſhed; the 4th column ſhews the Greek characters by which the ſtar is marked in the cœleſtial charts, or maps of the conſtellations; the 5th ſhews the magnitude of the ſtars; the 6th and 7th contain the right aſcenſion in time, reckoned from Aries, and the yearly variation in right aſcenſion; the 8th and 9th contain the declinations and the yearly variation in declination; where thoſe which are marked + are augmented by the yearly variation; but thoſe which have the mark — annexed, are to be diminiſhed by the variation: by the help of theſe yearly variations the right aſcenſions and declinations of theſe ſtars may be fitted for any diſtant year.

Precepts for finding the culminating of the ſtars are at articles 133, 134.

290. VIII. *Tables of the Equation of Time.*

In page 318 are three tables, articles 313, 314, 315: Article 313 is a table of the Sun's right aſcenſion in degrees, to each degree of longitude in the firſt quadrant of the ecliptic; and alſo the differences between thoſe longitudes and right aſcenſions. The table, art. 314, contains the ſaid differences turned into time (132), of minutes, ſeconds, and the tenth part of ſeconds: the numbers in this table are the differences between the mean and true noons, ariſing from the obliquity of the ecliptic (267); and the table, art. 315, is nothing more than the equations of the center, table art. 305, converted into time; and are the differences between the times of the mean and true noons, ariſing from the eccentricity of the Earth's orbit: theſe two equations of time, properly put together, conſtitute another table, art. 316, of the abſolute equation of time with relation to the place of the Sun's apogee.

291. *To conſtruct the table* 316, *of the abſolute Equation of Time.*

1ſt. To the given time find the Sun's true place, or aſſume a place.

2d. The difference between that place, and the place of the apogee, gives the Sun's true anomaly.

3d. From the true anomaly find the mean. . (294)

4th. In table I. 314, ſeek the equation of time to the Sun's place.

5th. In table II. 315, ſeek the equation of time to the mean anomaly.

6th. The ſum, or difference of theſe equations, according as their titles, or ſigns direct, will be the abſolute equation of time to the Sun's place found at firſt, or to the correſponding time.

The tables, articles 314, 315, are made only to whole degrees of longitude and anomaly; the proportional parts of the differences are to be taken for minutes or ſeconds, above whole degrees of the Sun's longitude and anomaly.

292. Exam. I. *What is the Equation of Time, when the Sun's longitude is 7ˢ 12°?*

In table, art. 316, against 12° in the outside column, and under ♏, or 7 ſ., ſtands —, 16 m. 12 ſ.; which ſhews that 16 m. 12 ſ. is to be ſubtracted from the apparent time; to give the mean time of apparent noon, or the time which ſhould be ſhewn by a good clock, when the Sun's center is on the meridian.

293. Exam. II. *What is the Equation of Time when the Sun's longitude is 4ˢ 24° 30′ 42″?*

The difference between the equation in table, art. 316, to 4ˢ 24° and 4ˢ 25°, is 13ˢ decreaſing; and 30′ 42″=30,7′.
Then 60′ : 30,7′ : : 13ˢ : 6,65 or 7ˢ, the proportional part decreaſing.
And + 3 m. 46 ſ. — 7 ſ. = + 3 m. 39 ſ., the equation ſought.
So 24 h. the apparent time of ſolar noon, increaſed by 3 m. 39 ſ. will give the mean time of noon.

If the time was given, viz. the month, day, hour, &c., to find the Equation.
To the given time find the Sun's longitude. (278)
Then to this longitude find the equation of time, as above.

294. *To find the mean anomaly from the true being given.*

Solution, Say, As the ſquare root of the perihelion diſtance,
To the ſquare root of the aphelion diſtance;
So the tangent of half the true anomaly,
To the tangent of half the excentric anomaly,
And As radius, to the ſign of the excentric anomaly,
So the degrees in an arc equal in length to the eccentricity,
To the degrees, &c. in the arc of correction.

The correction added to the excentric anomaly gives the mean anomaly.

295. Remarks. 1ſt. The greateſt equation of the center being taken at 1° 55′ 39″, the eccentricity (249) will be 0,01682; the aphelion diſtance will be 1,01682, and the perihelion 0,98318.

Hence the ratio of the ſquare root of the perihelion diſtance to the ſquare root of the aphelion diſtance will be expreſſed by the logarithm 0,00731; which conſtant logarithm, added to the logarithmic tangent of ½ the true anomaly, will give the logarithmic tangent of ½ the excentric anomaly.

296. 2d. In the 2d proportion, the arc equal to the length of the eccentricity 1682 is a conſtant quantity.
Now the radius, or mean diſtance, is equal to the length of an arc of 57°,29578 (249); then 100000 : 1682 : : 57°,29578 : 0°,96375, the length of the eccentricity in degrees; the conſtant logarithm of which is 9,98396, which added to the logarithmic ſine of the excentric anomaly, abating 10 in the index of the ſum, gives the logarithm of an arc, the degrees, minutes, and ſeconds of which being added to the excentric anomaly, give the mean anomaly.

297. IX. *Table of corrections for the middle time between equal altitudes of the Sun.* Art. 317.

This table, which is fitted to the latitudes of 30°, 40°, 50°, and 60°, will alſo ſerve, nearly, to all latitudes between 25° and 65°; by entering the table with the neareſt latitude to that given, and the given declination in degrees. It is conſtructed by art. 216.

EXAM. I. *In latitude 50° N., when the Sun's declination is 16° N., and the interval between the morning and afternoon obſervation is 5 hours: what correction muſt be applied to the middle time, to give the time of apparent noon?*

In the table, art. 317, againſt 16° of declination taken in the outſide column, and under 50° latitude, and 5 hours, with N. declination, ſtand 12 ſeconds; which 12 ſ. applied to the middle time between the obſervations, give the time when the Sun was on the meridian.
The correction is applied to the middle time by the precepts at the bottom of the table.

298. EXAM. II. *In latitude 50° N., on November 16th, 1761, obſervations at equal altitudes of the Sun were taken at the following times ſhewn by a clock, the equal altitude inſtrument having three horizontal wires.*

Morning obſervations.		Afternoon obſervations.	
⊙ preceding limb	⊙ following limb	⊙ preceding limb	⊙ following limb
$9^h\ 28^m\ 55''$	$9^h\ 35^m\ 21\frac{1}{2}''$	$1^h\ 46^m\ 43\frac{1}{2}''$	$1^h\ 53^m\ 30\frac{1}{2}''$
9 32 $46\frac{1}{2}$	9 39 $23\frac{1}{2}$	1 50 $53\frac{1}{2}$	1 57 $28\frac{1}{2}$
9 36 $44\frac{1}{2}$	9 43 30	1 54 56	2 1 $20\frac{1}{2}$

Now

$$\frac{9^h\ 28^m\ 55'' + 2^h\ 1^m\ 20\tfrac{1}{2}'' + 12^h}{2} = 11^h\ 45^m\ 7\tfrac{1}{4}''$$

$$\frac{9\ 32\ 46\tfrac{1}{2} + 1\ 57\ 28\tfrac{1}{2} + 12}{2} = 11\ 45\ 7\tfrac{1}{2}$$

$$\frac{9\ 36\ 44\tfrac{1}{2} + 1\ 53\ 30\tfrac{1}{2} + 12}{2} = 11\ 45\ 7\tfrac{1}{2}$$

the mean $= 11^h\ 45^m\ 7{,}6''$ by the preceding limb.

Again

$$\frac{9\ 35\ 21\tfrac{1}{2} + 1\ 54\ 56 + 12}{2} = 11\ 45\ 8\tfrac{3}{4}$$

$$\frac{9\ 39\ 23\tfrac{1}{2} + 1\ 50\ 53\tfrac{1}{2} + 12}{2} = 11\ 45\ 8\tfrac{1}{2}$$

$$\frac{9\ 43\ 30 + 1\ 46\ 43\tfrac{1}{2} + 12}{2} = 11\ 45\ 6\tfrac{3}{4}$$

the mean $= 11^h\ 45^m\ 8''$ by the following limb.

The mean time of obſervation from both limbs is 11 h. 45 m. 7,8 ſ.
The declination on the day of obſervation is 19° S. nearly; the interval between the obſervations is about 4 hours; and theſe give + 14 ſeconds for the correction of the middle time.
So the Sun was on the meridian when the clock ſhewed 11 h. 45 m. 21,8 ſ.
The Sun's place, at that time, was $7^s\ 24°\ 26'\ 46''$ nearly.
In table 316, to $7^s\ 24°$ the tabular difference is 12′, decreaſing.

Then

Then 60′ : 26,75′ : : 12 ſ. : 5,35 ſ.; and + 14 m. 56 ſ. — $5\frac{1}{3}$ ſ. = + 14 m. $50\frac{1}{3}$ ſ., which is the equation of time: hence 11 h. 45 m. 21,8 ſ. + 14 m. 50,6 ſ. = 12 h. 0 m. 12,4 ſ.
Which ſhews that the clock was 12 ſ., nearly, too faſt.

299. X. *Tables of Refraction and of the Sun's parallax.* (318,319)

Theſe tables are the reſult of the experience of ſome of the moſt eminent Aſtronomers. By the refraction of the atmoſphere, objects appear more elevated than they really are, and therefore the apparent altitude is to be diminiſhed by the refraction, which is greateſt near the horizon, and gradually diminiſhes towards the zenith, where there is no refraction. The parallax in altitude is the difference between the altitude of an object, as ſeen from the cente rand ſurface of the Earth, that from the center being the true altitude, and the greateſt, except at the zenith, where parallax vaniſhes; therefore the apparent altitude is to be augmented by the parallax.

EXAM. *The Sun's apparent altitude was obſerved to be* 18° 34′ 48″; *what was his true altitude?*

Apparent altitude	18°	34′	48″	Refraction	2′ 47″	—
Correction is —		2	38	Parallax	9	+
Sun's true altitude	18	32	10.			

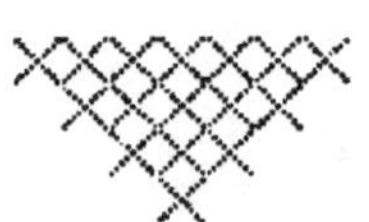

300.

ASTRONOMICAL TABLES,

Fitted, in general, to the meridian of GREENWICH.

The tables of the Sun's place, declination, and right aſcenſion, are fitted to the years 1792, 1793, 1794, 1795; and will ſerve in moſt nautical operations as well for the four years preceding, viz. 1788, 1789, 1790, 1791, and alſo for the four years following, viz. 1796, 1797, 1798, 1799, as is mentioned at the heads of thoſe tables. But as a Nautical Almanack is publiſhed yearly under the direction of the commiſſioners of longitude, the tables contained therein ſhould be conſulted in caſes where the utmoſt preciſion is neceſſary.

TABLES of the MEAN MOTIONS of the SUN and his APOGEE to MEAN SOLAR TIME.

301

For years absolute.							
Years.	M. lon. ☉ s	°	'	"	M. lon. ap. °	'	"
1	11	29	45	[illegible]		1	5
2	11	29	31	[illegible]		2	10
3	11	29	17	1		3	15
4	0	0	1	49		4	20
5	11	29	47	29		5	25
6	11	29	33	10		6	30
7	11	29	18	50		7	35
8	0	0	3	39		8	40
9	11	29	49	19		9	45
10	11	29	34	59		10	50
11	11	29	20	39		11	55
12	0	0	5	28		13	0
13	11	29	51	8		14	5
14	11	29	36	48		15	10
15	11	29	22	29		16	15
16	0	0	7	17		17	20
17	11	29	52	57		18	25
18	11	29	38	38		19	30
19	11	29	24	18		20	35
20	0	0	9	6		21	40
30	11	29	44	5		32	30
40	0	0	18	13		43	20
50	11	29	53	11		54	10
60	0	0	27	19	1	5	0
70	0	0	2	18	1	15	50
80	0	0	36	26	1	26	40
90	0	0	11	24	1	37	30
100	0	0	45	32	1	48	20
500	0	3	47	40	9	1	40
1000	0	7	35	20	18	3	20

302

For the radical years, new stile.																	
Years.	M. lon. ☉ s	°	'	"	M. lon. ap. s	°	'	"	Years.	M. lon. ☉ s	°	'	"	M. lon. ap. s	°	'	"
B 1752	9	10	31	29	3	8	38	45	1782	9	10	15	34	3	9	11	15
53		10	17	9			39	50	83		10	1	15			12	20
54		10	2	49			40	55	B 1784		10	46	3			13	25
55		9	48	30			42	0	85		10	31	43			14	30
B 1756		10	33	18			43	5	86		10	17	24			15	35
57		10	18	58			44	10	87		10	3	4			16	40
58	9	10	4	39	3	8	45	15	B 1788	9	10	47	53	3	9	17	45
59		9	50	19			46	20	89		10	33	33			18	50
B 1760		10	35	8			47	25	90		10	19	13			19	55
61		10	20	48			48	30	91		10	4	53			21	0
62		10	6	28			49	35	B 1792		10	49	42			22	5
63		9	52	8			50	40	93		10	35	22			23	10
B 1764	9	10	36	57	3	8	51	45	94	9	10	21	2	3	9	24	15
65		10	22	37			52	50	95		10	6	42			25	20
66		10	8	17			53	55	B 1796		10	51	31			26	25
67		9	53	58			55	0	97		10	37	11			27	30
B 1768		10	38	46			56	5	98		10	22	52			28	35
69		10	24	26			57	10	99		10	8	32			29	40
70	9	10	10	[illegible]	3	8	58	15	C 1800	9	9	54	12	3	9	30	45
71		9	55	47			59	20	B 1820		10	3	18			52	25
B 1772		10	40	35		9	0	25	B 1840		10	12	25	3	10	14	5
73		10	26	16			1	30	B 1860		10	21	31			35	45
74		10	11	56			2	35	B 1880		10	30	38			57	25
75		9	57	36			3	40	C 1900		9	40	36		11	19	5
B 1776	9	10	42	25	3	9	4	45	B 1920	9	9	49	42	3	11	40	45
77		10	28	5			5	50	B 1940		9	58	48		12	2	25
78		10	13	45			6	55	B 1960		10	7	55			24	5
79		9	59	25			8	0	B 1980		10	17	1			45	45
B 1780		10	44	14			9	5	B 2000		10	26	8		13	7	25
81		10	29	54			10	10	C 2100		10	12	31		14	55	45

303

For hours, minutes, and secs.							
H	Lon. ☉ '	"	‴	M	Lon. ☉ '	"	‴
1	2	27	51	31	1	16	23
2	4	55	42	32	1	18	51
3	7	23	32	33	1	21	19
4	9	51	23	34	1	23	47
5	12	19	14	35	1	26	15
6	14	47	5	36	1	28	42
7	17	14	56	37	1	31	10
8	19	42	47	38	1	33	38
9	22	10	37	39	1	36	6
10	24	38	28	40	1	38	34
11	27	6	19	41	1	41	2
12	29	34	10	42	1	43	30
13	32	2	1	43	1	45	57
14	34	29	52	44	1	48	25
15	36	57	42	45	1	50	53
16	39	25	33	46	1	53	21
17	41	53	24	47	1	55	49
18	44	21	15	48	1	58	17
19	46	49	6	49	2	0	44
20	49	16	56	50	2	3	12
21	51	44	47	51	2	5	40
22	54	12	38	52	2	8	8
23	56	40	29	53	2	10	36
24	59	8	20	54	2	13	4
25	61	36	11	55	2	15	32
26	64	4	1	56	2	17	59
27	66	31	52	57	2	20	27
28	68	59	43	58	2	22	55
29	71	27	34	59	2	25	23
30	73	55	25	60	2	27	51

TABLE of the MEAN MOTIONS of the SUN and APOGEE to MONTHS and DAYS.

…ry.	March.	April.	May.	June.	July.	August.	September.	October.	November.	December.	
…on.	☉ M. lon.	☉ M. lon.	☉ M. lon.	☉ M. lon.	☉ M. lon.	☉ M. lon.	☉ M. lon.	☉ M. lon.	☉ M. lon.	☉ M. lon.	Days.
′ ″	s ° ′ ″	s ° ′ ″	s ° ′ ″	s ° ′ ″	s ° ′ ″	s ° ′ ″	s ° ′ ″	s ° ′ ″	s ° ′ ″	s ° ′ ″	
2 27	1 29 8 20	2 29 41 38	2 29 15 48	4 29 49 6	5 29 23 16	6 29 56 34	8 0 29 52	9 0 4 2	10 0 37 20	11 0 11 30	1
1 35	2 0 7 28	3 0 40 46	4 0 14 56	5 0 48 14	6 0 22 24	7 0 55 42	1 29 1	1 3 11	1 36 29	1 10 39	2
0 43	1 6 36	1 39 55	1 14 4	1 47 23	1 21 33	1 54 51	2 28 9	2 2 19	2 35 37	2 9 47	3
9 52	2 5 45	2 39 3	2 13 13	2 46 31	2 20 41	2 53 59	3 27 17	3 1 27	3 34 45	3 8 55	4
9 0	3 4 53	3 38 11	3 12 21	3 45 39	3 19 49	3 53 7	4 26 26	4 0 36	4 33 54	4 8 4	5
8 8	4 4 1	4 37 20	4 11 29	4 44 48	4 18 58	4 52 16	5 25 34	4 59 44	5 33 2	5 7 12	6
7 16	5 3 10	5 36 28	5 10 38	5 43 56	5 18 6	5 51 24	6 24 42	5 58 52	6 32 10	6 6 20	7
6 25	6 2 18	6 35 36	6 9 46	6 43 4	6 17 14	6 50 32	7 23 51	6 58 1	7 31 19	7 5 29	8
5 33	7 1 26	7 34 45	7 8 55	7 42 13	7 16 22	7 49 41	8 22 59	7 57 9	8 30 27	8 4 37	9
4 41	8 0 35	8 33 53	8 8 3	8 41 21	8 15 31	8 48 49	9 22 7	8 56 17	9 29 36	9 3 45	10
3 50	8 59 43	9 33 1	9 7 11	9 40 29	9 14 39	9 47 57	10 21 16	9 55 26	10 28 44	10 2 54	11
2 58	9 58 51	10 32 10	10 6 19	10 39 38	10 13 48	10 47 6	11 20 24	10 54 34	11 27 52	11 2 2	12
2 6	10 58 0	11 31 18	11 5 28	11 38 46	11 12 56	11 46 14	12 19 32	11 53 42	12 27 0	12 1 10	13
1 15	11 57 8	12 30 26	12 4 36	12 37 54	12 12 4	12 45 22	13 18 41	12 52 51	13 26 9	13 0 19	14
0 23	12 56 16	13 29 35	13 3 44	13 37 3	13 11 13	13 44 31	14 17 49	13 51 59	14 25 17	13 59 27	15
9 31	13 55 25	14 28 43	14 2 53	14 36 11	14 10 21	14 43 39	15 16 57	14 51 7	15 24 25	14 58 35	16
8 40	14 54 33	15 27 51	15 2 1	15 35 19	15 9 29	15 42 47	16 16 6	15 50 16	16 23 34	15 57 44	17
7 48	15 53 4	16 27 0	16 1 9	16 34 28	16 8 38	16 41 56	17 15 14	16 49 24	17 22 42	16 56 52	18
6 56	16 52 50	17 26 8	17 0 18	17 33 36	17 7 46	17 41 4	18 14 22	17 48 32	18 21 50	17 56 0	19
6 5	17 51 58	18 25 16	17 59 26	18 32 44	18 6 54	18 40 12	19 13 31	18 47 40	19 20 59	18 55 9	20
5 13	18 51 6	19 24 25	18 58 34	19 31 53	19 6 3	19 39 21	20 12 39	19 46 49	20 20 7	19 54 17	21
4 21	19 50 15	20 23 33	19 57 43	20 31 1	20 5 11	20 38 29	21 11 47	20 45 57	21 19 15	20 53 25	22
3 30	20 49 23	21 22 41	20 56 51	21 30 9	21 4 19	21 37 37	22 10 56	21 45 5	22 18 24	21 52 34	23
2 38	21 48 31	22 21 50	21 55 59	22 29 18	22 3 28	22 36 46	23 10 4	22 44 14	23 17 32	22 51 42	24
1 40	22 47 40	23 20 58	22 55 8	23 28 26	23 2 36	23 35 54	24 9 12	23 43 22	24 16 40	23 50 50	25
0 55	23 46 48	24 20 6	23 54 16	24 27 34	24 1 44	24 35 2	25 8 21	24 42 30	25 15 49	24 49 59	26
0 3	24 45 56	25 19 15	24 53 24	25 26 43	25 0 52	25 34 11	26 7 29	25 41 39	26 14 57	25 49 7	27
9 11	25 45 5	26 18 23	25 52 33	26 25 51	26 0 1	26 33 19	27 6 37	26 40 47	27 14 5	26 48 15	28
	26 44 13	27 17 31	26 51 41	27 24 59	26 59 9	27 32 27	28 5 46	27 39 55	28 13 14	27 47 23	29
	27 43 21	28 16 40	27 50 49	28 24 8	27 58 17	28 31 36	29 4 54	28 39 4	29 12 22	28 46 32	30
	28 42 30		28 49 58		28 57 26	29 30 44		29 38 12		29 45 40	31
0 10	0 16	0 21	0 27	0 32	0 38	0 43	0 49	0 54	0 59	1 5	

305. TABLE of the EQUATION of the SUN's CENTER to each sign and degree of mean Anomaly.

Deg.	0 Subt. ° ′ ″	Diff. ′ ″	I. Subt. ° ′ ″	Diff. ′ ″	II. Subt. ° ′ ″	Diff. ′ ″	III. Subt. ° ′ ″	Diff. ′ ″	IV. Subt. ° ′ ″	Diff. ′ ″	V. Subt. ° ′ ″	Diff. ′ ″	Deg.
0	0 0 0	1 59	0 56 47	1 43	1 39 6	1 1	1 55 37	0 2	1 41 12	1 0	0 58 53	1 46	30
1	1 59	58	58 30	42	40 7	0 59	55 39	1	40 12	2	57 7	48	29
2	3 57	59	1 0 12	41	41 6	57	55 38	2	39 10	4	55 19	49	28
3	5 56	58	1 53	40	42 3	56	55 36	5	38 6	6	53 30	50	27
4	7 54	58	3 33	39	42 59	53	55 31	7	37 0	8	51 40	51	26
5	9 52	58	5 12	38	43 52	52	55 24	9	35 52	9	49 49	52	25
6	0 11 50	1 58	1 6 50	1 37	1 44 44	0 50	1 55 15	0 12	1 34 43	1 11	0 47 57	1 52	24
7	13 48	58	8 27	35	45 34	48	55 3	13	33 32	13	46 5	54	23
8	15 46	57	10 2	34	46 22	46	54 50	15	32 19	15	44 11	55	22
9	17 43	57	11 36	33	47 8	45	54 35	18	31 4	17	42 16	55	21
10	19 40	57	13 9	32	47 53	42	54 17	20	29 47	18	40 21	56	20
11	21 37	56	14 41	30	48 35	40	53 57	21	28 29	20	38 25	57	19
12	0 23 33	1 56	1 16 11	1 29	1 49 15	0 39	1 53 36	0 24	1 27 9	1 21	0 36 28	1 58	18
13	25 29	56	17 40	28	49 54	36	53 12	26	25 48	23	34 30	58	17
14	27 25	55	19 8	26	50 30	35	52 46	28	24 25	25	32 32	59	16
15	29 20	55	20 34	25	51 5	32	52 18	30	23 0	26	30 33	2 0	15
16	31 15	54	21 59	23	51 37	31	51 48	33	21 34	28	28 33	0	14
17	33 9	53	23 22	22	52 8	28	51 15	34	20 6	30	26 33	0	13
18	0 35 2	1 53	1 24 44	1 21	1 52 36	0 27	1 50 41	0 36	1 18 36	1 31	0 24 33	2 1	12
19	36 55	52	26 5	19	53 3	24	50 5	39	17 5	32	22 32	2	11
20	38 47	52	27 24	17	53 27	23	49 26	40	15 33	34	20 30	2	10
21	40 39	51	28 41	16	53 50	20	48 46	43	13 59	35	18 28	2	9
22	42 30	50	29 57	14	54 10	18	48 3	44	12 24	37	16 26	2	8
23	44 20	49	31 11	13	54 28	16	47 19	47	10 47	38	14 24	3	7
24	0 46 9	1 48	1 32 24	1 11	1 54 44	0 14	1 46 32	0 48	1 9 9	1 40	0 12 21	2 3	6
25	47 57	48	33 35	10	54 58	12	45 44	51	7 29	40	10 18	4	5
26	49 45	47	34 45	8	55 10	10	44 53	52	5 49	42	8 14	3	4
27	51 32	46	35 53	6	55 20	8	44 1	54	4 7	43	6 11	4	3
28	53 18	45	36 59	4	55 28	6	43 7	57	2 24	45	4 7	3	2
29	55 3	1 44	38 3	1 3	55 34	3	42 10	0 58	0 39	46	2 4	4	1
30	0 56 47		1 39 6		1 55 37		1 41 12		0 58 53		0 0 0		0
	XI. Add.	Diff.	X. Add.	Diff.	IX. Add.	Diff.	VIII. Add.	Diff.	VII. Add.	Diff.	VI. Add.	Diff.	

306. TABLE of the SUN's DECLINATION to each ſign and degree of longitude.

Deg.	♈ 0 ♎ 6 ⊙ decl. ° ′ ″	Diff. ′ ″	♉ 1 ♏ 7 ⊙ decl. ° ′ ″	Diff. ′ ″	♊ 2 ♐ 8 ⊙ decl. ° ′ ″	Diff. ′ ″	Deg.
0	0 0 0	23 53	11 29 5	21 1	20 10 25	12 32	30
1	0 23 53	23 54	11 50 6	20 50	20 22 57	12 10	29
2	0 47 47	23 52	12 10 56	20 38	20 35 7	11 48	28
3	1 11 39	23 51	12 31 34	20 25	20 46 55	11 25	27
4	1 35 30	23 50	12 51 59	20 13	20 58 20	11 1	26
5	1 59 20	23 48	13 12 12	20 0	21 9 21	10 38	25
6	2 23 8	23 46	13 32 12	19 46	21 19 59	10 14	24
7	2 46 54	23 43	13 51 58	19 32	21 30 13	9 50	23
8	3 10 37	23 40	14 11 30	19 18	21 40 3	9 26	22
9	3 34 17	23 37	14 30 48	19 4	21 49 29	9 1	21
10	3 57 54	23 33	14 49 52	18 45	21 58 30	8 36	20
11	4 21 27	23 30	15 8 40	18 33	22 7 6	8 11	19
12	4 44 57	23 25	15 27 13	18 17	22 15 17	7 46	18
13	5 8 22	23 20	15 45 30	18 1	22 23 3	7 21	17
14	5 31 42	23 15	16 3 31	17 45	22 30 24	6 54	16
15	5 54 57	23 9	16 21 16	17 28	22 37 18	6 29	15
16	6 18 6	23 3	16 38 44	17 11	22 43 47	6 3	14
17	6 41 9	22 57	16 55 55	16 53	22 49 50	5 37	13
18	7 4 6	22 51	17 12 48	16 35	22 55 27	5 11	12
19	7 26 57	22 43	17 29 23	16 17	23 0 38	4 44	11
20	7 49 41	22 36	17 45 40	15 58	23 5 22	4 17	10
21	8 12 17	22 28	18 1 38	15 40	23 9 39	3 50	9
22	8 34 45	22 20	18 17 18	15 20	23 13 29	3 24	8
23	8 57 5	22 11	18 32 38	15 0	23 16 53	2 57	7
24	9 19 17	22 2	18 47 38	14 40	23 19 50	2 30	6
25	9 41 19	21 53	19 2 18	14 19	23 22 20	2 2	5
26	10 3 12	21 44	19 16 37	13 58	23 24 22	1 35	4
27	10 24 56	21 34	19 30 35	13 38	23 25 57	1 8	3
28	10 46 30	21 23	19 44 13	13 17	23 27 5	0 41	2
29	11 7 53	21 12	19 57 30	12 55	23 27 46	0 14	1
30	11 29 5		20 10 25		23 28 0		0
D	♓ 11 ♍	Diff.	♒ 10 ♌ 4	Diff.	♑ 9 ♋ 3	Diff.	D

307. TABLE of the SUN's RIGHT ASCENSION to each ſign and degree of longitude.

Deg.	♈ 0 ♎ 6 ⊙ rt. aſ. h. m. ſ.	Diff. m. ſ.	♉ 1 ♏ 7 ⊙ rt. aſ. h. m. ſ.	Diff. m. ſ.	♊ 2 ♐ 8 ⊙ rt. aſ. h. m. ſ.	Diff. m. ſ.	♋ 3 ♑ 9 ⊙ rt. aſ. h. m. ſ.	Diff. m. ſ.	♌ 4 ♒ 10 ⊙ rt. aſ. h. m. ſ.	Diff. m. ſ.	♍ 5 ♓ 11 ⊙ rt. aſ. h. m. ſ.	Diff. m. ſ.	Deg.
0	0 0 0	3 40	1 51 37	3 50	3 51 15	4 10	6 0 0	4 22	8 8 45	4 9	10 8 23	3 49	0
1	3 40	3 40	55 27	3 50	55 25	4 11	4 22	4 21	12 54	4 9	12 12	3 48	1
2	7 20	3 41	59 17	3 51	59 36	4 12	8 43	4 22	17 3	4 8	16 0	3 48	2
3	11 1	3 40	2 3 8	3 51	4 3 48	4 12	13 5	4 21	21 11	4 8	19 48	3 47	3
4	14 41	3 40	6 59	3 52	8 0	4 13	17 26	4 21	25 19	4 7	23 35	3 47	4
5	18 21	3 41	10 51	3 53	12 13	4 13	21 47	4 22	27 26	4 6	27 22	3 46	5
6	22 2	3 40	14 44	3 53	16 26	4 14	26 9	4 21	33 32	4 5	31 8	3 46	6
7	0 25 42	3 41	2 18 37	3 54	4 20 40	4 15	6 30 30	4 21	8 37 37	4 4	10 34 54	3 46	7
8	29 23	3 41	22 31	3 54	24 55	4 15	34 51	4 20	41 41	4 4	38 40	3 45	8
9	33 4	3 41	26 25	3 55	29 10	4 16	39 11	4 20	45 45	4 3	42 25	3 44	9
10	36 45	3 41	30 20	3 56	33 26	4 16	43 31	4 20	49 48	4 3	46 9	3 44	10
11	40 26	3 42	34 16	3 57	37 42	4 17	47 51	4 20	51 51	4 1	49 53	3 44	11
12	44 8	3 42	38 13	3 57	41 59	4 17	52 11	4 19	57 52	4 1	53 37	3 43	12
13	0 47 50	3 42	2 42 10	3 58	4 46 16	4 18	6 56 30	4 19	9 1 53	4 0	10 57 20	3 43	13
14	51 32	3 42	46 8	3 59	50 34	4 18	7 0 49	4 19	5 53	4 0	11 1 3	3 43	14
15	55 14	3 43	50 7	4 0	54 52	4 19	5 8	4 18	9 53	3 59	4 46	3 42	15
16	58 57	3 43	54 7	4 0	59 11	4 19	9 26	4 18	13 52	3 58	8 28	3 42	16
17	1 2 40	3 43	58 7	4 1	5 3 30	4 19	13 44	4 17	17 50	3 57	12 10	3 42	17
18	6 23	3 44	3 2 8	4 1	7 49	4 20	18 1	4 17	21 47	3 57	15 52	3 42	18
19	1 10 7	3 44	3 6 9	4 3	5 12 9	4 20	7 22 18	4 16	9 25 44	3 56	11 19 34	3 41	19
20	13 51	3 45	10 12	4 3	16 29	4 20	26 34	4 16	29 40	3 55	23 15	3 41	20
21	17 36	3 45	14 15	4 4	20 49	4 20	30 50	4 15	33 35	3 54	26 56	3 41	21
22	21 21	3 45	18 19	4 4	25 9	4 21	35 5	4 15	37 29	3 54	30 37	3 41	22
23	25 6	3 46	22 23	4 5	29 30	4 21	39 20	4 14	41 23	3 53	34 18	3 40	23
24	28 52	3 46	26 28	4 6	33 51	4 21	43 34	4 13	45 16	3 53	37 58	3 41	24
25	1 32 38	3 47	3 30 34	4 7	5 38 12	4 22	7 47 47	4 13	9 49 9	3 52	11 41 39	3 40	25
26	36 25	3 47	34 41	4 8	42 34	4 21	52 0	4 12	53 1	3 51	45 19	3 41	26
27	40 12	3 48	38 49	4 8	46 55	4 22	56 12	4 12	56 52	3 51	59 0	3 40	27
28	44 0	3 48	42 57	4 9	51 17	4 21	8 0 24	4 11	10 0 43	3 50	52 40	3 40	28
29	47 48	3 49	47 6	4 9	55 38	4 22	4 35	4 10	4 33	3 50	56 20	3 40	29
30	51 37		51 15		6 0 0		8 45		8 23		12 0 0		30
D		Diff.		Diff.		Diff.		Diff.		Diff.		Diff.	D

A TABLE of the SUN'S LONGITUDE for the Years 1788, 1792, and 1796, being Leap Years.

Days.	January.	February.	March.	April.	May.	June
	s ° ′ ″	s ° ′ ″	s ° ′ ″	s ° ′ ″	s ° ′ ″	s ° ′ ″
1	9 10 51 0	10 12 24 16	11 11 38 33	0 12 25 13	1 11 41 51	2 11 31 22
2	11 52 20	13 25 6	12 38 38	13 24 15	12 39 56	12 28 47
3	12 53 31	14 25 55	13 38 39	14 23 13	13 38 0	13 26 12
4	13 54 42	15 26 42	14 38 39	15 22 11	14 36 2	14 23 35
5	14 55 53	16 27 30	15 38 38	16 21 6	15 34 1	15 20 57
6	15 57 4	17 28 15	16 38 34	17 20 0	16 31 59	16 18 19
7	16 58 15	18 28 59	17 38 28	18 18 52	17 29 57	17 15 40
8	17 59 25	19 29 41	18 38 21	19 17 41	18 27 53	18 13 0
9	19 0 34	20 30 22	19 38 12	20 16 29	19 25 49	19 10 20
10	20 1 44	21 31 1	20 38 1	21 15 14	20 23 39	20 7 39
11	21 2 53	22 31 39	21 37 47	22 13 58	21 21 30	21 4 56
12	22 4 1	23 32 16	22 37 31	23 12 39	22 19 19	22 2 14
13	23 5 8	24 32 51	23 37 13	24 11 19	23 17 7	22 59 31
14	24 6 15	25 33 24	24 36 54	25 9 56	24 14 54	23 56 48
15	25 7 22	26 33 56	25 36 33	26 8 32	25 12 39	24 54 3
16	26 8 28	27 34 27	26 36 9	27 7 6	26 10 24	25 51 18
17	27 9 35	28 34 56	27 35 43	28 5 38	27 8 6	26 48 32
18	28 10 41	29 35 22	28 35 16	29 4 7	28 5 48	27 45 47
19	29 11 45	11 0 35 47	29 34 46	1 0 2 36	29 3 28	28 43 2
20	10 0 12 48	1 36 12	0 0 34 14	1 1 2	2 0 1 7	29 40 16
21	1 13 50	2 36 34	1 33 40	1 59 27	0 58 44	3 0 37 30
22	2 14 53	3 36 55	2 33 4	2 57 49	1 56 20	1 34 44
23	3 15 54	4 37 13	3 32 26	3 56 9	2 53 55	2 31 55
24	4 16 53	5 37 30	4 31 47	4 54 28	3 51 30	3 29 6
25	5 17 52	6 37 45	5 31 5	5 52 45	4 49 3	4 26 19
26	6 18 51	7 37 58	6 30 21	6 51 1	5 46 34	5 23 33
27	7 19 47	8 38 10	7 29 35	7 49 14	6 44 6	6 20 44
28	8 20 43	9 38 20	8 28 46	8 47 26	7 41 35	7 17 57
29	9 21 38	10 38 28	9 27 54	9 45 37	8 39 3	8 15 8
30	10 22 32		10 27 1	10 43 44	9 36 30	9 12 20
31	11 23 24		11 26 8		10 33 57	

July.	August	September.	October.	November.	December.	Days.
s ° ′ ″	s ° ′ ″	s ° ′ ″	s ° ′ ″	s ° ′ ″	s ° ′ ″	
3 10 9 32	4 9 45 27	5 9 36 39	6 8 55 50	7 9 45 30	8 10 3 3	1
11 6 45	10 42 54	10 34 50	9 54 59	10 45 41	11 3 59	2
12 3 56	11 40 23	11 33 1	10 54 10	11 45 55	12 4 56	3
13 1 9	12 37 54	12 31 17	11 53 24	12 46 10	13 5 56	4
13 58 21	13 35 24	13 29 35	12 52 39	13 46 26	14 6 55	5
14 55 33	14 32 56	14 27 51	13 51 57	14 46 45	15 7 54	6
15 52 44	15 30 30	15 26 12	14 51 18	15 47 6	16 8 55	7
16 49 59	16 28 5	16 24 33	15 50 39	16 47 28	17 9 57	8
17 47 12	17 25 41	17 22 57	16 50 2	17 47 53	18 11 1	9
18 44 25	18 23 17	18 21 23	17 49 29	18 48 18	19 12 5	10
19 41 37	19 20 54	19 19 52	18 48 57	19 48 45	20 13 9	11
20 38 52	20 18 34	20 18 20	19 48 26	20 49 14	21 14 14	12
21 36 6	21 16 15	21 16 51	20 47 59	21 49 44	22 15 20	13
22 33 20	22 13 57	22 15 25	21 47 33	22 50 17	23 16 27	14
23 30 34	23 11 40	23 13 59	22 47 9	23 50 50	24 17 34	15
24 27 50	24 9 24	24 12 36	23 46 47	24 51 25	25 18 41	16
25 25 7	25 7 11	25 11 15	24 46 28	25 52 3	26 19 50	17
26 22 25	26 4 57	26 9 56	25 46 10	26 52 41	27 20 58	18
27 19 40	27 2 46	27 8 39	26 45 54	27 53 20	28 22 7	19
28 16 58	28 0 36	28 7 24	27 45 41	28 54 2	29 23 17	20
29 14 16	28 58 28	29 6 10	28 45 29	29 54 44	9 0 24 26	21
4 0 11 35	29 56 21	6 0 4 59	29 45 19	8 0 55 29	1 25 37	22
1 8 55	5 0 54 15	1 3 50	7 0 45 12	1 56 14	2 26 46	23
2 6 15	1 52 12	2 2 43	1 45 6	2 57 1	3 27 57	24
3 3 36	2 50 9	3 1 38	2 45 2	3 57 50	4 29 8	25
4 0 58	3 48 8	4 0 36	3 45 1	4 58 38	5 30 20	26
4 58 20	4 46 9	4 59 34	4 45 1	5 59 28	6 31 30	27
5 55 44	5 44 11	5 58 35	5 45 3	7 0 21	7 32 42	28
6 53 8	6 42 16	6 57 38	6 45 6	8 1 14	8 33 53	29
7 50 34	7 40 22	7 56 44	7 45 12	9 2 8	9 35 5	30
8 48 0	8 38 30		8 45 19		10 36 18	31

308 A TABLE of the SUN's LONGITUDE for the Years 1789, 1793, and 1797, being the first after Leap Year.

Days.	January.	February.	March.	April.	May.	June.	July.	August.	September.	October.	November.	December.	Days.
	s ° ′ ″	s ° ′ ″	s ° ′ ″	s ° ′ ″	s ° ′ ″	s ° ′ ″	s ° ′ ″	s ° ′ ″	s ° ′ ″	s ° ′ ″	s ° ′ ″	s ° ′ ″	
1	9 11 37 28	10 13 10 21	11 11 23 57	0 12 10 54	1 11 27 47	2 11 17 32	3 9 55 42	4 9 31 32	5 10 22 34	6 8 41 30	7 9 30 53	8 9 48 16	1
2	12 38 39	14 11 9	12 24 2	13 9 57	12 25 53	12 14 55	10 52 55	10 29 0	10 20 44	9 40 38	10 31 4	10 49 11	2
3	13 39 5	15 11 58	13 24 6	14 8 57	13 23 57	13 12 20	11 50 7	11 26 30	11 18 57	10 39 49	11 31 17	11 50 8	3
4	14 41 0	16 12 45	14 24 6	15 7 55	14 21 59	14 9 43	12 47 19	12 24 0	12 17 11	11 39 3	12 31 32	12 51 6	4
5	15 42 12	17 13 30	15 24 5	16 6 50	15 20 0	15 7 4	13 44 31	13 21 30	13 15 27	12 38 17	13 31 48	13 52 5	5
6	16 43 23	18 14 15	16 24 2	17 5 44	16 17 59	16 4 27	14 41 43	14 19 2	14 13 44	13 37 35	14 32 6	14 53 5	6
7	17 44 32	19 14 58	17 23 57	18 4 37	17 15 56	17 1 48	15 38 56	15 16 34	15 12 4	14 36 55	15 32 27	15 54 7	7
8	18 45 41	20 15 38	18 23 50	19 3 27	18 13 51	17 59 8	16 36 8	16 14 9	16 10 26	15 36 15	16 32 48	16 55 8	8
9	19 46 52	21 16 18	19 23 41	20 2 17	19 11 46	18 56 28	17 33 21	17 11 44	17 8 48	16 35 38	17 33 12	17 56 10	9
10	20 48 0	22 16 57	20 23 20	21 1 2	20 9 39	19 53 46	18 30 35	18 9 20	18 7 13	17 35 4	18 33 38	18 57 14	10
11	21 49 10	23 17 34	21 23 16	21 59 43	21 7 31	20 51 4	19 27 47	19 6 58	19 5 41	18 34 31	19 34 4	19 58 18	11
12	22 50 17	24 18 9	22 23 1	22 58 26	22 5 20	21 48 20	20 25 2	20 4 37	20 4 10	19 34 0	20 34 32	20 59 23	12
13	23 51 26	25 18 42	23 22 44	23 57 6	23 3 8	22 45 38	21 22 17	21 2 17	21 2 40	20 33 32	21 35 2	22 0 28	13
14	24 52 33	26 19 15	24 22 26	24 55 45	24 0 56	23 42 56	22 19 30	21 59 58	22 1 13	21 33 6	22 35 34	23 1 35	14
15	25 53 39	27 19 46	25 22 5	25 54 21	24 58 42	24 40 11	23 16 45	22 57 41	22 59 48	22 32 41	23 36 8	24 2 43	15
16	26 54 45	28 20 15	26 21 42	26 52 55	25 56 26	25 37 27	24 14 1	23 55 23	23 58 24	23 12 18	24 36 42	25 3 50	16
17	27 55 51	29 20 42	27 21 17	27 51 28	26 54 9	26 34 42	25 11 16	24 53 9	24 57 3	24 31 59	25 37 19	26 4 59	17
18	28 56 54	11 0 21 8	28 20 49	28 49 57	27 51 50	27 31 55	26 8 33	25 50 57	25 55 43	25 31 41	26 37 58	27 6 6	18
19	29 57 59	1 21 32	29 20 20	29 48 26	28 49 30	28 29 10	27 5 50	26 48 46	26 54 25	26 31 25	27 33 36	28 7 14	19
20	10 0 59 2	2 21 55	0 0 19 48	1 0 46 53	29 47 10	29 26 25	28 3 6	27 46 36	27 53 10	27 31 11	28 39 17	29 8 25	20
21	2 0 3	3 22 16	1 19 16	1 45 18	2 0 44 48	3 0 23 38	29 0 25	28 44 28	28 51 55	28 30 58	29 39 59	9 0 9 35	21
22	3 1 4	4 22 34	2 18 41	2 43 41	1 42 24	1 20 52	29 57 44	29 42 20	29 50 44	29 30 49	8 0 40 42	1 10 44	22
23	4 2 3	5 22 52	3 18 3	3 42 1	2 40 0	2 18 5	4 0 55 3	5 0 40 15	6 0 49 35	7 0 30 40	1 41 27	2 11 55	23
24	5 3 2	6 23 7	4 17 24	4 40 21	3 37 34	3 15 17	1 52 24	1 38 11	1 48 28	1 30 34	2 42 14	3 13 4	24
25	6 4 1	7 23 21	5 16 43	5 38 39	4 35 7	4 12 29	2 49 44	2 36 8	2 47 21	2 30 29	3 43 2	4 14 16	25
26	7 4 58	8 23 33	6 15 59	6 36 55	5 32 39	5 9 42	3 47 6	3 34 6	3 46 18	3 30 27	4 43 51	5 15 28	26
27	8 5 44	9 23 42	7 15 14	7 35 9	6 30 10	6 6 54	4 44 29	4 32 7	4 45 16	4 30 26	5 44 40	6 16 39	27
28	9 6 50	10 23 51	8 14 26	8 33 21	7 27 40	7 4 8	5 41 52	5 30 9	5 44 16	5 30 29	6 45 31	7 17 50	28
29	10 7 43		9 13 36	9 31 32	8 25 9	8 1 20	6 39 16	6 28 13	6 43 19	6 30 32	7 46 25	8 19 1	29
30	11 8 36		10 12 44	10 29 41	9 22 36	8 58 33	7 36 41	7 26 18	7 42 24	7 30 37	8 47 20	9 20 13	30
31	12 9 29		11 11 52		10 20 3		8 34 7	8 24 26		8 30 45		10 21 15	31

 A TABLE of the SUN'S LONGITUDE for the Years 1790, 1794, 1798, being the second after Leap Year.

Days	January.				February.				March.				April.				May.				June.			
	s	°	′	″	s	°	′	″	s	°	′	″	s	°	′	″	s	°	′	″	s	°	′	″
1	9	11	22	35	10	12	55	32	11	11	9	23	0	11	56	36	1	11	13	44	2	11	3	30
2		12	23	48		13	56	22		12	9	29		12	55	38		12	11	43		12	1	2
3		13	24	58		14	57	12		13	9	31		13	54	39		13	19	54		12	58	27
4		14	26	10		15	57	59		14	9	33		14	53	37		14	7	56		13	55	51
5		15	27	21		16	58	45		15	9	32		15	52	34		15	5	57		14	53	12
6		16	28	31		17	59	30		16	9	29		16	51	29		16	3	57		15	50	35
7		17	29	42		19	0	13		17	9	24		17	50	21		17	1	55		16	47	56
8		18	30	51		20	0	53		18	9	18		18	49	12		17	59	51		17	45	17
9		19	32	0		21	1	34		19	9	9		19	48	1		18	57	45		18	42	37
10		20	33	10		22	2	13		20	8	59		20	46	46		19	55	38		19	39	55
11		21	34	20		23	2	50		21	8	46		21	45	31		20	53	20		20	37	14
12		22	35	26		24	3	26		22	8	32		22	44	14		21	51	20		21	34	32
13		23	36	34		25	4	1		23	8	15		23	42	54		22	49	9		22	31	49
14		24	37	42		26	4	34		24	7	57		24	41	33		23	46	56		23	29	5
15		25	38	50		27	5	5		25	7	37		25	40	9		24	44	44		24	26	22
16		26	39	55		28	5	34		26	7	14		26	38	44		25	42	28		25	23	37
17		27	41	0		29	6	1		27	6	50		27	37	17		26	40	11		26	20	50
18		28	42	4	11	0	6	28		28	6	23		28	35	48		27	37	53		27	18	4
19		29	43	8		1	6	54		29	5	55		29	34	17		28	35	33		28	15	18
20	10	0	44	11		2	7	17	0	0	5	24	1	0	32	44		29	33	13		29	12	30
21		1	45	12		3	7	38		1	4	51		1	31	10	2	0	30	52	3	0	9	43
22		2	46	14		4	7	58		2	4	17		2	29	33		1	28	29		1	6	55
23		3	47	15		5	8	14		3	3	39		3	27	54		2	26	4		2	4	7
24		4	48	14		6	8	30		4	3	1		4	26	14		3	23	39		3	1	9
25		5	49	12		7	8	45		5	2	20		5	24	32		4	21	12		3	58	31
26		6	50	11		8	8	57		6	1	37		6	22	48		5	18	44		4	55	41
27		7	51	6		9	9	8		7	0	51		7	21	3		6	16	15		5	52	52
28		8	52	3		10	9	17		8	0	5		8	19	16		7	13	46		6	50	4
29		9	52	56						8	59	15		9	17	27		8	11	16		7	47	16
30		10	53	50						9	58	25		10	15	38		9	8	44		8	44	27
31		11	54	42						10	57	32						10	6	10				

Days	July.				August.				September.				October.				November.				December.			
	s	°	′	″	s	°	′	″	s	°	′	″	s	°	′	″	s	°	′	″	s	°	′	″
1	3	9	41	55	4	9	17	39	5	9	8	29	6	8	27	10	7	9	16	17	8	9	33	28
2		10	39	5		10	15	6		10	6	39		9	26	19		10	16	27		10	34	23
3		11	36	18		11	12	34		11	4	51		10	25	28		11	16	41		11	35	20
4		12	33	30		12	10	5		12	3	5		11	24	41		12	16	55		12	36	18
5		13	30	41		13	7	35		13	1	20		12	23	55		13	17	10		13	37	17
6		14	27	55		14	5	7		13	59	38		13	23	12		14	17	28		14	38	16
7		15	25	7		15	2	39		14	57	58		14	22	31		15	17	47		15	39	16
8		16	22	18		16	0	13		15	56	18		15	21	51		16	18	9		16	40	17
9		17	19	32		16	57	48		16	54	40		16	21	14		17	18	33		17	41	21
10		18	16	45		17	55	24		17	53	5		17	20	39		18	18	57		18	42	24
11		19	13	58		18	53	1		18	51	32		18	20	7		19	19	23		19	43	29
12		20	11	10		19	50	40		19	50	0		19	19	36		20	19	53		20	44	34
13		21	8	25		20	48	20		20	48	20		20	19	6		21	20	21		21	45	40
14		22	5	40		21	46	1		21	47	3		21	18	40		22	20	53		22	46	45
15		23	2	54		22	43	44		22	45	36		22	18	14		23	21	26		23	47	51
16		24	0	10		23	41	28		23	44	12		23	17	51		24	22	0		24	49	0
17		24	57	25		24	39	13		24	42	50		24	17	31		25	22	38		25	50	8
18		25	54	41		25	36	59		25	41	30		25	17	13		26	23	16		26	51	15
19		26	51	58		26	34	47		26	40	12		26	16	56		27	23	55		27	52	24
20		27	49	15		27	32	36		27	38	56		27	16	42		28	24	35		28	53	35
21		28	46	33		28	30	27		28	37	41		28	16	28		29	25	18		29	54	43
22		29	43	52		29	28	20		29	36	29		29	16	18	8	0	26	0	9	0	55	53
23	4	0	41	11	5	0	26	15	6	0	35	20	7	0	16	9		1	26	45		1	57	2
24		1	38	31		1	24	9		1	34	11		1	16	12		2	27	30		2	58	13
25		2	35	53		2	22	6		2	33	5		2	15	58		3	28	17		3	59	25
26		3	33	14		3	20	4		3	32	1		3	15	55		4	29	6		5	0	35
27		4	30	35		4	18	4		4	30	59		4	15	53		5	29	56		6	1	47
28		5	27	58		5	16	6		5	29	59		5	15	55		6	30	47		7	2	58
29		6	25	22		6	14	10		6	29	1		6	15	58		7	31	40		8	4	10
30		7	22	47		7	12	14		7	28	5		7	16	3		8	32	33		9	5	21
31		8	20	12		8	10	21						8	16	10						10	6	33

308. A TABLE of the SUN's LONGITUDE for the Years 1791, 1795, and 1799, being the third after Leap Year.

Days.	January. s ° ′ ″	February. s ° ′ ″	March. s ° ′ ″	April. s ° ′ ″	May. s ° ′ ″	June. s ° ′ ″
1	9 11 7 43	10 12 40 47	11 10 54 48	0 11 42 17	1 10 59 40	2 10 49 44
2	12 8 54	13 41 37	11 54 54	12 41 20	11 57 46	11 47 9
3	13 10 7	14 42 26	12 54 58	13 40 21	12 55 51	12 44 34
4	14 11 10	15 43 13	13 55 0	14 39 20	13 53 55	13 41 58
5	15 12 29	16 44 0	14 54 59	15 38 17	14 51 56	14 39 20
6	16 13 40	17 44 44	15 54 57	16 37 12	15 49 55	15 36 43
7	17 14 49	18 45 29	16 54 52	17 36 5	16 47 53	16 34 5
8	18 10 [illegible]	19 46 10	17 54 46	18 34 56	17 45 49	17 31 25
9	19 17 0	20 46 51	18 54 38	19 33 46	18 43 45	18 28 45
10	20 18 8	21 47 31	19 54 28	20 32 32	19 41 38	19 26 4
11	21 19 28	22 48 7	20 54 16	21 31 16	20 39 31	20 23 22
12	22 20 36	23 48 46	21 54 3	22 30 0	21 37 22	21 20 41
13	23 21 43	24 49 19	22 53 47	23 28 41	22 35 10	22 17 59
14	24 22 51	25 49 52	23 53 29	24 27 21	23 32 58	23 15 15
15	25 23 58	26 50 23	24 53 10	25 25 58	24 30 45	24 12 32
16	26 25 3	27 50 54	25 52 48	26 24 33	25 28 30	25 9 47
17	27 26 9	28 51 21	26 52 23	27 23 6	26 26 14	26 7 2
18	28 27 15	29 51 48	27 51 57	28 21 38	27 23 56	27 4 16
19	29 28 18	11 0 52 14	28 51 30	29 20 7	28 21 37	28 1 31
20	10 0 29 21	1 52 37	29 50 59	1 0 18 35	29 19 17	28 58 45
21	1 30 23	2 52 59	0 0 50 27	1 17 2	2 0 16 57	29 55 59
22	2 31 23	3 53 18	1 49 53	2 15 25	1 14 34	3 0 53 13
23	3 32 25	4 53 36	2 49 17	3 13 47	2 12 10	1 50 20
24	4 33 23	5 53 53	3 48 37	4 12 8	3 9 46	2 47 38
25	5 34 23	6 54 8	4 47 57	5 10 26	4 7 19	3 44 50
26	6 35 22	7 54 21	5 47 15	6 8 42	5 4 51	4 42 3
27	7 36 19	8 54 32	6 46 30	7 6 57	6 2 22	5 39 16
28	8 37 14	9 54 41	7 45 44	8 5 10	6 59 52	6 36 29
29	9 38 9		8 44 55	9 3 22	7 57 22	7 33 40
30	10 39 3		9 44 4	10 1 33	8 54 50	8 30 52
31	11 39 55		10 4 11		9 52 17	

Days.	July. s ° ′ ″	August. s ° ′ ″	September. s ° ′ ″	October. s ° ′ ″	November. s ° ′ ″	December. s ° ′ ″
1	3 9 28 3	4 9 3 46	5 8 54 24	6 8 12 51	7 9 1 41	8 9 18 40
2	10 25 14	10 1 12	9 52 35	9 11 58	10 1 51	10 19 34
3	11 22 28	10 58 41	10 50 47	10 11 7	11 2 4	11 20 31
4	12 19 39	11 56 11	11 48 59	11 10 20	12 2 17	12 31 29
5	13 16 52	12 53 41	12 47 14	12 9 34	13 2 32	13 22 27
6	14 14 2	13 51 12	13 45 31	13 8 49	14 2 50	14 23 28
7	15 11 17	14 48 44	14 43 50	14 8 8	15 3 9	15 24 28
8	16 8 28	15 46 17	15 42 10	15 7 28	16 3 30	16 25 29
9	17 5 41	16 43 52	16 40 33	16 6 51	17 3 52	17 26 32
10	18 2 55	17 41 28	17 38 55	17 6 14	18 4 18	18 27 34
11	19 0 8	18 39 5	18 37 21	18 5 41	19 4 44	19 28 38
12	19 57 22	19 36 43	19 35 50	19 5 10	20 5 12	20 29 43
13	20 54 36	20 34 23	20 34 20	20 4 39	21 5 40	21 30 48
14	21 51 49	21 32 4	21 32 51	21 4 12	22 6 11	22 31 55
15	22 49 4	22 29 46	22 31 24	22 3 48	23 6 44	23 33 0
16	23 46 18	23 27 30	23 30 0	23 3 23	24 7 17	24 34 7
17	24 43 34	24 25 15	24 28 36	24 3 3	25 7 53	25 35 17
18	25 40 51	25 23 2	25 27 16	25 2 44	26 8 31	26 36 25
19	26 38 8	26 20 48	26 25 57	26 2 26	27 9 9	27 37 32
20	27 35 26	27 18 36	27 24 41	27 2 12	28 9 49	28 38 41
21	28 32 43	28 16 28	28 23 26	28 1 57	29 10 31	29 39 51
22	29 30 1	29 14 20	29 22 13	29 1 46	8 0 11 13	9 0 41 1
23	4 0 27 19	5 0 12 13	6 0 21 3	7 0 1 37	1 11 58	1 42 11
24	1 24 40	1 10 9	1 19 55	1 1 29	2 12 44	2 43 20
25	2 22 0	2 8 6	2 18 49	2 1 24	3 13 32	3 44 32
26	3 19 21	3 6 3	3 17 44	3 1 21	4 14 19	4 45 44
27	4 16 44	4 4 3	4 16 42	4 1 20	5 15 8	5 46 55
28	5 14 7	5 2 3	5 15 40	5 1 21	6 15 59	6 48 6
29	6 11 30	6 0 6	6 14 41	6 1 22	7 16 52	7 49 17
30	7 8 54	6 58 10	7 13 46	7 1 27	8 17 46	8 50 29
31	8 6 20	7 56 17		8 1 33		9 51 42

309. A TABLE of the SUN's DECLINATION for the Years 1788, 1792, and 1796, being Leap Years.

	January. South.	February. South.	March. South.	April. North.	May. North.	June. North.	July. North.	August. North.	September. North.	October South.	Novemb. South.	December South	Days.
	° ′ ″	° ′ ″	° ′ ″	° ′ ″	° ′ ″	° ′ ″	° ′ ″	° ′ ″	° ″	° ′ ″	° ′ ″	° ′ ″	
1	23 1 21	17 6 0	7 12 17	4 54 48	15 21 38	22 11 26	23 4 3[illegible]	17 49 35	7 58 29	3 32 39	14 45 16	21 58 56	1
2	22 56 8	48 46	6 49 20	5 17 48	39 25	19 4	0 4	34 4	36 30	55 57	15 4 12	22 7 39	2
3	50 28	31 14	26 19	40 42	56 57	26 18	22 55 5	18 15	14 24	4 19 11	22 53	15 56	3
4	44 21	13 25	3 12	6 3 31	16 14 13	33 9	49 44	2 11	6 52 9	42 22	41 19	23 48	4
5	37 40	55 18	5 39 59	26 13	31 12	39 37	43 58	16 45 49	29 47	5 5 30	59 29	31 13	5
6	30 45	30 55	16 43	48 49	47 56	45 41	37 48	29 11	7 21	28 35	16 17 23	38 11	6
7	23 16	18 17	4 53 22	7 11 18	17 4 24	51 21	31 15	12 17	5 44 49	51 35	35 1	44 43	7
8	15 21	14 59 23	29 57	33 40	20 33	56 37	24 18	15 55 8	22 9	6 14 30	52 21	50 48	8
9	7 1	40 14	6 28	55 54	36 26	23 1 28	16 58	37 43	4 59 24	37 20	17 9 25	56 26	9
10	21 58 15	20 51	3 42 57	8 17 59	52 0	5 53	9 16	20 2	36 35	7 0 5	26 11	23 1 37	10
11	49 2	1 13	19 24	39 57	18 7 17	9 59	1 11	2 9	3 13 41	22 45	42 39	6 20	11
12	39 24	13 41 22	2 55 48	9 1 46	22 16	13 37	21 52 42	14 43 59	50 42	45 18	58 48	10 36	12
13	29 22	21 16	32 10	23 27	36 57	16 51	43 51	25 36	27 39	8 7 46	18 14 39	14 24	13
14	18 54	0 58	8 30	44 58	51 18	19 41	34 38	6 58	4 32	30 5	30 10	17 44	14
15	8 2	12 40 27	1 44 49	10 6 19	19 5 20	22 6	25 4	13 48 7	2 41 22	52 18	45 21	20 36	15
16	20 56 45	19 45	21 8	27 29	19 3	24 6	15 5	29 4	18 9	9 14 23	19 0 13	23 0	16
17	45 4	11 58 50	0 57 27	43 31	32 27	25 41	4 46	9 47	1 54 52	36 21	14 45	24 56	17
18	32 59	37 45	33 45	11 9 21	45 31	26 52	20 54 6	12 50 18	31 33	58 11	28 55	26 24	18
19	20 32	16 28	S. 10 3	30 0	58 15	27 38	43 5	30 37	8 14	10 19 51	42 44	27 24	19
20	7 41	10 55 0	N. 13 38	50 28	20 10 39	27 59	31 43	10 44	0 44 50	41 22	56 12	27 55	20
21	19 54 28	33 23	37 18	12 10 44	22 42	27 54	20 1	11 50 38	N. 21 26	11 2 43	20 9 18	27 58	21
22	40 53	11 35	1 0 56	30 49	34 23	27 26	7 56	30 23	S. 1 59	23 55	22 1	27 32	22
23	26 56	9 49 38	24 33	50 41	45 44	26 32	19 55 33	9 55	25 25	44 56	34 22	26 38	23
24	12 38	27 33	48 8	13 10 21	56 44	25 15	42 50	10 49 17	48 51	12 5 46	46 20	25 16	24
25	18 57 58	5 20	2 11 40	29 47	21 7 22	23 32	29 47	28 29	1 12 18	26 26	57 55	23 26	25
26	42 57	8 42 57	35 10	49 1	17 38	21 24	16 23	7 31	35 44	46 54	21 9 6	21 7	26
27	27 36	20 28	58 36	14 8 1	27 32	18 52	2 42	9 46 23	59 10	13 7 10	19 53	18 20	27
28	11 56	7 57 51	3 21 59	26 46	37 4	15 55	18 48 41	25 6	2 22 35	27 13	30 16	15 5	28
29	17 55 55	35 8	45 17	45 19	46 14	12 34	34 22	3 39	45 58	47 4	40 15	11 22	29
30	39 35		4 8 31	15 3 37	55 1	8 48	19 43	8 42 4	3 9 20	14 6 42	49 48	7 12	30
31	22 58		31 42		22 3 25		4 48	20 21		26 6		2 33	31

309. TABLE of the SUN's DECLINATION for the Years 1789, 1793, and 1797, being the first after Leap Year.

Days.	January.	February.	March.	April.	May.	June.	July.	August.	September.	October.	Novemb.	December	Days.
	South.	South.	South.	North.	North.	North.	North	North.	North.	South.	South.	South.	
	° ′ ″	° ′ ″	° ′ ″	° ′ ″	° ′ ″	° ′ ″	° ′ ″	° ′ ″	° ′ ″	° ′ ″	° ′ ″	° ′ ″	
1	22 57 27	16 52 59	7 17 51	4 49 12	15 17 17	22 9 32	23 5 41	17 53 17	8 3 47	3 27 0	14 40 39	21 56 45	1
2	51 54	35 31	6 54 56	5 12 14	35 8	17 15	1 12	37 51	7 41 50	50 17	59 37	22 5 34	2
3	45 52	17 45	31 55	35 10	52 44	24 35	22 56 18	22 6	19 44	4 13 33	15 18 22	13 58	3
4	39 24	15 59 43	8 49	58 0	16 10 4	31 32	51 4	6 5	6 57 33	36 45	36 54	21 56	4
5	32 28	41 25	5 45 3[illegible]	6 20 44	27 8	38 6	45 24	16 49 48	35 14	59 54	55 5	29 27	5
6	25 7	22 50	22 22	43 21	43 55	44 15	39 19	33 14	12 48	5 22 59	16 13 4	36 32	6
7	17 20	3 59	4 59 0	7 5 52	17 0 26	50 1	32 52	16 24	5 50 18	46 1	30 45	43 10	7
8	9 5	14 44 54	35 37	28 15	16 40	55 23	26 1	15 59 18	27 39	6 8 56	48 10	49 22	8
9	0 24	25 34	12 10	50 32	32 36	23 0 20	18 47	41 57	4 56	31 48	17 5 17	55 6	9
10	21 51 19	5 59	3 48 41	8 12 39	48 15	4 54	11 10	24 21	4 42 8	54 34	22 9	23 0 23	10
11	41 46	13 46 12	25 7	34 37	18 3 37	9 2	3 10	6 29	19 14	7 17 16	38 40	5 14	11
12	31 50	26 10	1 32	56 29	18 40	12 46	21 54 47	14 48 23	3 56 16	39 50	54 57	9 36	12
13	21 28	5 55	2 37 53	9 18 12	33 25	16 7	46 1	30 5	33 14	8 2 19	18 10 49	13 31	13
14	10 42	12 45 27	14 15	39 46	47 51	19 2	36 54	11 30	10 8	24 41	26 25	16 58	14
15	20 59 31	24 48	1 50 34	10 1 9	19 1 59	21 33	27 24	13 52 43	2 56 59	46 55	41 42	19 58	15
16	47 55	3 56	26 52	22 22	15 47	23 39	17 32	33 43	23 47	9 9 3	56 38	22 28	16
17	35 5[illegible]	11 42 52	3 11	43 26	29 15	25 20	7 18	14 29	0 31	31 3	19 11 15	24 31	17
18	23 3[illegible]	21 38	0 39 29	11 4 15	42 24	26 37	20 56 44	12 55 1	1 37 13	52 54	25 31	26 5	18
19	1[illegible] 50	0 14	S. 15 48	25 1	55 12	27 29	45 47	35 25	13 52	10 14 36	39 24	27 12	19
20	19 57 43	10 38 39	N. 7 53	45 32	20 7 41	27 56	34 30	15 34	0 50 30	36 10	53 0	27 50	20
21	44 13	16 5[illegible]	31 33	12 5 51	19 49	27 58	22 52	11 55 31	27 [illegible]5	57 34	20 6 [illegible]	28 0	21
22	30 22	9 55 0	55 12	25 5[illegible]	31 36	27 35	10 53	35 18	N. 3 41	11 18 47	18 58	27 41	22
23	16 8	32 56	1 18 49	45 5[illegible]	43 2	26 48	19 58 35	14 53	S. 19 45	39 51	31 24	26 53	23
24	1 3[illegible]	10 45	42 26	13 5 36	54 6	25 36	45 56	10 54 17	43 11	12 0 45	43 28	25 39	24
25	18 46 38	8 48 24	2 5 58	25 6	21 4 40	23 59	32 57	33 32	1 6 37	21 27	55 8	23 55	25
26	31 22	25 5[illegible]	29 29	44 23	15 11	21 57	19 39	12 37	30 4	41 57	21 6 25	21 44	26
27	15 46	3 2[illegible]	52 56	14 3 26	25 11	19 31	6 2	9 51 31	53 29	13 2 16	17 18	19 [illegible]3	27
28	17 59 51	7 40 39	3 16 19	22 16	34 48	16 40	18 52 5	30 16	2 16 54	22 23	27 47	15 55	28
29	43 35		39 39	40 51	44 3	13 25	37 51	8 51	40 17	42 16	37 51	12 19	29
30	27 2		4 2 54	59 12	52 56	9 45	23 18	8 47 18	3 3 40	14 1 57	47 31	8 15	30
31	10 9		26 6		22 1 23		8 27	25 36		21 25		3.43	31

309. A TABLE of the SUN's DECLINATION for the Years 1790, 1794, and 1798, being the second after Leap Year.

Days.	January.	February.	March.	April.	May.	June.	July.	August.	September.	October.	Novemb.	December.	Days.
	South.	South.	South.	North.	North.	North.	North.	North.	North.	South.	South.	South.	
	° ′ ″	° ′ ″	° ′ ″	° ′ ″	° ′ ″	° ′ ″	° ′ ″	° ′ ″	° ′ ″	° ′ ″	° ′ ″	° ′ ″	
1	22 53 44	16 57 11	7 23 23	4 43 37	15 12 56	22 7 36	23 6 42	17 56 59	8 9 5	3 21 21	14 35 59	21 54 33	1
2	53 16	39 48	6 0 29	5 6 40	30 51	15 25	2 20	41 36	7 47 10	44 40	55 3	22 3 28	2
3	47 22	22 6	37 28	29 37	48 29	22 51	22 57 33	25 57	25 7	4 7 56	15 13 51	11 58	3
4	41 1	4 7	14 25	52 28	16 5 53	29 54	52 23	10 0	2 56	31 9	32 24	20 2	4
5	34 13	15 45 53	5 51 16	6 15 14	23 1	36 33	46 48	16 53 46	6 40 38	54 18	50 41	27 40	5
6	26 57	27 22	28 1	37 53	39 53	42 48	40 49	37 16	18 14	5 17 23	16 8 43	34 51	6
7	19 15	8 36	4 42	7 0 25	56 28	48 40	34 28	20 30	5 55 43	40 26	26 29	41 36	7
8	11 8	14 49 35	4 41 19	22 51	17 12 46	54 7	27 43	3 28	33 8	6 3 24	43 58	47 54	8
9	2 34	30 19	17 53	45 8	28 46	59 10	20 34	15 46 11	10 27	26 16	17 1 11	53 45	9
10	21 53 33	10 47	3 54 23	8 7 18	44 30	23 3 50	13 2	28 38	4 47 39	49 4	18 5	59 9	10
11	44 8	13 51 2	30 50	29 20	59 56	8 4	5 7	10 51	24 45	7 11 47	34 41	23 4 6	11
12	34 18	31 3	7 15	51 13	18 15 3	11 55	21 56 51	14 52 48	1 50	34 23	51 0	8 35	12
13	24 1	10 52	2 43 38	9 12 58	29 52	15 21	48 10	34 32	3 38 47	56 53	18 6 59	12 37	13
14	13 21	12 50 27	19 58	34 34	44 23	18 22	39 9	16 1	15 44	8 19 17	22 40	16 11	14
15	2 16	29 50	1 56 18	55 59	58 36	21 0	29 43	13 57 17	2 52 36	41 34	38 1	19 16	15
16	20 50 46	9 1	32 37	10 17 15	19 12 28	23 12	19 57	38 20	29 24	9 3 43	53 3	21 54	16
17	38 54	11 48 1	8 56	38 21	26 1	24 59	9 49	19 9	6 9	25 43	19 7 44	24 4	17
18	26 38	26 49	0 45 14	59 16	39 15	26 21	20 59 19	12 59 47	1 42 51	47 37	22 4	25 45	18
19	13 58	5 26	S. 21 30	11 20 1	52 8	27 18	48 28	40 10	19 31	10 9 21	36 4	26 58	19
20	0 57	10 43 53	N. 2 9	40 34	20 4 42	27 51	37 16	20 22	0 56 9	30 57	49 43	27 43	20
21	19 47 33	22 10	25 49	12 0 57	16 55	28 0	25 43	0 24	32 47	52 23	20 3 0	28 0	21
22	33 46	0 18	49 29	21 7	28 47	27 43	13 49	11 40 12	N. 9 21	11 13 38	15 54	27 49	22
23	19 37	9 38 18	1 13 6	41 6	40 18	27 1	1 36	19 50	S. 14 4	34 46	28 25	27 8	23
24	5 8	16 8	36 42	13 0 51	51 27	25 55	19 49 1	10 59 18	37 30	55 41	40 35	26 0	24
25	18 50 18	8 53 50	2 0 16	20 24	21 2 16	24 25	36 7	38 36	1 0 57	12 16 27	52 20	24 23	25
26	35 6	31 23	23 47	39 44	12 43	22 29	22 54	17 42	24 23	37 0	21 3 43	22 18	26
27	19 35	8 50	47 14	58 50	22 48	20 9	9 22	9 56 39	47 49	57 22	14 42	19 45	27
28	3 45	7 46 10	3 10 37	14 17 43	32 31	17 24	18 55 30	35 25	2 11 14	13 17 32	25 17	16 43	28
29	17 47 34		33 59	36 22	41 51	14 15	41 19	14 2	34 38	37 29	35 28	13 14	29
30	31 5		57 17	54 47	50 49	10 41	26 49	8 52 32	58 0	57 12	45 13	9 17	30
31	14 17		4 20 30		59 24		12 4	30 53		14 16 43		4 52	31

A TABLE of the SUN's DECLINATION for the Years 1791, 1795, and 1799, being the third after Leap Year.

January.	February.	March.	April.	May.	June.	July.	August.	September.	October.	Novemb.	December	Days.
South.	South.	South.	North.	North.	North.	North.	North.	North.	South.	South.	South.	
° ′ ″	° ′ ″	° ′ ″	° ′ ″	° ′ ″	° ′ ″	° ′ ″	° ′ ″	° ′ ″	° ′ ″	° ′ ″	° ′ ″	
23 0 [illegible]	17 1 22	7 28 5[illegible]	4 38 1	15 8 34	22 5 39	23 7 42	17 0 39	8 14 23	3 15 42	14 31 20	21 52 19	1
54 3[illegible]	41 3	6 3	5 1 5	26 32	13 34	3 25	45 21	7 52 29	39 1	50 26	22 1 21	2
48 51	16 26 25	6 43 4	24 4	44 15	21 5	22 58 45	29 45	30 27	4 2 17	15 9 18	9 57	3
42 3[illegible]	8 31	20 1	46 57	16 1 43	28 14	53 39	13 52	8 18	25 31	27 55	18 7	4
35 5[illegible]	15 50 [illegible]	5 56 53	6 9 43	18 54	34 59	48 11	16 57 42	6 46 3	48 41	46 15	25 51	5
28 4[illegible]	31 5[illegible]	33 [illegible]	32 25	35 50	41 20	42 19	41 16	23 40	5 11 48	16 4 22	33 9	6
21 1	13 4[illegible]	10 22	54 58	52 28	47 17	36 2	24 34	1 11	34 51	22 12	40 0	7
13 [illegible]	14 54 [illegible]3	4 47 0	7 17 25	17 8 50	52 50	29 23	7 37	5 38 37	57 50	39 45	46 25	8
4 41	35 [illegible]	23 34	39 45	24 55	57 59	22 20	15 50 22	15 56	6 20 45	57 2	52 23	9
21 55 47	15 [illegible]2	3 0 5	8 1 56	40 43	23 2 44	14 53	32 54	4 53 11	43 32	17 14 0	57 53	10
46 2[illegible]	13 55 51	46 33	24 0	56 13	7 5	7 5	15 11	30 20	7 6 16	30 41	23 2 56	11
[illegible]6 43	35 [illegible]5	12 59	45 56	18 11 26	11 2	21 58 53	14 57 11	7 24	28 55	47 4	7 32	12
20 3[illegible]	15 [illegible]	2 49 22	9 7 42	26 19	14 33	50 19	38 58	3 44 24	51 26	18 3 8	11 41	13
15 7[illegible]	12 55 25	25 44	29 21	40 55	17 41	41 21	20 31	21 20	8 13 51	18 54	15 21	14
4 5[illegible]	34 51	2 3	50 49	55 11	20 23	32 3	1 50	2 58 12	36 10	34 20	18 33	15
19 53 3[illegible]	14 6	1 38 22	10 12 7	19 9 8	22 41	22 21	13 42 56	35 1	58 20	49 25	21 18	16
41 40	11 53 7	14 41	33 15	22 46	24 34	12 18	23 48	11 48	9 20 24	19 4 12	23 35	17
29 30	31 58	0 50 53	54 14	36 6	26 3	1 54	4 28	1 48 31	42 9	18 37	25 23	18
17 5	10 38	27 16	11 15 0	49 4	27 7	20 51 8	12 44 56	25 10	10 4 5	32 42	26 43	19
4 9	10 40 8	S. 3 35	35 37	20 1 42	27 46	40 0	25 12	1 50	25 43	46 27	27 35	20
19 50 5[illegible]	27 28	N. 20 5	56 2	14 0	28 0	28 32	5 15	0 38 27	47 11	59 48	27 58	21
37 [illegible]	5 39	43 44	12 16 16	25 57	27 49	16 44	11 45 6	N. 15 3	11 8 30	20 12 47	27 53	22
23 5	9 43 41	1 7 23	36 16	37 33	27 14	4 35	24 47	S. 8 23	29 39	25 25	27 20	23
8 41	21 32	30 58	56 6	48 48	26 14	19 52 5	4 17	31 49	50 37	37 40	26 19	24
18 53 56	8 59 15	54 33	13 15 42	59 42	24 48	39 16	10 43 36	55 16	12 11 25	49 31	24 49	25
38 50	36 51	2 18 5	35 4	21 10 13	22 59	26 8	22 45	1 18 43	32 1	21 0 59	22 51	26
23 23	14 20	41 34	54 14	20 23	20 45	12 40	1 44	42 9	52 26	12 3	20 24	27
7 38	7 51 41	5 0	14 13 10	30 11	18 5	18 58 52	9 40 34	2 5 33	13 12 39	22 45	17 30	28
17 51 32		3 28 22	31 52	39 37	15 2	44 46	19 14	28 57	32 38	33 12	14 8	29
35 7		51 38	50 20	48 41	11 34	30 22	8 57 45	52 21	52 26	42 53	10 17	30
18 21		4 14 56		57 22		15 40	36 8		14 12 0		5 59	31

310. A TABLE of the SUN's RIGHT ASCENSION for the Years 1788, 1792, and 1796, being Leap Years.

Days.	January	February.	March.	April.	May.	June.	July.	August.	Septemb.	October.	Novemb.	December	Days.
	h. m. s.	h. m. s.	h. m. s.	h. m. s.	h. m. s.	h. m. s.	h. m. s.	h. m. s.	h. m. s.	h. m. s.	h. m. s.	h. m. s.	
1	18 47 13	20 59 30	22 52 17	0 45 41	2 37 1	4 39 56	6 44 14	8 48 49	10 44 42	12 32 49	14 29 24	16 33 39	1
2	51 38	21 3 33	56 0	49 19	40 51	44 2	48 21	52 42	48 19	36 27	33 20	37 59	2
3	56 2	7 37	59 44	52 58	44 41	48 9	52 28	56 33	51 56	40 5	37 18	42 20	3
4	19 0 27	11 39	23 3 27	56 36	48 32	52 15	56 35	9 0 25	55 33	43 43	41 16	46 42	4
5	4 50	15 41	7 9	1 0 15	52 23	56 22	7 0 42	4 15	59 10	47 22	45 14	51 4	5
6	9 13	19 41	10 51	3 54	56 15	5 0 29	4 49	8 5	11 2 47	51 2	49 14	55 26	6
7	13 36	23 41	14 33	7 34	3 0 7	4 37	8 55	11 54	6 23	54 42	53 15	59 49	7
8	17 58	27 40	18 14	11 13	4 0	8 45	13 1	15 43	9 58	58 21	57 17	17 4 13	8
9	22 20	31 39	21 55	14 53	7 53	12 53	17 6	19 31	13 35	13 2 3	15 1 39	8 36	9
10	26 41	35 36	25 35	18 33	11 47	17 2	21 11	23 19	17 11	5 44	5 22	13 1	10
11	31 2	39 32	29 15	22 13	15 42	21 11	25 16	27 6	20 47	9 26	9 26	17 25	11
12	35 22	43 29	32 55	25 53	19 37	25 19	29 20	30 52	24 22	13 8	13 31	21 50	12
13	39 41	47 24	36 35	29 34	23 33	29 28	33 23	34 39	27 58	16 51	17 37	26 16	13
14	44 0	51 18	40 14	33 16	27 30	33 38	37 26	38 24	31 34	20 34	21 44	30 42	14
15	48 18	55 12	43 53	36 57	31 26	37 46	41 29	42 9	35 9	24 17	25 51	35 7	15
16	52 35	59 5	47 31	40 39	35 24	41 56	45 32	45 53	38 45	28 2	30 0	39 31	16
17	56 52	22 2 57	51 9	44 21	39 22	46 5	49 33	49 37	42 20	31 47	34 9	44 0	17
18	20 1 9	6 49	54 47	48 4	43 21	50 14	53 34	53 20	45 56	35 32	38 19	48 27	18
19	5 24	10 39	58 25	51 47	47 20	54 24	57 35	57 3	49 31	39 19	42 29	52 53	19
20	9 38	14 29	0 2 6	55 31	51 20	58 34	8 1 35	10 0 45	53 7	43 6	46 41	57 20	20
21	13 52	18 19	5 44	59 15	55 20	6 2 43	5 34	4 27	56 42	46 53	50 53	18 1 46	21
22	18 5	22 8	9 21	2 2 59	59 21	6 53	9 33	8 9	12 0 18	50 41	55 6	6 13	22
23	22 17	25 56	13 0	6 44	4 3 22	11 3	13 32	11 50	3 55	54 30	59 20	10 40	23
24	26 28	29 43	16 38	10 30	7 24	15 12	17 29	15 30	7 31	58 19	16 3 35	15 7	24
25	30 39	33 31	20 15	14 15	11 26	19 21	21 26	19 10	11 7	14 2 10	7 50	19 33	25
26	34 49	37 17	23 53	18 2	15 29	23 30	25 23	22 50	14 43	6 1	12 7	24 0	26
27	38 57	41 2	27 31	21 49	19 33	27 39	29 19	26 29	18 20	9 53	16 24	28 26	27
28	43 6	44 48	31 9	25 37	23 37	31 48	33 14	30 8	21 57	13 45	20 42	32 52	28
29	47 13	48 33	34 47	29 24	27 41	35 56	37 8	33 47	25 33	17 38	25 0	37 18	29
30	51 19		38 25	33 12	31 45	40 5	41 2	37 26	29 11	21 33	29 20	41 43	30
31	55 25		42 3		35 50		44 56	41 4		25 28		46 9	31

 A TABLE of the SUN's RIGHT ASCENSION for the Years 1789, 1793, and 1797, being the first after Leap Year.

Days.	January. h. m. s.	February. h. m. s.	March. h. m. s.	April. h. m. s.	May. h. m. s.	June. h. m. s.	July. h. m. s.	August. h. m. s.	Septemb. h. m. s.	October. h. m. s.	Novemb. h. m. s.	December. h. m. s.	Days.
1	18 50 34	21 2 35	22 51 23	0 44 48	2 36 6	4 38 56	6 43 13	8 47 53	10 43 49	12 31 55	14 28 26	16 32 36	1
2	54 58	6 38	55 6	48 26	39 55	43 3	47 21	51 45	47 27	35 34	32 22	36 56	2
3	59 23	10 41	58 49	52 5	43 45	47 9	51 28	55 37	51 4	39 12	36 20	41 16	3
4	19 3 46	14 42	23 2 32	55 44	47 36	51 15	55 35	59 29	54 41	42 50	40 18	45 38	4
5	8 10	18 43	6 15	59 22	51 27	55 22	59 42	9 3 19	58 18	46 30	44 16	50 0	5
6	12 32	22 44	9 57	1 3 1	55 19	59 29	7 3 49	7 9	11 1 54	50 9	48 16	54 22	6
7	16 55	26 43	13 39	6 40	59 11	5 3 37	7 56	10 59	5 30	53 49	52 17	58 45	7
8	21 17	30 41	17 20	10 20	3 3 3	7 45	12 1	14 47	9 7	57 29	56 18	17 3 8	8
9	25 38	34 38	21 1	14 0	6 57	11 53	16 7	18 36	12 43	13 1 9	15 0 20	7 32	9
10	29 59	38 36	24 42	17 39	10 51	16 1	20 12	22 24	16 19	4 50	4 23	11 58	10
11	34 19	42 31	28 22	21 19	14 45	20 10	24 16	26 11	19 55	8 32	8 27	16 21	11
12	38 39	46 27	32 2	25 0	18 40	24 20	28 21	29 58	23 30	12 14	12 31	20 51	12
13	42 58	50 22	35 42	28 40	22 36	28 28	32 26	33 44	27 5	15 56	16 37	25 11	13
14	47 16	54 15	39 22	32 22	26 33	32 37	36 28	37 29	30 42	19 39	20 43	29 37	14
15	51 33	58 8	43 0	36 4	30 29	36 46	40 31	41 14	34 17	23 24	24 50	34 3	15
16	55 50	22 2 1	46 39	39 46	34 27	40 56	44 33	44 59	37 52	27 7	28 59	38 28	16
17	20 0 6	5 52	50 18	43 28	38 24	45 5	48 35	48 42	41 28	30 52	33 8	42 55	17
18	4 22	9 47	53 56	47 10	42 23	49 15	52 36	52 26	45 4	34 38	37 18	47 21	18
19	8 30	13 34	57 35	50 53	46 22	53 23	56 36	56 9	48 39	38 25	41 29	51 48	19
20	12 50	17 24	0 1 12	54 37	50 21	57 33	8 0 36	59 12	52 15	42 11	45 40	56 15	20
21	17 3	21 12	4 51	58 20	54 22	6 1 42	4 36	10 3 34	55 50	45 58	49 52	18 0 41	21
22	21 15	25 0	8 29	2 2 6	58 22	5 52	8 35	7 15	59 26	49 46	54 5	5 8	22
23	25 27	28 48	12 7	5 50	4 2 24	10 2	12 34	10 56	12 3 1	53 34	58 19	9 34	23
24	29 38	32 15	15 45	9 35	6 25	14 11	16 31	14 37	6 38	57 25	16 2 33	14 1	24
25	33 48	36 22	19 23	13 21	10 27	18 20	20 29	18 17	10 14	14 1 15	6 48	18 28	25
26	37 57	40 8	23 0	17 7	14 30	22 28	24 25	21 57	13 50	5 5	11 4	22 55	26
27	42 6	43 53	26 38	20 53	18 34	26 39	28 22	25 36	17 27	8 57	15 21	27 21	27
28	46 13	47 38	30 17	24 41	22 37	30 48	32 18	29 16	21 4	12 49	19 39	31 47	28
29	50 20		33 55	28 29	26 42	34 56	36 12	32 55	24 41	16 42	23 57	36 13	29
30	54 25		37 32	32 17	30 46	38 4	40 7	36 33	28 18	20 36	28 16	40 39	30
31	58 30		41 10		34 51		44 0	40 11		24 31		45 4	31

 A TABLE of the SUN's RIGHT ASCENSION for the Years 1790, 1794, 1798, being the second after Leap Year.

Days.	January.			February.			March.			April.			May.			June.			July.			August.			Septemb.			October.			Novemb.			December			Days.
	h.	m.	s.	h.	m.	s.	h.	m.	s.	h.	m.	s.	h.	m.	s.	h.	m.	s.	h.	m.	s.	h.	m.	s.	h.	m.	s.	h.	m.	s.	h.	m.	s.	h.	m.	s.	
1	18	49	29	21	1	35	22	50	28	0	43	55	2	35	11	4	37	56	6	42	13	8	46	57	10	42	56	12	31	3	14	27	29	16	31	33	1
2		53	54		5	39		54	12		47	33		39	0		42	3		46	21		50	49		46	34		34	41		31	25		35	53	2
3		58	18		9	41		57	56		51	11		42	49		46	9		50	29		54	41		50	11		38	19		35	22		40	13	3
4	19	2	42		13	44	23	1	39		54	48		46	40		50	16		54	36		58	33		53	48		41	58		39	20		44	34	4
5		7	5		17	45		5	21		58	28		50	31		54	23		58	43	9	2	23		57	25		45	37		43	18		48	56	5
6		11	29		21	45		9	4	1	2	8		54	22		58	29	7	2	50		6	14	11	1	2		49	16		47	16		53	18	6
7		15	51		25	44		12	45		5	48		58	14	5	2	38		6	56		10	4		4	38		52	55		51	18		57	41	7
8		20	13		29	43		16	27		9	26	3	2	7		6	45		11	2		13	53		8	14		56	35		55	19	17	2	4	8
9		24	35		33	41		20	8		13	6		6	0		10	53		15	8		17	41		11	50	13	0	16		59	22		6	28	9
10		28	55		37	38		23	48		16	46		9	54		15	2		19	13		21	29		15	26		3	57	15	3	24		10	53	10
11		33	16		41	34		27	28		20	26		13	48		19	10		23	18		25	16		19	2		7	38		7	28		15	17	11
12		37	35		45	30		31	8		24	7		17	43		23	19		27	22		29	3		22	38		11	20		11	33		19	41	12
13		41	55		49	24		34	48		27	47		21	39		27	28		31	25		32	49		26	14		15	2		15	38		24	7	13
14		46	13		53	17		38	28		31	28		25	35		31	36		35	29		36	35		29	49		18	45		19	44		28	32	14
15		50	31		57	11		42	7		35	10		29	32		35	44		39	22		40	20		33	25		22	29		23	51		32	58	15
16		54	48	22	1	4		45	46		38	51		33	29		39	55		43	34		44	5		37	0		26	13		27	59		37	24	16
17		59	4		4	56		49	24		42	34		37	27		44	5		47	36		47	49		40	36		29	58		32	7		41	50	17
18	20	3	19		8	47		53	3		46	16		41	25		48	14		51	33		51	32		44	11		33	43		36	17		46	17	18
19		7	36		12	38		56	42		49	59		45	24		52	23		55	39		55	15		47	47		37	29		40	28		50	43	19
20		11	49		16	28	0	0	19		53	42		49	24		56	33		59	39		58	58		51	23		41	16		44	39		55	10	20
21		16	2		20	16		3	58		57	26		53	24	6	0	42	8	3	38	10	2	40		54	58		45	3		48	51		59	37	21
22		20	14		24	5		7	36	2	1	10		57	24		4	52		7	38		6	21		58	34		48	51		53	4	18	4	4	22
23		24	26		27	53		11	15		4	55	4	1	25		9	1		11	36		10	3	12	2	9		52	39		57	17		8	30	23
24		28	37		31	41		14	52		8	40		5	27		13	10		15	34		13	44		5	42		56	28	16	1	31		12	57	24
25		32	47		35	27		18	30		12	26		9	29		17	19		19	31		17	24		9	21	14	0	18		5	46		17	23	25
26		36	57		39	13		22	7		16	12		13	32		21	28		23	29		21	4		12	58		4	9		10	2		21	49	26
27		41	5		42	58		25	45		19	59		17	35		25	37		27	25		24	43		16	35		8	0		14	19		26	16	27
28		45	13		46	44		29	23		23	46		21	38		29	46		31	20		28	23		20	11		11	53		18	36		30	43	28
29		49	20					33	1		27	34		25	43		33	55		35	15		32	2		23	48		15	46		22	55		35	9	29
30		53	25					36	39		31	21		29	47		38	4		39	10		35	40		27	25		19	39		27	14		39	34	30
31		57	31					40	17					33	52					43	4		39	18					23	34					44	0	31

310. A TABLE of the SUN's RIGHT ASCENSION for the Years 1791, 1795, 1799, being the third after Leap Year.

Days	January.	February.	March.	April.	May.	June.	July.	August.	Septemb.	October.	Novemb.	December	Days.
	h. m. s.	h. m. s.	h. m. s.	h. m. s.	h. m. s.	h. m. s.	h. m. s.	h. m. s.	h. m. s.	h. m. s.	h. m. s.	h. m. s.	
1	18 48 26	21 0 36	22 49 33	0 43 2	2 34 15	4 36 58	6 41 13	8 46 0	10 42 3	12 30 11	14 26 32	30 30	1
2	52 50	4 40	53 17	46 40	38 4	41 4	45 21	49 53	45 41	33 48	30 28	34 50	2
3	57 14	8 43	57 1	50 19	41 54	45 9	49 29	53 46	49 19	37 27	34 25	39 10	3
4	19 1 38	12 45	23 0 45	53 57	45 44	49 16	53 36	57 37	52 56	41 5	38 23	43 31	4
5	6 2	16 46	4 27	57 36	49 35	53 23	57 43	9 1 28	56 33	44 43	42 20	47 52	5
6	10 25	20 47	8 10	1 1 15	53 27	57 29	7 1 50	5 18	11 0 9	48 22	46 19	52 15	6
7	14 47	24 46	11 51	4 54	57 19	5 1 37	5 56	9 8	3 46	52 2	50 19	56 37	7
8	19 10	28 45	15 32	8 33	3 1 11	5 45	10 3	12 57	7 22	55 42	54 20	17 1 0	8
9	23 31	32 43	19 14	12 13	5 4	9 53	14 9	16 45	10 58	59 22	58 22	5 23	9
10	27 52	36 40	22 55	15 53	8 57	14 1	18 14	20 34	14 34	13 3 3	15 2 25	9 48	10
11	32 13	40 37	26 35	19 33	12 51	18 9	22 18	24 22	18 10	6 45	6 28	14 12	11
12	36 33	44 33	30 15	23 13	16 46	22 19	26 22	28 8	21 45	10 26	10 33	18 37	12
13	40 52	48 27	33 55	26 54	20 41	26 28	30 27	31 54	25 21	14 9	14 38	23 2	13
14	45 10	52 22	37 35	30 35	24 38	30 36	34 30	35 40	28 57	17 51	18 44	27 28	14
15	49 28	56 15	41 14	34 16	28 35	34 45	38 33	39 25	32 32	21 35	22 51	31 54	15
16	53 45	22 0 8	44 53	37 58	32 33	38 55	42 36	43 10	36 8	25 19	26 58	36 19	16
17	58 2	4 0	48 31	41 39	36 29	43 4	46 38	46 54	39 44	29 3	31 7	40 46	17
18	20 2 18	7 51	52 10	45 21	40 28	47 14	50 39	50 38	43 19	32 48	35 16	45 12	18
19	6 33	11 42	55 49	49 5	44 26	51 23	54 40	54 22	46 54	36 34	39 26	49 39	19
20	10 47	15 32	59 27	52 48	48 26	55 33	58 41	58 4	50 30	40 20	43 37	54 6	20
21	15 0	19 21	0 3 5	56 32	52 26	59 43	8 2 41	10 1 46	54 6	44 8	47 49	58 32	21
22	19 13	23 10	6 43	2 0 16	56 26	6 3 52	6 40	5 28	57 42	47 55	52 2	18 2 59	22
23	23 25	26 58	10 21	4 1	4 0 27	8 2	10 33	9 9	12 1 17	51 43	56 15	7 25	23
24	27 36	30 46	14 1	7 46	4 29	12 11	14 37	12 50	4 53	55 33	16 0 30	11 51	24
25	31 47	34 32	17 37	11 31	8 31	16 20	18 34	16 31	8 29	59 22	4 44	16 19	25
26	35 56	38 18	21 15	15 17	12 33	20 29	22 31	20 11	12 6	14 3 13	9 0	20 45	26
27	40 5	42 4	24 53	19 4	16 36	24 38	26 28	23 50	15 42	7 4	13 16	25 12	27
28	44 12	45 49	28 31	22 51	20 39	28 47	30 23	27 30	19 19	10 56	17 34	29 38	28
29	48 19		32 8	26 38	24 43	32 56	34 18	31 8	22 57	14 48	21 52	34 3	29
30	52 26		35 46	30 26	28 47	37 4	38 13	34 47	26 33	18 42	26 10	38 30	30
31	56 32		39 24		32 53		42 7	38 26		22 37		42 55	31

311. TABLE for fitting the TABLES of the SUN's LONG. DECL. or RT. ASCEN. to any meridian: Or, for finding either quantity at any hour. Degrees of longitude from the Meridian of London: Or, time before and after noon.

Daily diff.	5 Deg. h. m. 0 20	10 D. h. m. 0 40	15 D. h. m. 1 0	20 D. h. m. 1 20	25 D. h. m. 1 40	30 D. h. m. 2 0	35 D. h. m. 2 20	40 D. h. m. 2 40	45 D. h. m. 3 0	50 D. h. m. 3 20	55 D. h. m. 3 40	60 D. h. m. 4 0	65 D. h. m. 4 20	70 D. h. m. 4 40	75 D. h. m. 5 0	80 D. h. m. 5 20	85 D. h. m. 5 40	90 D. h. m. 6 0	95 D. h. m. 6 20	100D. h. m. 6 40	105D. h. m. 7 0	110D. h. m. 7 20	115D. h. m. 7 40	120D. h. m. 8 0	Daily diff.
′ ″	′ ″	′ ″	′ ″	′ ″	′ ″	′ ″	′ ″	′ ″	′ ″	′ ″	′ ″	′ ″	′ ″	′ ″	′ ″	′ ″	′ ″	′ ″	′ ″	′ ″	′ ″	′ ″	′ ″	′ ″	′ ″
0 20	0 0	0 0	0 1	0 1	0 1	0 2	0 2	0 2	0 2	0 3	0 3	0 3	0 4	0 4	0 4	0 4	0 5	0 5	0 5	0 5	0 6	0 6	0 6	0 7	0 20
40	0 0	1	2	2	3	3	4	4	5	5	6	7	7	8	8	9	9	10	10	11	12	12	13	13	40
1 0	1	2	2	3	4	5	6	7	7	8	9	10	11	12	12	13	14	15	16	17	17	19	19	20	1 0
20	1	2	3	4	5	7	8	9	10	11	12	13	14	15	17	18	19	20	21	22	23	24	25	27	20
40	1	3	4	5	7	8	10	11	12	14	15	17	18	19	21	22	24	25	26	28	29	30	32	33	40
2 0	2	3	5	7	8	10	12	13	15	17	18	20	22	23	25	27	28	30	32	33	35	37	38	40	2 0
20	2	4	6	8	10	12	14	15	17	19	21	23	25	27	29	31	33	35	38	39	40	43	45	47	20
40	2	4	7	9	11	13	15	18	20	22	24	27	29	31	33	35	38	40	42	44	47	49	51	53	40
3 0	2	5	7	10	12	15	17	20	22	25	27	30	32	35	37	40	42	45	47	50	52	55	57	1 0	3 0
20	3	5	8	11	14	17	19	22	25	28	30	33	36	39	42	44	47	50	53	55	58	1 1	1 4	1 7	20
40	3	6	9	12	15	18	21	24	27	30	34	37	40	43	46	49	52	55	58	1 1	1 4	1 7	1 10	1 13	40
4 0	3	7	10	13	17	20	23	27	30	33	37	40	43	47	50	53	57	1 0	1 3	1 7	1 10	1 13	1 16	1 20	4 0
20	4	7	11	14	18	22	25	29	32	36	40	43	47	50	54	58	1 1	1 5	1 9	1 12	1 16	1 19	1 23	1 27	20
40	4	8	12	15	19	23	27	31	35	39	43	47	50	54	58	1 2	1 6	1 10	1 14	1 18	1 22	1 25	1 29	1 33	40
5 0	4	8	12	17	21	25	29	33	37	42	46	50	54	58	1 2	1 7	1 10	1 15	1 19	1 23	1 27	1 32	1 36	1 40	5 0
20	4	9	13	18	22	26	31	35	40	44	49	53	58	1 2	1 6	1 11	1 15	1 20	1 24	1 29	1 33	1 38	1 42	1 47	20
40	5	9	14	19	24	28	33	38	42	47	52	57	1 1	1 6	1 11	1 15	1 20	1 25	1 30	1 34	1 39	1 44	1 49	1 53	40
6 0	5	10	15	20	25	30	35	40	45	50	55	1 0	1 5	1 10	1 15	1 20	1 25	1 30	1 39	1 40	1 45	1 50	1 55	2 0	6 0
20	5	10	16	21	26	32	37	42	47	53	58	1 3	1 9	1 14	1 19	1 24	1 30	1 35	1 40	1 45	1 51	1 56	2 1	2 7	20
40	5	11	17	22	28	33	39	44	50	55	1 1	1 7	1 12	1 18	1 23	1 29	1 34	1 40	1 45	1 51	1 57	2 2	2 8	2 13	40
7 0	6	12	17	23	29	35	41	47	52	58	1 4	1 10	1 16	1 22	1 27	1 33	1 39	1 45	1 51	1 57	2 2	2 8	2 14	2 20	7 0
20	6	12	18	24	30	37	43	49	55	1 1	1 7	1 13	1 19	1 25	1 32	1 38	1 44	1 50	1 56	2 2	2 8	2 14	2 20	2 27	20
40	6	13	19	25	32	38	45	51	57	1 4	1 10	1 17	1 23	1 29	1 36	1 42	1 49	1 55	2 1	2 8	2 14	2 20	2 27	2 33	40
8 0	7	13	20	27	33	40	47	53	1 0	1 7	1 13	1 20	1 27	1 33	1 40	1 47	1 53	2 0	2 7	2 13	2 20	2 27	2 33	2 40	8 0
20	7	14	21	28	35	42	49	55	1 2	1 9	1 16	1 23	1 30	1 37	1 44	1 51	1 58	2 5	2 12	2 19	2 26	2 33	2 40	2 47	20
40	7	14	21	29	36	43	50	58	1 5	1 12	1 19	1 27	1 34	1 41	1 48	1 55	2 3	2 10	2 17	2 24	2 32	2 39	2 46	2 53	40
9 0	7	15	22	30	37	45	52	1 0	1 7	1 15	1 22	1 30	1 37	1 45	1 52	2 0	2 7	2 15	2 22	2 30	2 37	2 45	2 52	3 0	9 0
20	8	15	23	31	39	47	54	1 2	1 10	1 18	1 25	1 33	1 41	1 49	1 57	2 4	2 12	2 20	2 28	2 35	2 43	2 51	2 59	3 7	20
40	8	16	24	32	40	48	56	1 4	1 12	1 20	1 29	1 37	1 45	1 53	2 1	2 9	2 17	2 25	2 33	2 41	2 49	2 57	3 5	3 13	40
10 0	8	17	25	33	41	50	58	1 7	1 15	1 23	1 32	1 40	1 48	1 57	2 5	2 13	2 22	2 30	2 38	2 47	2 55	3 3	3 12	3 20	10 0
20	9	17	26	34	43	52	1 0	1 9	1 17	1 26	1 35	1 43	1 52	2 0	2 9	2 18	2 26	2 35	2 44	2 52	3 1	3 9	3 18	3 27	20
40	9	18	27	35	44	53	1 3	1 11	1 20	1 29	1 38	1 47	1 55	2 4	2 13	2 22	2 31	2 40	2 49	2 58	3 7	3 15	3 24	3 33	40
11 0	9	18	27	37	46	55	1 4	1 13	1 22	1 32	1 41	1 50	1 59	2 8	2 17	2 27	2 36	2 45	2 54	3 3	3 12	3 22	3 31	3 40	11 0
20	10	19	28	38	47	57	1 6	1 16	1 24	1 35	1 44	1 54	2 3	2 12	2 22	2 31	2 41	2 50	2 59	3 9	3 18	3 28	3 38	3 47	20
40	10	19	29	39	49	58	1 8	1 18	1 27	1 37	1 47	1 57	2 6	2 16	2 26	2 35	2 45	2 55	3 5	3 14	3 24	3 34	3 44	3 53	40

311. TABLE for fitting the SUN's LONGITUDE, DECLINATION, or RIGHT ASCENSION, to any meridian, continued.

Daily diff.	5 Deg. h. m. 0 20	10 D. h. m. 0 40	15 D. h. m. 1 0	20 D. h. m. 1 20	25 D. h. m. 1 40	30 D. h. m. 2 0	35 D. h. m. 2 20	40 D. h. m. 2 40	45 D. h. m. 3 0	50 D. h. m. 3 20	55 D. h. m. 3 40	60 D. h. m. 4 0	65 D. h. m. 4 20	70 D. h. m. 4 40	75 D. h. m. 5 0	80 D. h. m. 5 20	85 D. h. m. 5 40	90 D. h. m. 6 0	95 D. h. m. 6 20	100 D. h. m. 6 40	105 D. h. m. 7 0	110 D. h. m. 7 20	115 D. h. m. 7 40	120 D. h. m. 8 0	Daily diff.
′ ″	′ ″	′ ″	′ ″	′ ″	′ ″	′ ″	′ ″	′ ″	′ ″	′ ″	′ ″	′ ″	′ ″	′ ″	′ ″	′ ″	′ ″	′ ″	′ ″	′ ″	′ ″	′ ″	′ ″	′ ″	′ ″
12 0	10	20	30	40	50	1 0	1 10	1 20	1 30	1 40	1 50	2 0	2 10	2 20	2 30	2 40	2 50	3 0	3 10	3 20	3 30	3 40	3 50	4 0	12 0
20	10	20	31	41	52	1 2	1 12	1 23	1 32	1 43	1 53	2 3	2 14	2 24	2 34	2 45	2 55	3 5	3 15	3 25	3 35	3 46	3 57	4 7	20
40	11	21	31	42	53	1 3	1 14	1 25	1 34	1 45	1 56	2 7	2 18	2 28	2 38	2 49	2 59	3 10	3 20	3 31	3 41	3 52	4 3	4 14	40
13 0	11	22	32	43	54	1 5	1 16	1 27	1 37	1 48	1 59	2 10	2 21	2 32	2 42	2 53	3 4	3 15	3 26	3 37	3 47	3 58	4 9	4 20	13 0
20	11	22	33	44	55	1 7	1 18	1 20	1 40	1 51	2 2	2 13	2 24	2 35	2 47	2 58	3 9	3 20	3 31	3 42	3 53	4 4	4 15	4 27	20
40	11	23	34	45	57	1 8	1 20	1 31	1 43	1 54	2 5	2 16	2 28	2 39	2 51	3 3	3 14	3 25	3 37	3 47	3 59	4 11	4 22	4 34	40
14 0	12	23	35	47	58	1 10	1 22	1 33	1 45	1 57	2 8	2 20	2 32	2 43	2 55	3 7	3 18	3 30	3 42	3 53	4 5	4 17	4 28	4 40	14 0
20	12	24	36	48	59	1 11	1 24	1 35	1 48	1 59	2 11	2 24	2 35	2 47	2 59	3 11	3 23	3 35	3 46	3 59	4 11	4 23	4 35	4 47	20
40	12	24	37	49	1 0	1 13	1 25	1 38	1 50	2 2	2 14	2 27	2 39	2 51	3 3	3 15	3 28	3 40	3 52	4 4	4 17	4 29	4 41	4 53	40
15 0	12	25	37	50	1 2	1 15	1 27	1 40	1 52	2 5	2 17	2 30	2 42	2 55	3 7	3 20	3 32	3 45	3 57	4 10	4 22	4 35	4 47	5 0	15 0
20	13	25	38	51	1 3	1 16	1 29	1 43	1 55	2 8	2 20	2 33	2 46	2 59	3 12	3 25	3 37	3 50	4 3	4 16	4 28	4 41	4 54	5 7	20
40	13	26	39	52	1 5	1 18	1 31	1 45	1 58	2 11	2 24	2 37	2 50	3 3	3 16	3 29	3 42	3 55	4 8	4 21	4 34	4 47	5 0	5 14	40
16 0	13	27	40	53	1 7	1 20	1 33	1 47	2 0	2 13	2 27	2 40	2 53	3 7	3 20	3 33	3 47	4 0	4 13	4 27	4 40	4 53	5 7	5 20	16 0
20	14	27	41	54	1 8	1 22	1 35	1 49	2 2	2 16	2 30	2 43	2 57	3 10	3 24	3 38	3 51	4 5	4 19	4 32	4 46	4 59	5 13	5 27	20
40	14	28	41	56	1 10	1 23	1 37	1 51	2 5	2 19	2 33	2 47	3 1	3 14	3 28	3 42	3 56	4 10	4 24	4 38	4 52	5 6	5 20	5 34	40
17 0	14	29	42	57	1 11	1 25	1 39	1 53	2 7	2 21	2 36	2 50	3 4	3 18	3 32	3 47	4 0	4 15	4 29	4 44	4 58	5 12	5 26	5 40	17 0
20	14	29	43	58	1 12	1 27	1 41	1 55	2 10	2 24	2 39	2 53	3 8	3 22	3 37	3 51	4 5	4 20	4 34	4 49	5 3	5 18	5 32	5 47	20
40	15	30	44	59	1 14	1 28	1 43	1 58	2 12	2 27	2 42	2 57	3 11	3 26	3 41	3 56	4 10	4 25	4 39	4 55	5 9	5 24	5 38	5 54	40
18 0	15	30	45	1 0	1 15	1 30	1 45	2 0	2 15	2 30	2 45	3 0	3 15	3 30	3 45	4 0	4 15	4 30	4 45	5 0	5 15	5 30	5 45	6 0	18 0
20	15	30	46	1 1	1 16	1 32	1 47	2 2	2 17	2 33	2 48	3 3	3 19	3 34	3 49	4 4	4 20	4 35	4 50	5 6	5 21	5 36	5 51	6 7	20
40	15	31	47	1 2	1 18	1 33	1 49	2 4	2 20	2 35	2 51	3 7	3 22	3 38	3 53	4 9	4 24	4 40	4 55	5 11	5 27	5 42	5 58	6 13	40
19 0	16	31	47	1 3	1 19	1 35	1 51	2 7	2 23	2 38	2 54	3 10	3 26	3 42	3 58	4 14	4 29	4 45	5 0	5 17	5 33	5 49	6 5	6 20	19 0
20	16	32	48	1 4	1 20	1 36	1 53	2 9	2 25	2 41	2 57	3 13	3 29	3 45	4 2	4 18	4 34	4 50	5 6	5 22	5 38	5 55	6 11	6 27	20
40	16	32	49	1 5	1 21	1 38	1 55	2 11	2 27	2 44	3 0	3 16	3 33	3 49	4 6	4 22	4 39	4 55	5 12	5 28	5 44	6 1	6 17	6 34	40
20 0	17	33	50	1 7	1 23	1 40	1 57	2 13	2 30	2 47	3 3	3 20	3 37	3 53	4 10	4 27	4 43	5 0	5 17	5 33	5 50	6 7	6 23	6 40	20 0
20	17	33	50	1 8	1 25	1 42	1 59	2 16	2 33	2 50	3 6	3 23	3 40	3 57	4 14	4 31	4 48	5 5	5 22	5 39	5 56	6 13	6 29	6 47	20
40	17	34	51	1 9	1 26	1 43	2 1	2 18	2 35	2 52	3 9	3 26	3 43	4 1	4 18	4 35	4 53	5 10	5 27	5 44	6 1	6 19	6 36	6 54	40
21 0	17	35	52	1 10	1 27	1 45	2 2	2 20	2 37	2 55	3 12	3 30	3 47	4 5	4 22	4 40	4 57	5 15	5 32	5 50	6 7	6 25	6 42	7 0	21 0
20	18	35	53	1 11	1 29	1 47	2 4	2 22	2 40	2 58	3 15	3 33	3 51	4 9	4 27	4 44	5 2	5 20	5 38	5 55	6 13	6 31	6 49	7 7	20
40	18	36	54	1 12	1 30	1 49	2 6	2 24	2 43	3 0	3 19	3 36	3 55	4 13	4 31	4 48	5 7	5 25	5 43	6 1	6 19	6 37	6 55	7 13	40
22 0	18	37	55	1 13	1 32	1 50	2 8	2 27	2 45	3 3	3 22	3 40	3 58	4 17	4 35	4 53	5 12	5 30	5 48	6 7	6 25	6 43	7 2	7 20	22 0
20	18	37	56	1 14	1 33	1 52	2 10	2 29	2 48	3 6	3 25	3 44	4 2	4 21	4 39	4 58	5 17	5 35	5 54	6 13	6 31	6 49	7 8	7 27	20
40	19	38	57	1 15	1 34	1 53	2 12	2 31	2 50	3 9	3 28	3 47	4 5	4 24	4 43	5 2	5 21	5 40	5 59	6 18	6 37	6 55	7 14	7 33	40
23 0	19	38	58	1 17	1 36	1 55	2 14	2 33	2 52	3 12	3 31	3 50	4 9	4 28	4 47	5 7	5 26	5 45	6 4	6 23	6 42	7 2	7 21	7 40	23 0
27	19	39	59	1 18	1 38	1 57	2 17	2 36	2 55	3 15	3 35	3 54	4 14	4 33	4 53	5 12	5 32	5 52	6 11	6 30	6 49	7 9	7 29	7 49	27
54	20	40	1 0	1 20	1 39	1 59	2 19	2 39	2 59	3 19	3 39	3 59	4 19	4 39	4 59	5 19	5 38	5 58	6 18	6 38	6 58	7 18	7 38	7 58	54

312. TABLE of the RIGHT ASCENSIONS and DECLINATIONS of ſixty STARS in the Northern Hemiſphere; for the Year 1780.

Conſtellations.	Places of the Stars in the Conſtellations.	Names.	Marks	Magn.	Rt. Aſcen. in time. h.	m.	ſ.	Year. Var. ſ.	Declinat. North. °	'	"	Yearly Var. "
Pegaſus	Ending of the Wing		γ	2	0	1	56	3,08	13	57	36	20,04+
Caſſiopea	Breaſt	Schedar	α	3	0	28	8	3,31	55	19	46	19,91+
Pole Star		Alruccabah	α	2	0	47	43	10,05	88	7	57	19,69+
Andromeda	Girdle	Mirach	β	2	0	57	29	3,30	34	26	56	19,45+
Aries	Preceding Horn		β	3	1	42	32	3,28	19	43	32	18,10+
Andromeda	Foot	Almaach	γ	2	1	50	29	3,62	41	15	54	17,80+
Aries	Following Horn		α	3	1	54	49	3,34	22	24	52	17,64+
Whale	Following in the Check		γ	3	2	31	56	3,12	2	17	59	15,86+
	Jaw	Menkar	α	2	2	50	48	3,13	3	12	56	14,80+
Meduſa	Head	Algol	β	2	2	53	56	3,85	40	5	37	14,63+
Perſeus	Brighteſt	Algenib	α	2	3	8	43	4,20	49	3	44	13,72+
Taurus	Brighteſt in	Pleiades	η	3	3	34	27	3,55	23	24	38	12,00+
Perſeus	Knee		ε	3	3	43	08	3,94	38	21	24	11,41+
Taurus	Firſt of the	Hyades	γ	3	4	7	18	3,39	15	4	51	9,60+
	Northern Eye		ε	3	4	15	48	3,48	18	40	32	8,90+
	Southern Eye	Aldebaran	α	1	4	23	19	3,43	16	3	6	8,32+
Auriga	In the Goat	Capella	α	1	5	0	28	4,40	45	44	48	5,30+
Taurus	Northern Horn		β	2	5	12	24	3,79	28	24	13	4,26+
Orion	Weſt Shoulder	Bellatrix	γ	2	5	13	21	3,22	6	8	2	4,15+
	Eaſt Shoulder	Betelgueſe	α	1	5	43	16	3,25	7	20	56	1,58+
Auriga	In the Hand		θ	3	5	44	43	4,09	37	10	36	1,40+
Gemini	Foot of Pollux		γ	3	6	25	00	3,47	16	34	9	2,10—
	Knee of Pollux		ζ	3	6	51	3	3,58	20	52	31	4,33—
	Brighteſt in the Head	Caſtor	α	2	7	20	33	3,88	32	21	8	6,78—
Little Dog	Brighteſt	Procyon	α	1	7	27	48	3,20	5	46	56	7,40—
Gemini	Head of Pollux	Pollux	β	2	7	31	51	3,75	28	32	29	7,70—
Great Bear	North Paw		ι	3	8	44	4	4,25	48	53	29	13,00—
Cancer	In the Claw	Acubens	α	3	8	46	27	3,24	12	41	50	13,30—
Great Bear	Preceding Knee		θ	3	9	18	5	4,23	52	40	21	15,18—
Leo	North in the Head		μ	3	9	40	13	3,47	27	1	58	16,33—
	In the Heart	Regulus	α	1	9	56	39	3,24	13	2	6	17,16—
Great Bear	Lower Pointer		β	2	10	48	27	3,74	57	33	25	19,05—
	Upper Pointer	Dubhe	α	2	10	50	0	3,88	62	56	05	19,09—
Leo	In the Tail		β	2	11	37	50	3,10	15	48	8	19,95—
Great Bear	S following in the Square		γ	2	11	42	10	3,24	54	55	4	19,99—
	Laſt in the Square		δ	2	12	4	27	3,05	58	15	25	20,05—
	Firſt in the Tail	Alioth	ε	2	12	44	17	2,69	57	9	25	19,69—
	Middle of the Tail		ζ	2	13	15	2	2,44	56	4	46	19,01—
	Laſt in the Tail	Benetnach	η	2	13	38	52	2,41	50	25	03	18,24—
Dragon	In the Tail		α	2	13	58	27	1,63	65	25	54	17,46—
Bootes	Skirt of the Coat	Arcturus	α	1	14	5	40	2,82	20	20	39	17,16—
	In the following Thigh	Mirach	ε	3	14	35	28	2,63	28	0	37	15,67—
Crown	The brighteſt	Alphacca	α	2	15	25	23	2,54	27	28	00	12,60—
Serpent	In the Neck		α	2	15	33	27	2,94	7	7	48	12,03—
Hercules	Preceding Shoulder		β	3	16	20	46	2,59	21	58	52	8,51—
	Following at the Side		ε	3	16	51	52	2,29	31	15	43	5,96—
	The Head	Raſ. Algethi	α	2	17	4	38	2,74	14	39	18	4,87—
Ophiucus	The Head	Raſ. Alhague	α	2	17	24	43	2,75	12	44	8	3,15—
Dragon	In the Head	Raſtaben	γ	2	17	51	31	1,37	51	31	21	0,78—
Harp	The brighteſt	Vega	α	1	18	29	29	2,02	38	35	14	2,52+
	Following in Lozange		δ	3	18	46	49	2,11	36	37	48	3,97+
Eagle	Preceding Wing		δ	3	19	14	24	3,02	2	41	22	6,31+
	The brighteſt	Atair	α	2	19	40	02	2,90	8	17	53	8,40+
Swan	The Breaſt		γ	3	20	14	20	2,16	39	33	43	11,00+
	The Tail	Deneb	α	2	20	33	56	2,05	44	30	7	12,44+
Cepheus	Preceding Shoulder	Alderamin	α	3	21	13	19	1,44	61	39	32	14,95+
Pegaſus	The Neck		ζ	3	22	30	29	2,99	9	41	18	18,46+
	The Thigh	Scheat	β	2	22	53	8	2,88	26	53	32	19,18+
	The Wing	Markab	α	2	22	53	49	2,98	14	1	30	19,20+
Andromeda	The Head		α	2	23	57	3	3,07	27	52	22	20,05+

312. TABLE of the RIGHT ASCENSIONS and DECLINATIONS of sixty STARS in the Southern Hemisphere; for the Year 1780.

Constellations	Places of the Stars in the Constellations.	Names.	Marks.	Magn.	Rt. Ascen. in time. h.	m.	s.	Year. Var. s.	Declinat. South. °	′	″	Yearly Var.
Phenix	The Head		α	2	0	15	22	3,01	43	29	43	20,00—
Whale	Brightest in the Tail		β	2	0	32	32	3,01	19	11	50	19,86—
Phenix	Thigh		β	3	0	56	15	2,73	47	54	58	19,46—
	Following Wing		γ	3	1	18	49	2,67	44	26	52	18,90—
Eridanus	Source of the River	Achernar	α	1	1	29	31	2,25	58	21	35	18,56—
Whale	Preceding Jaw		δ	3	2	28	13	3,07	0	37	50	16,00—
Eridanus	Near the Whale		ζ	3	3	5	10	2,91	9	38	55	13,92—
	The following		δ	3	3	32	44	2,88	10	31	30	12,08—
	The fourth Bend		γ	3	3	47	46	2,80	14	8	47	11,01—
Goldfish	In the Tail		α	3	4	29	15	1,28	55	30	20	7,76—
Orion	Bright Foot	Rigel	β	1	5	3	58	2,89	8	28	11	4,94—
	Preceding in Belt		δ	2	5	20	47	3,07	0	28	40	3,50—
	Middle of Belt		ε	2	5	25	4	3,05	1	21	30	3,13—
	Last in the Belt		ζ	2	5	29	41	3,04	2	4	27	2,77—
Dove	Preceding of the brightest		α	2	5	31	43	2,20	34	12	6	2,56—
Orion	In the Knee		κ	3	5	37	20	2,85	9	45	35	2,10—
Dove	Following of brightest		β	3	5	43	13	2,11	35	51	51	1,65—
Argo	The brightest	Canopus	α	1	6	19	5	1,34	52	34	57	1,60+
Great Dog	The brightest	Syrius	α	1	6	35	28	2,69	16	25	8	3,10+
	In the Back		δ	2	6	59	27	2,45	26	3	37	5,08+
	In the Tail		η	2	7	15	24	2,38	28	53	5	6,42+
Argo	In the Poop		ζ	2	7	55	52	2,12	39	23	28	9,62+
	Preceding in the Hull		γ	2	8	2	46	1,85	46	41	40	10,16+
	Brightest in the Middle		δ	2	8	38	36	1,61	53	54	24	12,73+
	Bright among the Oars		β	1	9	10	44	0,75	68	48	50	14,79+
Female Hydra	The Heart	Alphard	α	2	9	16	47	2,96	7	42	51	15,13+
Argo	Northern in Section		κ	2	10	36	34	2,27	58	31	59	18,68+
Centaur	Preceding in the Crupper		δ	3	11	57	3	3,06	49	29	40	20,04+
Crofs	Preceding Arm		δ	3	12	3	35	3,10	57	31	31	20,04+
	The Foot		α	1	12	14	33	3,22	61	52	48	20,01+
	The Head		γ	2	12	19	4	3,24	55	52	42	19,98+
Centaur	Top of the Crupper		γ	2	12	29	30	3,27	47	44	50	19,89+
Crofs	Following Arm		β	2	12	35	2	3,42	58	29	3	19,83+
Female Hydra	The Tail		γ	3	13	7	00	3,22	22	0	22	19,22+
Virgo	The Sheaf	Virgins Spike	α	1	13	13	38	3,15	10	0	24	19,00+
Centaur	Preceding Leg		ε	2	13	48	30	4,09	59	17	59	17,91+
	South in the Shield		η	3	14	21	37	3,75	41	10	42	16,43+
	Bright in the Foot		α	1	14	25	2	4,41	59	55	17	16,26+
Libra	Southern Scale	Zubenesch	α	2	14	38	45	3,31	15	6	55	15,50+
Centaur	Following in the Head		κ	3	14	44	56	3,84	41	12	21	15,17+
Libra	Northern Scale	Zubenelg.	β	2	15	5	12	3,22	8	33	31	13,93+
Southern Δ	The Vertex		β	3	15	35	56	5,12	62	43	31	11,88+
Scorpio	Middle of the Forehead		δ	3	15	47	21	3,53	21	58	42	11,00+
	N. in the Forehead		β	2	15	52	41	3,47	19	11	14	10,70+
Ophiucus	Preceding Hand		δ	3	16	2	50	3,14	3	6	45	9,89+
Scorpio	The Heart	Antares.	α	1	16	15	57	3,66	25	55	32	8,90+
	First Joint in the Tail		ε	3	16	35	58	3,90	33	52	21	7,34+
Ophiucu	Following Knee		η	2	16	57	47	3,44	15	26	14	5,52+
Altar	In the Middle		α	3	17	14	52	4,61	49	40	36	4,12+
Scorpio	Bright at Tail's End		λ	3	17	18	42	4,08	36	55	22	3,77+
	Sixth Knot in the Tail		ι	3	17	32	13	4,18	40	1	7	2,60+
Sa[illegible]	S. End of the Bow		ε	2	18	9	35	4,00	34	27	58	0,72—
	Preceding Shoulder		σ	3	18	41	37	3,73	26	32	57	3,54—
	Following to the Head		τ	3	18	56	41	3,58	21	21	17	4,80—
Capricorn	In the Following Horn		α	3	20	5	54	3,35	13	12	45	10,40—
Peacock	The Eye		α	2	20	8	8	4,89	57	25	14	10,44—
Capricorn	In the Forehead		β	3	20	8	57	3,35	15	27	43	10,60—
Crane	Preceding Wing		α	2	21	54	18	3,92	48	0	51	17,00—
A[illegible]	Following Arm		γ	3	22	11	17	3,11	2	29	23	17,76—
S[illegible] Fish	The Brightest	Fomalhaut	α	1	22	45	27	3,33	30	46	55	18,97—

313. TABLE of the Sun's Right Ascension, in Degrees, &c. to each Deg. of Long. And of the Diff. between Long. and Rt. Ascen.

	0 S. or 6 S.		1 S. or 7 S.		2 S. or 8 S.		
	Add to { 0 / 180	Sub. from ☉'s Long.	Add to { 0 / 180	Sub. from ☉'s Long.	Add to { 0 / 180	Sub. from ☉'s Long.	
	° ′ ″	° ′ ″	° ′ ″	° ′ ″	° ′ ″	° ′ ″	
0	0 0 0	0 0 0	27 54 20	2 5 40	57 48 48	2 11 12	30
1	0 55 2	0 4 58	28 51 43	2 8 17	58 51 21	2 8 39	29
2	1 50 5	0 9 55	29 49 15	2 10 45	59 54 4	2 5 56	28
3	2 45 8	0 14 52	30 46 56	2 13 4	60 56 57	2 3 3	27
4	3 40 12	0 19 48	31 44 46	2 15 14	62 0 0	2 0 0	26
5	4 35 18	0 24 42	32 42 45	2 17 15	63 3 12	1 56 48	25
6	5 30 25	0 29 35	33 40 54	2 19 6	64 6 34	1 53 26	24
7	6 25 34	0 34 26	34 39 13	2 20 47	65 10 4	1 49 56	23
8	7 20 45	0 39 15	35 37 41	2 22 19	66 13 43	1 46 17	22
9	8 15 59	0 44 1	36 36 19	2 23 41	67 17 31	1 42 29	21
10	9 11 16	0 48 44	37 35 8	2 24 52	68 21 27	1 38 33	20
11	10 6 35	0 53 25	38 34 7	2 25 53	69 25 31	1 34 29	19
12	11 1 58	0 58 2	39 33 16	2 26 44	70 29 42	1 30 18	18
13	11 57 25	1 2 35	40 32 36	2 27 24	71 34 1	1 25 59	17
14	12 52 56	1 7 4	41 32 7	2 27 53	72 38 27	1 21 33	16
15	13 48 32	1 11 28	42 31 48	2 28 12	73 42 59	1 17 1	15
16	14 44 12	1 15 48	43 31 40	2 28 20	74 47 38	1 12 22	14
17	15 39 57	1 20 3	44 31 43	2 28 17	75 52 23	1 7 37	13
18	16 35 47	1 24 13	45 31 56	2 28 4	76 57 13	1 2 47	12
19	17 31 43	1 28 17	46 32 21	2 27 39	78 2 9	0 57 51	11
20	18 27 45	1 32 15	47 32 57	2 27 3	79 7 9	0 52 51	10
21	19 23 53	1 36 7	48 33 43	2 26 17	80 12 13	0 47 47	9
22	20 20 7	1 39 53	49 34 41	2 25 19	81 17 21	0 42 39	8
23	21 16 28	1 43 32	50 35 49	2 24 11	82 22 33	0 37 27	7
24	22 12 55	1 47 5	51 37 8	2 22 52	83 27 49	0 32 11	6
25	23 9 30	1 50 30	52 38 58	2 21 22	84 33 7	0 26 53	5
26	24 6 12	1 53 48	53 40 19	2 19 41	85 38 27	0 21 33	4
27	25 3 2	1 56 58	54 42 11	2 17 49	86 43 48	0 16 12	3
28	26 0 0	2 0 0	55 44 13	2 15 47	87 49 11	0 10 49	2
29	26 57 6	2 2 54	56 46 25	2 13 35	88 54 35	0 5 25	1
30	27 54 20	2 5 40	57 48 48	2 11 12	90 0 0	0 0 0	0
	Sub. from { 180 / 360	Add to ☉'s Long.	Sub. from { 180 / 360	Add to ☉'s Long.	Sub. from { 180 / 360	Add to ☉'s Long.	
	5 S. or 11 S.		4 S. or 10 S.		3 S. or 9 S.		

314. TABLE I. of the Equat. of Time on the Diff. betw. the Sun's Lon. and Rt. Asc.

Deg.	♈ ♎ 0 6 m. s.	♉ ♏ 1 7 m. s.	♊ ♐ 2 8 m. s.	Deg.
0	0 0,0	8 22,7	8 44,8	30
1	0 19,9	8 33,1	8 34,6	29
2	0 39,7	8 43,0	8 23,7	28
3	0 59,5	8 52,3	8 12,2	27
4	1 19,2	9 0,9	8 0,0	26
5	1 38,8	9 9,0	7 47,2	25
6	1 58,3	9 16,4	7 33,7	24
7	2 17,7	9 23,1	7 19,7	23
8	2 37,0	9 29,3	7 5,1	22
9	2 56,1	9 34,7	6 49,9	21
10	3 14,6	9 39,5	6 34,2	20
11	3 33,7	9 43,5	6 17,7	19
12	3 52,1	9 46,9	6 1,2	18
13	4 10,3	9 49,6	5 43,9	17
14	4 28,3	9 51,5	5 26,2	16
15	4 45,9	9 52,8	5 8,1	15
16	5 3,2	9 53,3	4 49,5	14
17	5 20,2	9 53,1	4 30,5	13
18	5 36,9	9 52,3	4 11,1	12
19	5 53,1	9 50,6	3 51,4	11
20	6 9,0	9 48,2	3 31,4	10
21	6 24,5	9 45,1	3 11,1	9
22	6 39,5	9 41,3	2 50,6	8
23	6 54,1	9 36,7	2 29,9	7
24	7 8,3	9 31,5	2 8,7	6
25	7 22,0	9 25,5	1 47,5	5
26	7 35,2	9 18,7	1 26,2	4
27	7 47,7	9 11,3	1 4,8	3
28	8 0,0	9 3,1	0 43,3	2
29	8 11,6	8 54,3	0 21,7	1
30	8 22,7	8 44,8	0 0,0	0
Deg.	♓ ♍ 11 5	♒ ♌ 10 4	♑ ♋ 9 3	Deg.

315. TABLE II. of the Equation of Time on the Sun's Anomaly; or the Equation of the Center turned into Time.

☉ Mea. An.	Sign 0 m. s.	Sign 1 m. s.	Sign 2 m. s.	Sign 3 m. s.	Sign 4 m. s.	Sign 5 m. s.	☉ Mea. An.
0	0 0	3 47	6 36	7 42	6 45	3 56	30
1	0 8	3 54	6 40	7 43	6 41	3 48	29
2	0 16	4 1	6 44	7 43	6 37	3 41	28
3	0 24	4 8	6 48	7 42	6 32	3 34	27
4	0 32	4 14	6 52	7 42	6 28	3 27	26
5	0 39	4 21	6 55	7 42	6 23	3 19	25
6	0 47	4 27	6 59	7 41	6 19	3 12	24
7	0 55	4 34	7 2	7 40	6 14	3 4	23
8	1 3	4 40	7 5	7 39	6 9	2 57	22
9	1 11	4 46	7 9	7 38	6 4	2 49	21
10	1 23	4 53	7 12	7 37	5 59	2 41	20
11	1 26	4 59	7 14	7 36	5 54	2 32	19
12	1 34	5 5	7 17	7 34	5 49	2 26	18
13	1 43	5 11	7 20	7 33	5 43	2 18	17
14	1 50	5 17	7 22	7 31	5-38	2 10	16
15	1 57	5 22	7 24	7 29	5 32	2 2	15
16	2 5	5 28	7 26	7 27	5 26	1 54	14
17	2 13	5 33	7 28	7 25	5 20	1 46	13
18	2 20	5 39	7 30	7 23	5 14	1 38	12
19	2 28	5 44	7 32	7 20	5 8	1 30	11
20	2 35	5 50	7 34	7 18	5 2	1 22	10
21	2 43	5 55	7 35	7 15	4 56	1 14	9
22	2 50	6 0	7 37	7 12	4 50	1 6	8
23	2 57	6 5	7 38	7 9	4 43	0 58	7
24	3 5	6 10	7 39	7 6	4 37	0 49	6
25	3 12	6 14	7 40	7 3	4 31	0 41	5
26	3 19	6 19	7 41	7 0	4 23	0 33	4
27	3 26	6 24	7 41	6 56	4 16	0 25	3
28	3 33	6 28	7 42	6 52	4 10	0 16	2
29	3 40	6 32	7 42	6 49	4 3	0 8	1
30	3 47	6 36	7 42	6 45	3 56	0 0	0
	11 Sign	10 Sign	9 Sign	8 Sign	7 Sign	6 Sign	

316. Table of the Abſolute Equation of Time, fitted to each Sign and Degree of the Ecliptic.

Place of the Apogee ♋ 9°. Obliquity of Ecliptic 23° 28′.

Deg.	♈ 0	♉ 1	♊ 2	♋ 3	♌ 4	♍ 5	♎ 6	♏ 7	♐ 8	♑ 9	♒ 10	♓ 11	Deg.
	+ —	—	— +	+	+	+ —	—	—	—	— +	+	+	
	m. ſ.	m. ſ.	m. ſ.	m. ſ.	m. ſ.	m. ſ.	m. ſ.	m. ſ.	m. ſ.	m. ſ.	m. ſ.	m. ſ.	
0	7 36	1 9	3 51	1 13	5 57	2 20	7 38	15 31	13 33	1 11	11 28	14 19	0
1	7 17	1 23	3 47	1 26	5 59	2 4	7 58	15 39	13 17	0 42	11 45	14 13	1
2	6 58	1 36	3 41	1 40	6 0	1 48	8 19	15 46	13 0	— 12	12 1	14 6	2
3	6 39	1 48	3 37	1 53	6 1	1 31	8 40	15 52	12 42	+ 17	12 17	13 59	3
4	6 20	2 0	3 32	2 7	6 1	1 14	9 1	15 57	12 23	0 46	12 32	13 51	4
5	6 1	2 11	3 26	2 20	6 0	0 56	9 21	16 2	12 4	1 16	12 46	13 43	5
6	5 42	2 22	3 19	2 33	5 59	0 38	9 41	16 6	11 44	1 45	12 59	13 34	6
7	5 24	2 32	3 12	2 45	5 57	0 20	10 1	16 9	11 23	2 14	13 12	13 24	7
8	5 5	2 42	3 4	2 58	5 54	+ 1	10 20	16 11	11 1	2 43	13 24	13 14	8
9	4 47	2 51	2 56	3 11	5 51	— 18	10 39	16 13	10 39	3 11	13 35	13 3	9
10	4 28	3 0	2 47	3 23	5 47	0 37	10 57	16 13	10 16	3 39	13 45	12 51	10
11	4 9	3 8	2 38	3 35	5 42	0 57	11 15	16 13	9 53	4 7	13 54	12 39	11
12	3 50	3 16	2 29	3 46	5 37	1 17	11 33	16 12	9 29	4 35	14 2	12 27	12
13	3 32	3 23	2 19	3 58	5 31	1 38	11 51	16 10	9 5	5 2	14 9	12 14	13
14	3 13	3 30	2 8	4 9	5 24	1 58	12 8	16 7	8 40	5 29	14 16	12 0	14
15	2 55	3 36	1 57	4 19	5 17	2 19	12 25	16 4	8 14	5 56	14 22	11 46	15
16	2 37	3 41	1 46	4 29	5 9	2 40	12 41	16 0	7 48	6 22	14 27	11 31	16
17	2 19	3 46	1 35	4 39	5 1	3 1	12 57	15 55	7 22	6 48	14 31	11 16	17
18	2 1	3 50	1 23	4 48	4 52	3 22	13 12	15 49	6 55	7 13	14 35	11 1	18
19	1 43	3 53	1 11	4 57	4 43	3 44	13 27	15 42	6 28	7 37	14 38	10 46	19
20	1 26	3 56	0 59	5 5	4 33	4 5	13 42	15 35	6 0	8 1	14 40	10 30	20
21	1 9	3 58	0 46	5 13	4 22	4 26	13 56	15 26	5 32	8 24	14 41	10 14	21
22	0 52	4 0	0 34	5 20	4 11	4 47	14 9	15 17	5 4	8 47	14 42	9 58	22
23	0 36	4 1	0 21	5 27	3 59	5 9	14 21	15 7	4 36	9 9	14 41	9 41	23
24	0 20	4 1	— 8	5 33	3 46	5 30	14 33	14 56	4 8	9 31	14 40	9 24	24
25	+ 4	4 1	+ 5	5 39	3 33	5 52	14 44	14 44	3 39	9 53	14 39	9 6	25
26	— 11	4 0	0 19	5 44	3 19	6 13	14 53	14 31	3 10	10 14	14 37	8 48	26
27	0 26	3 59	0 31	5 48	3 4	6 35	15 5	14 17	2 41	10 34	14 34	8 30	27
28	0 40	3 57	0 46	5 52	2 50	6 56	15 14	14 3	2 11	10 53	14 30	8 12	28
29	0 53	3 54	0 59	5 55	2 35	7 17	15 23	13 48	1 41	11 11	14 25	7 54	29
30	1 9	3 51	1 13	5 57	2 20	7 3	15 31	13 33	1 11	11 28	14 19	7 36	30

The equations with +, are to be added to the apparent time, to have the mean time; thoſe with —, are to be ſubtracted from apparent for mean time.

The preceding mark, whether + or —, at the head of any column, belongs to all equations in that column until the ſign changes; and thoſe columns having two ſigns at the head, ſhew that the preceding ſign changes to the following ſomewhere in that column.

317. Table

317. Table of Corrections for the Middle Time between the Equal Altitudes of the Sun.

Deg. of Declin.	Latitude 30 D.N.						Latitude 40 D.N.						Latitude 50 D.N.						Latitude 60 D.N.						Deg. of Declin.
	Hours bet. Obser.						Hours bet. Obser.						Hours bet. Obser.						Hours bet. Obser.						
	6	5	4	6	5	4	6	5	4	6	5	4	6	5	4	6	5	4	6	5	4	6	5	4	
	N. decl.			S. decl.			N. decl.			S. decl.			N. decl.			S. decl.			N. decl.			S. decl.			
	sec.	sec.	sec.	sec.	sec.	sec.	sec.	sec.	sec.	sec.	sec.	sec.	sec.	sec.	sec.	sec.	sec.	sec.	sec.	sec.	sec.	sec.	sec.	sec.	
0	9	9	8	9	9	8	14	13	13	14	13	13	20	19	18	20	19	18	28	28	27	28	28	27	0
1	9	9	8	9	9	9	14	13	12	14	13	13	19	19	18	20	19	18	28	27	27	29	28	27	1
2	9	8	8	9	9	9	13	13	12	14	14	13	19	18	18	20	19	18	28	27	26	29	28	27	2
3	8	8	7	10	9	9	13	12	12	14	14	13	18	18	17	20	19	18	28	27	26	29	28	27	3
4	8	8	7	10	10	9	13	12	12	14	14	13	18	17	17	20	19	19	27	26	25	29	29	28	4
5	8	7	7	10	10	10	12	12	11	15	14	14	18	17	17	20	19	19	27	26	25	29	29	28	5
6	8	7	6	10	10	10	12	11	11	15	14	14	17	17	16	20	20	19	27	25	24	29	29	28	6
7	7	7	6	10	10	10	12	11	11	15	14	14	17	16	16	20	20	19	26	25	24	29	28	27	7
8	7	7	6	10	10	10	11	11	10	15	14	14	17	16	16	20	20	19	26	24	23	29	28	27	8
9	7	6	6	10	10	10	11	10	10	15	15	14	16	15	15	20	20	19	25	23	23	28	28	27	9
10	7	6	5	10	10	10	11	10	10	15	15	14	16	15	15	20	19	19	24	23	22	28	28	27	10
11	6	6	5	10	10	10	10	10	9	14	14	14	15	15	14	19	19	18	23	22	22		27	27	11
12	6	6	5	10	10	10	10	9	9	14	14	14	15	14	14	19	19	18	22	21	21		27	26	12
13	6	5	5	10	10	9	9	9	8	14	14	14	14	14	13	19	19	18	21	21	20		26	26	13
14	5	5	4	10	9	9	9	8	8	14	14	14	13	13	12	18	18	17	20	20	19		25	25	14
15	5	5	4	9	9	9	8	8	7	14	14	13	13	12	12	18	18	17	19	19	18			24	15
16	5	4	4	9	9	9	8	7	7	13	13	13	12	12	11	17	17	17	18	18	17			23	16
17	4	4	3	9	9	8	7	7	6	12	12	12	11	11	10	16	16	16	17	17	16			22	17
18	4	3	3	9	8	8	6	6	5	12	12	12	10	10	9	15	15	15	16	15	15			21	18
19	3	3	2	8	8	8	6	5	5	11	11	11	9	9	8	14	14	14	15	14	13			19	19
20	3	2	2	8	7	7	5	5	4	10	10	10	8	8	7	13	13	13	14	13	12			17	20
21	2	2	1	7	7	7	4	3	3	9	9	9	7	6	6		11	11	12	11	10			14	21
22	1	1	0	6	6	5	3	2	2	7	7	7	5	5	5		9	9	8	8	8			11	22
23	0	0	0	3	3	3	2	1	0	4	4	4	3	2	2		5	5	5	5	4			7	23

The correction is ſubtractive from December 22 to June 21, or in aſcending ſigns; and additive from June 21 to December 22, or in deſcending ſigns.

318. A Table of Refractions.

Alt. Deg.	Refr. min.	Refr. sec.	Alt. Deg.	Refr. min.	Refr. sec.	Alt. Deg.	Refr. min.	Refr. sec.	Alt. Deg.	Refr. min.	Refr. sec.	Alt. Deg.	Refr. min.	Refr. sec.	Alt. Deg.	Refr. min.	Refr. sec.	Alt. Deg.	Refr. min.	Refr. sec.
0	33	00	4	11	51	14	3	45	26	1	56	38	1	13	50	0	48	62	0	30
0¼	30	35	4½	10	48	15	3	30	27	1	51	39	1	10	51	0	46	63	0	29
0½	28	22	5	9	54	16	3	17	28	1	47	40	1	8	52	0	44	64	0	28
0¾	26	21	5½	9	8	17	3	4	29	1	42	41	1	5	53	0	43	65	0	26
1	24	20	6	8	28	18	2	54	30	1	38	42	1	3	54	0	41	66	0	25
1¼	22	48	7	7	20	19	2	44	31	1	35	43	1	1	55	0	40	67	0	24
1½	21	15	8	6	29	20	2	35	32	1	31	44	0	59	56	0	38	68	0	23
1¾	19	51	9	5	48	21	2	27	33	1	28	45	0	57	57	0	37	69	0	22
2	18	35	10	5	15	22	2	20	34	1	24	46	0	55	58	0	35	70	0	21
2½	16	24	11	4	47	23	2	14	35	1	21	47	0	53	59	0	34	71	0	19
3	14	36	12	4	23	24	2	7	36	1	18	48	0	51	60	0	33	72	0	18
3½	13	6	13	4	3	25	2	2	37	1	16	49	0	49	61	0	32	73	0	17

319. *Of the Sun's Parallax.*

Altitudes	0°.	10°	20°	30°	40°	50°	60°	70°	80°	90°.
Parallax	9″	9″	8″	8″	6″	5″	3″	2″	1″	0″.

END of BOOK V.

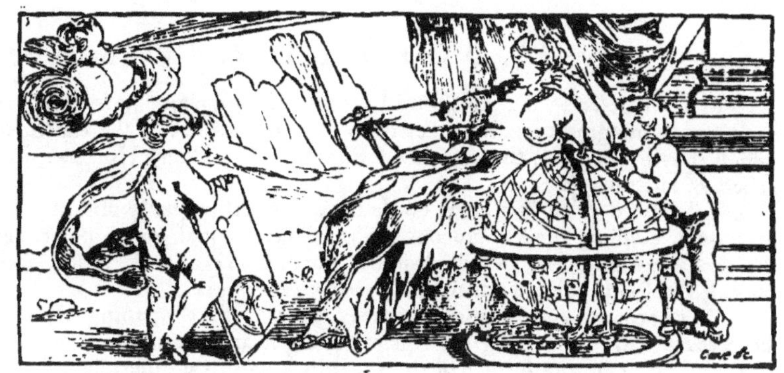

THE ELEMENTS OF NAVIGATION.

BOOK VI.

OF GEOGRAPHY.

SECTION I.

Definitions and *Principles.*

1. GEOGRAPHY is the art of defcribing the figure, magnitude, and pofitions of the feveral parts of the furface of the Earth.

2. The EARTH is a fpherical or globular figure *, and is ufually called the terraqueous globe.

3. There are two points on the furface of the terraqueous globe, called the POLES OF THE EARTH, which are diametrically oppofite to one another: one is called the *north pole*, and the other, the *fouth pole*.

---

* For in fhips at fea the firft parts of them that become vifible are the upper fails; and as they approach nearer, the lower fails appear; and fo on until they fhew their hulls.

Alfo fhips in failing from high capes, or head lands, lofe fight of thofe eminences gradually from the lower parts, until the top vanifhes.

Now as thefe appearances are the objects of our fenfes in all parts of the Earth,

Therefore the furface of the Earth muft be convex.

And this convexity is, at fea, obferved to be every where uniform.

But a body, the furface of which is every where uniformly convex, is a globe.

Therefore the figure of the Earth is globular.

In order to deſcribe the poſitions of places, Geographers have found it neceſſary to imagine certain circles drawn on the ſurface of the Earth, to which they have given the names of Equator, Meridian, Horizon, Parallels of latitude, *&c.*

4. The **Equator** is a great circle on the Earth, equally diſtant from each pole, dividing the terraqueous globe into two equal parts; one called the *northern hemiſphere*, in which is the north pole; and the other, containing the ſouth pole, is called the *ſouthern hemiſphere.*

5. **Meridians** are imaginary circles on the Earth paſſing through both the poles, and cutting the equator at right angles.

Every point on the ſurface of the Earth has its proper meridian.

6. **Latitude** is the diſtance of a place from the equator, reckoned in degrees and parts of degrees on a meridian.

On the north ſide of the equator it is north latitude; and on the ſouth ſide it is ſouth latitude.

As latitude begins at the equator, where it is nothing; ſo it ends at the poles, where the latitude is greateſt, or 90 degrees.

7. **Parallels of Latitude** are circles parallel to the equator.

Every place on the Earth has its parallel of latitude.

Difference of Latitude is an arc of a meridian, or the leaſt diſtance of the parallels of latitude of two places; ſhewing how far one of them is to the northward, or ſouthward, of the other.

The difference of latitude can never exceed 180 degrees.

8. In north latitudes, if about the middle of the months of March and September a perſon looks towards the Sun at noon, the ſouth is before him, the north behind, the weſt on the right hand, and the eaſt on the left: and in ſouth latitudes, if the face is turned toward the Sun at the ſame times, the north is before, the ſouth behind, the eaſt to the right, and the weſt on the left.

In latitudes greater than $23\frac{1}{2}$ degrees, theſe poſitions, found at noon, will hold good on any day of the year.

9. **Longitude** of any place on the Earth is expreſſed by an arc of the equator, ſhewing the eaſt or weſt diſtance of the meridian of that place from ſome fixed meridian, where longitude is reckoned to begin.

10. **Difference of Longitude** is an arc of the equator, intercepted between the meridians of two places, ſhewing how far one of them is to the eaſtward, or weſtward, of the other.

As longitude begins at the meridan of ſome place, and is counted from thence both eaſtward and weſtward, till they meet at the ſame meridian on the oppoſite point of the equator; therefore the difference of longitude can never exceed 180 degrees.

11. When two places have latitudes both north, or both ſouth; or have longitudes both eaſt, or both weſt, they are ſaid to be of the ſame, or of like name: but when one has north latitude, and the other ſouth; or if one has eaſt longitude, and the other weſt, then they are ſaid to have contrary, or different, or unlike names.

12. The **Horizon** is that apparent circle which limits, or bounds, the view of a ſpectator on the ſea, or on an extended plain; the eye of the ſpectator being always ſuppoſed in the center of his horizon.

When the Planets or Stars come above the eastern part of the horizon, they are said to rise; and when they descend below the western part, they are said to set.

When a ship is under the equator, both the poles appear in the horizon; and in proportion as she falls towards either, or increases her latitude, that pole is seen proportionally higher above the horizon, and the other disappears as much: but when a ship is sailing towards the equator, or decreases her latitude, she depresses the elevated pole; that is, its distance from the horizon decreases.

Of the division of the Earth into Zones.

13. A Zone is a broad space on the Earth, included between two parallels of latitude.

There are five zones: namely, one *Torrid*, two *Frigid*, and two *Temperate*; these names arise from the degree of heat or cold, to which their situations are liable.

14. The Torrid Zone is that portion of the Earth, over every part of which the Sun is perpendicular at one time of the year or other.

This zone is about 47 degrees in breadth, extending to about 23½ degrees on each side of the equator; the parallel of latitude terminating the limits in the northern hemisphere, is called the *Tropic of Cancer*; and in the southern hemisphere, the limiting parallel is called the *Tropic of Capricorn*.

15. The Frigid Zones are those regions about the poles, where the Sun does not rise for some days, nor set for some days, of the year.

These zones extend round the poles to the distance of about 23½ degrees: that in the northern hemisphere is called the north frigid zone, and is bounded by a parallel of latitude, called the *Arctic polar circle*: and the other, in the southern hemisphere, the south frigid zone; the parallel of latitude bounding it, being called the *Antarctic polar circle*.

16. The Temperate Zones are the spaces between the Torrid and the Frigid zones.

Of the division of the Earth by Climates.

17. A Climate, in a geographical sense, is that space of the Earth contained between two parallels of latitude, when the difference between the longest day in each parallel is half an hour.

These climates are narrower the farther they are from the equator; therefore, supposing the equator to be the beginning of the first climate, the polar circle will be the end of the 24th climate; for afterwards the longest day does dot increase by half hours, but by days and months.

SECTION II.

Of the natural diviſion of the Earth.

18. By the natural diviſion of the Earth is meant the parts on its ſurface formed by nature; ſuch as *Continents*, *Oceans*, *Iſlands*, *Seas*, *Rivers*, *Mountains*, &c.

The ſurface of the Earth is naturally divided into Land and Water.

Land is divided into	1. Continents.	4. Iſthmuſes.
	2. Iſlands.	5. Promontaries.
	3. Peninſulas.	6. Mountains.

Water is divided into	1. Oceans.	4. Straits.
	2. Seas.	5. Lakes.
	3. Gulfs.	6. Rivers.

19. A CONTINENT, or, as it is frequently called, the *main land*, is a very large track, comprehending ſeveral contiguous Countries, Kingdoms, and States.

20. An OCEAN is a vaſt collection of ſalt water, ſeparating the continents from one another.

21. An ISLAND is a part of dry land, ſurrounded with water.

22. A SEA is a branch of the Ocean, flowing between ſome parts of the Continent, or ſeparating an Iſland from the Continent.

23. A PENINSULA is a part of dry land encompaſſed by water, except a narrow neck which joins it to ſome other land.

24. An ISTHMUS is the neck joining the peninſula to the adjacent land, and forms the paſſage between them.

25. A MOUNTAIN is a part of the land more elevated than the adjacent country, and to be ſeen at a greater diſtance than the neighbouring lower lands.

26. A PROMONTORY is a mountain ſtretching itſelf into the ſea; the extremity of which is called a *Cape*, or *Head-land*.

27. A HILL is a ſmall kind of mountain: A *Cliff* is a ſteep ſhore, hill, or mountain: And *Rocks* are great ſtones, riſing like hills above the dry land, or above the bottom of the ſea.

28. A GULF, or BAY, is a part of the Ocean, or Sea, contained between two ſhores: and is every where environed with land, except at its entrance, where it communicates with other Bays, Seas, or Oceans.

29. A STRAIT is a narrow paſſage, by which there is a communication between a Gulf and its neighbouring ſea, or which joins one part of the ſea, or ocean, with another.

30. A LAKE is a collection of Waters contained in ſome hollow or cavity, in an inland place, of a large extent, and every where ſurrounded with land, having no viſible communication with the Ocean.

31. RIVERS are ſtreams of Water, flowing chiefly from the Mountains, and running in long narrow channels, or cavities, through the land, 'till they fall into the ſea, or into other rivers, which at laſt run into the ſea.

32. There

32. There are generally reckoned four Continents, namely, EUROPE, ASIA, AFRICA, and AMERICA.

To these may be added the *Terra arctica*, or nothern continent, and the *Terra antarctica*, or lands detached from *Asia*, towards the south.

The continent of *America* is usually divided into two parts, called *North* and *South America*; they are joined together by the *Isthmus* of *Darien*. Also the continents of *Asia* and *Africa* are joined together by the *Isthmus* of *Sues*.

The *Terra arctica*, *Europe*, and *Asia*, lie all within the northern hemisphere; and also part of *Africa* and *America*: The other parts of these two continents, together with the *Terra antarctica*, lie in the southern hemisphere.

33. There are five Oceans, namely, the NORTHERN, the ATLANTIC, the PACIFIC, the INDIAN, and the SOUTHERN.

The *Atlantic ocean* is usually divided into two parts, one called the *north Atlantic ocean*, and the other the *south Atlantic*, or *Ethiopic ocean*.

The *Northern ocean* stretches to the northward of Europe, Asia, and America, towards the north pole.

The *Atlantic ocean* lies between the continents of Europe and Africa on the east, and America on the west.

That part of the north Atlantic ocean, lying between Europe and America, is frequently called the *Western ocean*.

The *Pacific ocean*, or, as it is sometimes called, the *South Sea*, is bounded by the western and north-west shores of America, and by the eastern and north-east shores of Asia.

The *Indian ocean* washes the shores of the eastern coasts of Africa, and the south of Asia; and is bounded on the east by the Indian islands, New Holland, and New Zeeland.

The *Southern ocean* extends to the southward of Africa and America towards the south pole.

The northern and southern continents not being sufficiently known to Geographers, all that need be said of them is, that the Terra Arctica, or land to the northward of Hudson's Bay and Greenland, is in general too cold for the residence of mankind; and that the lands formerly supposed to be parts of the southern continent, are found to be very large islands: *viz.* New Zeland is much larger than Great Britain, and has a strait dividing it into two islands. New Holland is an island as large as Europe. New Guinea is a very large island; and New Britain is a cluster of large and small islands, and are thought by some to be the islands hitherto called the Solomon's islands.

SECTION III.

Of the Political division of the Earth.

34. By the political division of the Earth is meant the different Countries, Empires, Kingdoms, States, and other denominations established by men, either from the ambition of tyrants, or for the sake of good government.

OF EUROPE.

Europe is bounded on the north by the northern, or frozen, ocean; on the east by Asia; on the south by the Mediterranean Sea, separating Europe from Africa; and by the north Atlantic, or western ocean, on the west. It lies between the latitudes of 36 and 72 degrees of north latitude; and between the longitudes of 10 degrees west, and 65 degrees east from London; is about 3000 miles long, reckoning from the N. E. to the S. W. and about 2500 miles broad.

35. The countries, their position, with regard to the middle parts of Europe, the chief cities, principal rivers, with their courses, and the most noted mountains, and what quarter of the country they are in, are exhibited in the following table; where E. stands for empire, K. for kingdom, R. for republic, Nd. for northward, &c.

Countries.	Position.	Chief Cities.	Rivers.	Course.	Mountains.
E. Turky	S. E.	Constantinople	Danube	E.	Argentum Nd.
K. Poland	Mid.	Warsaw	Vistula	N. N. W.	Carpathian Sd.
E. Muscovy } E. Russia }	N. E.	Moscow / Petersburg	Volga	E. to S.	Boglowy Sd.
			Niaper	S.	Riphean Wd.
K. Sweden	N.	Stockholm	Dalecarlia	E.	Dofrine Wd.
K. Norway	N. N. W.	Bergen	Glama	S.	Dofrine Ed.
K. Denmark	N. W.	Copenhagen	Eyder	W.	
K. Hungary	Mid.	Presburg	Danube	S. E.	Carpathian Nd.
E. Germany	Mid.	Vienna	Danube	E.	Alps Sd.
Italy	S.	Rome	Po	E.	Alps Nd.
			Tyber	S.	Apennine Mid.
R. Switzerland	Mid.	Bern	Rhine	W.	Alps Sd.
Netherlands	W.	Brussels	Maese	N.	
R. Holland	W.	Amsterdam	Rhine	N. N. W.	
K. France	W.	Paris	Loire	N. to W.	Pyrenees S. W.
			Rhone	S.	Alps Ed.
K. Spain	S. W.	Madrid	Tagus	W.	Pyrenees N. E.
K. Portugal	S. W.	Lisbon	Tagus	W.	C. Rocca W.
K. England	W.	London	Thames	E.	Malvern N. W.
K. Scotland	W.	Edinburgh	Forth	E,	Grampian Nd.
K. Ireland	W.	Dublin	Shannon	S. W.	Knockpatric W

There are in Europe four Kingdoms beside those enumerated above; but they are contained in the forenamed Countries.

The Kingdom of Prussia, which is part of Poland; the King's residence is at Berlin, a city in Germany.

The

The Kingdom of Bohemia, a part of Germany; the chief city is Prague.

The Kingdom of Sardinia, an Italian island; the King resides at Turin, a city in Italy.

The Kingdom of the Sicilies, appending to Italy; the King resides at Naples, a city in Italy.

In some of the forenamed countries are several dominions independent one of the other; particularly in Germany and Italy.

The principal states in Germany are the following 12; where D. stands for duchy, El. for electorate, P. for principality.

States Ch.cities	D. Austria Vienna	K. Bohemia Prague	El. Bavaria Munich	El. Brandenburg Berlin
States Ch.cities	El. Saxony Dresden	El. Hanover Hanover	El. Palatine Manheim	El. Mentz Mentz
States Ch.cities	El. Triers Triers	El. Cologne Cologne	P. HesseCassel Cassel	D. Wurtemburg Stutgard

The principal states in Italy are the following 12.

States Ch.cities	D. Savoy Chamberry	P. Piedmont Turin	D. Milanese Milan	D. Parmesan Parma
States Ch.cities	D. Modenese Modena	D. Mantuan Mantua	R. Venice Venice	R. Genoa Genoa
States Ch.cities	D. Tuscany Florence	Patriarchate Rome	R. Lucca Lucca	K. Naples Naples

36. *The principal Seas, Gulfs and Bays in Europe, are*

The *Mediterranean Sea*, having Europe on the N. and Africa on the S.
The *Adriatic Sea*, between Italy and Turky.
The *Euxine*, or *Black Sea*, in Turky, between Europe and Asia.
The *White Sea*, in the N. N. W. parts of Muscovy.
The *Baltic Sea*, between Sweden, Denmark, and Poland.
The *German Ocean*, or Sea, between Germany and Britain.
The *English Channel*, between England and France.
St. George's Channel, between Britain and Ireland.
The *Bay of Biscay*, formed between France and Spain.
The *Gulf of Bothnia*, in the N. E. parts of Sweden.
The *Gulf of Finland*, between Sweden and Russia.
The *Gulf of Venice*, the N. W. end of the Adriatic Sea

37. *The principal Islands in Europe, are*

The *British Isles*, viz. Great Britain, Ireland, Orkneys, and Western Isles.
The *Spanish Isles*; Majorca, Minorca, Ivica, in the Medit. Sea.
Turkish Isles; Sicily, Sardinia, Corsica, Lipari, in the Medit. Sea.
Italian Isles; Candia, Archipelago Isles, in the Medit. Sea.
Swedish Isles; Gothland, Oeland, Alan, Rugen, in the Baltic Sea.
Danish Isles; Zeland in the Baltic Sea; and Iceland, Faro Isles, E. and W. Greenlands in the Northern ocean.
Azores Isles in the Atlantic ocean, belonging to Portugal.

OF ASIA.

38. The continent of Aſia is bounded on the north by the Northern or frozen ocean, on the eaſt by the Pacific ocean, on the ſouth by the Indian ocean, and by Africa and Europe on the weſt. It lies, including its Iſlands, between the latitudes of 10 degrees ſouth, and 72 degrees north; and is between the longitudes of 25 and 148 degrees eaſt of London; its length, excluſive of the iſles, being about 4800 miles, and breadth about 4300 miles.

39. The poſitions and names of the chief countries, cities, rivers, and mountains, are contained in the following table.

Countries.	Poſition.	ChiefCities.	Rivers.	Courſe.	Mountains.
E. China	S. E.	Pekin	Yellow R.	S. to E.	Ottorocoran Nd.
		Nankin	Kiam	E	Damaſian Wd.
		Canton	Ta	S. E.	
K. Korea	E.	Kingkitau	Yalu	S.	Shanalin
ChineſeTartary	E.	Chynian	Yamour	N.E.to E.	Fongwanſhan
Mongalia	Mid.	Kudak	Yellow R.	N. to W.	
K. Thibet	Mid.	Eſkerdu	Yaru	E.	Kantes
Bukharia, or Uſbecs	Mid.	Samarkand	Amu	N. W.	Belurlag
Karazm	Mid.	Urjenz	Amu	S. W.	Irder
Kalmucks	Mid.		Tekis		Tubratubuſluk
E. Siberia	N.	Tobolſki	Oby	N.	Stolp
		Aſtracan	Jeniſka	N. N. W.	
E. Turky	W.	Smyrna	Euphrates	S. E.	Taurus
K. Syria	W.	Aleppo	Euphrates	S.	Lebanon
Arabia	S. W.	Medina	Euphrates	S. E.	Gabel el ared
E. Perſia	S.	Iſpahan	Oxus	W.	Caucaſus
			Araxes	S. W.	Taurus
India Weſt of the Ganges	S.	Agra	Indus	S. W.	Caucaſus
		Delli	Ganges	S. W.	Balagate
India Eaſt of the Ganges	S.	Ava	Domea	S.	Damaſcene
		Pegu	Mecon	S.	
		Siam	Menan	S.	
		Cambodia	Ava	S.	

Some of theſe countries contain ſeveral others.

Aſiatic Turky contains

Countries	Georgia N.	Turcomania E. or Armenia	Curdiſtan E. or Aſſyria	Diarbec E.
Ch. cities	Teflis	Erzerum	Betlis	Mouſol
Countries	Eyraca S.E.	Arabia deſert S.	Natolia W.	Syria W.
Ch. cities	Bagdat		Smyrna	Aleppo

India

India west of the Ganges contains

Northern Parts	Countries	Indostan N.	Cambaya S. W. or Guzarat	Bengala S.E.
	Ch. cities	Delli	Surat	Patna
Malabar Coast	Countries	Decan or Visapour	Bisnagar W. or Carnate	
	Ch. cities	Goa	Calcut and Cochin	
Coromandel Coast	Countries	Bisnagar Carnate, E. side	K. Golconda	K. Orixa
	Ch. cities	Madras	Golconda	Orixa

India east of the Ganges contains

Countries	K. Ava N. W.	K. Pegu W	K. Siam S.	K. Malacca S.
Ch. cities	Ava	Pegu	Siam	Malacca
Countries	K. Cambodia S.	K. Cochin China E.	K. Laos N.	K. Tonquin N. E.
Ch. cities	Cambodia	Thoanoa	Lanchan	Keccio

40. *The principal Seas, Gulfs and Bays in Asia, are*

Caspian Sea, quite surrounded by Siberia on the north, Korazm east, by Persia on the south, and by Georgia on the west.
Korean Sea, between Korea and the islands of Japan.
Yellow Sea, between China and the Japan isles.
Gulf of Cochin China, on the borders of Tonquin and Cochin China.
Bay of Siam, formed by the countries of Siam and Malacca.
Bay of Bengal, between India east, and India west of the Ganges.
Gulf of Persia, having Persia on the N. E. and Arabia on the S. W.

41. *The principal Islands belonging to Asia, are*
Ladrone, or *Marian Isles*, whose chief island is Guam.

Japan Isles	Ch. isles	Japan	Bongo	Tonsa
	Ch. cities	Jeddo	Bongo	Tonsa
Philippines	Ch. isles	Luconia	Mindanao	Samar
	Ch. cities	Manilla	Mindanao	
Chinese Isles	Ch. isles	Formosa	Ainan	Makao
	Ch. cities	Taywansu	Tan	Makau
Moluccos	Ch. isles	Celebes	Gilolo	Ceram
	Ch. cities	Macasser	Gilolo	Ambay
Sunda Isles	Ch. isles	Borneo	Sumatra	Java
	Ch. cities	Banjar	Achin	Batavia

The *Andaman Isles* to the west of Siam.
Nicobar Islands west of Malacca.
Maldive Islands to the S. W. of Bisnagar.

The *Island of Ceylon* S. E. of Bisnagar; the chief city is Candy, or Candy Uta.

OF

42. This large continent is a peninsula, joined to Asia by the Isthmus of Suez. On the N. E. it is separated from Asia by the Red Sea; it has the Indian Ocean on the east, the Southern on the south, the Atlantic on the west, and the Mediterranean Sea on the north, which separates it from Europe. It is situated between the latitudes of 37 degrees N. and 35 degrees S; and between the longitude of 18 degrees W. and 50 degrees E. from London; is about 4300 miles long, and 4200 miles broad.

43. The positions and names of the chief countries, cities, rivers, and mountains, are contained in the following table.

Countries.	Position.	Chief Cities.	Rivers.	Course.	Mountains.
E. Morocco	N. W.	Fez	Mulvia	N.	Atlas
K. Algiers	N.	Algiers	Saffran	N.	Atlas
K. Tunis	N.	Tunis	Megrada	N.	Atlas
K. Tripoli	N.	Tripoli	Salines	N. E.	Atlas
K. Barca	N.	Docra			Meies
K. Egypt	N. E.	Cairo	Nile	N.	Gianadel
E. Abyssinia or Ethiopia	E.	Ambamarjam	Nile	N.	
Ajan	E.	Adea	Madadoxa	S.	
Zanguebar	E.	Melinda	Cuama	E. S. E.	
Sofala	S. E.	Sofala	Amara	E.	Amara
Terra de Natal	S. E.	Natal	St. Esprit	E.	Amara
Cafraria	S.	Cape Town	St. Christopher	E.	Table
Mataman	S. S. W.		Angri	W.	Sunda
K. Benguela	S. S. W.	Benguela	Negros	W.	Sunda
K. Angola	S. W.	Loando	Coanza	W.	Sunda
K. Congo	S. W.	St. Salvador	Zaara	S. W.	Sunda
K. Loango	S. W.	Loango	Zette	S. W.	St. Esprit
Biafara	S. W.	Biafara	Camerones	S. W.	St. Esprit
K. Benin	S. W.	Benin	Formosa	S. W.	
Guinea	S. W.	Cape Coast	Volta	S.	Sierra Leon
Mandinga	W.	James Fort	Gambia	W.	C. Verd
Sanhaga	W.	Sanhaga	Senegal	N. W.	
Biledulgerid	Mid. N.	Dara	Dara	S.	Atlas
Zara	Mid.	Zeenzega	Nubia	E.	
Nubia	Mid.	Nubia	Nubia	E.	
Negroland	Mid.	Tombute	Niger	W.	
Ethiopia inter	Mid.	Chaxumo	Niger	W.	Luna
Monoemugi	Mid. S.	Merango	Cuama	E. S. E	Luna
E. Monomotapa	Mid. S.	Morgar	Amara	S. E.	Amara

Many parts of the coasts of Africa are subject to the European nations: Thus the Kingdoms of Algiers, Tunis, Tripoli, Barca, and Egypt, are either subject to the Ottoman, or Turkish empire, or acknowledge themselves under its protection.

Abyſſinia is governed by its own Emperor.

Ajan or Anian is peopled by a few wild Arabs.

In Zanguebar and Sofala, the Portugueſe have many black Princes tributary to them.

Cafraria, or the country of the Hottentots, belongs to the Dutch.

The ſea coaſts of Guinea are uſually diſtinguiſhed by the names of the *Slave Coaſt*, *Gold Coaſt*, *Ivory Coaſt*, *Grain Coaſt*, and *Sierra Leon*.

The Engliſh, Dutch, French, Portugueſe, and others, have ſeveral ſettlements along theſe coaſts, and even many miles up the country, particularly the Engliſh on the rivers Gambia and Senegal.

In the general table the countries are taken in a very large ſenſe; for many of them contain a great number of ſtates independent one of the other, the particulars of which are not known to Geographers.

44. *The principal Seas, Gulfs, and Bays in Africa, are*

The *Red Sea*, between Africa and Aſia: It waſhes the coaſt of Arabia on the Aſiatic ſide, and the coaſts of Egypt and Abyſſinia on the African ſide.

Moſambique Sea, between Africa and the iſland of Madagaſcar eaſtward.

Saldanna Bay in Cafraria, on the Ethiopic Ocean.

Bight of Benin on the coaſt of Guinea, in the Ethiopic Ocean.

45. *The principal African Iſlands, are*

	Chief iſle.	Chief Town.	Situation.
Madeira iſles	Madeira	Funchal	N. Atlantic Ocean
Canary iſles	Canaria	Palma	N. Atlantic Ocean
C. Verd iſles	St. Jago	St. Jago	N. Atlantic Ocean
Ethiopian iſles	St. Helena		Ethiopic Ocean
Komora iſles	Johanna	Demani	Indian Ocean
Sokotora iſles	Zocotora	Calanſia	Indian Ocean
Almirante iſles	But little	known	Indian Ocean

The iſland of *Madagaſcar*, one of the largeſt in the world, lies in the Indian Ocean: It is divided into a multitude of little ſtates; ſome of them formed by the European privateers, and their ſucceſſors deſcended from a mixture with the natives.

The iſlands of *Bourbon* and *Mauritius* lie in the Indian Ocean, to the eaſt of Madagaſcar: theſe belong to the French.

The Madeiras, and Cape de Verd Iſles, belong to the Portugueſe.

The Canary Iſles to Spain; St. Helena to England.

OF AMERICA.

46. This vaſt continent, called by ſome the new world, having been diſcovered by the Europeans ſince the year 1492, is uſually divided into two parts, one called North, and the other South America, being joined to one another by the Iſthmus of Darien.

North America lies between the latitudes of 10 degrees and 80 degrees north; and chiefly between the longitudes of 50 degrees and 130 degrees weſt of London; is about 4200 miles from north to ſouth, and about 4800 from eaſt to weſt. It is bounded on the eaſt by the north Atlantic Ocean, by the Gulf of Mexico on the ſouth, on the weſt by the Pacific Ocean, and by the Northern continent and ocean to the northward.

South America is bounded on the eaſt by the ſouth Atlantic Ocean, by the Southern Ocean to the ſouth, by the Pacific Ocean on the weſt, and on the north by the Caribbean Sea. It lies between the latitudes of 12 degrees north, and 56 degrees ſouth; and between the longitudes of 45 degrees and 83 degrees weſt from London; is about 4200 miles long, and about 2200 miles in breadth.

47. The poſitions and names of the chief countries, cities, rivers, and mountains, in North America, are in the following table.

Countries.	Poſition.	Chief Cities.	Rivers.	Courſe.	Mountains.
California	W.	St. Juan.			
New Mexico	S.	Sante Fe	N. River	S. S. E.	
Old Mexico	S. W.	Mexico	Panuco	E.	
Louiſiana	S.	New Orleans	Miſſiſſipi	S.	
Florida	S.	St. Auguſtine	St. John	N. to E.	Apalachian
Georgia	S. S. E.	Savannah	Alatamaha	E. S. E.	Apalachian
Carolina	S. E.	Charles Town	Aſhly	S. E.	Apalachian
Virginia	E.	James Town	Powtomack	S. E.	Apalachian
Maryland	E.	Annapolis	Powtomack	S. E.	Apalachian
Penſylvania	E.	Philadelphia	Delawar	S.	Apalachian
Jerſeys	E.	New York	Albany	S.	
New England	E.	Boſton	Connecticut	S.	
Nova Scotia	N. E.	Halifax	St. John	S. S. E.	Ladies
Canada	Mid.	Quebec	St. Lawrence	N. E.	
New Britain	N. N. E.	Fort Rupert	Rupert	W.	
New Wales	N.	York Fort	Nelſon	W.	

California, Old Mexico, and New Mexico, belong to Spain.

Louiſiana, to the weſt of the river Miſſiſſippi, was poſſeſſed by the French at the end of the late war; but is now transferred to Spain.

All the other countries are in the hands of the Engliſh.

In

In South America the poſition and names of the chief countries, cities, rivers, and mountains, are as follow:

Countries.	Poſition.	Chief Cities.	Rivers.	Courſe.	Mountains.
Terra Firma.	N.	Panama	Oronoque	N. E.	
Peru	W.	Lima	Chuquimayo	W. N. W.	Andes
Chili	S. W.	St. Jago	Valpariſo	W.	Andes
Patagonia	S.		Deſaguadero	S.	Andes
La Plata	S. E.	Buenos Ayres	La Plata	S.	Andes
Paraguay	Mid.	Aſſumption	Paragua	S.	
Braſil	E.	St. Salvador	Rio Real	N. E.	
Amazonia	Mid.		Amazons	E.	
Guiana	N. E.	Surinam	Eſquebe	N. N. E.	

Terra Firma, Peru, Chili, La Plata, and Paraguay, are in the poſſeſſion of the Spaniards.

Braſil belongs to the Portugueſe.

Patagonia, Amazonia, and Guiana, are poſſeſſed by the native Indians, except ſome parts of the coaſts of Guiana, in the hands of the Dutch and French.

48. *The principal Seas, Gulfs, and Bays in America.*

The Caribbean Sea, bounded by Terra Firma on the ſouth, and a range of iſlands on the north and eaſt.

Gulf of Mexico, formed by Old Mexico, Louiſiana, and Florida.

Bay of Campeachy, part of the Gulf of Mexico, on the Mexican coaſt.

Bay of Honduras, part of the Caribbean Sea, next to Mexico.

Bay of Panama, in the Pacific Ocean, next the Iſthmus of Darien.

Bay of California, in the Pacific Ocean, having California on the weſt.

Bay of Fundy, in Nova Scotia, north Atlantic Ocean.

Gulf of St. Lawrence, in the North Atlantic Ocean, bounded by Nova Scotia, New Britain, and ſome iſlands eaſtward and ſouth-eaſtward.

Hudſon's Bay, between New Britain E. and New Wales W.

49. *The chief American Iſlands in the Atlantic Ocean.*

Newfoundland, and *Cape Breton*, eaſt of the Gulf of St. Lawrence.

Bermudas, or *Summer Iſlands*, eaſt of Carolina.

Bahama Iſles, ſouth eaſt of Florida.

Great Antilles	Cuba	ch. town Havanna	lying E. of the Mexican Gulf, and N. of the Car. Sea.
	Hiſpaniola	ch. town St. Domingo	
	Jamaica	ch. town Kingſton	

Caribbee Iſles, bounding the Caribbean Sea on the E. and N. E.

Leſſer Antilles, on the N. N. E. of Terra Firma, in the Caribbee Sea.

Terra del Fuego on the ſouth of Patagonia, in the Southern Ocean.

Gallipago Iſles, lying N. W. of Peru in the Pacific Ocean.

SECTION

SECTION IV.

Geographical Problems.

50. Problem I. *Given the latitudes of two places: Required their difference of latitude.*

Case I. When the latitudes of the given places have the same name:

Rule. Subtract the lesser latitude from the greater, the remainder is the difference of latitude.

Exam. I. *What is the difference of latitude between London and Rome?*

London's lat.	51° 32′ N.	
Rome's lat.	41 54 N.	
Diff. lat.	9 38	
	60	
	578 miles.	

Exam. II. *What is the difference of latitude between the Lizard and the Island of Madeira?*

Lizard's lat.	49° 57′ N.
Madeira's lat.	32 36 N.
Diff. lat.	17 21=1041m.

Exam. III. *What is the difference of latitude between the Island of St. Helena and the Cape of Good Hope?*

C. Good Hope's lat.	34° 29′ S.
St. Helena's lat.	15 55 S.
Diff. lat.	18 34=1114m.

Exam. IV. *A ship from the latitude of 43° 18′ N. is come to the lat. of 34° 49′ N. Required the diff. of latitude.*

Lat. from	43° 18′ N.
Lat. in	34 49 N.
Diff. lat.	8 29=509m.

Case II. When the latitudes of the given places have contrary names:

Rule. Add the latitudes together, and the sum will be the difference of latitude.

Exam. I. *Required the diff. of lat. between C. Finisterre and C. St. Roque.*

C. Finisterre lat.	42° 57′ N.
C. St. Roque lat.	5 00 S.
Diff. lat.	47 57
	60
	2877 miles.

Exam. II. *What is the difference of latitude between the Island of Barbadoes and C. Negro?*

I. of Barbadoes's lat.	13° 00′ N.
C. Negro's lat.	16 30 S.
Diff. lat.	29 30=1770m.

Exam. III. *Required the difference of latitude between Cape Horn and Cape Corientes in Mexico.*

Cape Horn's lat.	55° 59′ S.
C. Corientes's lat.	20 18 N.
Diff. lat.	76 17=4577m.

Exam. IV. *A ship from the lat. of 8° 28′ S. has sailed north to the lat. 6° 45′ N. Required the diff. of latitude.*

Lat. from	8° 28′ S.
Lat. in	6 45 N.
Diff. lat.	15 13=913m.

The situation of about 1500 particular places are contained in a Geographical Table, art. 137, at the end of this book; where the latitudes and longitudes of places are to be sought, as they follow in alphabetical order.

51. Pro-

51. **Problem II.** *Given the latitude of one place and the difference of latitude between it and another place: Required the latitude of the latter place.*

Case I. When the given latitude and difference of latitude have the ſame name:

Rule. To the given latitude add the degrees and minutes in the diff. of latitude, that ſum is the other latitude of the ſame name.

Exam. I. *A ſhip from the latitude of 38° 14′ N. ſails north till her difference of latitude is 12° 32′: What latitude is ſhe come to?*

Lat. from	38° 14′ N.
Diff. lat.	12 32 N.
Lat. in	50 46 N.

Exam. II. *A ſhip from the iſland of Aſcenſion runs ſouth till her diff. of latitude is 5° 37′: What is the preſent latitude of the ſhip?*

I. Aſcenſion's lat.	7° 59′ S.
Diff. lat.	5 37 S.
Ship's lat.	13 36 S.

Exam. III. *A ſhip from the iſland of Madeira ſails N. 675 miles: What lat. is ſhe in?*

I. Madeira's lat.	32° 36′ N.
Diff. lat. $\frac{675}{60}$ (I. 22) =	11 15 N.
Ship's lat.	43 51 N.

Exam. IV. *Three days ago we were in the latitude of the Cape of Good Hope, and have run each day 92 miles directly S. What is our preſent latitude?*

C. Good Hope's lat.	34° 29′ S.
Diff. lat. $\frac{92 \times 3}{60}$ (I. 22) =	4 36 S.
Preſent latitude	39 05 S.

Case II. When the given latitude and difference of latitude have contrary names:

Rule. Take the difference between the given latitude and the degrees and minutes in the diff. of latitude, the remainder is the other latitude, of the ſame name with the greater.

Exam. I. *A ſhip from the latitude of 38° 14′ N. ſails ſouth till her difference of latitude is 12° 32′: What latitude is ſhe come to?*

Lat. from	38° 14′ N.
Diff. lat.	12 32 S.
Lat. in	25 42 N.

Exam. II. *A ſhip from the iſland of Aſcenſion runs north till her diff. lat. is 5° 37′: What is the preſent latitude of the ſhip?*

I. Aſcenſion's lat.	7° 59′ S.
Diff. lat.	5 37 N.
Ship's lat.	2 22 S.

Exam. III. *A ſhip from Sierra Leon ſails S. 839 miles: What latitude is ſhe in?*

Sierra Leon's lat.	8° 30′ N.
Diff. lat. $\frac{839}{60}$ (I. 22) =	13 59 S.
Ship's lat.	5 29 S.

Exam. IV. *Four days ago we were in the latitude of the iſland of St. Matthew, and ſailed due north 6 miles an hour: What latitude is the ſhip in?*

St. Matthew's lat.	1° 23′ S.
Diff. lat. $\frac{6 \times 24 \times 4}{60}$ (I. 22) =	9 36 N.
Ship's latitude	8 13 N.

52. Pro-

52. PROBLEM. III. *Given the longitudes of two places: Required their difference of longitude.*

RULE. If the longitudes are of the same name, their difference is the difference of longitude required.

But if the longitudes are of different names, their sum gives the difference of longitude.

And if this sum exceeds 180 degrees, take it from 360 degrees, and there remains the difference of longitude.

EXAM. I. *Required the difference of longitude between London and Naples?*

London's long.	00° 00′
Naples' long.	14 19 E.
Diff. longitude	14 19
	60
	859

EXAM. II. *A ship in longitude 14° 45′ W. is bound to a port in longitude 48° 18′ west: What diff. of longitude must she make?*

Ship's long.	14° 45′ W.
Long. bound to	48 18 W.
Diff. longitude	33 33
	60
	2013 miles.

EXAM. III. *What is the difference of longitude between Cape Gardafuir and Cape Comorin?*

C. Gardafuir's long.	50° 25′ E.
C. Comorin's long.	78 17 E.
Diff. longitude	27 52
	60
	1672 miles.

EXAM. IV. *Required the difference of longitude between St. Christopher's and Cape Negro.*

St. Christopher's long.	62° 54′ W.
C. Negro's long.	11 30 E.
Diff. longitude	74 24
	60
	4464 miles.

EXAM. V. *A ship in longitude 140° 20′ W. is bound to a place in longitude 139° 25′ E. what diff. of longitude must she make?*

Ship's long.	140° 20′ W.
Long. bound to	139 25 E.
	279 55
	360 00
Diff. longitude	80 05

EXAM. VI. *What is the difference of longitude between Cape Horn and Manila?*

Cape Horn's long.	67° 26′ W.
Manila's long.	120 25 E.
	187 51
	360 00
Diff. longitude	172 09

Sometimes the diff. lon. between two places is estimated by the diff. of time, allowing an hour to every 15 degrees of longitude, and one min. of time for every 15 min. of a deg. or a deg. for every 4 min. of time.

EXAM. *At 6 h. 48 m. P. M. having observed at sea a certain appearance in the heavens, which I knew was seen the same instant at 3 h. 25 m. P. M. in London: Required the diff. longitude between the places of observation.*

From	6 h. 48 m.		3 h. =	45 deg.
Take	3 35		13 m. =	3 15′
Remain	3 13 = diff. time.		Sum	48 15 = Diff. long.

And because the hour of appearance at London was least, therefore I know myself to be to the eastward of London.

53. PRO-

53. **Problem IV.** *Given the longitude of one place, and the difference of longitude between that and another: Required the longitude of the second place.*

Rule. If the given longitude and difference of longitude are of a contrary name, their difference is the longitude required; and is of the same name with the greater.

But if the given longitude and difference of longitude are of the same name, the sum is the longitude sought, of the same name with the given place.

And if the sum is greater than 180 degrees, take it from 360 degrees, remains the longitude required, of a contrary name to that of the given place.

Exam. I. *A ship from the longitude of 41° 12′ E. sails westward until her difference of longitude is 15° 47′: What is her present longitude?*

Ship's longitude	41°	12′	E.
Diff. long.	15	47	W.
Pres. long.	25	25	E.

Exam. II. *A ship from Cape Charles in Virginia sails eastward until she has altered her longitude 22° 53′: What longitude is she in?*

C. Charles's long.	76°	07′	W.
Diff. long.	22	53	E.
Ship's long.	53	14	W.

Exam. III. *Four days ago I departed from C. St. Sebastian in Madagascar, and I have made each day 75 miles of east longitude: Required the longitude the ship is in?*

75
4

6,0)30,0

5°

C. Sebas. long.	49°	13′	E.
Diff. long.	5	00	E.
Ship's long.	54	13	E.

Exam. IV. *A ship from Cape Finisterre sails westward, and finds she has altered her longitude 587 miles: What longitude is she arrived in?*

C. Finisterre's long.	9°	36′	W.
Diff. lon. $\frac{587}{60}$	9	47	W.
Long. in.	19	23	W.

Exam. V. *A ship from Cape St. Lucar in California has made 87° 18′ of west longitude: What longitude is she in?*

C. St. Lucar's long.	109°	40′	W.
Diff. long.	87	18	W.
	196	58	W.
	360	00	
Ship's longitude	163	02	E.

Exam. VI. *Seven days ago my longitude was 172° 17′ W. and I have made each day 132 miles of west longitude: Required my present longitude?*

132
7

6,0)92,4

15 24

Departed long.	172°	17′	W.
Diff. long.	15	24	W.
	187	41	
	360	00	
Present long.	172	19	E.

SECTION V.

54. *Of the Use of the Globes.*

By the globes are here meant two ſpherical bodies, called the Terreſtrial and Celeſtial Globes, the convex ſurfaces of which are ſuppoſed to to give a true repreſentation of the earth and heavens.

The TERRESTRIAL GLOBE has delineated on its convexity the whole furface of the *earth* and *ſea* in their relative ſize, form, and ſituation.

The CELESTIAL GLOBE has drawn on its ſurface the images of the ſeveral conſtellations and ſtars; the relative magnitude and poſition which the ſtars are obſerved to have in the heavens, being preſerved on this globe.

The globes are fitted up with certain machinery, by means of which a great variety of uſeful problems are neatly ſolved.

The BRAZEN MERIDIAN is that ring, or hoop, in which the globe hangs on its axis; which is repreſented by two wires paſſing through its poles. This circle is divided into four quarters, of 90° each; in one ſemicircle the diviſions begin at each pole, and end at 90°, where they meet: In the other ſemicircle, the diviſions begin at the middle, and proceed thence towards each pole, where they end at 90 degrees. The graduated ſide of this brazen circle ſerves as a meridian for any point on the ſurface of the earth, the globe being turned about till that point comes under the circle.

The HOUR CIRCLE is a ſmall circle of braſs, which is divided into 24 hours, the quarters and half quarters. It is fixed on the brazen meridian, equally diſtant from the north end of the axis, to which an index is fitted, that points out the diviſions of the hour circle as the globe is turned about.

The HORIZON is repreſented by the upper ſurface of the wooden circular frame encompaſſing the globe about its middle. On this wooden frame is a kind of perpetual calender, contained in ſeveral concentric circles: The inner one is divided into four quarters, of 90 degrees each; the next circle is divided into the twelve months, with the days in each according to the new ſtyle; the next contains the 12 equal ſigns of the zodiac, each being divided into 30 degrees: the next is the 12 months and days according to the old ſtyle; and there is another circle, containing the 32 winds, with their halves and quarters. Although theſe circles are on all horizons, yet their diſpoſition is not always the ſame.

The QUADRANT of ALTITUDE is a thin ſtreight ſlip of braſs, one edge of which is graduated into 90 degrees and their quarters, equal to thoſe of the meridian. To one end of this is fixed a braſs nut and ſcrew, by which it is put on, and faſtened to the meridian: and if it is fixed to the zenith, or pole of the horizon, then the graduated edge repreſents a vertical circle paſſing through any point.

Beſides theſe, there are ſeveral circles deſcribed on the ſurfaces of both globes; ſuch as the equinoctial, ecliptic, circles of longitude and right aſcenſion, the tropics, polar circles, parallels of lat. and decl., on the celeſtial globe; and on the terreſtrial, the equator, ecliptic, tropics, polar circles, parallels of latitude, hour circles, or meridians to every 15 degrees, and the ſpiral rhumbs flowing from ſeveral centers, called Flies.

55. PROBLEM I.

To find the latitude and longitude of any place on the terreſtrial globe.

1ſt. Bring the given place under that ſide of the graduated brazen meridian where the degrees begin at the equator, by turning the globe about.
2d. Then the degree of the meridian over it ſhews the latitude.
3d. And the degree of the equator under the merid., ſhews the long.

On ſome globes the longitude is reckoned on the equator from the meridian where it begins, eaſtward only, until it ends at 360°: On ſuch globes, when the longitude of a place exceeds 180°, take it from 360, and call the remainder the longitude weſtward.

56. PROBLEM II.

To find any place on the globe, the latitude and longitude of which are given.

1ſt. Bring the given longitude, found on the equator, to the meridian.
2d. Then under the given latitude, found on the meridian, is the place ſought.

57. PROBLEM III.

To find the diſtance and bearing of any two given places on the globe.

1ſt. Lay the graduated edge of the quadrant of altitude over both places, the beginning, or 0 degree, being on one of them, and the degrees between them ſhew their diſtance; theſe degrees multipled by 60 give ſea miles, and by 70 give the diſtance in land miles nearly; or multiplied by 20 give leagues.
2d. Obſerve, while the quadrant lies in this poſition, what rhumb of the neareſt fly, or compaſs, runs moſtly parallel to the edge of the quadrant, and that rhumb ſhews the bearing ſought, nearly.

58. PROBLEM IV.

To find the Sun's place and declination on any day.

1ſt. Seek the given day in the circle of months on the horizon, and right againſt it in the circle of ſigns is the Sun's place.
Thus it will be found that the Sun enters

The ſpring ſigns,	Aries,	March	20.	Taurus,	April 20.	Gemini,	May 21.
The ſummer ſigns,	Cancer.	June	21.	Leo,	July 23.	Virgo,	Aug. 23.
Autumnal ſigns,	Libra,	Sept.	22.	Scorpio,	Oct. 23.	Sagittar.	Nov. 22.
The winter ſigns,	Capric.	Dec.	21.	Aquarius,	Jan. 20.	Piſces,	Feb. 18.

2d. Seek the Sun's place in the ecliptic on the globe, bring that place to the meridian, and the diviſion it ſtands under is the Sun's declination on the given day.

On the globes, the ecliptic is readily diſtinguiſhed from the equator, not only by the different colours they are ſtained with, but alſo by the ecliptic's approaching towards the poles, after its interſection with the equator. The marks of the ſigns are alſo put along the ecliptic, one at the beginning of every ſucceſſive 30 degrees.

59. PROBLEM V.

To rectify the globe for the latitude, zenith, and noon.

1ſt. Set the globe upon an horizontal plane with its parts anſwering to thoſe of the world; move the meridian in its notches, by raiſing or depreſſing the pole, until the degrees of latitude cut the horizon; then is the globe rectified for the latititude.

2d. Reckon the latitude from the equator towards the elevated pole, there ſcrew the bevil edge of the nut belonging to the quadrant of altitude, and the rectification is made for the zenith.

3d. Bring the Sun's place (found by the laſt problem) to the meridian, ſet the index to the XII at noon, or upper XII, and the globe is rectified for the Sun's ſouthing, or noon.

60. PROBLEM VI.

To find where the Sun is vertical, at any given time, in a given place.

1ſt. Bring the Sun's place, found for the given day (58), to the meridian, and note the degree over it.

2d. Bring the place, for which the time is given, to the meridian, and ſet the index to the given hour.

3d. Turn the globe till the index comes to 12 at noon, then the place under the ſaid noted degree has the Sun in the zenith at that time.

4th. All the places that paſs under that degree, while the globe is turned round, will have the Sun vertical to them on that day.

61. PROBLEM VII.

To find on what days the Sun will be vertical, at any given place, in the torrid zone.

1ſt. Note the latitude of the given place on the meridian.

2d. Turn the globe, and note what two points of the ecliptic paſs under the latitude noted on the meridian.

3d. Seek thoſe points of the ecliptic in the circle of ſigns on the horizon, and right againſt them, in the circle of months, ſtand the days required.

In this manner it will be found, that the Sun will be vertical to the Iſland of St. Helena on the 6th of November, and on the 4th of February. And at Barbadoes on the 24th of April, and the 18th of Auguſt.

62. PROBLEM VIII.

At any given hour in a given place, to find what hour it is in any other place.

1ſt. Bring the place where the time is given to the meridian, and ſet the index to the given hour.

2d. Bring the other given place to the meridian, and the index ſhews the hour correſponding to the given time.

63. PRO-

63. PROBLEM IX.

At any given time to find all those places of the Earth where the Sun is then rising or setting, and where it is mid-day or midnight.

Find the place where the Sun is vertical at the given time (60), rectify the globe for the latitude of that place, and bring it to the meridian.

Then all those places, that are in the western half of the horizon, have the Sun rising; and those in the eastern half have it setting.

Those under the meridian, above the horizon, have the Sun culminating, or noon; and those under the meridian, below the horizon, have midnight.

Those above the horizon have day; those below it have night.

64. PROBLEM X.

To find the angle of position of two places, or the angle made by the meridian of one place, and a great circle passing through both places.

Rectify for the latitude of one of the given places, and bring it to the meridian; there fix the quadrant of altitude, and set its graduated edge to the other place: then will that edge of the quadrant cut the horizon in the degree of position sought.

Thus, the angle of position at the Land's End to Barbadoes is south $71\frac{1}{2}^{\circ}$ westerly: but the angle of position at Barbadoes to the Land's End is north $37\frac{1}{2}$ degrees easterly.

Hence neither of those positions can be the true bearing; for the rhumb passing through both places, will be opposite one way to what it is the other.

65. PROBLEM XI.

The latitude of any place not within the polar circle being given, to find the time of sun-rising and setting, and the length of the day and night.

Rectify for the latitude and the noon; bring the Sun's place to the eastern side of the horizon, and the index shews the time of rising: the Sun's place being brought to the western side of the horizon, the index gives the setting.

Or, the time of rising taken from 12 hours gives the time of setting.

The time of setting being doubled gives the length of the day.

And the time of rising being doubled gives the length of the night.

Thus, at London, on April 15th, the day is $13\frac{1}{2}$ hours; the night $10\frac{1}{2}$ hours.

66. PROBLEM XII.

To find the length of the longest and shortest days in any given place.

Rectify for the latitude; bring the solstitial point of that hemisphere to the eastern part of the horizon, set the index to 12 at noon, turn the globe till the solstitial point comes to the western side of the horizon, the hours past over by the index give the length of the longest day, or night; and its complement to 24 hours gives the length of the shortest night, or day.

67. PROBLEM XIII.

A place being given in either frigid or frozen zone, to find the time when the Sun begins to appear at, or depart from, that place: alſo how many ſucceſſive days he is preſent to, or abſent from, that place.

Rectify for the latitude, turn the globe, and obſerve what degrees in the firſt and ſecond quadrants of the ecliptic are cut by the north point of the horizen, the latitude being ſuppoſed to be north.

Find thoſe degrees in the circle of ſigns on the horizon, and their correſponding days of the month; and all the time between thoſe days the Sun will not ſet in that place.

Again. Obſerve what degree in the third and fourth quadrants of the ecliptic will be cut by the ſouth point of the horizon, and the days anſwering: then the Sun will be quite abſent from the given place during the intermediate days; that day in the third quadrant ſhews when he begins to diſappear; and that in the fourth quadrant ſhews when he begins to ſhine in the place propoſed.

Thus at the North cape, in lat. 71°, the Sun never ſets from May 15 to July 28, which is 74 days; and never riſes from November 16 to January 24, which is 69 days.

68. PROBLEM XIV.

To find the antœci, periœci, and antipodes of any place.

Bring the given place to the meridian, tell as many degrees of latitude on the contrary ſide of the equator, and it gives the place of the antæci; that is, of thoſe who have oppoſite ſeaſons of the year, but the ſame times of the day.

The given place being under the meridian, ſet the index to 12 at noon, turn the globe until the index points to 12 at night, and the point under the meridian in the given latitude is the place of the periœci; that is, of thoſe who have the ſame ſeaſons of the year, but oppoſite times of the day.

The globe remaining in this poſition, ſeek on the contrary ſide of the equator for the degrees of latitude given, and the point under the meridian, thus found, will be the antipodes to the given place; that is, there the ſeaſons of the year and times of the day are directly oppoſite to thoſe of the given place.

69. PROBLEM XV.

To find the beginning and end of the twilight in any place.

Rectify the globe for the latitude, zenith, and noon. (59)

Seek the point of the ecliptic oppoſite to the Sun's place, turn the globe and quadrant of altitude, till the ſaid oppoſite point of the ecliptic ſtands againſt 18 degrees on the quadrant of altitude; then will the index ſhew the beginning or end of the twilight; that is, the beginning in the morning, when thoſe points meet in the weſtern hemiſphere; or the end in the evening, when the ſaid points meet in the eaſtern hemiſphere.

70. PRO-

70. PROBLEM XVI.

The latitude of a place and day of the month being given, to find the Sun's declination, meridian altitude, right ascension, amplitude, oblique ascension, ascensional difference; and thence the time of rising, setting, length of the day and night.

Rectify for the latitude and noon. Then,

The degree of the meridian over the Sun's place is the declination.

The meridian altitude is shewn by the degrees the Sun is above the horizon; and is equal to the sum or diff. of the co-lat. and decl.

The Sun's right ascen. is that degree of the equator under the meridian.

Bring the Sun's place to the eastern part of the horizon. Then,

The amplitude is that degree of the horizon opposite the Sun.

The oblique ascension is that degree of the equator cut by the horizon.

The ascen. diff. is the diff. between the right and oblique ascensions.

The ascen. diff. converted into time, will give the time the Sun rises before or after the hour of six, according as his amplitude is to the northward or southward of the east point of the horizon.

71. PROBLEM XVII.

Given the latitude of the place and day of the month, to find the Sun's altitude and azimuth, either when he is due east or west, at 6 o'clock, or at any other hour while he is above the horizon.

Rectify the globe for the latitude, zenith, and noon.

Set the quadrant of altitude to the east point of the horizon, turn the globe till the Sun's place comes to the quadrant's edge, and it shews the altitude, his azimuth being now 90°, and the index shews the hour.

Turn the globe till the index points at 6, there stay it, and move the quadrant until its edge cuts the Sun's place; then the degrees at the Sun shew its altitude, and the degrees cut by the quadrant in the horizon shew the azimuth, reckoning from the north.

In like manner, the globe being turned till the index is against any other hour, suppose 10 in the forenoon; then,

The graduated edge of the quadrant of altitude being turned to cut the Sun's place, will give both the altitude and azimuth at that time.

72. PROBLEM XVIII.

Given the latitude, day of the month, and Sun's altitude, to find the azimuth and hour of the day.

Rectify the globe for the latitude, zenith, and noon.

Turn the globe and quadrant, until the Sun's place coincide with the altitude on the graduated edge of the quadrant.

Then will that edge of the quadrant cut the degrees of azimuth on the horizon, reckoned from the north; and the index will shew the hour of the day.

73. PROBLEM XIX.

To represent the appearance of the heavens at any time in a given place.

Rectify the celestial globe for the latitude, zenith, and noon, and turn the globe till the index points at the given hour. Then,

The stars in the eastern half of the horizon are rising; those in the western are setting: and those on the meridian are culminating.

The quadrant being set to any given star will shew its altitude, and at the same time its azimuth, reckoned on the horizon.

Now by turning the globe round it will readily appear, what stars never set in that place, and what never rise: those of perpetual apparition never go below the horizon, those of perpetual absence never come above it.

74. PROBLEM XX.

To find the latitude and longitude of any star.

Put the center of the quadrant of altitude on the pole of the ecliptic, and its graduated edge on the given star. Then,

The latitude is shewn by the degrees between the ecliptic and star.

The longitude is the degrees cut on the ecliptic by the quadrant.

75. PROBLEM XXI.

To find the declination and right ascension of a star.

Bring the star to the meridian, the degree over it is the declination; and the degree of the equator under the meridian is the right ascension.

76. PROBLEM XXII.

On any day, and in any given place, to find when a proposed star rises, sets, or culminates.

Rectify the globe for the latitude and noon.

Bring the star to the eastern side of the horizon, and the index shews the time of its rising.

Turn the globe till the star comes to the meridian, and the index shews the time of its culminating; and in like manner when it sets, the time will be shewn by the index.

Its meridian altitude, oblique ascension, and ascensional difference, are found in the same manner as for the Sun, at art. 70.

SECTION VI.

Of Winds.

77. A FLUID is a body, the particles of which readily give way to any impreſſed force; and by this readineſs of yielding, the particles are eaſily put into motion.

Thus, not only liquids, but ſtreams or vapours, ſmoke or fumes, and others of the like kind, are reckoned as fluids.

From all parts of the Earth vapours and fumes are conſtantly ariſing to ſome diſtance from its ſurface.

This is known by obſervation; it is cauſed chiefly by the heat of the Sun, and ſometimes by ſubterraneous fires ariſing from the accidental mixing of ſome bodies.

78. AIR is a fine inviſible fluid ſurrounding the globe of the Earth, and extended to ſome miles above its ſurface.

The ATMOSPHERE is that collection of air, and of bodies contained in it, which circumſcribes the Earth.

79. From a multitude of experiments, air is found to be both heavy and ſpringy.

By its weight it is capable of ſupporting other bodies, ſuch as vapours and fumes, in the ſame manner as wood is ſupported by water.

By its ſpringineſs or elaſticity a quantity of air is capable of being expanded, or of ſpreading itſelf ſo as to fill a larger ſpace *; and of being compreſſed or confined in a ſmaller compaſs †.

80. Air is compreſſed or condenſed by cold, and expanded or rarefied by heat.

This is evident from a multitude of experiments.

An alteration being made by heat or cold in any part of the atmoſphere, its neighbouring parts will be put in motion, by the endeavour which the air always makes to reſtore itſelf to its former ſtate.

For experiments ſhew, that condenſed or rarefied air will return to its natural ſtate, when the cauſe of that condenſation or rarefaction is removed.

81. WIND is a ſtream or current of air which may be felt; it uſually blows from one part of the horizon to its oppoſite part.

82. The *horizon*, beſide being divided into 360 degrees, like all other circles, is by mariners ſuppoſed to be divided into four *quadrants*, called the north-eaſt, north-weſt, ſouth-eaſt and ſouth-weſt quarters; each of theſe quarters they divide into eight equal parts, called points, and each point into four equal parts, called quarter-points.

So that the horizon is divided into 32 points, which are called *rhumbs*, or *winds*; to each wind is aſſigned a name, which ſhews from what point of the horizon the wind blows.

The points of North, South, Eaſt, and Weſt, are called *cardinal points*; and are at the diſtance of 90 degrees, or 8 points, from one another.

---

* Near 14000 times. *Wallis*'s Hydroſ. p. 13.

† Into the [illegible] part. Phil. Tranſ. Nº 181.

83. Winds

83. Winds are either conftant or variable, general or particular.

Conftant winds are fuch as blow the fame way, at leaft for one or more days; and *variable winds* are fuch as frequently fhift within a day.

A *general wind* is that which blows the fame way over a large tract of the Earth, almoft the whole year.

A *particular wind* is that which blows in any place, fometimes one way, and fometimes another, indifferently.

If the wind blows gently, it is called a breeze; if it blows harder, it is called a gale, or a ftiff gale; and if it blows very hard, it is called a ftorm *.

84. The following obfervations on the wind have been made by fkillful feamen; and particularly by the great Dr. Halley.

1ft. Between the limits of 60 degrees, namely, from 30° of north latitude to 30° of fouth latitude, there is a conftant eafterly wind throughout the year, blowing on the Atlantic and Pacific Oceans; and this is called the *trade-wind.*

For as the Sun, in moving from eaft to weft, heats the air more immediately under him, and thereby expands it; the air to the eaftward is conftantly rufhing towards the weft to reftore the equilibrium, or natural ftate of the atmofphere; and this occafions a perpetual eafterly wind in thofe latitudes.

2d. The trade-winds near the northern limits blow between the north and eaft; and near the fouthern limits they blow between the fouth and eaft.

For as the air is expanded by the heat of the Sun near the equator; therefore the air from the northward and fouthward will both tend towards the equator to reftore the equilibrium. Now thofe motions from the north and fouth, joined with the foregoing eafterly motion, will produce the motions obferved near the faid limits between the north and eaft, and between the fouth and eaft.

3d. Thefe general motions of the wind are difturbed on the continents, and near their coafts.

For the nature of the foil may caufe the air to be either heated or cooled; and hence will arife motions that may be contrary to the foregoing general one.

4th. In fome parts of the Indian ocean there are periodical winds, called Monsoons; that is, fuch as blow one half the year one way, and the other half-year the contrary way.

For air that is cool and denfe, will force the warm and rarefied air in a continual ftream upwards, where it muft fpread itfelf to preferve the equilibrium: So that the upper courfe or current of the air fhall be contrary to the under current; for the upper air muft move from thofe parts where the greateft heat is; and fo, by a kind of circulation, the N. E. trade-wind below will be attended with a S. W. above; and a S. E. below with a N. W. above: And this is confirmed by the experience of feamen, who, as foon as they get out of the trade-winds, immediately find a wind blowing from the oppofite quarter.

* The fwiftnefs of the wind in a ftorm is not more than 50 or 60 miles in an hour; and a common brifk gale is about 15 miles an hour.

5th. In

5th. In the Atlantic Ocean near the coasts of Africa, at about 100 leagues from the shore, between the latitudes of 28° and 10° north, seamen constantly meet with a fresh gale of wind blowing from the N. E.

6th. Those bound to the Caribee Islands, across the Atlantic Ocean, find, as they approach the American side, that the said N. E. wind becomes easterly; or seldom blows more than a point from the east, either to the northward or southward.

These trade-winds, on the American side, are extended to 30, 31, or even to 32° of N. latitude; which is about 4° farther than what they extend to on the African side. Also to the southward of the equator, the trade-winds extend 3 or 4 degrees farther towards the coast of Brasil on the American side, than they do near the Cape of Good Hope on the African side.

7th. Between the latitudes of 4° North, and 4° South, the wind always blows between the south and east: On the African side the winds are nearest to the south; and on the American side nearest to the east. In these seas Dr. Halley observed, that when the wind was eastward, the weather was gloomy, dark, and rainy, with hard gales of wind: but when the wind veered to the southward, the weather generally became serene with gentle breezes next to a calm.

These winds are somewhat changed by the seasons of the year; for when the Sun is far northward, the Brasil S. E. wind gets to the south, and the N. E. wind to the east; and when the Sun is far south, the S. E. wind gets to the east, and the N. E. winds on this side of the equator veer more to the north.

8th. Along the coast of Guinea, from Sierra Leon to the Island of St. Thomas (under the equator) which is above 500 leagues, the southerly and south-west winds blow perpetually. For the S. E. trade-wind having passed the equator, and approaching the Guinea coast within 80 or 100 leagues, inclines towards the shore, and becomes south, then S. E. and by degrees, as it comes near the land, it veers about to south, S. S. W. and in with the land it is S. W. and sometimes W. S. W. This tract is troubled with frequent calms, violent sudden gusts of wind, called Tornadoes, blowing from all points of the horizon.

The reason why the wind sets in west on the coast of Guinea, is, in all probability, owing to the nature of the coast, which being greatly heated by the Sun, rarefies the air exceedingly; and consequently the cool air from off the sea will keep rushing in to restore the equilibrium.

9th. Between the 4th and 10th degrees of north latitude, and between the longitudes of Cape Verd, and the eastermost of the Cape Verd Isles, there is a tract of sea which seems to be condemned to perpetual calms, attended with terrible thunder and lightnings, and such frequent rains, that this part of the sea is called the *Rains*. Ships in sailing these 6 degrees have been sometimes detained whole months, as it is reported.

The cause of this seems to be, that the westerly winds setting in on this coast, and meeting the general easterly wind in this tract, balance each other, and so cause the calms; and the vapours carried thither by each wind meeting and condensing, occasion the almost constant rains.

The last three observations shew the reason of two things which mariners experience in sailing from Europe to India, and in the Guinea trade

First. The difficulty which ships in going to the southward, especially in the months of July and August, find in passing between the coast of Guinea and Brasil, notwithstanding the width of this sea is more than 500 leagues. This happens, because the S. E. winds at that time of the year commonly extend some degrees beyond the ordinary limits of 4° N. latitude; and besides come so much southerly, as to be sometimes south, sometimes a point or two to the west; it then only remains to ply to windward. And if, on the one side, they steer W. S. W. they get a wind more and more easterly; but then there is a danger of falling in with the Brasilian coast, or shoals; and if they steer E. S. E. they fall into the neighbourhood of the coast of Guinea, from whence they cannot depart without running easterly as far as the island of St. Thomas; and this is the constant practice of all the Guinea ships.

Secondly. All ships departing from Guinea for Europe, their direct course is northward; but on this course they cannot go, because the coast bending nearly east and west, the land is to the northward: Therefore as the winds on this coast are generally between the S. and W. S. W. they are obliged to steer S. S. E. or south, and with these courses they run off the shore; but in so doing they always find the winds more and more contrary; so that when near the shore, they can lie south, at a greater distance they can make no better than S. E., and afterwards E. S. E.; with which courses they commonly fetch the island of St. Thomas and Cape Lopez, where finding the winds to the eastward of the south, they sail westerly with it, until they come to the latitude of 4 degrees south, where they find the S. E. wind blowing perpetually.

On account of these general winds, all those who use the West India trade, even those bound to Virginia, reckon it their best course to get as soon as they can to the southward, that so they may be certain of a fair and fresh gale to run before to the westward. And for the same reason the homeward bound ships from America endeavour to gain the latitude of 30 degrees, where they first find the winds begin to be variable; though the most ordinary winds in the north Atlantic Ocean come from between the south and west.

10th. Between the southern latitudes of 10 and 30 degrees in the Indian Ocean, the general trade-wind about the S. E. by S. is found to blow all the year long in the same manner, as in the like latitude in the Ethiopic Ocean: and during the six months from May to December, these winds reach to within 2 degrees of the equator; but during the other six months, from November to June, a N. W. wind blows in the tract lying between the 3d and 10th degrees of southern latitude, in the meridian of the north end of Madagascar: and between the 2d and 12th degree of south latitude, near the longitude of Sumatra and Java.

11th. In

11th. In the tract between Sumatra and the African coast, and from 3 degrees of south latitude quite northward to the Asiatic coasts, including the Arabian Sea and the Gulf of Bengal, the Monsoons blow from September to April on the N. E.; and from March to October on the S. W. In the former half year the wind is more steady and gentle, and the weather clearer than in the latter six months; and the wind is more strong and steady in the Arabian Sea than in the Gulf of Bengal.

12th. Between the Island of Madagascar and the coast of Africa, and thence northward as far as the equator, there is a tract, where from April to October there is a constant fresh S. S. W. wind; which to the northward changes into the W. S. W. wind, blowing at that time in the Arabian Sea.

13th. To the eastward of Sumatra and Malacca, on the north of the equator, and along the coasts of Cambodia and China, quite through the Phillippines as far as Japan, the Monsoons blow northerly and southerly, the northern setting in about October or November, and the southern about May; the winds are not quite so certain as those in the Arabian Seas.

14th. Between Sumatra and Java to the west, and New Guinea to the east, the same northerly and southerly winds are observed; but the first half year Monsoon inclines to the N. W. and the latter to the S. E. These winds begin a month or six weeks after those in the Chinese Seas set in, and are quite as variable.

15th. These contrary winds do not shift from one point to its opposite all at once; in some places the time of the change is attended with calms, in others by variable winds. And it often happens on the shores of Coromandel and China towards the end of the Monsoons, that there are most violent storms, greatly resembling the hurricanes in the West Indies; when the wind is so vastly strong, that hardly any thing can resist its force.

All navigation in the Indian Ocean must necessarily be regulated by these winds; for if mariners should delay their voyages till the contrary Monsoon begins, they must either sail back, or go into harbour, and wait for the return of the trade-wind.

SECTION VII.

Of the Tides.

85. A TIDE is that motion of the waters in the ſeas and rivers, by which they are found regularly to riſe and fall.

The general cauſe of the tides was diſcovered by Sir Iſaac Newton, and is deduced from the following conſiderations.

86. Daily experience ſhews, that all bodies thrown upwards from the Earth, fall down to its ſurface in perpendicular lines; and as lines perpendicular to the ſurface of a ſphere tend towards the center, therefore the lines, along which all heavy bodies fall, are directed towards the Earth's center.

As theſe bodies apparently fall by their weight, or gravity; therefore the law by which they fall, is called the LAW OF GRAVITATION.

87. A piece of glaſs, amber, or ſealing-wax, and ſome other things, being rubbed againſt the palm of a hand, or againſt a woollen cloth, until they are warmed, will draw bits of paper, or other light ſubſtances, towards them, when held ſufficiently near thoſe ſubſtances.

Alſo a magnet, or loadſtone, being held near the filings of iron or ſteel, or other ſmall pieces of theſe metals, will draw them to itſelf; and a piece of hammered iron or ſteel, that has been rubbed by a magnet, will have a like property of drawing iron or ſteel to itſelf. And this property is called ATTRACTION.

88. Now as bodies by their gravity fall towards the Earth, it is not improper to ſay the Earth attracts thoſe bodies; and therefore in reſpect to the earth, the words gravitation and attraction may be uſed one for the other, as by them is meant no more than the power, or law, by which bodies tend towards its center.

And it is likely, that this is the cauſe, why the parts of the Earth adhere and keep cloſe to one another.

89. The incomparable Sir Iſaac Newton, by a ſagacity peculiar to himſelf, diſcovered from many obſervations, that this law of gravitation or attraction was univerſally diffuſed throughout the ſolar ſyſtem; and that the regular motions obſerved among the heavenly bodies were governed by this ſame principle; ſo that the Earth and Moon attracted each other, and both of them are attracted by the Sun. He diſcovered alſo that the force of attraction, exerted by theſe bodies one on the other, was leſs and leſs as the diſtance increaſed, in proportion to the ſquares of thoſe diſtances; that is, the power of attraction at double the diſtance was four times leſs, at triple the diſtance nine times leſs, at quadruple the diſtance ſixteen times leſs, and ſo on.

90. Now as the Earth is attracted by the Sun and Moon, therefore all the parts of the Earth will not gravitate towards its center in the ſame manner, as if thoſe parts were not affected by ſuch attractions. And it is very evident that, were the Earth entirely free from ſuch actions of the Sun and Moon, the ocean being equally attracted towards its center, on all ſides, by the force of gravity, would continue in a perfect ſtagnation without ever ebbing or flowing. But ſince the caſe is otherwiſe, the water in the ocean muſt needs riſe higher in thoſe places where the Sun and Moon

Moon diminiſh its gravity, or where the Sun and Moon have the greateſt attraction.

As the force of gravity muſt be diminiſhed moſt in thoſe parts of the Earth to which the Moon is neareſt, that is, where ſhe is in the ZENITH, or vertical, and, conſequently, where her attraction is moſt powerful; therefore the waters in ſuch places will riſe higheſt, and it will be *full ſea* or *flood* in ſuch places.

91. *The parts of the Earth directly under the Moon, and alſo thoſe in her* NADIR, *viz. ſuch places as are diametrically oppoſite to thoſe where the Moon is in the Zenith, will have the flood, or high water, at the ſame time.*

FOR either half of the Earth would gravitate equally towards the other half, were they free from all external attraction.

But by the action of the moon, the gravitation of one half-earth towards its center is diminiſhed, and of the other is increaſed.

Now in the half-earth next the Moon, the parts in the zenith being moſt attracted, and thereby their gravitation towards the Earth's center diminiſhed, the waters in theſe parts muſt be higher than in any other part of this half-earth.

And in the half-earth fartheſt from the Moon, the parts in the nadir being leſs attracted by the Moon than the parts nearer to her, gravitate leſs towards the Earth's center, and conſequently the waters in theſe parts muſt be higher than they are in any other part of this half-earth.

92. *Thoſe parts of the Earth, where the Moon appears in the horizon, or is 90 degrees diſtant from the zenith and nadir, will have the ebbs or loweſt waters.*

For as the waters in the zenith and nadir riſe at the ſame time, the waters in their neighbourhood will preſs towards thoſe places to maintain the equilibrium; and to ſupply the places of theſe, others will move the ſame way, and ſo on to places of 90° diſtant from the ſaid zenith and nadir; conſequently, in thoſe places where the Moon appears in the horizon, the waters will have more liberty to deſcend towards the center; and therefore in thoſe places they will be the loweſt.

93. Hence it plainly follows, that the ocean, if it covered the ſurface of the Earth, muſt put on a ſpheroidal, or egg-like figure; in which the longeſt diameter paſſes through the place where the Moon is vertical; and the ſhorteſt diameter, will be, in the horizon of that place. And as the Moon apparently ſhifts her poſition from eaſt to weſt in going round the Earth every day, the longer diameter of the ſpheroid following her motion, will occaſion the two floods and ebbs obſervable in about every 25 hours, which is about the length of a lunar day, or the time ſpent between the Moon's leaving the meridian of any place, and coming to it again.

94. Hence the greater the Moon's meridian altitude is at any place, the greater theſe tides will be which happen when ſhe is above the horizon; and the greater her meridian depreſſion is, the greater will thoſe tides be which happen while ſhe is below the horizon.

Moreover the ſummer day, and the winter night-tides have a tendency to be higheſt, becauſe the Sun's ſummer altitude and his winter depreſſion are greateſt, but this is more eſpecially to be noted when the

Moon

Moon has north declination in summer, and south declination in winter.

95. *The time of high water is not precisely at the time of the Moon's coming to the meridian, but about an hour after.*

For the moon acts with some force after she has past the meridian, and by that means adds to the libratory, or waving motion, which she had put the water into, whilst she was in the meridian; in the same manner as a small force applied upwards to a ball, already raised to some height, will raise it still higher.

96. *The tides are greater than ordinary twice every month; that is, about the times of new and full Moon: these are called* SPRING-TIDES.

For at these times the actions of both Sun and Moon concur to draw in the same right line; and therefore the sea must be more elevated. In *conjunction*, or when the Sun and moon are on the same side of the Earth, they both conspire to raise the water in the zenith, and consequently in the nadir. And when the Sun and Moon are in *opposition*, that is, when the Earth is between them, whilst one makes high water in the zenith and nadir, the other does the same in the nadir and zenith.

97. *The tides are less than ordinary twice every month; that is, about the times of the first and last quarters of the Moon: and these are called* NEAP TIDES.

BECAUSE in the quarters of the Moon the Sun raises the water where the Moon depresses it; and depresses where the Moon raises the water; so that the tides are made only by the difference of their actions.

It must be observed, that the spring tides happen not directly on the new and full moons, but rather a day or two after, when the attractions of the Sun and moon have conspired together for a considerable time. In like manner the neap-tides happen a day or two after the quarters, when the moon's attraction has been lessened by the Sun for several days together.

98. *When the Moon is in her* PERIGÆUM, *or nearest approach to the Earth, the tides increase more than in the same circumstances at other times.*

FOR according to the laws of gravitation, the Moon must attract most when she is nearest to the Earth.

99. *The spring-tides are greater about the time of the* EQUINOXES, *that is, about the latter ends of March and September, than at other times of the year; and the neap-tides then are less.*

BECAUSE the longer diameter of the spheroid, or the two opposite floods, will at that time be in the Earth's equator; and consequently will describe a great circle of the Earth; by the diurnal rotation of which those floods will move swifter, describing a great circle in the same time they used to describe a lesser circle parallel to the equator, and consequently the waters being thrown more forcibly against the shores, must rise higher.

100. The following observations have been made on the rise of the tides.

1st. The morning tides generally differ in their rise from the evening-tides.

2d. The new and full Moon spring-tides rise to different heights.

3d. In winter the morning-tides are highest.

4th. In

4th. In summer the evening-tides are highest.

So that after a period of about six months the order of the tides are inverted; that is, the rise of the morning and evening-tides will change places, the winter morning high-tides becoming the summer evening high-tides.

Some of these effects arise from the different distances of the Moon from the Earth after a period of six months, when she is in the same situation with respect to the Sun; for, if she is in perigee at the time of new moon, in about six months after she will be in perigee about the time of full Moon.

These particulars being known, a pilot may chuse that time, which is most convenient for conducting a ship in or out of a port, where there is not sufficient depth at low-water.

Small inland seas, such as the Mediterranean and Baltic, are little subject to tides; because the action of the Sun and Moon is always nearly equal at both extremities of such seas. In very high latitudes the tides are also very inconsiderable. For the Sun and Moon acting towards the equator, and always raising the water towards the middle of the torrid zone, the neighbourhood of the poles must consequently be deprived of those waters, and the sea must, within the frigid zones, be low, with relation to other parts.

101. All the things hitherto explained would exactly obtain, were the whole surface of the Earth covered with sea. But since it is not so, and there being a multitude of islands, besides continents, lying in the way of the tide, which interrupt its course; therefore in many places near the shores, there arises a great variety of other appearances beside the foregoing ones which require particular solutions, in which the situations of the shores, straits, shoals, winds, and other things, must necessarily be considered. For instance:

102. As the sea * has no visible passage between Europe and Africa, let them be supposed to be one continent, extending from 78 degrees north to 34 degrees south, the middle between these two would be in latitude 19 degrees north, near Cape Blanco, on the west coast of Africa. But it is impossible that the flood-tide should set to the westward upon the western coast of Africa (for the general tide following the course of the Moon must set from east to west), because the continent, for above 50 degrees, both northward and southward, bounds that sea on the east; therefore if any regular tide, proceeding from the motion of the sea, from east to west, should reach this place, it must come either from the north of Europe southward, or from the south of Africa northward, to the said latitude upon the west coast of Africa.

103. This opinion is further corroborated, or rather fully confirmed by common experience, which shews that the flood-tide sets to the southward along the west coast of Norway, from the north cape to the Naze, or entrance of the *Baltic Sea*, and so proceeds to the southward along the east coast of *Great Britain*, and in its passage supplies all those ports with the tides [illegible], the coast of *Scotland* having the tide first, be-

* *Varen.* Geogr. p. 81[illegible]. Edit. 1734.

cauſe it proceeds from the northward to the ſouthward; and thus on the days of the full, or change, it is high-water at *Aberdeen* at 12 h. 45 m. but at *Tinmouth Bar*, the ſame day, not till 3 h. From thence rolling to the ſouthward, it makes high-water at the *Spurn* a little after 5 h.; but not till 6 h. at *Hull*, by reaſon of the time required for its paſſage up the river; from thence paſſing over the *Welbank* into *Yarmouth Road*, it makes high-water there a little after 8 h. but in the *Pier* not till 9 h., and it requires near an hour more to make high-water at *Yarmouth* town; in the mean time ſetting away to the ſouthward, it makes high-water at *Harwich* at 10 h. 30 m., at the *Nore* at 12, at *Graveſend* 1 h. 30 m., and at *London* at 3 h. all on the ſame day. And although this may ſeem to contradict that hypotheſis of the natural motion of the tide being from eaſt to weſt, yet as no tide can flow weſt from the main continent of *Norway* or *Holland*, or out of the *Baltic*, which is ſurrounded by the main continent, except at its entrance, it is evident that the tide we have been now tracing by its ſeveral ſtages from *Scotland* to *London*, is ſupplied by the tide, the original motion of which is from eaſt to weſt; yet as water always inclines to the level, it will in its paſſage fall towards any other point of the compaſs, to fill up vacancies where it finds them, and yet not contradict, but rather confirm, the firſt hypotheſis.

104. While the tide, or high-water, is thus gliding to the ſouthward along the eaſt coaſt of *England*, it alſo ſets to the ſouthward along the weſt coaſts of *Scotland* and *Ireland*, a branch of it falls into *St. George*'s channel, the flood running up north-eaſt, as may be naturally inferred from its being high-water at *Waterford* above three hours before it is high-water at *Dublin*, or thereabout, on that coaſt; and it is three quarters of an hour ebb at *Dublin* before it is high-water at the *Iſle of Man*, &c.

But not to proceed farther in particulars than to our own, or the *Britiſh* channel, we find the tides ſet to the ſouthward from the coaſt of *Ireland*, and in their paſſage a branch falls into the *Britiſh* channel between the *Lizard* and *Uſhant*; this progreſs to the ſouthward may be eaſily proved, by its being high-water on the day of the full and changes at *Cape Clear* a little after 4 h., and at *Uſhant* about 6 h., and at the *Lizard* after 7 h. The *Lizard* and *Uſhant* may properly be called the chaps of the *Britiſh* channel, between which the flood ſets to the eaſtward along the coaſts of *England* and *France*, till it comes to the *Goodwin* or *Galloper*, where it meets the tide before mentioned, which ſets to the ſouthward along the eaſtern coaſt of *England* to the *Downs*, where theſe two tides meeting, contribute very much towards ſending a powerful tide up the river *Thames* to *London*. And when the natural courſe of theſe two tides has been interrupted by a ſudden ſhift of the wind, by which means that tide was accelerated which had before been retarded, and that driven back which was before hurried in by the wind, it has been known to occaſion twice high-water in 3 or 4 hours, which, by thoſe who did not conſider this natural cauſe, was looked upon as a prodigy.

105. But now it may be objected, that this courſe of the flood-tide, E. E., or eaſt-north-eaſt, up the channel, is quite contrary to the hypotheſis of the general motion of the tides being from eaſt to weſt, and conſequently of its being high-water where the moon is vertical, or any where elſe in the meridian.

In

In anſwer. This particular direction of any branch of the tide does not at all contradict the general direction of the whole; a river, with a weſtern courſe, may ſupply canals which wind north, ſouth, or even eaſt, and yet the river keep its natural courſe; and if the river ebbs and flows, the canals ſupplied by it would do the ſame, although they did not keep exact time with the river, becauſe it would be flood, and the river advanced to ſome height, before the flood reached the farther part of the canals; and the more remote the canals are, the longer time it would require; and it may be added, that if it was high-water in the river juſt when the moon was on the meridian, ſhe would be far paſt it before it could be high-water in the remoteſt part of thoſe canals, or ditches, and the flood would ſet according to the courſe of thoſe canals that received it, and could not ſet weſt up a canal of a different poſition; and as *St. George*'s channel, the *Britiſh* channel, &c. are no more in proportion to the vaſt ocean, than theſe canals are to a large navigable river; it will evidently follow, that among thoſe obſtructions and confinements the flood may ſet upon any other point of the compaſs as well as weſt, and may make high-water at any other time as well as when the Moon is upon the meridian, and yet no way contradict the general theory of the tides before aſſerted.

106. When the time of high-water at any place is, in general, mentioned, it is to be underſtood on the days of the ſyzygies, or days of new and full Moon, when the Sun and Moon paſs the meridian of that place at the ſame time. Among pilots it is cuſtomary to reckon the time of flood, or high-water, by the point of the compaſs the Moon is on at that time, allowing $\frac{3}{4}$ of an hour for each point: Thus on the full and change days, in places where it is flood at noon, the tide is ſaid to flow north and ſouth, or at 12 o'clock; in other places, on the ſame days, where the Moon bears 1, 2, 3, 4, or more points to the eaſt or weſt of the meridian, when it is high-water, the tide is ſaid to flow on ſuch point: Thus, if the Moon bears S. E. at flood, it is ſaid to flow S. E. and N. W., or 3 hours before the meridian, that is, at 9 o'clock; if it bears S. W., it flows S. W. and N. E., or at 3 hours after the meridian; and in like manner for other points of the Moon's bearing.

107. In ſome places it is high water on the ſhore, or by the ground, while the tide continues to flow in the ſtream, or offing; and according to the length of time it flows longer in the ſtream than on the ſhore, it is ſaid to flow tide, and ſuch part of tide; allowing 6 hours to a tide; Thus 3 hours longer in the offing than on the ſhore, make tide and half-tide; an hour and half longer makes tide and quarter-tide; three quartees of an hour longer make tide and half-quarter tide; &c.

108. Along an extent of coaſt next to the ocean, ſuch as the weſtern coaſt of Africa, and the eaſtern and weſtern coaſts of South America, it is generally high-water about the ſame hour. But ports on the coaſts of narrow ſeas, or within land, have the times of their high-water ſooner or later on the ſame day, according as thoſe ports are farther removed from the tide's way, or have their entrances more or leſs contracted.

109. The times of high-water, in any place, fall about the ſame hours after a period of 15 days nearly, which is the time between one ſpring-

tide and another: and during that period, the times of high-water fall each day later by about 48 minutes.

110. From the obſervations of different perſons, the times when it is high-water on the days of the new and full Moon, on moſt of the ſea-coaſts of Europe, and many other places, have been collected. Theſe times are uſually put in a table againſt the names of the places, digeſted in an alphabetical order; the like is followed in this work, only they are not given in a table by themſelves, but make a column in the table of the latitudes and longitudes of places; which column is not filled up againſt many of the names in that table, for want of a ſufficient collection of obſervations. This may be ſupplied by thoſe who have opportunity and inclination.

The uſe of ſuch a table is to find the time when it is high-water at any of the places mentioned in it. But as this depends upon knowing the time when the Moon comes to the meridian, and this on the Moon's age, and this on the knowledge how to find ſome of the common notes in the Calendar; therefore it was thought convenient to introduce in this place a compendium of Chronology, containing the ſeveral articles above mentioned.

SECTION VIII.

Of Chronology.

111. CHRONOLOGY is the art of eſtimating, and comparing together, the times when remarkable events have happened, ſuch as are related in hiſtory.

An ÆRA, or EPOCHA, is a time when ſome memorable tranſaction occurred; and from which ſome nations date and meaſure their computations of time.

	Years of the Julian Period.	Years before Chriſt.
Some have dated their events from the creation of the world, and ſuppoſe it to have happened	710	4004
Others, from the deluge, or flood — —	2366	2348
The Greeks, from their Olympiads of 4 years each — — — —	3938	776
The Romans, from the building of Rome —	3961	753
The Aſtronomers, from Nabonaſſar king of Babylon — — — —	3967	747
Some Hiſtorians, from the death of Alexander the Great — — — —	4390	324
The Chriſtians, from the birth of Chriſt —	4713	A. D.
The Mahometans, from the flight of Mahomet, called the Hegira — — —	5335	622

In

In order to aſſign the diſtance between theſe, and other events, the ancients found it neceſſary to have a large meaſure of time, the limits of which were naturally pointed out to them by the return of the ſeaſons and this interval they called a year.

112. The moſt natural diviſion of the year appeared to them to be the returns of the new Moon; and as they obſerved 12 new moons to happen within the time of the general return of the ſeaſons, they therefore firſt divided the year into 12 equal parts, which they called months; and as they reckoned about 30 returns of morning and evening between the times of the new moon and new moon, therefore they reckoned their month to conſiſt of 30 days, and their year, or 12 months, to contain 360 days; and this is what is generally underſtood by the lunar year of the ancients.

113. But in length of time it was found, that this year did not agree with the courſe of the ſun, the ſeaſons gradually falling later in the year than they had been formerly obſerved; this put them upon correcting the method of eſtimating their year, which they did from time to time, by taking a day or two from the month, as often as they found it too long for the courſe of the moon; and by adding a month, called an intercalary month, as often as they found 12 lunar months to be too ſhort for the return of the four ſeaſons and fruits of the Earth. This kind of year, ſo corrected from time to time by the prieſts, whoſe buſineſs it was, is what is to be underſtood by the *luni-ſolar* year; which was anciently uſed in moſt nations, and is ſtill among the *Arabs* and *Turks*.

As a great variety of methods was uſed in different countries to correct the length of the year, ſome by intercalating days in every year, and others by inſerting months and days in certain returns, or periods of years; and theſe different methods being obſerved by ſome eminent men to create a conſiderable difference in the accounts of time kept by neighbouring nations, introducing a confuſion in the chronological order of times, they therefore invented certain periods of years, called *cycles*, with which they compared the moſt memorable occurrences.

114. At length *Julius Cæſar* obſerving the confuſion which this variety of accounts occaſioned, and knowing that his order, as Emperor of the Romans, would be followed by a very conſiderable part of the world; he therefore, about 40 years before the birth of Chriſt, decreed that every fourth year ſhould conſiſt of 366 days, and the other three of 365 days each. This he did in conſequence of the information given him by *Soſigenes*, an eminent mathematician of Alexandria in Egypt; for at that time the philoſophers of the Alexandrinian ſchool knew from a length of experience, that the year conſiſted of about 365 days and a quarter; and this was the reaſon of ordering every fourth year to conſiſt of 366 days, thereby compenſating for the quarter day omitted in each of the preceding three years. This method, called the *Julian Account*, or *Old Stile*, continued to be uſed in moſt Chriſtian ſtates until the year 1582.

The Aſtronomers, ſince the time of *Julius Cæſar*, have found that the true length of the ſolar year, or common year, is 365 days, 5 hours, 48 minutes, 55 ſeconds, nearly; being leſs than the Julian, of 365 days, 6 hours, by about 11 minutes, 5 ſeconds, which is about the 130th part of 86400, the seconds contained in a day; so that in 130 Julian years there would be one day gained above 130 solar years; and in 400 Julian years there would be gained 3 days, 1 hour, 53 minutes, 20 seconds; consequently one day omitted in every 130 common years, would bring the current account of time to agree very nearly with the motion of the Sun.

115. In the year of our Lord 325, when the *Council of Nice* settled the day for the celebration of Easter, the *Vernal Equinox* (that is, the day in the spring when the Sun rose at six and set at six) happened on the 21st of March; but about the year 1580 the *Vernal Equinox* fell on the 11th of March, making a difference of about 10 days. Now *Gregory* the XIIIth, who was Pope at that time, observing that this difference of time in the falling out of the *Equinox* would affect the intention of the *Nicene Council*, concerning the time of the year appointed by them for the celebration of Easter; he therefore, in the year 1581, published a *Bull*, ordering that in the year 1582, the 5th of October should be called the 15th, and so on; thus the 10 days taken off would cause the time of the *Vernal Equinox* to fall on the 21st of March, as at the time of the *Nicene Council*: and because a little more than three days were gained in every 400 years by the *Julian* account; therefore to prevent any future difference, every century, or number of 100 years, not divisible by 4, such as 17 hundred, 18 hundred, 19 hundred, &c., should contain only 365 days, which, by the *Julian* account, should have contained 366; and the centuries divisible by 4, such as 16 hundred, 20 hundred, 24 hundred, &c. should be leap-years of 366 days; and thus the three days would be omitted, which the anticipation of the equinoxes would gain in 400 years; the small excess of 1 hour, 53 minutes, 20 seconds, not amounting to a whole day in less than 5082 years, being rejected as inconsiderable; the intermediate years to be reckoned as they used to be in the *Julian* or *Old Stile*. This Pope's alteration, called the *Gregorian* or *New Stile*, was received in most of the Christian states: But some at that time chose to continue the *Julian*; among whom were the English; and they, in the year 1752, reformed their account, and introduced among themselves a new one, that nearly corresponds with the *Gregorian*.

A certain length of the year being once settled, and a regular account of time in consequence of it being so fitted, as to conform invariably to the seasons; it was natural for the States who received such account, to fit to it a register of the days in each month, and to note the days when any remarkable occurrence was to be commemorated; and such register has obtained the name of *Calendar*.

116. The Calendar now in use among most of the Christian states consists of 12 months, called *January*, *February*, *March*, *April*, *May*, *June*, *July*, *August*, *September*, *October*, *November*, *December*; these months are called *civil*, the number of days in each may be readily remembered by the following rule.

117. Thirty days has *September*, *April*, *June*, and *November*;
February has twenty-eight alone: All the rest have thirty-one;

When the year consists of 365 days: But in every fourth, which consists of 366 days, *February* has 29. This additional day was intercalated

lated after the 24th of *February*, which in the Old Roman Calendars was called the *ſixth of the calends of March*, and being this year reckoned twice over, the year was called *Biſſextilis*, or LEAP-YEAR.

Beſide the months, time is alſo divided into weeks, days, hours, minutes, &c. a year containing 52 weeks, a week 7 days, a day 24 hours, an hour 60 minutes, &c.

In the Calendars it has been uſual to mark the ſeven days of the week with the ſeven firſt letters of the alphabet, always calling the firſt of January A, the 2d B, the 3d C, the 4th D, the 5th E, the 6th F, and the 7th G, and ſo on, throughout the year: and that letter anſwering to all the Sundays for a year, is called the DOMINICAL LETTER.

According to this diſpoſition, the letters anſwering to the firſt day of every month in the year, will be known by the following rule:

118. At Dover Dwells George Brown, Eſquire,
Good Caleb Finch, and David Frier;

Where the firſt letter of each word anſwers to the letter belonging to the firſt day of the months in the order from January to December.

119. A year of 365 days contains 52 weeks and 1 day; and a leap-year has 52 weeks and 2 days; therefore the firſt and laſt days of a common year fall on the ſame week-day, ſuppoſe it *Monday*; then the next year begins on a *Tueſday*, the next year on *Wedneſday*, and ſo on to the eighth year, which would be on *Monday* again, did every year contain 365 days; alſo the Dominical letter would run backwards through all the ſeven letters. But this round of ſeven years is interrupted by the leap-years; for then *February* having a 29th day annexed, the firſt Dominical letter in *March* muſt fall a day ſooner than in the common year; ſo that leap-year has two Dominical letters, the one (ſuppoſing G) ſerving for *January* and *February*, and the other, which is the preceding letter (F) ſerves for the reſt of the Sundays in that year.

120. The SOLAR CYCLE, or cycle of the Sun, is a period of 28 years, in which all the varieties of the Dominical letters will have happened, and they will return in the ſame order as they did 28 years before. At the birth of Chriſt 9 years had paſt in this cycle.

For the changes, were all the years common ones, would be 7;
But the interruptions by leap-year being every fourth year;
Therefore the changes will be 4 times 7, or 28 years.

This return of the Dominical letter is conſtant in the *Julian* account. But in the *Gregorian*, where among the complete centuries, or hundredth years, only every fourth is leap-year; the other three hundred years, which according to the *Julian*, would be leap-years, are by the *Gregorian* only common years of 365 days: in theſe all the letters muſt be removed one place forwards in a direct order; and either year, inſtead of having two Dominical letters (as ſuppoſe D, C), will have only one (as D), the Dominical letters moving retrograde.

121. The LUNAR CYCLE, or cycle of the Moon (and ſometimes called the *Metonic Cycle*, from *Meton*, an Athenian who invented it about 432 years before the time of *Chriſt*), is a period of nineteen years, containing all the variations of the days on which the new and full Moons happen; after which they fall on the ſame days they did 19 years before.

The PRIME, or GOLDEN NUMBER, is the number of years elapsed in this cycle.

At the birth of *Christ* the golden number was 2.

For many years after the *Nicene Council*, it was thought that 19 solar years, or 228 solar months, were exactly equal to 235 synodical, or lunar, months: and that the same yearly *golden number* set in their calendars against the days when the new Moons happened throughout one lunar cycle, would invariably serve for the new Moons of corresponding years throughout every successive lunar cycle. But later observations shew, that this cycle is less than 19 years, by a little more than one hour, twenty-eight minutes; therefore, the new Moons will, in a little less than 311 years, happen a day earlier than by the Metonic account; and consequently all the festivals depending on the new Moons, will in time be removed into other seasons of the year than those which they fell in at their first institution: thus the new Moons in the year 1750 happened above $4\frac{1}{2}$ days earlier than the times shewn by the calendar. But were the golden numbers, when once prefixed to the proper new Moon days in a Metonic period, to be set a day earlier at the end of every 310,7 years, a pretty regular correspondence might be preserved between the solar and lunar years.

122. The EPACT of any year is the Moon's age the beginning of that year; that is, the days past since the last new Moon.

The time between new Moon and new Moon is in the nearest round numbers $29\frac{1}{2}$ days; therefore the lunar year consisting of 12 lunations must be equal to 354 days, which is 11 days less than the solar year of 365 days. Now supposing the solar and lunar years to begin together, the epact is 0; the beginning of the next solar year, the epact is 11; the 3d year the epact is 22; the fourth 33, &c. But when the epact exceeds 30, an intercalary month of 30 days is added to the lunar year, making it consist of 13 months; so that the epact at the beginning of the 4th year is only 3, the 5th 14, the 6th 25, the 7th 36, or only 6, on account of the intercalary month; and so on to the end of the cycle of 19 years; at the expiration of which the same epacts would run over again, were the cycle perfect; and the epact would always be 11 times the prime.

123. By the Nicene Council it was enacted,

1st. That Easter-day should be celebrated after the vernal equinox, which at that time happened on the 21st of March.

2d. That it should be kept after the full, or 14th day of that Moon which happened first after the 21st of March in common years, and first after the 20th of March in leap-years.

3d. That the Sunday next following the 14th, or day of full Moon, should be Easter-Sunday: which must always fall between the 20th or 21st of March, and 25th of April.

124. The MOON'S SOUTHING at any place is the time when she comes to the meridian of that place, which is every day later by about $\frac{4}{5}$ of an hour; because 24, the hours in a day, being divided by 30, the number of times which she passes the meridian between new Moon and new Moon, will give $\frac{4}{5}=48'$ for the retardation of her passage over the meridian in one day.

The Sun and Moon come to the meridian at the ſame time on the day of the change, or at new Moon; alſo the Moon comes to the oppoſite part of the ſame meridian, when ſhe is in oppoſition, or at full Moon. Hence between new and full ſhe comes to the meridian in the afternoon; at full ſhe comes to the meridian at mid-night; and when paſt the full, after mid-night, or in the morning.

125. The ROMAN INDICTION is a cycle of 15 years, uſed by the ancient Romans for the times of taxing the provinces. Three years of this cycle were elapſed at the birth of Chriſt.

The DIONYSIAN PERIOD is a cycle of 532 years, ariſing by multiplying together 28 and 19, the ſolar and lunar cycles; it was contrived by *Dionyſius Exiguus*, a Roman abbot, about the year of Chriſt 527, as a period for comparing chronological events.

The JULIAN PERIOD contains 7980 years; it ariſes by multiplying together 28, 19, 15, the cycles of the Sun, Moon, and Indiction. This was alſo contrived as a period for chronological matters; and its beginning falls 710 years before the uſual date of the creation.

On the principles laid down in the preceding articles depend the ſolution of the following problems.

126. PROBLEM I. *To find whether any given year is leap-year.*

RULE. Divide the given year by 4; if 0 remains, it is leap-year; if 1, 2, or 3 remains, it is ſo many years after.

Obſerving that the years 1800, 1900, 2100, &c. are common years.

EXAM. I. *Is 1788 leap-year?*	EXAM. II. *Is 1787 leap-year?*
4)1788(447	4)1787(446
0	Remains 3 years paſt leap-year.
Remains 0, ſo it is leap-year.	

127. PROBLEM II. *To find the years of the ſolar, lunar, and indiction cycles.*

RULE. To the given year add 9 for the ſolar, 1 for the lunar, 3 for the indiction: Divide the ſums in order by 28, 19, 15; the remainder in each ſhews the year of its reſpective cycle.

EXAM. *Required the years of the ſolar, lunar, and indiction cycles for the year 1787?*

1787	1787	1787
9	1	3
28)1796(64	19)1788(94	15)1790(119
Remains 4=ſolar cycle.	2=lunar cyc. or golden N.	5=indict. cycle.

Whereby it appears that the year 1787 is the { 4th year of the 65th ſolar cycle; 2d year of the 95th lunar cycle; 5th year of the 120th indiction cycle } ſince the birth of Chriſt.

128. PROBLEM III. *To find the Dominical letter till the year* 1800.

RULE. To the given year add its fourth part, divide the sum by 7; the remainder taken from 7 leaves the index of the letter in common years, reckoning A 1, B 2, C 3, &c.

But in leap-year, this letter and its preceding one (in the retrograde order which these letters take), are the Dominical letters.

EXAM. I. *For the year* 1787.

```
4)1787
   446
7)2233(319
      0
```

Remains 0. Then 7—0=7=G.
So G is the Dominical letter.

EXAM. II. *For the year* 1788.

```
4)1788
   447
7)2235(319
      2
```

Remains 2. Then 7—2=5=E
So F and E are the Dominical letters.

And in this manner were the following numbers computed.

For the Dominical letters during the 18th century.

Solar cycles	1	2	3	4	5	6	7	8	9	10	11	12	13	14
Dom. letters	DC	B	A	G	FE	D	C	B	AG	F	E	D	CB	A
Solar cycles	15	16	17	18	19	20	21	22	23	24	25	26	27	28
Dom. letters	G	F	ED	C	B	A	GF	E	D	C	BA	G	F	E

The year 1800 being a common year, stops the above order, and the following are the Dominical letters for the 19th century.

Solar cycles	1	2	3	4	5	6	7	8	9	10	11	12	13	14.
Dom. letters	ED	C	B	A	GF	E	D	C	BA	G	F	E	DC	B
Solar cycles	15	16	17	18	19	20	21	22	23	24	25	26	27	28
Dom. letters	A	G	FE	D	C	B	AG	F	E	D	CB	A	G	F

129. PROBLEM IV. *To find the Epact till the year* 1900.

RULE. Multiply the golden number for the given year by 11, and divide the product by 30; from the remainder take 11, and it will leave the epact.

If the remainder is less than 11, add 19 to it, and it gives the epact

Ex. I. *To find the epact for* 1783.

```
The Golden number is 17.   (127)
Multiply by              11
                   30)187(6
                      180
Remains                 7
Add                    19
Consequently the Epact is 26
```

Ex. II. *To find the epact for* 1786.

```
The Golden number is 01   (127)
Multiply by               11
                          11
Subtract                  11
Remains the Epact        =00
```

And thus might the following numbers be found.

Gold. N°	1	2	3	4	5	6	7	8	9	10	11	12	13	14	15	16	17	18	19.
Epacts	29	11	22	3	14	25	6	17	28	9	20	1	12	23	4	15	26	7	18.

The epacts here proceed by the difference 11, rejecting thirties.

130. PRO-

130. PROBLEM V. *To find the Moon's age.*

RULE. To the epact add the number and day of the month; their sum, if under 30, is the Moon's age; but if it be above 30, take 30 from it, and the remainder will be the Moon's age, or days since the last conjunction.

The numbers of the months, or monthly epacts are the Moon's age at the beginning of each month, when the solar and lunar years begin together;

And are	0	2	1	2	3	4	5	6	7	8	9	10.
	Jan.	Feb.	Mar.	Apr.	May,	June,	July,	Aug.	Sept.	Oct.	Nov.	Dec.

EXAM. I. *What is the Moon's age on the 14th of October, 1787?*

The epact is	2	(129)
The N° of month	8	
The day of the month	14	
The sum is	24 the Moon's age.	

EXAM. II. *What is the Moon's age on the 29th of March, 1786?*

The epact is 0. (129)
Then $0+1+29=30$ is the sum of the epact, number and day of the month.
And $30-30=0$ is the Moon's age.

131. The day of next new Moon is readily found by taking her age from 30.

The day of new Moon in any month is equal to the difference between the sum of the year's and month's epacts, and 30. Thus;

On March 29, the Moon is 0 days old.
So that new Moon is on the 29th.
Now $0+1=1$, is the sum of the epacts.
Then $30-1=29$, the day of new Moon, as it should be.

132. PROBLEM VI. *The day of the month in any year being given, to know on what week-day it will fall.*

RULE. Find the Dominical letter (128): also the week day on which the first of the proposed month falls (118); and hence the name of the proposed day of the month will be known; observing that the 1st, 8th, 15th, 22d, and 29th days of any month fall on the same week-days.

Ex. I. *On what day of the week does the 14th of Oct. fall, in 1787?*

The Dominical letter is G. (128)
The 1st of October is A, (118)
Therefore October 7th is Sunday.
Consequently 14th is also Sunday.

Ex. II. *In 1788, on what week-day does the 20th of March fall?*

The Dominical letter is E. (128)
The 1st of March is D. (118)
Then March 2d is Sunday.
And so March 20th is Thursday.

133. PROBLEM VII. *To find when Easter-day will fall in any year between 1700 and 1899.*

RULE. Find what day that new Moon falls on which is nearest to the 21st of March in common years, or to the 20th in leap-years; then the Sunday next after the full, or 15th day of that new Moon, will be Easter-day.

If the 15th day fall on a Sunday, the next Sunday is Easter-day.

Ex. I. *When does Easter-day fall in the year 1787?*
The Dominical letter is G. (128)
March 21, Moon's age is 3. (130)
New Moon on March 18.
The 15th day is April 2.
April the 1st is G, on Sunday.
Then Easter-Sunday is April 8th.

Ex. II. *Required the time of Easter-day in the year 1788?*
The Dominical letter is E. (128)
March 20, Moon's age 13. (130)
New Moon on March 7th.
Full Moon on March 22.
March 1st is D, on Saturday.
Then Easter-Sunday is March 23d.

134. Easter-day is always found by the Paschal full Moons, and these are readily found in the following curious table, which was communicated to the Royal Society in the year 1750, by the Earl of Macclesfield, and published in the Philosophical Transactions for the same year; and its use shewn in the following precepts.

"To find the day, on which the Paschal limit, or full Moon, falls in "any given year; look, in the column of golden numbers belonging to "that period of time wherein the given year is contained, for the golden "number of that year; over-against which, in the same line continued "to the column intitled Paschal full Moons, you will find the day of the "month, on which the Paschal limit, or full Moon, happens in that "year. And the Sunday next after that day is Easter-day in that year, "according to the Gregorian account."

His Lordship also gave with the following table an account of the principles upon which he constructed it; and which the more inquisitive readers may consult, if they please.

A TABLE,

A Table, ſhewing, by means of the Golden Numbers, the ſeveral days on which the Paſchal limits, or full Moons, according to the Gregorian account, have already happened, or will hereafter happen; from the Reformation of the Calendar in the year 1582, to the year 4199, incluſive.

Golden Numbers from the year 1583 to 1699, and ſo on to 4199, all incluſive.																Paſchal full Moons.
1583 to 1699	1700 to 1899	1900 to 2199	2200 to 2299	2300 to 2399	2400 to 2499	2500 to 2599	2600 to 2899	2900 to 3099	3100 to 3399	3400 to 3499	3500 to 3599	3600 to 3699	3700 to 3799	3800 to 4099	4100 to 4199	Days of the month and Sun. letters.
3	14	—	6	17	6	17	—	9	—	1	12	1	12	—	4	March 21 C
—	3	14	—	6	—	6	17	—	9	—	1	—	1	12	—	22 D
11	—	3	14	—	14	—	6	17	—	9	—	9	—	1	12	23 F
—	11	—	3	14	3	14	—	6	17	—	9	—	9	—	1	24 F
19	—	11	—	3	—	3	14	—	6	17	—	17	—	9	—	25 G
8	19	—	11	—	11	—	3	14	—	6	17	6	17	—	9	26 A
—	8	19	—	11	—	11	—	3	14	—	6	—	6	17	—	27 B
16	—	8	19	—	19	—	11	—	3	14	—	14	—	6	17	28 C
5	16	—	8	19	8	19	—	11	—	3	14	3	14	—	6	29 D
—	5	16	—	8	—	8	19	—	11	—	3	—	3	14	—	30 E
13	—	5	16	—	16	—	8	19	—	11	—	11	—	3	14	31 F
2	13	—	5	16	5	16	—	8	19	—	11	—	11	—	3	April 1 G
—	2	13	—	5	—	5	16	—	8	19	—	19	—	11	—	2 A
10	—	2	13	—	13	—	5	16	—	8	19	8	19	—	11	3 B
—	10	—	2	13	2	13	—	5	16	—	8	—	8	19	—	4 C
18	—	10	—	2	—	2	13	—	5	16	—	16	—	8	19	5 D
7	18	—	10	—	10	—	2	13	—	5	16	5	16	—	8	6 E
—	7	18	—	10	—	10	—	2	13	—	5	—	5	16	—	7 F
15	—	7	18	—	18	—	10	—	2	13	—	13	—	5	16	8 G
4	15	—	7	18	7	18	—	10	—	2	13	2	13	—	5	9 A
—	4	15	—	7	—	7	18	—	10	—	2	—	2	13	—	10 B
12	—	4	15	—	15	—	7	18	—	10	—	10	—	2	13	11 C
1	12	—	4	15	4	15	—	7	18	—	10	—	10	—	2	12 D
—	1	12	—	4	—	4	15	—	7	18	—	18	—	10	—	13 E
9	—	1	12	—	12	—	4	15	—	7	18	7	18	—	10	14 F
—	9	—	1	12	1	12	—	4	15	—	7	—	7	18	—	15 G
17	—	9	—	1	—	1	12	—	4	15	—	15	—	7	18	16 A
6	17	17	9	—	9	—	1	12	12	4	15	4	15	15	7	17 B
14	6	6	17	9	17	9	9	1	1	12	4	12	4	4	15	18 C

135. Problem VIII. *To find the time of the Moon's ſouthing on a given day.*

Rule. The Moon's age in days, multiplied by 0,8, gives the time of her ſouthing, nearly, in hours and tenth parts.

That time, if leſs than 12 hours, is the time after mid-day.

But if greater, the exceſs is the time after laſt midnight.

Ex. I. *At what time does the Moon come to the meridian of London, on the 14th of October, 1787?*

The Moon's age is 3 days.
Which multiplied by 0,8

Moon So. $2^h\ 24^m = 2{,}4$

Ex. II. *Required the time of the Moon's ſouthing on the 20th of March, 1788?*

The Moon's age 13 days. (130)
Which multiplied by 0,8

Moon So. $10^h\ 24^m = 10{,}4$

Each tenth part of an hour being 6 minutes, any number of ſuch tenth parts multiplied by 6, produces minutes.

136. PROBLEM IX. *To find the time of high-water at any place.*

RULE. To the time of the Moon's ſouthing add the time the Moon has paſſed the meridian on the full and change days to make high-water at that place; the ſum ſhews the time of high-water on the given day.

The time of high-water, on the full and change days, is found in the right-hand column of the geographical table, art. 137, againſt the name of the place.

Ex. I. *On the 14th of October 1787, at what time will it be high-water at London?*

Moon ſouths at	2h.	24m.	(135)
H.W. at Lond.	3	0 on ſyzygies	
Sum	5	24	
H. W. at	5h	24m. P. M. on the day propoſed.	

Ex. II. *Required the time when it will be high-water at Uſhant on March 20th, 1788.*

Moon ſouths at	10h.	24m.	(135)
High-water at Uſhant	4	30	P. M.
	14	54	
Subtract	12	00	
High-water at	2	54	A. M. on the day propoſed.

The V. VIII. IX. problems preceding have ſolutions, ſuch as are common in books of pilotage, and which in ſome caſes will produce concluſions conſiderably wide of the truth; it has therefore been judged neceſſary to conſider theſe articles in a more accurate manner in Book IX. of Days works.

SECTION IX.

137. *A Geographical Table.*

Containing the latitudes and longitudes of the chief towns, iſlands, bays, capes, and other parts of the ſea-coaſts in the known world, collected from the moſt authentic obſervations and charts extant; with the times of high-water on the days of the new and full Moon.

The longitudes are reckoned from the meridian of London. By the latitude and longitude of an iſland, or harbour, is meant the middle of that place.

Note. B. ſtands for bay; C. for cape; R. for river; P. for port; Pt. for point; I. for Iſle; St. for ſaint; G. for gulf; M. for mount; Eu. for Europe; Am. for America; Atl. for the Atlantic; Ind. for Indian; Med. Sea for Mediterranean Sea; Wh. Sea for White Sea; Archip. for Archipelago; Nov. Sco. for Nova Scotia; Phil. I. for Philippine Iſles; Adriat. for Adriatic; Eng. for England; D. Neth. for the Dutch Netherlands: Beſides other contractions which will be eaſily underſtood.

Names

Names of Places.	Cont.	Countries.	Coaſt.	Latitude.	Longitude.	H. Water.
A				° ′	° ′	
I. Abacco, or Lucayos { N. point S. point	Am.	Bahama I.	Atl. Ocean	{ 27 12 N. 26 15 N.	77 05 W. 77 01 W.	
Abbreviak	Eu.	France	Eng. Channel	48 32 N.	4 15 W.	4h. 30m.
St. Abbſhead	Eu.	Scotland	Germ. Ocean	55 55 N.	1 56 W.	
I. Abdeleur	Africa	Anian	Indian Sea	11 55 N.	51 45 E.	
Aberdeen	Eu.	Scotland	Germ. Ocean	57 06 N.	01 44 W.	0 45
Abo	Eu.	Finland	Baltic Sea	60 27 N.	22 15 E.	
Abrolhos Bank	Am.	Braſil	Atl. Ocean	18 22 S.	38 45 W.	
Abrollo Bank, N. part	Am.	Bahama	Atl. Ocean	21 33 N.	69 50 W.	
Achen	Aſia	I. Sumatra	Indian Ocean	5 22 N.	95 40 E.	
Aden	Aſia	Arabia	Indian Sea	12 55 N.	45 35 E.	
I. Admiralties	Eu.	Nova Zem.	North Ocean	75 05 N.	52 50 E.	
Adventure Iſland	Aſia	Soc. Iſles	Pacif. Ocean	17 6 S.	144 18 W.	
I. Agalega, or Gallega	Africa	Madagaſcar	Indian Ocean	10 15 S.	54 46 E.	
C. St. Agnes	Am.	Patagonia	S. Atl. Ocean	53 55 S.	66 29 W.	
Agra	Aſia	India	Mogul's	26 43 N.	76 49 E.	
I. St. Aguſta	Eu.	Dalmatia	Adriatic Sea	42 40 N.	18 57 E.	
C. Ajuga	Am.	Peru	Pacif. Ocean	6 38 S.	80 50 W.	
B. Alagoa	Africa	Caffers	Indian Ocean	25 30 S.	33 33 E.	
Iſ. Aland	Eu.	Sweden	Baltic Sea	60 20 N.	21 30 E.	
R. Albany	Am.	New S. Wales	Hud. Bay	52 35 N.	85 18 W.	
I. Alboran	Africa	Algiers	Medit. Sea	36 00 N.	2 27 W.	
Aldborough	Eu.	England	Germ. Ocean	52 20 N.	1 25 E.	9 45
I. Alderney	Eu.	England	Eng. Channel	49 48 N.	2 11 W.	12 00
Aleppo	Aſia	Syria	Medit. Sea	35 45 N.	37 25 E.	
Alexandretta	Aſia	Syria	Medit. Sea	36 35 N.	36 20 E.	
Alexandria	Africa	Egypt	Medit. Sea	31 11 N.	30 17 E.	
I. Algeranca	Africa	Canaries	Atl. Ocean	29 23 N.	15 53 W.	
Algiers	Africa	Algiers	Medit. Sea	36 49 N.	2 18 E.	
Alicant	Eu.	Spain	Medit. Sea	38 34 N.	0 07 W.	
I. Alicur, Lipari Iſ.	Eu.	Italy	Medit. Sea	38 31 N.	14 37 E.	
Aikoſir	Africa	Egypt	Red Sea	26 20 N.	34 41 E.	
B. All Saints, or Todos Sanctos	Am.	Braſil	Atl. Ocean	13 05 S.	38 45 W.	
Almeria	Eu.	Spain	Medit. Sea	36 51 N.	2 15 W.	
Iſ. Almirante, limits	Africa	Zanguebar	Indian Sea	{ 5 45 S. 4 30 S.	52 30 E. 55 40 E.	
St. Alphonſo's Iſ.	Am.	T. del Fuego	Pacif. Ocean	55 51 S.	69 28 W.	
Altur	Aſia	Arabia	Red Sea	28 20 N.	34 19 E.	
R. Amazons, mouths	Am.	Terra Firma	Atl. Ocean	0 30 S.	{ 47 35 W. 49 20 W.	6 00
I. Amboyna	Aſia	Molucca I.	Indian Ocean	4 25 N.	127 25 E.	
Ambrym	Aſia	N. Hebrides	Pacif. Ocean	16 10 S.	168 12 E.	
Iſ. Ambroſi	Am.	Chili	Pacif. Ocean	26 40 S.	82 30 W.	
I. Ameyland	Eu.	D. Neth.	Germ. Ocean	53 30 N.	6 20 E.	7 30
I. Amoy	Aſia	China	Pacif. Ocean	24 30 N.	118 45 E.	
Amſterdam	Eu.	D. Neth.	Germ. Ocean	52 23 N.	04 52 E.	3 00
I. Amſterdam	Aſia	Madagaſcar	Indian Ocean	37 55 S.	75 15 E.	
I. Amſterdam, or Tonga-Tabu	Aſia	Friendly Iſ.	Pacif. Ocean	21 09 S.	174 41 W.	8 30
I. Anabona	Africa	Eth. Coaſt	Atl. Ocean	2 36 S.	5 35 E.	
Ancona	Eu.	Italy	Mediterran.	43 38 N.	13 31 E.	
Iſ. Andaman, limits	Aſia	India	B. Bengal	{ 14 00 N. 10 08 N.	93 03 E. 93 35 E.	
I. Andiro	Aſia	India	Indian Ocean	10 00 N.	73 40 E.	
I. St. Andero, Sotovento	Am.	Mexico	Atl. Ocean	12 30 N.	81 35 W.	
C. St. Andrea	Africa	Madagaſcar	Indian Ocean	15 46 S.	45 22 E.	
St. Andrews	Eu.	Scotland	Germ. Ocean	56 18 N.	2 37 W.	2 15
Iſ. Androſ. { N. point S. point	Am.	Bahama I.	Atl. Ocean	{ 25 00 N. 23 30 N.	77 58 W. 77 00 W.	
Iſ. Angaſay	Africa	Madagaſcar	Indian Ocean	17 00 S.	58 40 E.	
C. St. Angelo	Eu.	Turkey	Archipelago	36 27 N.	33 38 E.	

Mount

Names of Places.	Cont.	Countries.	Coast.	Latitude.	Longitude.	H. Water.
				° ′	° ′	
Mount St. Angelo	Eu.	Italy	Medit. Sea	41 42 N.	16 16 E.	
R. d'Angra	Africa	Ethiopia	N. Atl. Ocean	01 00 N.	9 35 E.	
C. d'Anguilhas	Africa	Caffers	Indian Ocean	34 50 S.	20 06 E.	
I. Anguilla	Am.	Antilles If.	Atl. Ocean	18 15 N.	62 57 W.	
C. Anguille	Am.	Newfoundl.	Atl. Ocean	47 55 N.	59 11 W.	
I. Anholt	Eu.	Denmark	Sound	56 40 N.	12 00 E.	oh. oom.
C. Anne	Am.	New Eng.	Weft. Ocean	42 50 N.	70 27 W.	
C. Queen Anne	Am.	Greenland	North Ocean	64 15 N.	50 30 W.	
Q. Anne's Foreland	Am.	N. Main	Hudfon's Str.	64 08 N.	74 36 W.	
Annamocka, or Rotterdam	Afia	Friendly If.	Pacif. Ocean	20 16 S.	174 30 W.	
Annapolis Royal	Am.	Nova Scotia	B. Fundy	44 52 N.	64 00 W.	
I. Antego	Am.	Caribbee If.	Atl. Ocean	16 57 N.	61 56 W.	
Antibes	Eu.	France	Medit. Sea	43 35 N.	7 09 E.	
I. Ante-cost { W. point	Am.	Canada	B. St. Laurence	49 52 N.	64 04 W.	
I. Ante-cost { E. point				49 10 N.	61 42 W.	
Antiochetta	Afia	Syria	Medit. Sea	36 08 N.	36 17 E.	
C. d'Antifer	Eu.	France	Eng. Channel	49 47 N.	0 34 E.	
C. Antonio	Am.	Ifle Cuba	Atl. Ocean	21 45 N.	84 05 W.	
I. St. Antonio	Africa	Cape Verd	Atl. Ocean	17 00 N.	25 02 W.	
C. St. Antony	Am.	Magellan	Atl. Ocean	54 46. S.	63 42 W.	
Antwerp	Eu.	Flanders	R. Scheld	51 13 N.	4 24 E.	6 00
B. Apalaxy	Am.	Florida	G. Mexico	30 00 N.	83 53 W.	
I. Apalioria	Afia	India	Indian Ocean	9 08 S.	79 40 E.	
Aquapulco	Am.	Mexico	Pacif. Ocean	17 10 N.	101 40 W.	
Aquatulco	Am.	Mexico	Pacif. Ocean	15 27 N.	96 03 W.	
Archangel	Eu.	Ruffia	White Sea	64 34 N.	38 59 E.	6 00
I. d'Areas	Am.	Mexico	G. Mexico	20 45 N.	92 35 W.	
Arica	Am.	Peru	Pacif. Ocean	18 27 S.	71 05 W.	
I. Arran	Eu.	Ireland	St. Geo. Ch.	54 48 N.	8 59 W.	11 00
I. Afcenfion	Am.	Brafil	Atl. Ocean	7 56 S.	14 18 W.	
I. Afinaria, Sardinia	Eu.	Italy	Medit. Sea	41 06 N.	8 36 E.	
R. Afhley	Am.	Carolina	Atl. Ocean	33 22 N.	79 50 W.	0 45
R. Affene	Africa	Guinea	Atl. Ocean	5 30 N.	2 20 W.	
I. Aftores	Africa	Madagafcar	Indian Ocean	10 22 S.	53 25 E.	
Athens	Eu.	Turkey	Archipelago	38 5 N.	23 52 E.	
Atkin's Key	Am.	Bahama Ifles	Atl. Ocean	22 07 N.	74 26 W.	
Atwood's Keys	Am.	Bahama Ifles	Atl. Ocean	21 22 N.	72 04 W.	
C. Ava	Afia	Japan	Pacif. Ocean	34 45 N.	141 00 E.	
If. Aves, Sotovento	Am.	Terra Firma	Atl. Ocean	15 26 N.	66 15 W.	
C. St. Auguftine	Am.	Brafil	Atl. Ocean	8 48 S.	35 00 W.	
C. St. Auguftine	Afia	Mindanao	Pacif. Ocean	6 40 N.	126 25 E.	
St. Auguftine	Am.	Florida	Atl. Ocean	30 10 N.	81 29 W.	7 30
Aurora	Afia	N. Hebrides	Pacif. Ocean	15 8 S.	168 17 E.	
Aydhab	Africa	Egypt	Red Sea	21 53 N.	36 26 E.	
Aylah	Afia	Arabia	Red Sea	29 08 N.	35 41 E.	
B						
Babelmondel Straits	Africa	Abyffinia	Red Sea	12 50 N.	43 50 E.	
C. Baba	Afia	Natolia	Archipelago	39 33 N.	26 22 E.	
I. Bachian	Afia	Moluccalfies	Pacif. Ocean	00 40 N.	123 00 E.	
I. Bahama	Am.	Bahama Ifles	Atl. Ocean	26 45 N.	78 35 W.	
Bahama Bank, N. pt.	Am.	Bahama Ifles	Atl. Ocean	27 50 N.	78 43 W.	
C. Bajador	Africa	Negroland	Atl. Ocean	26 29 N.	14 36 W.	0 00
Baker's Dozen	Am.	Labrador	Hudfon's Bay	57 0 N.		
Balafor	Afia	India	B. Bengal	21 20 N.	86 00 E.	
Baldivia	Am.	Chili	Pacif. Ocean	39 38 S.	73 20 W.	
I. Bali	Afia	Sunda Ifles	Indian Ocean	8 05 S.	114 30 E.	
Baltimore	Eu.	Ireland	Weft. Ocean	51 16 N.	9 26 W.	4 30
I. Banca { S. end	Afia	Sunda Ifles	Indian Ocean	3 15 S.	107 10 E.	
I. Banca { N.W. end				1 50 S.	105 30 E.	
I. Banda	Afia	Moluccalfles	Indian Ocean	4 30 N.	127 25 E.	

Banjar

Names of Places.	Cont.	Countries.	Coaft.	Latitude.	Longitude.	H. Water.
				° ′	° ′	
Banjar	Afia	I. Borneo	Indian Ocean	2 27 S.	113 50 E.	
Banks's Ifle	Afia	N. Zealand	Pacif. Ocean	43 45 S.	172 40 E.	
Bantam	Afia	I. Java	Indian Ocean	6 15 S.	106 25 E.	
B. Bantry	Eu.	Ireland	Atl. Ocean	51 45 N.	10 46 W.	
I. Barbadoes, Bridge-town	Am.	CaribbeeIfles	Atl. Ocean	13 05 N.	59 36 W.	
C. Barbas	Africa	Sanaga	N. Atl. Ocean	21 50 N.	16 26 W.	
I. Barbuda	Am.	CaribbeeIfles	Atl. Ocean	17 46 N.	61 47 W.	
C. Barcam	Eu.	Greenland	North Ocean	78 18 N.	20 06 E.	
Barcelona	Eu.	Spain	Medit. Sea	41 26 N.	2 18 E.	
C. Barfleur	Eu.	France	Eng. Channel	49 38 N.	1 16 W.	7h. 30m.
Bargazar Point	Eu.	Iceland	North Ocean	66 30 N.	17 12 W.	
I. Bardfey	Eu.	Wales	St. Geo. Cha.	52 44 N.	5 00 W.	
C. Barfo	Eu.	Ruffia	White Sea	66 30 N.	38 00 E.	
I. Bartholomew	Am.	CaribbeeIfles	Atl. Ocean	17 56 N.	63 11 W.	
I. de Bas	Eu.	France	Eng. Channel	48 50 N.	4 00 W.	3 45
Baffora	Afia	Arabia	Perfian Gulf	29 45 N.	47 40 E.	
C. Baffos, or Baxos	Africa	Anian	Indian Sea	4 12 N.	47 07 E.	
Baffos de Banhos	Africa	Zanguebar	Indian Ocean	5 00 S.	48 08 E.	
Baffos de Chagos	Afia	India	Indian Ocean	6 42 S.	68 20 E.	
I. Baffus des Indes	Africa	Zanguebar	Indian Ocean	21 19 S.	41 43 E.	
Batavia	Afia	I. Java	Indian Ocean	6 12 S.	106 45 E.	
Bayonne	Eu.	France	B. Bifcay	43 30 N.	1 30 W.	3 30
Bayona Ifles	Eu.	Spain	Atl. Ocean	41 45 N.	9 01 W.	
Beachy Head	Eu.	England	Eng. Channel	50 44 N.	0 25 E.	0 00
Bear-bay	Eu.	Greenland	North Ocean	79 10 N.	24 15 E.	
N. Bear, S. Bear	Am.	Labradore	Hudfon's Bay	54 40 N. / 54 25 N.	80 0 W.	12 00
I. Beerenberg	Eu.	———	North Ocean	71 45 N.	4 30 E.	
Belcher's Ifles	Am.	Labradore	Hudfon's Bay	56 0 N.	83 4 W.	
Belfaft	Eu.	Ireland	Irifh Sea	54 43 N.	5 52 W.	10 0
Belleifle	Eu.	France	B. Bifcay	47 21 N.	3 13 W.	3 30
Belleifle	Am.	Newfound.	Atl. Ocean	51 55 N.	55 25 W.	
Bembridge Point	Eu.	Ifle Wight	Eng. Channel	50 41 N.	1 5 W.	
Straits of Belleifle	Am.	Newfoundl.	Atl. Ocean	51 48 N.	56 00 W.	
Bell Sound	Eu.	Greenland	North Ocean	77 15 N.	12 40 E.	
Bencoolin	Afia	I. Sumatra	Indian Ocean	3 49 S.	102 5 E.	
[illegible]	Afia	India	B. Bengal	22 00 N.	92 45 E.	
Bergen	Eu.	Norway	Weftern Oc.	60 10 N.	6 14 E.	
Berlin	Eu.	Germany	R. Elbe	52 33 N.	13 26 E.	
I. Berm[illegible]	Am.	Bahama Ifles	Atl. Ocean	32 35 N.	63 23 W.	7 00
I. Be[illegible]	Am.	Mexico	G. Mexico	21 40 N.	92 53 W.	
Berwick	Eu.	England	Germ. Ocean	55 45 N.	1 50 W.	2 30
B[illegible] Point	Eu.	England	Eng. Channel	50 37 N.	3 49 W.	
Bird Ifland	Am.	Acadia	G. St. Lawr.	47 44 N.	60 24 W.	
B[illegible]	Eu.	Spain	B. Bifcay	43 26 N.	3 18 W.	
I. [illegible] Bic	Am.	Acadia	R. St. Lawr.	48 30 N.	68 36 W.	2 0
Bl[illegible]	Eu.	England	Germ. Ocean	53 [illegible] N.	0 55 E.	6 00
Black P[illegible]	Eu.	Greenland	North Ocean	75 00 N.	10 50 E.	
Black I[illegible]	Eu.	Nova Zem.	North Ocean	72 52 N.	52 35 E.	
C. Blanco	Africa	Negroland	Atl. Ocean	20 55 N.	17 5 W.	9 45
C. Blanco	Am.	Patagonia	Atl. Ocean	47 20 S.	64 37 W.	
C. Blanco	Eu.	Greenland	North Ocean	77 58 N.	20 04 E.	
C. Blanco	Am.	Mexico	Pacif. Ocean	9 42 N.	85 55 W.	
I. B[illegible], S[illegible]	Am.	Terra Firma	Atl. Ocean	11 42 N.	64 20 W.	
B[illegible] R[illegible]	Eu.	France	Eng. Channel	49 42 N.	2 08 W.	0 00
B[illegible]	Eu.	Ireland	Atl. Ocean	52 00 N.	10 56 W.	
[illegible] Port Louis	Eu.	France	B. Bifcay	47 45 N.	3 13 W.	3 0
[illegible]	Am.	Terra Firma	Carib. Sea	10 [illegible] N.	75 30 W.	
[illegible]	Afia	Society If.	Pacif. Ocean	16 33 S.	151 52 W.	
R. B[illegible]	Afia	[illegible]	Pacif. Ocean	52 43 N.	157 00 E.	
I. B[illegible]	Afia	India	Indian Ocean	18 57 N.	72 43 E.	

Names of Places.	Cont.	Countries.	Coast.	Latitude.	Longitude.	H. Water.
				° ′	° ′	
Bona	Africa	Tunis	Mediterran.	37 08 N.	7 10 E.	
C Bona	Africa	Tunis	Mediterran.	37 10 N.	10 00 E.	
C Bona vista	Am.	Newfoundl.	Atl. Ocean	48 54 N.	52 33 W.	
I. Bena vista	Africa	C. Verd Isles	Atl. Ocean	16 05 N.	22 42 W.	
C. Bona fortuna	Eu.	Russia	White Sea	65 35 N.	38 25 E.	
I. Bonayre, Sotovento	Am.	Terra Firma	Atl. Ocean	11 52 N.	67 20 W.	
B. Bonaventura	Am.	Terra Firma	Pacif. Ocean	3 18 N.	76 50 W.	
C. Bon Esperance	Africa	Caffers	Indian Ocean	34 29 S.	18 23 E.	3h. 00m.
Bourdeaux	Eu.	France	B. Biscay	44 50 N.	0 30 W.	3 00
I. Borneo — East point	Asia		Indian Ocean	1 12 N.	117 10 E.	
I. Borneo — West point	Asia		Indian Ocean	3 15 N.	108 57 E.	
I. Borneo — North point	Asia		Indian Ocean	7 05 N.	113 40 E.	
I. Borneo — South point	Asia		Indian Ocean	3 32 S.	112 05 E.	
I. Borneo — Borneo	Asia		Indian Ocean	5 00 N.	112 15 E.	
I. Borneo — Succadano	Asia		Indian Ocean	0 50 S.	108 35 E.	
I. Bornholm	Eu.	Sweden	Baltic Sea	55 12 N.	15 50 E.	
Boston	Eu.	England	Germ. Ocean	53 10 N.	0 25 E.	
Boston	Am.	New Eng.	Atl. Ocean	42 25 N.	70 32 W.	
Botany Isle	Asia	N. Caledonia	Pacif. Ocean	22 27 S.	167 12 E.	
Botany Bay	Asia	N. Holland	Pacif. Ocean	34 00 S.	151 28 E.	
Boulogne	Eu.	France	Eng. Channel	50 44 N.	1 40 E.	10 30
I. Bourbon, St. Den.	Africa	Madagascar	Indian Ocean	20 52 S.	55 35 E.	
I. St. Brandon	Africa	Madagascar	Indian Ocean	16 45 S.	64 48 E.	
B. Brandwyns	Eu.	Greenland	North Ocean	79 50 N.	26 20 E.	
I. Bravas	Africa	C. Verd	Atl. Ocean	14 54 N.	24 45 W.	
Bremen	Eu.	Germany	R. Weser	53 30 N.	9 00 E.	6 00
Breefound, a sand	Eu.	D. Neth.	Germ. Ocean	53 12 N.	5 15 E.	4 30
Breslau	Eu.	Silesia	R. Oder	51 03 N.	17 13 E.	
Brest	Eu.	France	B. Biscay	48 23 N.	4 26 W.	3 45
P. Brest	Am.	New Britain	West. Ocean	52 10 N.	52 30 W.	
Cape Bret	Asia	N. Zealand	Pacif. Ocean	35 07 S.	173 52 E.	
Bridge Town	Am.	I. Barbadoes	Atl. Ocean	13 05 N.	59 36 W.	
Bridlington Bay	Eu.	England	Germ. Ocean	54 07 N.	00 04 E.	3 45
Brill	Eu.	D. Neth.	Germ. Ocean	51 56 N.	4 10 E.	1 30
Brion Isle	Am.	Acadia	G. St. Lawr.	47 50 N.	60 47 W.	
Bristol	Eu.	England	St. Geo. Ch.	51 28 N.	2 30 W.	6 45
C. Bristol	Am.	Sandwich L.	Atl. Ocean	59 2 S.	26 46 W.	
I. Cape Britain — Louisbourgh	Am.	Acadia	Atl. Ocean	45 54 N.	59 55 W.	
I. Cape Britain — I. Scateri	Am.	Acadia	Atl. Ocean	46 01 N.	61 57 W.	
I. Cape Britain — North Cape	Am.	Acadia	Atl. Ocean	47 05 N.	60 8 W.	
New Britain — I. Mathias	Asia	New Guinea	Pacif. Ocean	2 00 S.	147 50 E.	
New Britain — North point	Asia	New Guinea	Pacif. Ocean	2 30 S.	148 40 E.	
New Britain — S. W. point	Asia	New Guinea	Pacif. Ocean	6 00 S.	146 37 E.	
New Britain — Strait Dampier	Asia	New Guinea	Pacif. Ocean	6 15 S.	146 15 E.	
New Britain — C. St. George	Asia	New Guinea	Pacif. Ocean	5 30 S.	150 55 E.	
New Britain — I. St. John	Asia	New Guinea	Pacif. Ocean	4 20 S.	152 40 E.	
Buchaness	Eu.	Scotland	Germ. Ocean	57 29 N.	1 23 W.	3 00
Buenos Ayres	Am.	Brasil	Atl. Ocean	34 35 S.	58 26 W.	
C. Buller	Am.	S. Georgia	Atl. Ocean	53 58 S.	37 40 W.	
B[illegible] point	Eu.	Iceland	North Ocean	66 03 N.	16 34 W.	
Burgeo Isles	Am.	Newfoundl.	Atl. Ocean	47 36 N.	57 31 W.	
Burlings, rocks	Eu.	Portugal	Atl. Ocean	39 20 N.	9 32 W.	
Burlington	Eu.	England	Germ. Ocean	54 00 N.	0 08 E.	
Button's Isles	Am.	New Britain	Hudf. Straits	60 35 N.	65 20 W.	6 50
Cape Byron	Asia	N. Zealand	Pacif. Ocean	28 39 S.	153 31 E.	
Byron's Isle	Asia		Pacif. Ocean	1 18 S.	170 6 W.	
C						
I. Cabrera	Eu.	Italy	Mediterran.	43 10 N.	9 11 E.	
Cadiz	Eu.	Spain	Atl. Ocean	36 31 N.	6 07 W.	4 30
Caen	Eu.	France	Eng. Channel	49 11 N.	0 17 W.	9 00
Cagliari, I. Sardinia	Eu.	Italy	Medit. Sea	39 25 N.	9 38 E.	
Cajaneburg	Eu.	Finland	Baltic Sea	64 13 N.	27 51 E.	

Isle:

Names of Places.	Cont.	Countries.	Coaſt.	Latitude.	Longitude.	H. Water.
				° ′	° ′	
Iſles Caicos, or Cankroſs, from	Am.	Bahama Iſles	Atl. Ocean	21 27 N. 22 5 N.	71 24 W. 72 15 W.	
Calabar { Old New	Africa	Guinea	Eth. Ocean	4 30 N. 5 00 N.	8 10 E. 7 00 E.	
C. Calaberno	Aſia	Natolia	Archipelago	38 42 N.	26 44 E.	
Calais	Eu.	France	Eng. Channel	50 58 N.	01 51 E.	11h. 30m.
C. Calamadon	Aſia	India	B. Bengal	10 22 N.	80 40 E.	
Calcutta	Aſia	India	B. Bengal	22 35 N.	88 34 E.	
Caldera	Aſia	I. Mindano	Pacif. Ocean	7 00 N.	121 25 E.	
I. Caldy	Eu.	England	St. Geo. Ch.	51 33 N.	5 14 W.	5 15
Calecut	Aſia	India	Indian Ocean	11 15 N.	75 39 E.	
Cairo	Africa	Egypt	R. Nile	30 02 N.	31 26 E.	
Callao	Am.	Peru	Pacif. Ocean	12 2 S.	76 53 W.	
I. Great Camanis	Am.	Weſt Indies	Atl. Ocean	19 18 N.	80 29 W.	
I. Little Camanis	Am	Weſt Indies	Atl. Ocean	19 42 N.	79 20 W.	
Camboida	Aſia	India	Indian Ocean	10 35 N.	104 45 E.	
Cambridge	Eu.	England	———	52 13 N.	0 9 E.	
Cambridge	Am.	N. England	———	42 25 N.	71 5 W.	
C. Cambron, or Carbon	Africa	Algiers	Medit. Sea	37 18 N.	4 58 E.	
C. Cameron	Am.	New Spain	Atl. Ocean	15 35 N	83 29 W.	
R. Camerones	Africa	Guinea	Atl. Ocean	3 30 N.	9 10 E.	
B. Camerones	Am.	Magellan	Atl. Ocean	44 50 S.	67 10 W.	
Camfer, a ſand	Eu.	D. Neth.	Germ. Ocean	53 33 N.	5 30 E.	1 30
Camin	Eu.	Germany	Baltic	54 04 N.	15 40 E.	
C. Campbell	Aſia	N. Zealand	Pacif. Ocean	41 51 S.	174 41 E.	
Compeachy	Am.	Yucatin	Atl. Ocean	19 36 N.	90 53 W.	
I. Canaria	Africa	Canaries	Atl. Ocean	28 01 N.	15 0 W.	3 0
C. Candenoſe	Eu.	Ruſſia	North Ocean	69 25 N.	45 30 E.	
I. Candia { C. St. John, W. end Candia C. Salomon, E. end	Eu.	Turkey	Medit. Sea	35 12 N. 35 19 N. 34 57 N.	23 54 E. 25 23 E. 27 06 E.	
Candia	Aſia	I. Ceylon	Indian Ocean	7 54 N.	81 53 E.	
Candlemas Iſles	Am.	Sandwich L.	Atl. Ocean	57 10 S.	27 13 W.	
I. Ca[illegible]	Aſia	India	Indian Ocean	7 30 S.	77 55 E.	
C. Can[illegible]	Am.	Nova Scotia	Atl. Ocean	45 18 N.	60 48 W.	
Canſo Paſſage	Am.	Nova Scotia	Atl. Ocean	45 30 N.	61 00 W.	
C. Cantin	Africa	Barbary	Atl. Ocean	32 41 N.	9 01 W.	0 00
Cantire, Mul	Eu.	Scotland	Weſt Ocean	55 22 N.	5 45 W.	
Can[illegible]	Aſia	China	Pacif. Ocean	23 08 N.	113 07 E.	
Cape Town	Africa	Caffers	Atl. Ocean	33 55 S.	18 23 E.	2 30
I. C[illegible]	Eu.	Italy	Medit. Sea	40 34 N.	14 11 E.	
I. C[illegible]	Eu.	Italy	Medit. Sea	43 03 N.	10 15 E.	
C. C[illegible]	Aſia	India	B. Bengal	19 22 N.	86 05 E.	
[illegible]	Am.	Terra Firma	Atl. Ocean	10 06 N.	66 45 W.	
[illegible] Iſle	Am.	Greenland	Baffin's Bay	77 15 N.	62 00 W.	
[illegible]	Am.	California	Pacif. Ocean	38 24 N.	124 25 W.	
[illegible]	Eu.	Sweden	Baltic	56 20 N.	15 31 E.	
[illegible]	Eu.	England	Iriſh Sea	54 47 N.	2 35 W.	
C. C[illegible]	Aſia	Syria	Levant	33 08 N	35 35 E.	
[illegible] Iſles, Limits	Aſia	———	Pacif. Ocean	7 10 N. 12 00 N.	137 25 E. 127 2[illegible] E.	
[illegible]	Africa	Barbary	Medit. Sea	36 52 N.	[illegible] 31 E.	
[illegible]	Am.	Terra Firma	Caribbean Sea	1[illegible] 27 N.	75 22 W.	
[illegible]	Eu.	Spain	Medit. Sea	37 37 N.	1 [illegible] W.	
[illegible] Iſle	Aſia	New Britain	Pacif. Ocean	8 26 S.	159 14 E.	
[illegible] Swan Neſt	Am.	———	Hudſon's Bay	62 [illegible] N.	83 30 W.	
[illegible]	Eu.	I. Guernſey	Eng. Channel	49 5[illegible] N	2 20 W.	8 15
C. C[illegible]	Eu.	Turkey	Archipelago	4[illegible] [illegible]2 N.	2[illegible] 41 E.	
I. St. Catharine's	Am.	Braſil	Atl. Ocean	27 35 N	4[illegible] 12 W.	

Names of Places.	Cont.	Countries.	Coast.	Latitude.	Longitude.	H. Water.
				° ′	° ′	
Cat Isle { N. point	Am.	Bahama	Atl. Ocean	{ 24 50 N.	75 38 W.	
Cat Isle { S. point				{ 23 48 N.	75 35 W.	
Cathness Point } Dinnet Head }	Eu.	Scotland	West. Ocean	58 42 N.	3 17 W.	9h. com.
Catenea	Eu.	I. Sicily	Medit. Sea	42 40 N.	20 30 E.	
C. Catocha	Am.	New Spain	Caribbean Sea	20 48 N.	86 35 W.	
I. Cayenne	Am.	Terra Firma	Atl. Ocean	4 56 N.	52 10 W.	
I. Celebes { N. E. point	Asia	Spice Isles	Indian Ocean	{ 1 48 N.	124 37 E.	
W. point				3 00 S.	117 55 E.	
S. W. point Macasser				5 11 S.	117 50 E.	
S. point				5 40 S.	119 55 E.	
S. E. point				5 20 S.	121 58 E.	
I. Cephalonia	Eu.	Turkey	Medit. Sea	38 20 N.	20 11 E.	
Ceuta	Africa	Barbary	Medit. Sea	35 49 N.	5 25 W.	
I. Ceylon { Infanapatam, N. point	Asia	India	Indian Ocean	{ 9 47 N.	80 55 E.	
Trinquemale, S. E. end				8 40 N.	81 40 E.	
C. Gallo, S. West end				6 27 N.	82 10 E.	
				6 15 N.	80 20 E.	
Chain Island	Asia	Society Isles	Pacif. Ocean	17 25 S.	145 30 W.	
Chandernagar	Asia	Bengal	River Ganges	22 51 N.	88 34 E.	
Charles Town	Am.	Carolina	Ashley River	33 22 N.	79 50 W.	3 0
C. Charles	Am.	Virginia	Atl. Ocean	37 11 N.	76 07 W.	
I. of Charles } East end	Am.	Labradore	Hudson's Str.	{ 62 46½ N.	74 15 W.	
I. of Charles } West end				{ 62 48 N.	75 30 W.	10 15
C. Charles	Am.	New Britain	West Ocean	51 50 N.	51 10 W.	
Charlotte's Isles	Asia	Guadalcanal	Pacif. Ocean	11 0 S.	164 0 E.	
C. Charlotte	Am.	S. Georgia	Atl. Ocean	54 32 S.	36 12 W.	
Q. Charlotte's Sound	Asia	N. Zealand	Pacif. Ocean	41 6 S.	174 19 E.	9 00
Q. Charlotte's Foreld.	Asia	N. Caledonia	Pacif. Ocean	22 15 S.	167 18 E.	
I. Charlton	Am.	New Wales	Hudson's Bay	52 03 N.	79 00 W.	
Chatteaux Bay	Am.	Labradore	Atl. Ocean	52 1 N.	55 50 W.	
B. Chebucto	Am.	Nova Scotia	Atl. Ocean	44 45 N.	63 18 W.	
Chegnecto	Am.	Nova Scotia	B. Fundy	46 15 N.	63 11 W.	0 45
Cherbourgh	Eu.	France	Eng. Channel	49 38 N.	01 33 W.	7 30
Cherry Isle	Eu.	Greenland	North Ocean	74 35 N.	18 05 E.	
Chester	Eu.	England	Irish Sea	53 10 N.	2 25 W.	
Chiddock	Eu.	England	Eng. Channel	50 47 N.	3 00 W.	
C. Chidley	Am.	New Britain	Hudf. Straits	60 22 N.	65 00 W.	
I. Chiloe { N. point	Am.	Patagonia	Pacif. Ocean	{ 41 45 S.	73 05 W.	
I. Chiloe { S. point				{ 43 50 S.		
C. Chickotskago	Asia	Siberia	North Ocean	64 00 N.	174 45 W.	
Christiana	Eu.	Norway	Sound	59 25 N.	10 30 E.	
Christianople	Eu.	Sweden	Baltic Sea	55 55 N.	15 10 E.	
Christianstadt	Eu.	Sweden	G. Bothnia	62 47 N.	22 50 E.	
Christmas Sound	Am.	T. del Fuego	Pacif. Ocean	55 22 S.	70 01 W.	2 30
I. St. Christopher's	Am.	Carib. Isles	Atl. Ocean	17 15 N.	62 38 W.	
R. St. Christopher's	Africa	Caffers	Indian Ocean	32 47 S.	30 00 E.	
C. Chukchenfe	Asia	Siberia	North Ocean	66 30 N.	171 10 W.	
C. Churchill }	Am.	New Wales	Hudson's Bay	{ 58 48 N.	93 10 W.	
R. Churchill }				{ 58 47½ N.	94 03 W.	7 20
I. Chusan	Asia	China	Chinese Sea	30 00 N.	121 50 E.	
Civita Vecchia	Eu.	Italy	Medit. Sea	42 5 N.	11 51 E.	
C. Clear	Eu.	Ireland	West. Ocean	51 18 N.	9 50 W.	4 30
Clerk's Isles	Am.	S. Georgia	Atl. Ocean	55 6 S.	34 57 W.	
I. C[illegible]te	Asia	India	Indian Ocean	22 00 S.	95 40 E.	
Cochin	Asia	India	Indian Ocean	9 50 N.	76 05 E.	
I. C[illegible]os	Asia	India	Indian Ocean	12 20 S.	98 10 E.	
I. Cocos	Am.	Mexico	Pacif. Ocean	5 00 N.	88 45 W.	
C. Cod	Am.	New Eng.	Atl. Ocean	42 15 N.	69 27 W.	

Names of Places.	Cont.	Countries.	Coast.	Latitude.	Longitude.	H. Water.
				° ′	° ′	
Colchester	Eu.	England	Germ. Ocean	52 00 N.	0 58 E.	
C. Cold	Eu.	Greenland	North Ocean	79 00 N.	10 00 E.	
C. Colnet	Asia	N. Caledonia	Pacif. Ocean	20 30 S.	164 56 E.	
R. Colerado	Am.	New Spain	G. California	31 40 N.	115 25 W.	
I. Colgau	Eu.	Russia	North Ocean	69 20 N.	45 00 E.	
Collioure	Eu.	Spain	Medit. Sea	42 31 N.	3 10 E.	
C. Colone	Eu.	Turkey	Archipelago	37 43 N.	24 41 E.	
C. Colone	Asia	Natolia	Archipelago	39 10 N.	27 04 E.	
C. Colonni	Eu.	Italy	Medit. Sea	38 56 N.	18 05 E.	
C. Colville	Asia	N. Zealand	Pacif. Ocean	36 27 S.	174 48 E.	
Comana	Am.	Terra Firma	Atl. Ocean	10 00 N.	65 07 W.	
C. Comarin	Asia	India	Indian Ocean	7 55 N.	78 7 E.	
C. Comfort	Am.	New Wales	Hudson's Bay	64 45 N.	82 30 W.	
Concarneau	Eu.	France	B. Biscay	47 54 N.	3 50 W.	3h. 00m.
C. Conception	Am.	Calefornia	Pacif. Ocean	35 40 N.	120 01 W.	
B. Conception Entra	Am.	Newfoundl.	Atl. Ocean	48 25 N.	50 07 W.	
Conception	Am.	Chili	Pacif. Ocean	36 43 S.	73 13 W.	
R. Congo	Africa	Congo	Eth. Ocean	5 45 S.	11 53 E.	
I. Coningen	Asia	N. Zealand	Pacif. Ocean	34 30 S.	164 25 E.	
Coningsburgh	Eu.	Poland	Baltic Sea	54 44 N.	21 53 E.	
Conquet	Eu.	France	Eng. Channel	48 30 N.	4 35 W.	2 15
C. Conquibaco	Am.	Terra Firma	Atl. Ocean	12 15 N.	69 57 W.	
Constantinople	Eu.	Turkey	Archipelago	41 00 N.	28 53 E.	
Cook's Straits	Asia	N. Zealand	Pacif. Ocean	41 6 S.	174 30 E.	
Cooper's Isle	Am.	S. Georgia	Atl. Ocean	54 57 S.	36 0 W.	
Copenhagen	Eu.	Denmark	Baltic Sea	55 41 N.	12 40 E.	
[illegible]	Eu.	Norway	Sound	59 20 N.	10 10 E.	
I. Copland	Eu.	Ireland	Irish Sea	54 40 N.	6 40 W.	
I. Coquet	Eu.	England	Germ. Ocean	55 20 N.	1 25 W.	3 00
R. Coquimbo	Am.	Chili	Pacif. Ocean	29 54 S.	71 10 W.	
C. Corbau	Asia	Natolia	Archipelago	38 03 N.	26 58 E.	
Cordoue	Eu.	France	B. Biscay	45 30 N.	01 10 W.	
Corea, South limit	Asia	China	Pacif. Ocean	34 50 N.	124 25 E. / 127 25 E.	
I. Corfu	Eu.	Turkey	Mediterran.	39 50 N.	19 48 E.	
C. Corientes	Africa	Caffres	Indian Ocean	24 08 S.	36 49 E.	
C. Corientes	Am.	Mexico	Pacif. Ocean	20 18 N.	108 00 W.	
Corinth	Eu.	Turkey	Archipelago	37 30 N.	23 00 E.	
Corke	Eu.	Ireland	St. Geo. Ch.	51 54 N.	8 30 W.	6 30
C. Coronation	Asia	N. Caledonia	Pacif. Ocean	22 5 S.	167 8 E.	
C. [illegible]	Africa	Guinea	Eth. Sea	5 12 N.	0 23 W.	3 30
Corsica: C. Corse, North point	Eu.	Italy	Mediterran.	42 53 N.	9 40 E.	
Corsica: Bonifacio, South point	Eu.	Italy	Mediterran.	41 22 N.	9 26 E.	
I. Corvo	Eu.	Azores	Atl. Ocean	39 42 N.	31 02 W.	
I. Cosmoledo	Africa	Madagascar	Indian Ocean	10 28 S.	51 40 E.	
I. Coudre	Am.	Canada	R. St. Lawr.	47 31 N.	69 2 W.	
Cow and Calf	Eu.	Ireland	West. Ocean	51 22 N.	10 30 W.	
I. Cozumel	Am.	Yucatan	Atl. Ocean	19 36 N.	86 35 W.	
R. [illegible]	Asia	China	B. Nankin	34 06 N.	120 10 E.	
Cromer	Eu.	England	Germ. Ocean	53 05 N.	0 56 E.	7 00
Crooked I. N. point	Am.	Bahama	Atl. Ocean	22 47 N.	73 50 W.	
[illegible]	Eu.	Russia	White Sea	66 31 N.	39 33 E.	
[illegible] Point	Eu.	Nova Zem.	North Ocean	72 00 N.	53 12 E.	
[illegible]	Africa	Barbary	Atl. Ocean	30 36 N.	9 35 W.	
I. St. [illegible]	Am.	Antilles I.	Atl. Ocean	17 53 N.	64 55 W.	
Cuba: C. [illegible] Antonio, W. point	Am.	Antilles I.	Atl. Ocean	21 45 N.	84 05 W.	
Cuba: P. [illegible] Maisi, E. point	Am.	Antilles I.	Atl. Ocean	20 03 N.	74 52 W.	
Cuba: [illegible] Cape	Am.	Antilles I.	Atl. Ocean	19 42 N.	77 25 W.	

Isl.

Names of Places.	Cont.	Countries.	Coast.	Latitude.	Longitude.	H. Water.
				° ′	° ′	
Isl. Cuba: St. Jago	Am.	Antilles I.	Atl. Ocean	20 03 N.	75 51 W.	
Isl. Cuba: St. Mary	Am.	Antilles I.	Atl. Ocean	21 26 N.	78 10 W.	
Isl. Cuba: Le St. Esprit	Am.	Antilles I.	Atl. Ocean	21 56 N.	79 50 W.	
Isl. Cuba: Havannah	Am.	Antilles I.	Atl. Ocean	23 12 N.	81 45 W.	
Isl. Cuba: B. Hondy	Am.	Antilles I.	Atl. Ocean	22 54 N.	82 40 W.	
Cubbs Isles	Am.	New Wales	Hudson's Bay	54 15 N.	82 34 W	
Cubello	Asia	Ind. Malab.	Indian Ocean	7 50 N.	71 55 E.	
C. Cumberland	Asia	N. Hebrides	Pacif. Ocean	14 40 S.	166 47 E.	
Cumberland Isles	Asia	Society Isles	Pacif. Ocean	19 18 S.	140 36 E.	
B. Cumberland	Am.	North Main	Davis's Str.	66 40 N.	65 20 W.	
Curassoa	Am.	Terra Firma	Atl. Ocean	11 56 N.	68 20 W.	
I. Cuzzola	Eu.	Turkey	Medit. Sea	42 50 N.	16 55 E.	
Cusco	Am.	Peru	Inland	12 25 S.	73 35 W.	
I. Cypress: C. Bassa, W. end	Asia	Syria	Medit. Sea	35 04 N.	33 04 E.	
I. Cypress: C. St. Andr. E. end	Asia	Syria	Medit. Sea	35 40 N.	35 08 E.	
I. Cypress: C. de Gasse, S. point	Asia	Syria	Medit. Sea	34 35 N.	33 41 E.	
I. Cypress: C. Grego, S. E. point	Asia	Syria	Medit. Sea	34 57 N.	34 36 E.	
D.						
Dabul	Asia	India	Arabian Sea	18 24 N.	73 33 E.	
Dahlak	Asia	Arabia	Red Sea	15 50 N.	41 44 F.	
Isles of Danger	Asia	Society Isles	Pacif. Ocean	10 15 S.	165 50 W.	
I. Dagerort Light-house	Eu.	Livonia	Baltic Sea	58 55 N.	22 32 E.	
Dantzic	Eu.	Poland	Baltic Sea	54 22 N.	18 36 E.	
Str. Dardanels	Eu.	Turkey	Archipelago	40 10 N.	26 26 E.	
Gulph Darien	Am.	Terra Firma	Caribbean Sea	8 45 N.	76 35 W.	
Dartmouth	Eu.	England	Eng. Channel	50 27 N.	3 36 W.	6h. 30m.
I. Dauphin	Am.	Louisiana	G. Mexico	29 40 N.	87 53 W.	
St. David's Head	Eu.	Wales	St. Geo. Ch.	51 55 N.	5 22 W.	6 00
Fort St. David's	Asia	India	Corom. Coast	12 05 N.	80 55 E.	
I. Deseada	Am.	Carib. Isles	Atl. Ocean	16 36 N.	61 10 W.	
C. Deseada	Am.	T. del Fuego	Pacif. Ocean	53 4 S.	74 13 W.	
C. Desire	Eu.	Nova Zem.	North Ocean	77 45 N.	79 20 E.	
C. Desolation	Am.	Greenland	North Ocean	61 45 N.	47 00 W.	
Devil's Isles	Eu.	Greenland	North Ocean	80 00 N.	11 43 E.	
Dewpoint	Asia	India	B. Bengal	16 07 N.	81 47 E.	
I. Diego Rayes	Asia	Ind. Malab.	Indian Ocean	0 45 S. / 0 30 N.	70 25 E.	
I. Diego Garcia	Africa	India	Indian Ocean	8 45 S.	68 10 E.	
Str. Diemen	Asia	Japan Isles	Pacif. Ocean	31 12 N.	130 55 E.	
I. Dieu	Eu.	France	Bay of Biscay	46 26 N.	2 20 W.	
Dieppe	Eu.	France	Eng. Channel	49 55 N.	1 12 E.	10 30
Digge's, or Dudley's Cape	Am.	Greenland	Baffin's Bay	76 48 N.	59 07 W.	
C. Diggs	Am.	Labradore	Hudson's Bay	62 45 N.	78 50 W.	
Po. Diu	Asia	India	Indian Ocean	21 37 N.	70 28 E.	
C. Dobbs	Am.	North Wales	Hudson's Bay	65 10 N.	86 25 W.	
Dofar	Asia	Arabia	Indian Ocean	16 24 N.	53 40 E.	
St. Domingo Hispaniola	Am.	Antilles	Atl. Ocean	18 25 N.	69 30 W.	
I. Dominico	Am.	Caribbee	Atl. Ocean	15 18 N.	61 28 W.	
Dordrecht	Eu.	D. Neth.	R. Maes	52 00 N.	4 26 E.	
C. Dorfui	Africa	Ajan	Indian Ocean	10 15 N.	50 44 E.	
C. Doro	Eu.	Turkey	Archipelago	38 02 N.	25 12 F.	
Dort	Eu.	D. Neth.	Germ. Ocean	51 47 N.	4 40 E.	3 00
I. Dofel	Eu.	Livonia	Baltic Sea	58 20 N.	23 00 E.	
I. Dos Banhos	Africa	Zanguebar	Indian Ocean	5 15 N.	49 24 E.	
Dover	Eu.	England	Eng. Channel	51 07 N.	1 19 E.	11 30
Downs	Eu.	England	Germ. Ocean	51 25 N.	1 27 E.	1 15

P..

Names of Places.	Cont.	Countries.	Coast.	Latitude.	Longitude.	H. Water.
				° ′	° ′	
Po. Dradate	Africa	Egypt	Red Sea	19 56 N.	37 40 E.	
Po. Drake, sir Francis	Am.	California	Pacif. Ocean	38 45 N.	128 35 W.	
Drontheim	Eu.	Norway	North Ocean	63 26 N.	11 08 E.	
Dublin	Eu.	Ireland	Irish Sea	53 21 N.	6 5 W.	9h. 15m
Dunbar	Eu.	Scotland	Germ. Ocean	55 58 N.	2 22 W.	2 30
Dundalk	Eu.	Ireland	Irish Sea	53 57 N.	6 28 W.	
Dundee	Eu.	Scotland	Germ. Ocean	56 26 N.	2 48 W.	2 15
Dungarven	Eu.	Ireland	Atl. Ocean	51 57 N.	7 55 W.	4 30
Dungeness	Eu.	England	Eng. Channel	50 53 N.	0 59 E.	9 45
Duncansby Head	Eu.	Scotland	Germ. Ocean	58 40 N.	2 57 W.	
Dunkirk	Eu.	France	Germ. Ocean	51 02 N.	2 27 E.	0 00
Dunnose	Eu.	I. White	Eng. Channel	50 34 N.	1 15 W.	9 45
Durazzo	Eu.	Turkey	Medit. Sea	41 58 N.	25 00 E.	
Dusky Bay	Asia	N. Zealand	Pacif. Ocean	45 47 S.	166 23 E.	10 57
E						
C. East	Am.	Statenland	Stra. le Maire	54 54 S.	64 47 W.	
Easter Isl.	Am.	Chili	Pacif. Ocean	27 7 S.	109 42 W.	2 00
Edinburgh	Eu.	Scotland	Germ. Ocean	55 58 N.	3 7 W.	4 30
Edystone	Eu.	England	Eng. Channel	50 8 N.	4 20 W.	5 30
Egmont Isle	Asia	Society Isles	Pacif. Ocean	19 20 S.	138 30 W.	
C. Egmont	Asia	N. Zealand	Pacif. Ocean	39 20 S.	173 45 E.	
I. Elba	Eu.	Italy	Mediterran.	42 52 N.	10 38 E.	
R. Elbe mouth	Eu.	Germany	Germ. Ocean	54 18 N.	7 10 E.	0 00
Elbing	Eu.	Poland	Baltic Sea	54 12 N.	20 35 E.	
Elsingburgh	Eu.	Sweden	Baltic Sea	56 00 N.	13 35 E.	
Elsinore	Eu.	Denmark	Baltic Sea	56 00 N.	13 23 E.	
I. Elutheria { N. point	Am.	Bahama	Atl. Ocean	25 45 N.	76 42 W.	
I. Elutheria { S. point				24 57 N.	75 53 W.	
Emblen	Eu.	Germany	Germ. Ocean	53 05 N.	7 26 E.	0 00
R. Ems mouth	Eu.	Germany	Germ. Ocean	53 10 N.	7 20 E.	7 30
Enchuysen	Eu.	D. Neth.	Zuyder Sea	52 43 N.	5 06 E.	0 00
Endeavour R.	Asia	N. Holland	Pacif. Ocean	15 26 S.	145 12 E.	
I. Engano, or Trompouse	Am.	Sumatra	Indian Ocean	6 00 S.	102 35 E.	
B. Enhora	Eu.	Greenland	North Sea	78 45 N.	26 05 E.	
Ephesus	Asia	Natolia	Archipelago	38 00 N.	27 53 E.	
Erramanga	Asia	N. Hebrides	Pacif. Ocean	18 44 S.	169 20 E.	
Estaples	Eu.	France	Eng. Channel	50 34 N.	1 42 E.	11 00
Eustatia	Am.	Caribbee	Atl. Ocean	17 30 N.	63 14 W.	
I. Exuma	Am.	Bahama	Atl. Ocean	23 25 N.	75 35 W.	
F						
Fairhead	Eu.	Ireland	West. Ocean	55 19 N.	6 20 W.	
C. Falcon	Africa	Barbary	Medit. Sea	36 03 N.	0 14 W.	
I. Falkland { E. end	Am.	Patagonia	Atl. Ocean	51 05 S.	56 40 W.	
I. Falkland { [illegible]				52 27 S.	61 53 W.	
Falmouth	Eu.	England	Eng. Channel	50 8 N.	5 0 W.	5 30
C. Fa[illegible]	Eu.	Turkey	Archipelago	40 12 N.	24 27 E.	
C. Fa[illegible]	Africa	Caffers	Indian Ocean	34 16 S.	18 44 E.	
C. Fa[illegible]	Africa	Zanguebar	Indian Ocean	8 52 S.	59 55 E.	
Fal[illegible]	Eu.	Sweden	Baltic Sea	55 20 N.	13 36 E.	
I. Fa[illegible]	Eu.	Turkey	Medit. Sea	40 14 N.	19 32 E.	
R. Fa[illegible]	Africa	Egypt	Red Sea	21 40 N.	36 29 E.	
Fa[illegible]	Eu.	Scotland	West. Ocean	58 40 N.	4 5[illegible] W.	
C. F[illegible]	Asia	N. Zealand	Pacif. Ocean	40 35 S.	172 4[illegible] E.	
C. F[illegible]	Am.	Greenland	North Ocean	59 37 N.	42 [illegible] W.	
C. F[illegible]	Asia	Arabia	Indian Ocean	15 41 N.	[illegible] E.	
C. F[illegible]	Am.	Carolina	Atl. Ocean	34 04 N.	78 [illegible] W.	
I. F[illegible]	Am.	Brasil	Atl. Ocean	[illegible] 5[illegible] S.	[illegible] 23 W.	
I. F[illegible]	Eu.	Italy	Medit. Sea	38 33 N.	14 51 E.	
I. F[illegible]	Eu.	Turkey	Archipelago	37 24 N.	25 05 E.	
I. F[illegible]	Africa	Guinea	Atl. Ocean	3 0[illegible] N.	[illegible] E.	

I. Ferro

Names of Places.	Cont.	Countries.	Coast.	Latitude.	Longitude.	H. Water.
				° ′	° ′	
I. Ferro	Africa	Canaries	Atl. Ocean	27 48 N.	17 40 W.	
C. Finisterre	Eu.	Spain	Atl. Ocean	42 52 N.	9 16 W.	
I. Fironda	Asia	Corea	Pacif. Ocean	33 30 N.	127 25 E.	
Flamborough Head	Eu.	England	Germ. Ocean	54 08 N.	0 11 E.	4h. oom.
I. Flores	Eu.	Azores	Atl. Ocean	39 34 N.	30 59 W.	
C. Florida	Am.	Florida	G. Mexico	25 50 N.	80 20 W.	7 30
Flushing	Eu.	D. Neth.	Germ. Ocean	51 33 N.	3 20 W.	0 45
I. Fly	Eu.	D. Neth.	Germ. Ocean	53 16 N.	5 35 E.	7 30
Forbisher's Straits	Am.	Greenland	Atl. Ocean	62 05 N.	47 18 W.	
North Foreland	Eu.	England	Germ. Ocean	51 28 N.	1 25 E.	9 45
South Foreland	Eu.	England	Eng. Channel	51 12 N.	1 24 E.	9 45
Foreland Fair	Eu.	Ireland	North Ocean	55 05 N.	6 30 W.	
Foreland Fair	Eu.	Greenland	North Ocean	79 18 N.	10 50 E.	
Foreland Merchants	Am.	Greenland	North Ocean	63 20 N.	17 05 W.	
I. Formentaria	Eu.	Spain	Medit. Sea	38 33 N.	1 15 E.	
I. Formigas	Eu.	Azores	Atl. Ocean	37 17 N.	24 43 W.	
C. Formosa	Africa	Guinea	Eth. Sea	4 22 N.	5 43 E.	
R. Formosa	Africa	Guinea	Eth. Sea	6 10 N.	4 49 E.	
I. Formosa { N. point	Asia	China	Indian Ocean	21 25 N.	121 25 E.	
I. Formosa { S. point				22 00 N.	120 40 E.	
I. Forteventura, S. W. end	Africa	Canaries	Atl. Ocean	28 35 N.	14 04 W.	
Foulness	Eu.	England	Germ. Ocean	52 57 N.	0 58 E.	6 45
Foulsound	Eu.	Greenland	North Ocean	77 30 N.	12 50 E.	
Fowey	Eu.	England	Eng. Channel	50 25 N.	4 30 W.	5 15
I. France, P. Louis	Africa	Madagascar	Indian Ocean	20 10 S.	57 33 E.	
C. St. Francis	Am.	Peru	Pacif. Ocean	0 30 N.	80 35 W.	
I. St. Francisco	Africa	Zanguebar	Indian Ocean	6 23 S.	53 22 E.	
R. St. Francisco	Am.	Brasil	Atl. Ocean	10 55 S.	36 30 W.	
C. Francois	Am.	Domingo	Atl. Ocean	19 47 N.	72 15 W.	
Frederickstadt	Eu.	Norway	Sound	59 00 N.	11 10 E.	
French Keys	Am.	Bahama	Atl. Ocean	21 30 N.	72 10 W.	
Fretum Borough	Eu.	Russia	North Ocean	70 00 N.	61 20 E.	
C. Frio	Am.	Brasil	Atl. Ocean	23 00 S.	40 11 W.	
R. Fugor	Africa	Zanguebar	Indian Ocean	00 10 N.	42 05 E.	
I. Fuego	Africa	De Verd	Atl. Ocean	14 55 N.	24 28 W.	
Furneaux Island	Asia	Soc. Isles	Pacif. Ocean	17 11 S.	143 07 W.	
B. Fushan	Asia	China	Pacif. Ocean	23 00 N.	112 35 E.	
I. Fyal	Eu.	Azores	Atl. Ocean	38 32 N.	28 36 W.	2 20
G						
I. Galla	Am.	Terra Firma	Pacif. Ocean	2 40 N.	79 35 W.	
R. Gallega	Am.	Patagonia	Atl. Ocean	51 37 S.	65 35 W.	
I. Gallego	Am.	Terra Firma	Pacif. Ocean	1 40 N.	104 35 W.	
Gallipoli	Eu.	Italy	Medit. Sea	40 19 N.	18 08 E.	
Gallipoly	Eu.	Turkey	Archipelago	40 36 N.	27 02 E.	
I. Gallita	Africa	Barbary	Medit. Sea	37 42 N.	9 03 E.	
C. Gallo	Asia	I. Ceylon	Indian Ocean	6 15 N.	80 20 E.	
Is. Gallepago	Am.	Peru	Pacif. Ocean	{ 2 00 N. 2 00 S.	89 00 W.	
Gally Head	Eu.	Ireland	West. Ocean	52 40 N.	9 30 W.	
Galway	Eu.	Ireland	West. Ocean	53 10 N.	10 03 W.	
R. Gambia	Africa	Negroland	Atl. Ocean	13 00 N.	14 58 W.	
I. Gamo	Asia	India	Indian Ocean	3 05 S.	77 25 E.	
C. Gardafui	Africa	Anian	Indian Ocean	11 48 N.	50 25 E.	
R. Garronne	Eu.	France	B. Biscay	45 30 N.	1 05 W.	3 00
Gaspey Bay	Am.	Acadia	G. St. Lawr.	48 49 N.	63 34 W.	1 30
C. de Gatt	Eu.	Spain	Medit. Sea	36 32 N.	2 05 W.	
C. Gear	Africa	Barbary	Atl. Ocean	30 35 N.	10 01 W.	
Genoa	Eu.	Italy	Medit. Sea	44 25 N.	8 41 E.	
C. St. George	Am.	Newfoundl.	Atl. Ocean	48 28 N.	57 43 W.	
C. G[illegible]	Am.	S. Georgia	Atl. Ocean	54 17 S.	36 33 W.	
B. St. George	Am.	Newfoundl.	Atl. Ocean	48 19 N.	57 30 W.	

Names of Places.	Cont.	Countries.	Coast.	Latitude.	Longitude.	H. Water.
				° ′	° ′	
I. St. George	Asia	Natolia	Archipelago	38 47 N.	25 07 E.	
I. St. George	Eu.	Azores	Atl. Ocean	38 39 N.	28 00 W.	
St. George's Fort	Asia	India	B. Bengal	13 05 N.	80 34 E.	
Gibraltar	Eu.	Spain	Medit. Sea	36 05 N.	5 17 W.	0h. 00m.
Gilbert's Island	Am.	T. del Fuego	Pacif. Ocean	55 13 S.	71 4 W.	
I. Gilolo { N. point S. point	Asia	Spice Islands	Indian Ocean	{ 2 30 N. 1 30 S.	128 00 E. 129 25 E.	
Glasgow	Eu.	Scotland	R. Clyde	55 52 N.	4 10 W.	
Gloucester Isles	Asia	Society Isles	Pacif. Ocean	19 11 S.	140 4 W.	
Gloucester Isles	Asia	Society Isles	Indian Ocean	20 36 S.	146 7 W.	
Goa	Asia	India	Malabar	15 31 N.	73 50 E.	
Goes	Eu.	D. Neth.	Germ. Ocean	51 39 N.	4 05 E.	
Golfe triste	Am.	Terra Firma	Carrib. Sea	10 20 N.	67 40 W.	
Gombroon	Asia	Persia	Persian Gulf	27 40 N.	55 20 E.	
I. Gomero	Africa	Canaries	Atl. Ocean	28 06 N.	17 03 W.	
C. Gondewar	Asia	India	B. Bengal	16 55 N.	82 55 E.	
C. Good Hope	Africa	Caffers	Indian Ocean	34 29 S.	18 28 E.	3 00
I. Gorea	Africa	Negroland	Atl. Ocean	14 40 N.	17 20 W.	
I. Gorgona	Eu.	Italy	Medit. Sea	43 21 N.	9 11 E.	
I. Goth- { N. end land { S. end Wisby	Eu.	Sweden	Baltic Sea	{ 58 00 N. 56 58 N. 57 40 N.	20 15 E. 19 37 E. 19 50 E.	
I. Goto	Asia	Corea	Pacif. Ocean	34 25 N.	125 50 E.	
Gottenberg	Eu.	Sweden	Sound	57 42 N.	11 44 E.	
Gottingen	Eu.	Germany	Inland	51 32 N.	9 58 E.	
Gower's Isle	Asia	N. Britain	Pacif. Ocean	7 56 S.	158 56 E.	
R. Grand	Am.	Paraguay	Atl. Ocean	31 58 S.	50 35 W.	
Granville	Eu.	France	Eng. Channel	48 50 N.	1 32 W.	7 00
C. De Grat	Am.	Newfoundl.	Atl. Ocean	51 36 N.	55 33 W.	
I. Gratiosa	Africa	Canaries	Atl. Ocean	29 15 N.	13 07 W.	
I. Gratiosa	Eu.	Azores	Atl. Ocean	39 02 N.	27 53 W.	
C. Gratios a Dios	Am.	New Spain	Carribbe. Sea	14 48 N.	82 15 W.	
Graveline	Eu.	France	Eng. Channel	50 59 N.	2 1? E.	0 00
Gravesend	Eu.	England	R. Thames	51 35 N.	0 20 E.	1 30
I. Grenada	Am.	Caribbee	Atl. Ocean	11 52 N.	61 39 W.	
Greenwich	Eu.	England	R. Thames	51 29 N.	0 05 E.	
C. Germa	Eu.	Turkey	Archipelago	40 33 N.	26 20 E.	
Gripswald	Eu.	Germany	Baltic Sea	54 04 N.	13 43 E.	
Grimsby	Eu.	England	Germ. Ocean	53 30 N.	0 56 E.	
Groin, or C. Corunna	Eu.	Spain	B. Biscay	43 28 N.	9 20 W.	3 00
I. Grey	Am.	Newfoundl.	Atl. Ocean	50 56 N.	55 35 W.	
I. Guadaloupe	Am.	Carribbee	Atl. Ocean	16 00 N.	61 55 W.	
Guayaquil	Am.	Peru	Pacif. Ocean	2 10 S.	81 05 W.	
I. Guernsey	Eu.	England	Eng. Channel	49 30 N.	2 47 W.	1 30
Gult	Eu.	England	St. Geo. Ch.	50 06 N.	6 00 W.	
Gurief	Asia	Astracan	Caspian Sea	47 7 N.	52 02 E.	
H						
Hacluit's Headland	Eu.	Greenland	North Ocean	79 55 N.	12 00 E.	
I. Hai- } N. E. point nam } S. W. point	Asia	China	Indian Ocean	{ 19 45 N. 18 22 N.	110 13 E. 108 13 E.	
Halifax	Am.	Nova Scotia	Western Oc.	44 46 N.	63 2? W.	3[illegible]
I. Hal[illegible]	Am.	Greenland	Atl. Ocean	63 56 N.	44 26 W.	
[illegible]	Eu.	Iceland	North Ocean	64 30 N.	27 15 W.	
Hamburgh	Eu.	Germany	R. Elbe	53 ?4 N.	9 55 E.	
Hare Isle	Am.	Canada	R. St. Lawr.	48 00 N.	6? 26 W.	
[illegible]	Eu.	D. Neth.	Germ. Ocean	52 ?4 N.	4 [illegible]	
Hartland Point	Eu.	England	Bristol Chan.	51 00 N.	4 [illegible]	
[illegible]	Eu.	England	Germ. Ocean	[illegible]	[illegible]	
[illegible]	Eu.	England	Germ. Ocean	[illegible]	1 ?8	
C. Hatteras	Am.	Carolina	Atl. Ocean	[illegible]	[illegible]	
[illegible]	Am.	I. Cuba	Atl. Ocean	[illegible]	[illegible]	
[illegible]	Eu.	France	Eng. Channel	49 [illegible] N.	[illegible]	

Names of Places.	Cont.	Countries.	Coast.	Latitude.	Longitude.	H. Water.
				° ′	° ′	
Hawke's Bay	Asia	N. Zealand	Pacif. Ocean	39 30 S.	177 6 E.	
I. St. Helena	Africa	Caffers	Atl. Ocean	15 55 S.	5 44 W.	
Helie's Sound	Eu.	Greenland	North Ocean	79 15 N.	12 50 E.	
Is. Heligh's Land	Eu.	Norway	North Ocean	65 15 N.	9 30 E.	
C. Henlopen	Am.	Maryland	Atl. Ocean	38 48 N.	75 08 W.	
C. Henrietta Maria	Am.	New Wales	Hudson's Bay	55 10 N.	84 00 W.	12h. com.
C. Henry	Am.	Virginia	Atl. Ocean	37 00 N.	76 23 W.	11 15
Hervey's Isle	Asia	Society Isles	Pacif. Ocean	19 17 S.	158 43 W.	
I. Heys	Eu.	France	B. Biscay	46 24 N.	2 14 W.	
High Mount	Eu.	Greenland	North Ocean	83 23 N.	26 40 E.	
Hinchingbrook I.	Asia	N. Hebrides	Pacif. Ocean	17 23 S.	168 38 E.	
Isl. Hispaniola { C. Tiberoon, W. pt.				18 17 N.	74 24 W.	
S. Louis				18 19 N.	73 11 W.	
C. St. Nichol. N. W. pt.	Am.	Antilles	Atl. Ocean	19 50 N.	73 18 W.	
Po. Grave				18 28 N.	72 42 W.	
St. Domingo				18 25 N.	69 30 W.	
C. Raphael N. E. pt.				19 05 N.	68 30 W.	
Hogsties	Am.	Bahama	Atl. Ocean	21 41 N.	73 25 W.	
New Holland { W. limit	Asia	———	Indian Ocean	25 30 S.	111 10 E.	
N. Ditto				12 35 S.	141 31 E.	
S. Ditto				43 38 S.	146 00 E.	
E. Ditto				27 10 S.	153 39 E.	
Holy Cape	Asia	Siberia	North Ocean	72 32 N.	179 45 E.	
Holy Head	Eu.	Wales	Irish Sea	53 23 N.	4 40 W.	1 30
C. Honduras	Am.	New Spain	Caribbean Sea	16 18 N.	85 23 W.	
B. Hondy, I. Cuba	Am.	Antilles	Atl. Ocean	22 54 N.	82 40 W.	
Honfleur	Eu.	France	R. Seine	49 24 N.	0 20 E.	9 00
Hood's Isle	Asia	Marquesas	Pacif. Ocean	9 26 S.	138 47 W.	
Hope Isle	Eu.	Greenland	North Ocean	76 22 N.	23 40 E.	
C. Horn	Am.	T. del Fuego	Pacif. Ocean	55 59 S.	67 21 W.	
Hornsound	Eu.	Greenland	North Ocean	76 41 N.	13 36 E.	
La Hogue	Eu.	France	Eng. Channel	49 45 N.	1 52 W.	
Howe's Isle	Asia	Society's Is.	Pacif. Ocean	16 46 S.	154 2 W.	
C. How	Asia	N. Holland	Pacif. Ocean	37 24 S.	150 00 E.	
R. Hughly	Asia	India	B. Bengal	21 45 N.	89 15 E.	
Hull	Eu.	England	R. Humber	53 50 N.	0 28 W.	6 00
R. Humber, Ent.	Eu.	England	Germ. Ocean	53 55 N.	0 24 E.	5 13
I. Hyneago	Am.	Bahama	Atl. Ocean	21 27 N.	73 29 W.	
I						
Jado	Asia	Japan	Pacif. Ocean	36 00 N.	139 40 E.	
C. Jaffanapatan	Asia	I. Ceylon	Indian Ocean	9 47 N.	80 55 E.	
I. Jago	Africa	C. Verd	Atl. Ocean	15 07 N.	23 30 W.	
Jakutskoi	Asia	Siberia	Pacif. Ocean	62 2 N.	129 52 E.	
I. Jam. { West end				18 45 N.	78 00 W.	
Port Royal	Am.	West Indies	Atl. Ocean	18 00 N.	76 40 W.	
East End				17 58 N.	76 05 W.	
James Town	Am.	Virginia	B. Chesapeak	37 30 N.	76 05 W.	
R. Janeiro	Am.	Brasil	Atl. Ocean	22 54 S.	42 44 W.	
Japan Isles	Asia	———	Pacif. Ocean	40 40 N. 31 45 N.	141 25 E. 126 10 E.	
Java I. { C. Delo, W. pt.	Asia	Siam	Indian Ocean	6 50 S. 7 00 S.	105 15 E.	
East limit				8 30 S.	115 55 E.	
Ice Cove	Am.	N. Main	Huds. Straits	62 20 N.	69 00 W.	10 00
Ice Point	Eu.	Nova Zem.	North. Ocean	77 40 N	69 10 E.	
Ice Sound	Eu.	Greenland	North Ocean	78 13 N.	12 00 E.	
I. Jersey	Eu.	England	Eng. Channel	49 07 N.	2 26 W.	
Jerusalem	Asia	Palestine	Inland	31 55 N.	35 25 E.	
I. Hay, S. pt.	Eu.	Scotland	West. Ocean	[illegible] 39 N.	6 20 W.	

R. Indus

Names of Places.	Cont.	Countries.	Coast.	Latitude.	Longitude.	H. Water.
				° ′	° ′	
R. Indus	Asia	India	Indian Ocean	25 50 N.	66 33 E.	
Inverness	Eu.	Scotland	Germ. Ocean	57 33 N.	4 02 W.	
I. Joanna	Africa	Zanguebar	Indian Ocean	12 05 S.	45 45 E.	
Juddah	Asia	Arabia	Red Sea	22 00 N.	39 27 E.	
C. St. John	Am.	Newfoundl.	Atl. Ocean	50 08 N.	55 32 W.	
C. St. John	Africa	Maiumbo	Eth. Ocean	1 17 N.	9 34 E.	
St. John's	Am.	Newfoundl.	Atl. Ocean	47 34 N.	52 18 W.	6h. 0m.
I. St. John { E. pt.	Am.	Canada	Bay St. Laurence	46 30 N.	62 03 W.	
I. St. John { N. pt.				47 07 N.	64 05 W.	
I. St. John de Nova	Africa	Madagascar	Indian Ocean	17 00 S.	44 02 E.	
St. John de Luz	Eu.	France	B. Biscay	43 10 N.	1 38 W.	3 30
Cape Jones	Am.	New Britain	Hudson's Bay	58 50 N.	79 00 W.	
Joppa	Asia	Syria	Levant	32 45 N.	36 00 E.	
Jones Sound	Am.	Greenland	Baffin's Bay	71 07 N.	91 30 W.	
St. Joseph	Am.	California	Pacif. Ocean	23 3 S.	109 35 W.	
Ipswich	Eu.	England	Germ. Ocean	52 14 N.	1 00 E.	
Ispahan	Asia	Persia	R. Zenduro	32 25 N.	52 55 E.	
C. St. Juan	Am.	Statenland	Atl. Ocean	54 47 S.	63 42 W.	
I. Juan Fernandez	Am.	Chili	Pacif. Ocean	33 45 S.	78 37 W.	
Port. St. Julian	Am.	Patagonia	S. Atl. Ocean	49 10 S.	66 10 W.	4 45
I. Ivica	Eu.	Spain	Medit. Sea	38 54 N.	1 15 E.	
K						
Kalmer	Eu.	Sweden	Baltic Sea	56 40 N.	17 25 E.	
Kambaya	Asia	India	Indian Ocean	23 36 N.	72 50 E.	
Kamtschatka { Lower	Asia	Siberia	Pacif. Ocean	56 11 N.	159 25 E.	
Kamtschatka { Upper				54 48 N.	157 25 E.	
L. Karaghinskoy	Asia	Siberia	Pacif. Ocean	58 00 N.	162 10 E.	
I. St. Katharine's	Am.	Brasil	Atl. Ocean	27 35 S.	49 12 W.	
Keo	Asia	Tonquin	Indian Ocean	21 55 N.	106 10 E.	
Kegor	Eu.	Muscovy	North Ocean	70 18 N.	34 00 E.	
R. Kennebeck	Am.	N. England	Atl. Ocean	44 00 N.	69 45 W.	
Kentish Knock, a sand	Eu.	England	Germ. Ocean	51 42 N.	1 45 E.	0 00
I. St. Kilda	Eu.	Scotland	West. Ocean	57 44 N.	8 18 W.	
I. Kilduin	Eu.	Lapland	North Ocean	69 30 N.	31 20 E.	7 30
Kinsale	Eu.	Ireland	Atl. Ocean	51 32 N.	9 01 W.	5 15
Klip	Eu.	Greenland	North Ocean	80 10 N.	12 22 E.	
R. Kola	Eu.	Lapland	North Ocean	68 53 N.	33 08 E.	
C. Kol	Eu.	Sweden	Sound	56 50 N.	13 13 E.	
Port Komel	Africa	Abyssinia	Red Sea	22 30 N.	36 17 E.	
Komero Isles	Africa	Zanguebar	Indian Ocean	10 48 S.	44 45 E.	
				13 10 S.	46 22 E.	
R. Kowima	Asia	Siberia	North Ocean	70 40 N.	159 00 E.	
L						
Ladrone, or Marian Isles	Asia	———	Pacif. Ocean	21 00 N.	144 00 E.	
				13 15 N.	142 55 E.	
C. L'Aiguille	Africa	Caffraria	Indian Ocean	34 50 S.	20 06 E.	
Lancaster	Eu.	England	St. Geo. Ch.	54 42 N.	4 36 W.	
I. Lancerota	Africa	Canaries	Atl. Ocean	29 10 N.	13 20 W.	
Land's End	Eu.	England	St. Geo. Ch.	50 06 N.	5 50 W.	7 30
Langeness	Eu.	Nova Zem.	North Ocean	74 4[illegible] N.	53 30 E.	
I. Lambay	Eu.	Ireland	Irish Sea	53 2[illegible] N.	7 3[illegible] W.	3 15
I. Lampadosa	Africa	Tunis	Medit. Sea	35 [illegible] N.	12 45 E.	
R. St. Lazarus	Am.	Patagonia	Pacif. Ocean	48 42 S.	73 35 W.	
C. Ledo	Africa	Angola	Atl. Ocean	9 24 S.	12 [illegible] E.	
Leith	Eu.	Scotland	Germ. Ocean	55 5[illegible] N.	2 [illegible] W.	4 30
Leghorn	Eu.	Italy	Medit. Sea	[illegible] N.	[illegible] E.	
I. Lemnos	Asia	Natolia	Archipelago	[illegible] N.	25 [illegible] E.	
C. Lingua	Eu.	Turkey	Medit. Sea	[illegible] N.	[illegible] E.	
Leostoff	Eu.	England	Germ. Ocean	52 [illegible] N.	1 54 E.	9 45
Lepanto	Eu.	Turkey	Medit. Sea	38 [illegible] N.	22 [illegible] E.	
Leper's Isle	Asia	N. Hebrides	Pacif. Ocean	15 [illegible] S.	[illegible] E.	

Names of Places.	Cont.	Countries.	Coast.	Latitude.	Longitude.	H. Water.
				° ′	° ′	
I. Lefow	Eu.	Denmark	Sound	57 05 N.	11 06 E.	
Liverpool	Eu.	England	Irish Sea	53 22 N.	3 10 W.	11h. 15m.
I. Lewes, N. point	Eu.	Scotland	West. Ocean	58 35 N.	6 37 W.	6 30
Liampo, or Ningpo	Asia	China	Pacif. Ocean	29 58 N.	120 23 E.	
Lima	Am.	Peru	Pacif. Ocean	12 01 S.	76 44 W.	
Lime	Eu.	England	Eng. Channel	50 45 N.	3 15 W.	7 00
Limerick	Eu.	Ireland	R. Shannon	52 22 N.	10 00 W.	
I. Limosa	Eu.	Italy	Medit. Sea	36 08 N.	13 01 E.	
I. Lipari	Eu.	Italy	Medit. Sea	38 35 N.	15 31 E.	
I. Liqueo	Asia	Japan	Pacif. Ocean	28 00 N.	127 30 E.	
Lisbon	Eu.	Portugal	R. Tagus	38 42 N.	9 4 W.	2 15
Lisbon Rock	Eu.	Portugal	West. Ocean	38 42 N.	9 25 W.	
C. Lisburne	Asia	N. Hebrides	Pacif. Ocean	15 41 S.	166 57 W.	
I. Lissa	Eu.	Dalmatia	Adriatic Sea	42 56 N.	18 32 E.	
Lizard	Eu.	England	Eng. Channel	49 57 N.	5 10 W.	7 30
Isles Loffout { S. W. end	Eu.	Norway	North Ocean	68 15 N.	10 20 E.	
Isles Loffout { N. E. end				69 00 N.	12 00 E.	
R. Loire, Ent.	Eu.	France	B. Biscay	47 07 N.	2 05 W.	3 00
London	Eu.	England	R. Thames	51 32 N.	0 00	3 00
New London	Am.	N. England	West. Ocean	41 50 N.	72 14 W.	1 30
Londonderry	Eu.	Ireland	West. Ocean	55 01 N.	[illegible] 11 W.	
Long Isle	Am.	N. England	West. Ocean	41 00 N.	{ 71 59 W. 74 20 W.	3 00
I. Longo	Eu.	Dalmatia	Adriat. Sea	43 45 N.	17 58 E.	
Longsand Head	Eu.	England	Germ. Ocean	51 47 N.	1 41 E.	10 30
Lookout Point	Eu.	Greenland	North Ocean	76 40 N.	16 25 E.	
C. Lopas	Africa	Loango	Atl. Ocean	0 47 S.	8 30 E.	
B. St. Louis	Am.	Louisiana	G. Mexico	28 50 N.	97 08 W.	
Louisbourg	Am.	C. Breton	B. St. Law.	45 54 N.	59 50 W.	
Lubec	Eu.	Germany	Baltic Sea	54 00 N.	11 40 E.	
C. St. Lucar	Am.	California	Pacif. Ocean	23 15 N.	109 40 W.	
R. Lucia	Africa	Caffers	Indian Ocean	27 52 S.	33 28 E.	
I. St. Lucia	Africa	C. de Verd	Atl. Ocean	16 43 N.	24 33 W.	
I. St. Lucia	Am.	Caribbee	Atl. Ocean	13 25 N.	60 46 W.	
I. Luconia { N. E. point	Asia	Phil. Isles	Pacif. Ocean	19 25 N.	121 45 E.	
I. Luconia { C. Bajador				18 50 N.	120 25 E.	
I. Luconia { Manilla				14 36 N.	120 58 E.	
I. Luconia { S. W. point				13 30 N.	119 35 E.	
I. Luconia { E. point				14 00 N.	124 00 E.	
Lunden	Eu.	Sweden	Baltic Sea	55 42 N.	13 26 E.	
I. Lundy	Eu.	England	St. Geo. Ch.	51 20 N.	4 04 W.	5 15
Lupis's Head	Eu.	Ireland	West. Ocean	52 24 N.	10 15 W.	
Lynn	Eu.	England	Germ. Ocean	52 46 N.	0 32 E.	6 45
M						
C. Mabo	Asia	New Guinea	Pacif. Ocean	0 40 S.	170 05 E.	
Macao, or Makau	Asia	China	Pacif. Ocean	22 12 N.	113 46 E.	
Macassar	Asia	I. Celebes	Pacif. Ocean	5 09 S.	119 50 E.	
C. Machian	Eu.	Spain	B. Biscay	43 44 N.	3 05 W.	
I. Madagascar { C. St. Mary, S. point	Africa	—	Indian Ocean	2[illegible] 24 S.	45 53 E.	
I. Madagascar { B. St. Augustine				2[illegible] 35 S.	4[illegible] 13 E.	
I. Madagascar { Terra de Gada				10 36 S.	[illegible] 26 E.	
I. Madagascar { C. St. Andrew				15 46 S.	[illegible] E.	
I. Madagascar { C. St. Sebastian				12 3[illegible] S.	[illegible] E.	
I. Madagascar { C. de Ambre N. point				12 [illegible] S.	[illegible] 15 E.	
I. Madagascar { B. d'Antongil				[illegible] S.	4[illegible] E.	
I. Madagascar { Antavare				20 5[illegible] S.	[illegible] E.	
I. Madagascar { Ft. Dauphin				24 [illegible] S.	[illegible] E.	
I. Madeira { Funchal	Africa	Canaries	Atl. Ocean	32 3[illegible] N.	[illegible] W.	12 4
I. Madeira { W. end				32 2[illegible] N.	[illegible] W.	12 0
[illegible]	Asia	India	Ind. Ocean	13 [illegible] N.	[illegible] 34 E.	

Madrid

Names of Places.	Cont.	Countries.	Coaft.	Latitu de.	Longitude.	H. Water.
				° ′	° ′	
Madrid	Eu.	Spain	R. Manzana	40 25 N.	03 21 W.	
Madura	Afia	India	Indian Ocean	10 15 N.	78 35 E.	
R. Maes, Mouth	Eu.	D. Neth.	Germ. Ocean	52 06 N.	3 50 E.	1h. 30m.
Str. Le Maire	Am.	Patagonia	Atl. Ocean	54 51 S.	65 00 W.	
Magadoxa	Africa	Zanguebar	Indian Ocean	2 53 N.	45 25 E.	
Str. Magellan, E. ent.	Am.	Patagonia	Atl. Ocean	52 30 S.	67 50 W.	
Str. Magellan, W. ent.	Am.	Patagonia	Pacif. Ocean	52 55 S.	74 18 W.	
Magifiland	Afia	India	Malabar Coa.	12 10 N.	74 14 E.	
I. Maguana	Am.	Bahama I.	Atl. Ocean	22 36 N.	72 25 W.	
P. Mahon, Ifle Minorca	Eu.	Spain	Medit. Sea	39 51 N.	3 53 E.	
Majorca, Ifl. Majorca	Eu.	Spain	Medit. Sea	39 35 N.	2 35 E.	
C. Mala	Eu.	Turkey	Archipelago	37 20 N.	24 07 E.	
Malacca	Afia	India	Str. Malacca	2 12 N.	102 10 E.	
Malaga	Eu.	Spain	Medit. Sea	36 43 N.	4 02 W.	
Ifles Maldive, N. end	Afia	India	Indian Ocean	7 20 N.	73 03 E.	
Ifles Maldive, S. end	Afia	India	Indian Ocean	0 20 S.	76 10 E.	
Maleftroom Whirlpool	Eu.	Norway	Weft. Ocean	68 08 N.	10 40 E.	
I. Malique	Afia	Maldive I.	Indian Ocean	7 45 N.	72 40 E.	
St. Maloes	Eu.	France	Eng. Channel	48 39 N.	1 57 W.	6 00
I. Malta	Eu.	Italy	Medit. Sea	35 54 N.	14 28 E.	
I. Man, W. end	Eu.	England	Irifh Sea	53 45 N.	5 00 W.	9 00
Mangalore	Afia	India	Indian Ocean	13 02 N.	75 10 E.	
Manilla	Afia	I. Luconia	Pacif. Ocean	14 36 N.	120 58 E.	
I. Mansfield, N. pt.	Am.	New Britain	Hudfon's Bay	62 38 N.	80 33 W.	
I. Mantia	Africa	Zanguebar	Indian Ocean	8 36 S.	40 40 E.	
I. Mardou	Eu.	Norway	Sound	58 14 N.	8 55 E.	
I. Margarita	Am.	Terra Firma	Atl. Ocean	11 15 N.	63 35 W.	
R. Maragnon	Am.	Brafil	Atl. Ocean	1 48 S.	44 17 W.	
Margate	Eu.	England	Eng. Channel	51 29 N.	1 10 E.	11 15
C. St. Maria	Eu.	Portugal	Atl. Ocean	36 45 N.	7 45 W.	
C. St. Maria, or Lucia	Eu.	Italy	Medit. Sea	40 04 N.	18 31 E	
Marian or Ladrone Ifles, N. lim.	Afia	———	Pacif. Ocean	21 00 N.	144 00 E.	
Marian or Ladrone Ifles, S. lim.	Afia	———	Pacif. Ocean	13 15 N.	142 55 E.	
I. St. Maries	Eu.	Azores	Atl. Ocean	37 00 N.	25 00 W.	
St. Maries	Eu.	I. Scilly	Eng. Channel	49 57 N.	6 38 W.	
I. Marigalante	Am.	Weft Indies	Atl. Ocean	16 00 N.	61 [illegible] W.	
I. Maritimo, Sicily	Eu.	Italy	Medit. Sea	38 04 N.	12 33 E.	
Marquefa If.	Afia	———	Pacif. Ocean	9 56 N.	139 00 W.	2 30
C. Martello	Eu.	Turkey	Medit. Sea	38 00 N.	26 00 E.	
St. Martha	Am.	Terra Firma	Atl. Ocean	11 26 N.	74 00 W.	
I. St. Martin	Am.	Weft Indies	Atl. Ocean	18 06 N.	63 06 W.	
C. St. Martin	Africa	Caffers	Atl. Ocean	32 08 S.	18 58 E.	
C. St. Martin	Eu.	Spain	Medit. Sea	38 44 N.	0 25 E.	
I. Martinique, Port Royal	Am.	Weft Indies	Atl. Ocean	14 36 N.	61 04 W.	
Marfeilles	Eu.	France	Medit. Sea	43 18 N.	5 27 E.	
C. St. Mary	Am.	Newfoundl.	Atl. Ocean	46 52 N.	54 01 W.	
C. St. Mary	Am.	Brafil	Atl. Ocean	34 52 S.	52 55 W.	
C. St. Mary	Afia	Natolia	Archipelago	37 46 N.	27 21 E.	
C. St. Mary	Eu.	Spain	N. Atl. Ocean	36 46 N.	7 49 W.	
C. Virgin Mary	Am.	Patagonia	S. Atl. Ocean	52 23 S.	68 [illegible] W.	
[illegible]	Am.	Chili	Pacif. Ocean	33 45 S.	[illegible] 31 W.	
I. M[illegible]	Africa	Zanguebar	Indian Ocean	[illegible] 52 S.	[illegible] 35 E.	
I. M[illegible]	Am.	Peru	Pacif. Ocean	1 [illegible] S.	[illegible] W.	
M[illegible]	Afia	Arabia	Indian Ocean	23 1[illegible] N.	57 40 E.	
M[illegible]	[illegible]	N. Hebrides	Pacif. Ocean	16 32 S.	[illegible] 59 E.	
M[illegible]	Eu.	Sweden	Sound	57 [illegible] N.	12 [illegible] E.	
M[illegible]	Afia	India	B. Bengal	15 [illegible] N.	81 40 E.	

Names of Places.	Cont.	Countries.	Coast.	Latitude.	Longitude.	H. Water.
				° ′	° ′	
C. Matapan	Eu.	Turkey	Archipelago	36 25 N.	22 40 E.	
I. Matbare	Asia	Japan	Pacif. Ocean	26 30 N.	137 00 E.	
I. St. Mathew's	Africa	Guinea	Eth. Ocean	1 23 S.	6 11 W.	
I. Mauritius	Africa	Madagascar	Indian Ocean	20 10 S.	57 33 E.	
Maurua	Asia	Society Isles	Pacif. Ocean	16 26 S.	152 33 W.	
I. May	Africa	C. Verd	Atl. Ocean	15 10 N.	23 00 W.	
C. May	Am.	Pensilvania	Atl. Ocean	39 15 N.	74 43 W.	
I. Mayette	Africa	Madagascar	Indian Ocean	12 53 S.	46 10 E.	
Mecca	Asia	Arabia	Red Sea	21 40 N.	41 00 E.	
Medina	Asia	Arabia	Red Sea	24 58 N.	39 53 E.	
I. Melada	Eu.	Dalmatia	Adriat. Sea	42 40 N.	19 34 E.	
Melinde	Africa	Zanguebar	Indian Ocean	3 07 S.	39 40 E.	
I. Melo	Eu.	Turkey	Archipelago	36 41 N.	25 05 E.	
Memel	Eu.	Courland	Baltic Sea	55 48 N.	22 23 E.	
Memissan	Eu.	France	B. Biscay	44 20 N.	1 23 W.	3h. 30m.
I. Menado	Asia	I. Celebes	Pacif. Ocean	1 36 N.	122 25 E.	
C. Mendozin	Am.	California	Pacif. Ocean	41 20 N.	130 15 W.	
Mercury Bay	Asia	N. Zealand	Pacif. Ocean	36 50 S.	175 12 E.	
R. Metaparvous	Am.	Bahama	Atl. Ocean	21 58 N.	74 13 W.	
Messina	Eu.	I. Sicily	Medit. Sea	38 21 N.	16 21 E.	
C. Mesurato	Africa	Tripoli	Medit. Sea	32 18 N.	16 36 E.	
I. Metylene — C. Sigre	Asia	Natolia	Archipelago	39 21 N.	26 08 E.	
I. Metylene — Metylene				39 11 N.	26 47 E.	
I. Metylene — Po. Olivica				39 00 N.	26 50 E.	
I. Meun	Eu.	Denmark	Baltic Sea	55 00 N.	13 15 E.	
Mexico	Am.	Mexico	Inland	19 54 N.	100 01 W.	
Miatea	Asia	Society Isles	Pacif. Ocean	17 52 S.	148 1 W.	
I. St. Michael	Eu.	Azores	Atl. Ocean	37 45 N.	25 38 W.	
Middleburgh	Eu.	D. Neth.	Germ. Ocean	51 37 N.	3 58 E.	
Middleburgh, or Eaoowe	Asia	Friendly Isl.	Pacif. Ocean	21 21 S.	174 34 W.	
Milford	Eu.	Wales	St. Geo. Ch.	51 45 N.	5 15 W.	5 15
Milo, I. Milo	Asia	Turkey	Archipelago	36 41 N.	25 05 E.	
Mill Isles	Am.	North Main	Hudson's Bay	64 36 N.	80 30 W.	
I. Mindanao — N. point	Asia	Spice Islands	Pacif. Ocean	9 40 N.	124 25 E.	
I. Mindanao — S. E. pt. C. St. Augustine				6 40 N.	126 25 E.	
I. Mindanao — S. W. pt. Caldera				7 00 N.	121 25 E.	
I. Mindanao — S. point				3 50 N.	124 43 E.	
I. Mindora	Asia	Philip. Isles	Pacif. Ocean	13 00 N.	119 37 E.	
I. Minorca — N. W. pt.	Eu.	Spain	Mediterran.	39 58 N.	3 54 E.	
I. Minorca — S. E. pt.				40 24 N.	4 18 E.	
G. Miquelon	Am.	Newfoundl.	Atl. Ocean	47 3 N.	56 13 W.	
L. Miquelon	Am.	Newfound.	Atl. Ocean	46 50 N.	56 13 W.	
I. Misco	Am.	Nova Scotia	G. St. Lawr.	48 04 N.	64 19 W.	
C. Miserata	Africa	Guinea	Atl. Ocean	6 25 N.	9 35 W.	
R. Mississippi, mouth	Am.	Louisiana	G. Mexico	29 00 N.	89 17 W.	
Mizen Head	Eu.	Ireland	Atl. Ocean	51 16 N.	10 20 W.	
Mocha	Asia	Arabia	Red Sea	13 45 N.	44 04 E.	
Modon	Eu.	Turkey	Medit. Sea	36 55 N.	21 03 E.	
I. Mohilla	Africa	Zanguebar	Indian Ocean	11 55 S.	45 00 E.	
I. Monserat	Am.	West Indies	Atl. Ocean	16 48 N.	62 12 W.	
Montagu Isle	Asia	N. Hebrides	Pacif. Ocean	17 26 S.	168 36 E.	
Montreal	Am.	Canada	R. St. Lawr.	45 52 N.	73 11 W.	
I. Monte Christo	Eu.	Italy	Medit. Sea	42 17 N.	10 28 E.	
C. Monte Sancto	Eu.	Turkey	Archipelago	40 27 N.	24 39 E.	
Monument	Asia	N. Hebrides	Pacif. Ocean	17 14 S.	168 38 E.	
Mount St. Michael	Eu.	France	Eng. Channel	48 39 N.	1 35 W.	
I. Mergo	Asia	Natolia	Archipelago	36 55 N.	26 30 E	
Morlaix	Eu.	France	Eng. Channel	48 30 N.	3 50 W.	
Mort Point	Eu.	England	St. Geo. Ch.	51 12 N.	4 40 W.	

Names of Places.	Cont.	Countries.	Coast.	Latitude.	Longitude.	H. Water.
				° ′	° ′	
Mosambique	Africa	Zanguebar	Indian Ocean	15 00 S.	41 40 E.	
Moscow	Eu.	Russia	R. Moscow	55 45 N.	37 51 E.	
Mosquitos Bank	Am.	Mexico	Atl. Ocean	14 45 N.	80 05 W.	
C. Mount	Africa	Guinea	Atl. Ocean	7 12 N.	10 44 W.	
Mount's Bay	Eu.	England	Eng. Channel	50 05 N.	5 45 W.	4h. 30m.
Mouse River	Am.	New Wales	Hudson's Bay	51 25 N.	85 15 W.	
C. Musaldon	Asia	Arabia	Persian Gulf	26 04 N.	55 22 E.	
N						
C. Nabo	Asia	Japan	Pacif. Ocean	40 35 N.	141 25 E.	
Nangasack	Asia	Japan	Pacif. Ocean	32 32 N.	128 50 E.	
Nankin	Asia	China	Pacif. Ocean	32 07 N.	118 35 E.	
Nantes	Eu.	France	B. Biscay	47 13 N.	1 29 W.	3 00
Nantucket Isle	Am.	New Eng.	West. Ocean	41 34 N.	69 40 W.	
Naples	Eu.	Italy	Medit. Sea	40 51 N.	14 19 E.	
Narbonne	Eu.	France	Medit. Sea	43 11 N.	3 05 E.	
Narsinga	Asia	India	B. Bengal	18 05 N.	85 20 E.	
Narva	Eu.	Livonia	G. Finland	59 08 N.	29 18 E.	
I. Nassau	Asia	Sumatra	Indian Ocean	3 00 S.	100 25 E.	
C. Nassau	Am.	Terra Firma	Atl. Ocean	7 53 N.	58 07 W.	
Nassau Str.	Eu.	Russia	North Ocean	69 55 N.	57 30 E.	
B. Natal	Africa	Caffers	Indian Ocean	29 25 S.	33 10 E.	
I. Naxos	Eu.	Turkey	Archipelago	37 06 N.	25 58 E.	
Naze	Eu.	Norway	West. Ocean	57 50 N.	7 32 E.	11 15
Needles	Eu.	England	Eng. Channel	50 41 N.	1 28 W.	10 15
C. Negrailles	Asia	Pegu	B. Bengal	16 20 N.	94 15 E.	
C. Negro	Africa	Caffers	Atl. Ocean	16 30 S.	11 30 E.	
C. Negro	Africa	Barbary	Medit. Sea	37 17 N.	9 09 E.	
Negropont	Eu.	Turkey	Archipelago	38 30 N.	24 05 E.	
Port Nelson	Am.	New Wales	Hudson's Bay	57 07 N.	92 37 W.	
Port Nelson's Shoals	Am.	New Wales	Hudson's Bay	57 35 N.	92 07 W.	8 20
I. Nevis	Am.	Caribbee Isles	Atl. Ocean	17 11 N.	62 52 W.	
Newcastle	Eu.	England	Germ. Ocean	55 03 N.	1 28 W.	3 15
R. Nicaragua	Am.	New Spain	Atl. Ocean	11 40 N.	82 47 W.	
Nice	Eu.	Italy	Medit. Sea	43 42 N.	7 22 E.	
I. Nicobar	Asia	Siam	B. Bengal	7 22 N.	94 40 E.	
I. St. Nicholas	Africa	C. Verd I.	Atl. Ocean	16 35 N.	24 06 W.	
Nicotera	Eu.	Italy	Medit. Sea	38 33 N.	16 30 E.	
Nieuport	Eu.	Flanders	Germ. Ocean	51 08 N.	2 50 E.	12 00
Ninhay	Asia	China	Pacif. Ocean	37 10 N.	122 25 E.	
Ningpo, or Liampo	Asia	China	Pacif. Ocean	29 58 N.	120 23 E.	
I. Nio	Eu.	Turkey	Archipelago	36 48 N.	26 02 E.	
I. Noel	Asia	India	Indian Ocean	10 30 S.	105 25 E.	
C. Noir	Am.	T. del Fuego	Pacif. Ocean	54 32 S.	73 3 W.	
Norfolk Isle	Asia	N. Holland	Pacif. Ocean	29 2 S.	168 15 E.	
C. de Non	Africa	Barbary	Atl. Ocean	28 04 N.	10 32 W.	
Nombre de Dios	Am.	Terra Firma	Caribbe. Sea	9 43 N.	78 35 W.	
Nore	Eu.	England	R. Thames	51 28 N.	0 48 E.	0 00
Noriton	Am.	Pensylvania	Inland	40 10 N.	75 17 W.	
C. North	Am.	Terra Firma	Atl. Ocean	1 45 N.	49 00 W.	
C. North	Am.	C. Breton	Atl. Ocean	47 5 N.	60 8 W.	
C. North	Am.	S. Georgia	Atl. Ocean	54 5 S.	38 10 W.	
N. Cape, I. Maggeroe	Eu.	Lapland	North Ocean	71 10 N.	26 02 E.	3 00
N[illegible]	Eu.	Norway	North Ocean	62 15 N.	6 15 E.	
N[illegible]	Am.	North Main	Hudson's Str.	62 30 N.	7? 59 W.	
I. N[illegible], E[illegible]	Am.	New Britain	Hudson's Str.	63 35 N.	7? 48 W.	10 00
O						
O[illegible] Bay	Asia	Otaheite	Pacif. Ocean	17 46 S.	149 9 W.	
O[illegible]	Eu.	Turkey	Black Sea	45 12 N.	3? 40 E.	
I. O[illegible] { S[illegible] / N[illegible] }	Eu.	Sweden	Baltic Sea	{ 56 15 N. / [illegible] 23 N. }	{ 18 35 E. / 17 [illegible] E. }	
O[illegible] Bay	Asia	Society Isles	Ulietea	16 4? S.	1?? ?3 W.	11 20
[illegible]	Eu.	Ireland	Atl. Ocean	51 3? N.	[illegible] W.	

Names of Places.	Cont.	Countries.	Coast.	Latitude.	Longitude.	H. Water.
				° ′	° ′	
I. Oleron	Eu.	France	B. Biscay	46 03 N.	1 20 W.	
Olinde	Am.	Brasil	S. Atl. Ocean	8 13 S.	35 00 W.	
Oliva	Eu.	Germany	Baltic Sea	54 20 N.	18 30 E.	
Ollone	Eu.	France	B. Biscay	46 32 N.	1 36 W.	3h. 45m.
Oneglia	Eu.	Italy	Medit. Sea	43 57 N.	7 52 E.	
Oporto	Eu.	Portugal	Atl. Ocean	41 10 N.	8 22 W.	
Oran	Africa	Barbary	Medit. Sea	35 45 N.	0 00	
C. Orange	Am.	Terra Firma	Atl. Ocean	4 27 N.	50 50 W.	
Orbitello	Eu.	Italy	Medit. Sea	42 30 N.	12 00 E.	
I. Orchillo	Am.	Terra Firma	Carribean Sea	11 32 N.	65 25 W.	
Orenburg	Asia	Astracan	Inland	51 46 N.	55 14 E.	
Orfordness	Eu.	England	Germ. Ocean	52 17 N.	1 11 E.	9 45
Orkney Isles, limits	Eu.	Scotland	West. Ocean	{ 59 24 N. 58 44 N.	3 23 W. 2 11 W.	3 00
New Orleans	Am.	Louisiana	R. Missisipi	30 00 N.	89 54 W.	
I. Ormus	Asia	Persia	G. Persia	27 30 N.	55 17 E.	
C. del Oro, or Olerada	Africa	Negroland	Atl. Ocean	23 30 N.	14 31 W.	
R. Oronoque	Am.	Terra Firma	Atl. Ocean	8 08 N.	59 50 W.	
C. Oropeso	Eu.	Spain	Medit. Sea	40 20 N.	0 49 E.	
Orsk	Asia	Astracan	Inland	51 12 N.	58 37 E.	
C. Ortegal	Eu.	Spain	B. Biscay	43 47 N.	8 32 W.	
Ortona	Eu.	Italy	Medit. Sea	42 19 N.	14 37 E.	
I. Oruba	Am.	Terra Firma	Caribbean Sea	12 03 N.	69 03 W.	
Osnaburg Isle	Asia	Society Isles	Pacif. Ocean	22 00 S.	141 34 W.	
Ostend	Eu.	Flanders	Germ. Ocean	51 14 N.	3 00 E.	12 00
C. Otranto	Eu.	Italy	Medit. Sea	40 23 N.	17 41 E.	
Owharre Bay	Asia	Huaheine	Pacif. Ocean	16 44 S.	151 3 W.	
Ozaca	Asia	Japan	Pacif. Ocean	35 10 N.	134 05 E.	
P						
C. Padron	Africa	Congo	Atl. Ocean	6 00 S.	11 40 E.	
Paita	Am.	Peru	Pacif. Ocean	5 20 S.	80 35 W.	
C. Paillouri	Eu.	Turkey	Archipelago	39 59 N.	24 03 E.	
Palermo, I. Sicily	Eu.	Italy	Medit. Sea	38 10 N.	13 43 E.	
Paliakate	Asia	India	B. Bengal	13 40 N.	80 50 E.	
Palliser's Isles	Asia	Society Isles	Pacif. Ocean	15 38 S.	146 25 W.	
C. Palliser	Asia	N. Zealand	Pacif. Ocean	41 40 S.	175 28 E.	
I. Palma	Africa	Canaries	Atl. Ocean	28 36 N.	17 45 W.	
I. Palmaria	Eu.	Italy	Medit. Sea	41 00 N.	13 03 E.	
Palmerston's Isle	Asia	Society Isles	Pacif. Ocean	18 00 S.	162 52 W.	
C. Palmiras	Asia	India	B. Bengal	20 40 N.	87 35 E.	
C. Palmas	Africa	Guinea	Atl. Ocean	4 26 N.	5 56 W.	
Panama	Am.	Mexico	Pacif. Ocean	8 45 N.	80 16 W.	
I. Panaria	Eu.	Italy	Medit. Sea	38 40 N.	15 41 E.	
Panorma	Eu.	Turkey	Medit. Sea	40 05 N.	21 40 E.	
I. Pantalaria	Eu.	Italy	Medit. Sea	36 55 N.	12 31 E.	
R. Panuco	Am.	Mexico	G. Mexico	24 02 N.	100 13 W.	
R. Paraiba	Am.	Brasil	Atl. Ocean	21 26 S.	39 50 W.	
Paris	Eu.	France	R. Seine	48 50 N.	2 25 E.	
C. Passero	Eu.	I. Sicily	Medit. Sea	36 35 N.	15 22 E.	
C. Patam	Asia	Malacca	Indian Ocean	7 27 N.	101 20 E.	
I. Patmos	Asia	Natolia	Archipelago	37 22 N.	26 48 E.	
R. Pattapan	Asia	I. Sumatra	Str. Malacca	0 28 N.	102 25 E.	
C. Paul	Eu.	Spain	Medit. Sea	37 50 N.	0 15 W.	
I. St. Paul	Am.	Newfoundl.	B. St. Lawr.	47 12 N.	59 59 W.	
I. St. Paul	Asia	Madagascar	Indian Ocean	37 51 S.	77 53 E.	
St. Paul de Leon	Eu.	France	Eng. Channel	48 41 N.	3 55 W.	4 00
I. Paxeros	Am.	California	Pacif. Ocean	30 18 N.	120 45 W.	
I. Pearl, or Serana	Am.	West Indies	Atl. Ocean	14 55 N.	79 00 W.	
Pegu	Asia	India	B. Bengal	17 00 N.	96 58 E.	
Pekin	Asia	China	Inland	39 55 N.	116 29 E.	
I. Pelugosa	Eu.	Italy	Adriatic Sea	42 20 N.	18 32 E.	
I. Pemba	Africa	Zanguebar	Indian Ocean	5 38 S.	40 00 E.	

C. Pembroke

Names of Places.	Cont.	Countries.	Coast.	Latitude.	Longitude.	H. Water.
				° ′	° ′	
C. Pembroke	Am.	New Wales	Hudson's Bay	63 12 N.	82 54 W.	
I. Pengwin	Am.	Newfoundl.	Atl. Ocean	47 23 N.	56 56 W.	
Penmark	Eu.	France	B. Biscay	47 50 N.	4 20 W.	
R. Penobscot	Am.	New Eng.	Atl. Ocean	44 40 N.	68 52 W.	
Pernambuco	Am.	Brasil	S. Atl. Ocean	8 30 S.	35 07 W.	
Petapoli	Asia	India	B. Bengal	16 14 N.	81 10 E.	
I. St. Peter	Am.	Newfoundl.	Atl. Ocean	46 46 N.	56 5 W.	
Petersburg	Eu.	Russia	Baltic Sea	59 56 N.	30 24 E.	
C. Petra	Asia	Natolia	Archipelago	37 02 N.	27 38 E.	
Peverel Point	Eu.	England	Eng. Channel	50 34 N.	1 22 W.	
Philadelphia	Am.	Pensilvania	R. Delawar	39 57 N.	75 8 W.	
St. Philip	Africa	Benguela	Atl. Ocean	12 22 S.	13 20 E.	
I. Pianosa	Eu.	Italy	Medit. Sea	42 46 N.	10 34 E.	
Isle of Pines	Asia	N. Caledonia	Pacif. Ocean	22 38 S.	167 43 E.	
I. Pico (Pike)	Eu.	Azores	Atl. Ocean	38 29 N.	28 19 W.	
C. Pinas	Eu.	Spain	B. Biscay	43 51 N.	6 14 W.	
Pickersgill's I.	Am.	S. Georgia	Atl. Ocean	54 42 S.	36 53 W.	
Mo. Pintados, or St. Martin	Am.	California	Pacif. Ocean	27 30 N.	117 15 W.	
Piscadore Isles	Asia	China	Pacif. Ocean	23 30 N.	119 25 E.	
Pitcairn's Isles	Am.	Chili	Pacif. Ocean	25 2 S.	133 21 W.	
Placentia	Am.	Newfoundl.	Atl. Ocean	47 15 N.	53 43 W.	9h. 0m.
R. Plata	Am.	La Plata	Atl. Ocean	36 00 S.	57 40 W.	
R. Platewrack	Am.	Bahama Isles	Atl. Ocean	20 04 N.	68 37 W.	
Plymouth	Eu.	England	Eng. Channel	50 22 N.	4 10 W.	6 00
Policastro	Eu.	Italy	Medit. Sea	40 18 N.	15 45 E.	
Is. Polsapate	Asia	Cambaya	Indian Ocean	9 45 N.	109 55 E.	
I. Poma	Eu.	Dalmatia	Adriat. Sea	42 57 N.	18 14 E.	
Pondicherry	Asia	India	B. Bengal	11 42 N.	79 58 E.	
Pontorson	Eu.	France	Eng. Channel	48 33 N.	1 27 W.	
Ponoi	Eu.	Lapland	North Sea	67 5 N.	38 48 E.	
I. Ponza	Eu.	Italy	Medit. Sea	40 53 N.	13 09 E.	
Pool	Eu.	England	Eng. Channel	51 00 N.	1 50 W.	
Porto Port	Eu.	Portugal	Atl. Ocean	41 10 N.	8 22 W.	
Port Mahon	Eu.	Spain	Medit. Sea	39 51 N.	3 53 E.	
Portland	Eu.	England	Eng. Channel	50 30 N.	2 48 W.	8 15
Port l'Orient	Eu.	France	B. Biscay	47 47 N.	3 13 W.	
Porto Bello	Am.	New Spain	Carrib. Sea	9 33 N.	79 45 W.	
Porto Praya	Africa	Cape Verd	Atl. Ocean	14 54 N.	23 24 W.	11 00
I. Porto Rico — E. point				18 35 N.	65 58 W.	
I. Porto Rico — Port Rico	Am.	Antilles	Atl. Ocean	18 29 N.	66 35 W.	
I. Porto Rico — W. point				18 34 N.	67 51 W.	
I. Porto Sancto	Africa	Canaries	Atl. Ocean	32 58 N.	16 20 W.	
Portsall	Eu.	France	Eng. Channel	48 36 N.	4 43 W.	
Portsmouth. R. Aca.	Eu.	England	Eng. Channel	50 48 N.	1 01 W.	11 15
Praken	Asia	Coch. Chi.	Indian Ocean	17 15 N.	106 15 E.	
Prenau	Eu.	Livonia	Baltic Sea	58 26 N.	24 58 E.	
I. Princes	Africa	Guinea	Atl. Ocean	1 47 N.	6 39 E.	
C. Prior	Eu.	Spain	Atl. Ocean	43 29 N.	8 15 W.	
I. Providence	Am.	Bahama	Atl. Ocean	24 51 N.	77 01 W.	
I. Providence, or St. Catherine	Am.	Mexico	Atl. Ocean	13 26 N.	80 42 W.	
Pudyoua	Asia	N. Caledonia	Pacif. Ocean	20 18 S.	164 46 E.	6 00
I. Pulo condor	Asia	Cambaya	Indian Ocean	8 40 N.	107 25 E.	
Q						
Quaqua, or Ivory Coast	Africa	Guinea	Eth. Sea	5 00 N.	4 00 W.	
Quebec	Am.	Canada	R. St. Lawr.	46 55 N.	69 48 W.	7 30
Querda	Asia	Malaya	B. Bengal	6 15 N.	100 12 E.	
I. Quelpert	Asia	Korea	Pacif. Ocean	33 32 N.	128 04 E.	
Quiloa	Africa	Zanguebar	Indian Ocean	9 30 S.	39 09 E.	

Names of Places.	Cont.	Countries.	Coaſt.	Latitude.	Longitude.	H. Water.
				° ′	° ′	
Quimper	Eu.	France	B. Biſcay	47 58 N.	4 02 W.	
Quinam	Aſia	Coch. Chi.	Indian Ocean	12 52 N.	109 10 E.	
Quiraba Iſles	Africa	Zanguebar	Indian Ocean	11 00 N.	41 39 E.	
C. Quiros	Aſia	N. Hebrides	Pacif. Ocean	14 56 S.	167 15 W.	
Quito	Am.	Peru	Inland	0 13 S.	77 50 W.	
R						
C. Race	Am.	Newfoundl.	Atl. Ocean	46 40 N.	52 38 W.	
Raguſa	Eu.	Dalmatia	Medit. Sea	42 45 N.	20 00 E.	
Rajapour	Aſia	India	Indian Ocean	17 19 N.	73 50 E.	
Ramſgate	Eu.	England	Downs	51 20 N.	1 22 E.	
Ramhead	Eu.	England	Eng. Channel	50 19 N.	4 15 W.	
C. Raſalgate	Aſia	Arabia	Indian Ocean	22 46 N.	58 48 E.	
Ravenna	Eu.	Italy	Medit. Sea	44 26 N.	12 21 E.	
C. Ray	Am.	Newfoundl.	Atl. Ocean	47 37 N.	59 8 W.	
I. Rhee	Eu.	France	B. Biſcay	46 15 N.	1 28 W.	3h. 00m.
Regio	Eu.	Italy	Mediterran.	38 22 N.	16 37 E.	
Cape Reſolution	Am.	N. Main	Hudſon's Str.	61 29 N.	65 10 W.	
Reſolution Bay	Aſia	Marqueſas	Pacif. Ocean	9 55 S.	139 4 W.	
Reſolution Iſland	Aſia	Society Iſles	Pacif. Ocean	17 23 S.	141 40 W.	
Revel	Eu.	Livonia	Baltic Sea	59 22 N.	25 33 E.	
Rhodes Iſle { Rhodes, N. end	Aſia	Natolia	Archipelago	36 27 N.	28 36 E.	
Rhodes Iſle { C. Tranquil, S. end				35 55 N.	28 23 E.	
Riga	Eu.	Livonia	Baltic Sea	56 55 N.	24 51 E.	
Ripraps, a ſand	Eu.	England	Straits Dover	51 53 N.	1 25 E.	
Robin Hood's Bay	Eu.	England	Germ. Ocean	54 25 N.	0 08 W.	3 00
I. Rocca	Am.	Terra Firma	Atl. Ocean	11 21 N.	66 17 W.	
Rochefort	Eu.	France	B. Biſcay	46 03 N.	0 54 W.	4 15
Rochel	Eu.	France	Bay Biſcay	46 10 N.	1 5 W.	3 45
Rocheſter	Eu.	England	R. Medway	51 26 N.	0 30 E.	0 45
I. Rodrigue	Aſia	Madagaſcar	Indian Ocean	19 41 S.	62 45 E.	
C. Romain	Am.	Terra Firma	Atl. Ocean	11 40 N.	69 05 W.	
Rome	Eu.	Italy	Medit. Sea	41 54 N.	12 34 E.	
I. Roncadore	Am.	Mexico	Atl. Ocean	13 30 N.	78 53 W.	
Rood Bay	Eu.	Greenland	North Ocean	79 53 N.	14 00 E.	
C. Roque	Am.	Braſil	Atl. Ocean	5 00 S.	35 43 W.	
I. Roquepiz	Africa	Madagaſcar	Indian Ocean	9 51 S.	64 30 E.	
G. Roſes	Eu.	Spain	Medit. Sea	42 10 N.	3 18 E.	
Roſtock	Eu.	Germany	Baltic Sea	54 10 N.	12 50 E.	
I. Rotterdam	Aſia	Friendly Is.	Pacif. Ocean	20 16 S.	174 25 W.	
Rotterdam	Eu.	D. Neth.	Germ. Ocean	51 56 N.	4 33 E.	3 00
Rouen	Eu.	France	R. Seine	49 27 N.	1 10 E.	1 15
C. Roxent	Eu.	Portugal	Atl. Ocean	38 45 N.	9 30 W.	
C. Roxo	Africa	Negroland	Atl. Ocean	11 42 N.	14 33 W.	
Po. Royal	Am.	I. Jamaica	Caribbean Sea	17 40 N.	76 37 W.	
C. Rozier	Am.	Nova Scotia	G. St. Law.	48 55 N.	63 36 W.	
I. Rugen	Eu.	Germany	Baltic Sea	54 32 N.	14 30 E.	
I. Rum Key, or Samana	Am.	Bahama	Atl. Ocean	23 00 N.	74 20 W.	
R. Rupert	Am.	New Britain	Hudſon's Bay	51 45 N.	78 40 W.	
C. R[illegible]	Africa	Barca	Medit. Sea	32 53 N.	20 41 E.	
R[illegible] Iſles	Eu.	Norway	North Sea	67 40 N.	10 25 E.	
Rye	Eu.	England	Eng. Channel	51 03 N.	0 45 E.	11 15
S						
C. Sable	Am.	Nova Scotia	Atl. Ocean	43 24 N.	65 35 W.	
I. Sable, W. end	Am.	Nova Scotia	Atl. Ocean	44 09 N.	60 29 W.	
I. Saddle back	Am.	North Main	Hudſ. Strait	62 07 N.	68 13 W.	10 00
Saffia	Africa	Barbary	Atl. Ocean	32 30 N.	8 50 W.	
I. S[illegible]	Africa	Egypt	Red Sea	27 05 N.	34 40 E.	
B. Saldanna	Africa	Caffers	Atl. Ocean	32 35 S.	19 30 E.	

I. Sal

Names of Places.	Cont.	Countries.	Coaſt.	Latitude.	Longitude.	H. Water.
				° ′	° ′	
I. Sal	Africa	C. Verd	Atl. Ocean	16 38 N.	22 51 W.	
Salerno	Eu.	Italy	Medit. Sea	40 39 N.	14 48 E.	
I. Salini, Lipari Iſl.	Eu.	Italy	Medit. Sea	38 39 N.	15 24 E.	
I. Saliſbury	Am.	N—Main	Hudſon's Bay	63 29 N.	76 47 W.	
Sallee	Africa	Barbary	Atl. Ocean	33 58 N.	6 20 W.	
Solomon Iſles	Aſia	———	Pacif. Ocean	{ 5 50 S. 11 15 S.	171 05 W. 178 35 W.	
Salonechi	Eu.	Turkey	Archipelago	40 41 N.	23 13 E.	
I. Salvages	Africa	Canaries	N. Atl. Ocean	30 00 N.	15 49 W.	
I. Salvages { Upper Lower }	Am.	North Main	Hudſ. Straits	{ 61 48 N. 62 32½N.	66 20 W. 70 48¼W	9h. 00m. 11 10
I. Samos	Aſia	Natolia	Archipelago	37 46 N.	27 13 E.	
C. Sambrough	Am.	Nova Scotia	Weſtern Oc.	44 33 N.	63 20 W.	
Sandwich	Eu.	England	Downs	51 20 N.	1 20 E.	11 30
Sandwich Iſland	Aſia	N. Hebrides	Pacif. Ocean	17 41 S.	168 38 E.	
Sandwich Harbour	Aſia	Malicola	Pacif. Ocean	16 25 S.	167 58 E.	
Sandwich's Bay	Am.	St. Georgia	Atl. Ocean	54 42 S.	36 4 W.	
I. Sanguin	Aſia	Philip. Iſles	Pacif. Ocean	3 50 N.	122 30 E.	
I. Sanien	Eu.	Norway	North Ocean	69 30 N.	14 30 E.	
Santa Cruz	Africa	Barbary	Atl. Ocean	30 30 N.	9 35 W.	
I. Sardinia { N. limit				41 15 N.	9 31 E.	
S. pt. C. Tavolaro	Eu.	Italy	Medit. Sea	38 54 N.	9 15 E.	
Cagliari				39 25 N.	9 38 E.	
Oriſtagni				39 53 N.	9 01 E.	
Sarena	Am.	Chili	Pacif. Ocean	29 40 S.	71 15 W.	
Saunders's Iſle	Am.	Sandwich L.	Atl. Ocean	58 00 S.	26 53 W.	
C. Saunders	Am.	St. Georgia	Atl. Ocean	54 6 S.	36 53 W.	
Scanderoon	Aſia	Syria	Levant	36 35 N.	36 25 E.	
Scarborough head	Eu.	England	Germ. Ocean	54 18 N.	00 00	3 45
I. Scarpanto	Aſia	Natolia	Archipelago	35 45 N.	27 40 E.	
I. Scatarie, N. E. pt.	Am.	Acadia	Weſt. Ocean	46 01 N.	61 57 W.	
Scaw	Eu.	Denmark	Sound	57 34 N.	10 54 E.	
I Schelling	Eu.	D. Neth.	Germ. Ocean	53 27 N.	5 30 E.	
I. Scio { C. St. Nicholas				{ 38 38 N.	26 12 E.	
Scio	Aſia	Natolia	Archipelago	38 24 N.	26 29 E.	
C. Blanco				38 08 N.	26 20 E.	
Scilly Iſles	Eu.	England	St. Geo. Ch.	50 00 N.	6 45 W.	3 45
Scolt Head	Eu.	England	Germ. Ocean	53 00 N.	0 44 E.	6 20
Scots Settlement	Am.	Terra Firma	Carribbe. Sea	8 45 N.	76 35 W.	
I. Sea	Eu.	Turkey	Archipelago	37 38 N.	24 53 E.	
Seane	Eu.	France	B. Biſcay	48 00 N.	4 51 W.	
I. Sebaldes	Am.	Patagonia	S. Atl. Ocean	50 53 S.	59 35 W.	
C. Sebaſtian	Am.	California	Pacif. Ocean	43 00 N.	126 00 W.	
C. St. Sebaſtian	Africa	Madagaſcar	Indian Ocean	12 30 S.	46 30 E.	
St. Sebaſtian	Eu.	Spain	B. Biſcay	43 16 N.	2 05 W.	
Port Segura	Am.	Braſil	Atl. Ocean	16 57 S.	39 45 W.	
R. Senegal	Africa	Negroland	Atl. Ocean	15 53 N.	16 26 W.	10 30
I. Serranilha	Am.	Weſt Indies	Atl. Ocean	16 20 N.	79 40 W.	
I. Serigo	Eu.	Turkey	Archipelago	36 09 N.	23 24 E.	
I. Sertes	Africa	Canaries	Atl. Ocean	32 35 N.	16 20 W.	
R. Settos	Africa	Guinea	Atl. Ocean	5 48 N.	8 13 W.	
Seven Capes	Africa	Barbary	Medit. Sea	37 30 N.	6 15 W.	
Seven Stones, or Iſles	Eu.	England	St. Geo. Ch.	50 10 N.	6 40 W.	4 30
R. Severn, Ent.	Eu.	England	St. Geo. Ch.	51 41 N.	3 05 W.	6 0
R. Severn	Am.	New Wales	Hudſon's Bay	56 12 N.	88 57 W.	
R. Seyn, Ent.	Eu.	France	Eng. Channel	49 36 N.	0 30 E.	9 00
Seynhead	Eu.	France	Eng. Channel	49 44 N.	0 34 E.	
Sheerneſs	Eu.	England	R. Thames	51 25 N.	0 50 E.	0 00
Shepherd's Iſles	Aſia	N. Hebrides	Pacif. Ocean	17 00 S.	168 4[illegible] E.	
Siam	Aſia	Indin	Bay Siam	14 18 N.	[illegible] 55 E.	
R. Siam Ent.	Aſia	India	Bay Siam	13 15 N.	[illegible] 4[illegible] E.	

Names of Places.	Cont.	Countries.	Coast.	Latitude.	Longitude.	H. Water.
Siara	Am.	Brasil	Atl. Ocean	3 18 S.	39 50 W.	
I. Sicily: E. end, Messina	Eu.	Italy	Medit. Sea	38 10 N.	15 58 E.	
Catanea				37 22 N.	15 21 E.	
Syracuse				37 04 N.	15 31 E.	
S. end, C. Passara				36 35 N.	15 22 E.	
Alicata				37 11 N	14 07 E.	
W. end, C. Bocco				37 51 N.	21 43 E.	
Palermo				38 10 N.	13 43 E.	
Sierra Leona	Africa	Guinea	Atl. Ocean	8 30 N.	12 07 W.	8h. 15m.
Sillabar Road	Asia	I. Sumatra	Indian Ocean	4 00 S.	102 50 E.	
Str. Sincapore	Asia	Malacca	Indian Ocean	1 00 N.	104 30 E.	
R. Sinda, or Indus, mouth	Asia	India	Indian Ocean	24 30 N. 25 45 N.	63 10 E. 62 40 E.	
Po. Shabak	Africa	Abyssinia	Red Sea	18 58 N.	38 24 E.	
Shark, or Seahorse point	Am.	New Wales	Hudson's Bay	64 05 N.	82 12 W.	
Shields	Eu.	England	Germ. Ocean	55 02 N.	1 20 W.	
Shelvock's Isle	Am.	California	Pacif. Ocean	23 15 N.	117 35 W.	
Shillocks	Eu.	Ireland	West. Ocean	51 30 N.	11 05 W.	5 0
I. Shetland, limits	Eu.	Scotland	West. Ocean	60 47 N. 59 54 N.	0 10 W. 1 31 W.	3 00
Shoreham	Eu.	England	Eng. Channel	50 55 N.	00 17 E.	10 30
I. Sky, N. point	Eu.	Scotland	West. Ocean	57 50 N.	6 30 W.	
I. Sky, S. point				57 15 N.	6 16 W.	5 30
Sleepers Isles	Am.	New Britain	Hudson's Bay	60 00 N. 58 35 N.	81 30 W.	
Great Sleeper				60 10 N.	82 00 W.	
The Sleepers lie in a chain from the Great Sleeper down to Lat. 58° 50′ N & Long. 82° 20′ W.						
Sline Head	Eu.	Ireland	West. Ocean	53 20 N.	2 15 W.	
R. Slude	Am.	New Britain	Hudson's Bay	53 24 N.	78 50 W.	
Sluyce	Eu.	D. Neth.	Germ. Ocean	51 19 N.	3 50 E.	
C. Smith	Am.	Labradore	Hudson's Bay	60 48 N.	80 55 W.	
Smyrna	Asia	Natolia	Archipelago	38 28 N.	27 25 E.	
I. Socatora	Africa	Anian	Indian Ocean	12 15 N.	52 55 E.	
C. Solomon	Eu.	I. Candia	Medit. Sea	34 57 N.	27 06 E.	
R. Somme	Eu.	France	Eng. Channel	50 18 N.	1 40 E.	11 00
Sound Royal	Eu.	Iceland	North Ocean	66 22 N.	15 15 W.	
Southampton	Eu.	England	Eng. Channel	50 55 N.	1 00 W.	0 00
C. Southampton	Am.	New Wales	Hudson's Bay	61 54 N.	86 14 W.	
South Cape	Asia	Diemen's la.	Pacif. Ocean	42 40 S.	130 05 E.	
C. Spartivento	Eu.	Italy	Medit. Sea	37 50 N.	16 41 E.	
C. Spartel	Africa	Barbary	Atl. Ocean	35 46 N.	5 53 W.	
I. Spirito Sancto	Am.	Brasil	Atl. Ocean	20 24 S.	39 55 W.	
Spurn	Eu.	England	Germ. Ocean	53 35 N.	0 30 E.	5 15
I. Stampalia	Asia	Natolia	Archipelago	36 25 N.	26 55 E.	
I. Sancho	Asia	Natolia	Archipelago	36 50 N.	27 30 E.	
Start point	Eu.	England	Eng. Channel	50 09 N.	3 46 W.	6 45
I. States: C. St. John	Am.	Patagonia	Atl. Ocean	54 45 S.	60 35 W.	
C. St. Bartholomew				55 08 S.	60 45 W.	
Stavenger	Eu.	Norway	West. Ocean	58 47 N.	6 45 E.	
C. Stephens	Asia	N. Zealand	Pacif. Ocean	40 36 S.	174 05 E.	
Stetin	Eu.	Germany	Baltic Sea	53 36 N.	15 25 E.	
C. Stillo	Eu.	Italy	Medit. Sea	38 23 N.	17 07 E.	
Port Steven	Am.	Chili	Pacif. Ocean	46 50 S.	82 36 W.	

Names of Places.	Cont.	Countries.	Coaſt.	Latitude.	Longitude.	H. Water.
				° ′	° ′	
Stockholm	Eu.	Sweden	Baltic Sea	59 22 N.	18 12 E.	
Stockton	Eu.	England	Germ. Ocean	54 33 N.	1 15 W.	5h. 15m.
Straelſund	Eu.	Germany	Baltic Sea	54 23 N.	14 10 E.	
Strangford Bay	Eu.	Ireland	Iriſh Sea	54 23 N.	5 40 W.	10 30
I. Stromboli	Eu.	Italy	Medit. Sea	38 42 N.	15 48 E.	
Succeſs Bay	Am.	T. del Fuego	Atl. Ocean	54 50 S.	65 20 W.	
Suez Town	Africa	Egypt	Red Sea	29 50 N.	33 27 E.	
Sukadana	Aſia	I. Borneo	Indian Ocean	1 00 S.	110 40 E.	
I. Suma-tra { NW. end	Aſia	India	Indian Ocean	{ 5 15 N.	95 55 E.	
{ SE. end				5 07 S.	106 20 E.	
Sunderland	Eu.	England	Germ. Ocean	54 55 N.	1 00 W.	3 30
Str. Sunda	Aſia	Siam	Indian Ocean	6 10 S.	105 35 E.	
Surinam	Am.	Terra Firma	Atl. Ocean	6 30 N.	55 30 W.	
Surat	Aſia	India	Indian Ocean	21 10 N.	72 25 E.	
I. Surroy	Eu.	Lapland	North Ocean	71 00 N.	22 00 E.	
Swaken	Africa	Abyſſinia	Red Sea	19 30 N.	37 38 E.	
Swally Road	Aſia	India	Arabian Sea	21 55 N.	72 00 E.	
Swanſey	Eu.	Wales	St. Geo. Cha.	51 40 N.	4 25 W.	
Sweetnoſe	Eu.	Lapland	North Ocean	68 08 N.	34 42 E.	
Swin, a ſand	Eu.	England	Ent. Thames	51 37 N.	1 12 E.	12 00
Syracuſe	Eu.	I. Sicily	Medit. Sea	37 04 N.	15 31 E.	
Syriam	Aſia	Pegu	B. Bengal	16 00 N.	96 40 E.	
T						
Tadouſac Fort	Am.	Canada	R. St. Lawr.	48 00 N.	67 35 W.	
I. Tamarica	Am.	Braſil	Atl. Ocean	7 56 S.	35 05 W.	
Tamarin Town	Africa	I. Socatora	Indian Ocean	12 30 N.	53 14 E.	9 00
B. Tanaſſarin	Aſia	Malacca	B. Bengal	12 00 N.	98 48 E.	
I. Tandoxima	Aſia	Japan	Pacif. Ocean	30 30 N.	130 40 E.	
Tangier	Africa	Barbary	Atl. Ocean	35 55 N.	5 45 W.	
Tanna	Aſia	N. Hebrides	Pacif. Ocean	19 32 S.	169 45 E.	3 00
Taoukaa	Aſia	Society Iſles	Pacif. Ocean	14 31 S.	145 4 W.	
Tarento	Eu.	Italy	Medit. Sea	40 43 N.	17 31 E.	
C. Tat'nam	Am.	New Wales	Hudſon's Bay	57 35 N.	91 30 W.	
R. Tees, mouth	Eu.	England	Germ. Ocean	54 36 N.	0 52 W.	3 00
Tegoantepec	Am.	Mexico	Pacif. Ocean	14 45 N.	96 23 W.	
Tellichery	Aſia	India	Malabar Coaſt	11 42 N.	75 30 E.	
C. Telling	Eu.	Ireland	Weſt. Ocean	54 40 N.	10 07 W.	
I. Tenedos	Aſia	Natolia	Archipelago	39 57 N.	26 14 E.	
I. Teneriff (Peak)	Africa	Canaries	Atl. Ocean	28 13 N.	16 24 W.	3 00
C. Tenes	Africa	Barbary	Medit. Sea	36 26 N.	1 53 E.	
I. Tercera	Eu.	Azores	Atl. Ocean	38 45 N.	27 01 W.	
Terra Nieva	Am.	N— Main	Hudſ. Straits	62 4 N.	67 2 W.	9 50
Tervere	Eu.	D. Neth.	Germ Ocean	51 38 N.	3 35 E.	0 45
Tetuan	Africa	Barbary	Medit. Sea	35 27 N.	4 50 W.	
I. Texel	Eu.	D. Neth.	Germ. Ocean	53 10 N.	4 59 E.	7 30
C. St. Thadæus	Aſia	Siberia	North Ocean	62 10 N.	175 05 E.	
R. Thames, mouth	Eu.	England	Germ. Ocean	51 28 N.	1 10 E.	1 30
C. St. Thomas	Africa	Caffers	Atl. Ocean	24 54 S.	15 25 E.	
I. St. Thomas	Africa	Guinea	Atl. Ocean	00 00	1 00 E.	
St. Thomas	Aſia	India	B. Bengal	13 00 N.	80 00 E.	
C. Three Points	Am.	Terra Firma	Atl. Ocean	10 51 N.	62 41 W.	
C. Three Points	Africa	Guinea	Atl. Ocean	4 48 N.	1 21 W.	
South Thule	Am.	Sandwich la.	Atl. Ocean	59 34 S.	27 45 W.	
I. Tidore	Aſia	Molucca Is.	Indian Ocean	0 35 N.	126 40 E.	
I. Timor { NE. pt.	Aſia	Molucca Is.	Indian Ocean	{ 8 20 S.	127 40 E.	
{ SW. pt.				10 23 S.	123 55 E.	
Tinmouth	Eu.	England	Germ. Ocean	55 03 N.	1 17 W.	3 00
I. Tino	Eu.	Turkey	Archipelago	37 33 N.	25 43 E.	
I. Tobago	Am.	Carribbee	Atl. Ocean	11 15 N.	60 27 W.	
Tobolſki	Aſia	Siberia	Inland	58 12 N.	68 20 E.	
B. Todos Sanctos	Am.	Braſil	Atl. Ocean	13 05 S.	38 45 W.	

Tonquin

Names of Places.	Cont.	Countries.	Coaſt.	Latitude.	Longitude.	H. Water.
				° '	° '	
Tonquin	Aſia	India	Pacif. Ocean	20 50 N.	105 55 E.	
Tonſberg	Eu.	Norway	Sound	58 50 N.	10 05 E.	
Topſham	Eu.	England	Eng. Channel	50 37 N.	3 27 W.	6h. oom.
Torbay	Eu.	England	Eng. Channel	50 34 N.	3 36 W.	5 15
Tornea	Eu.	Sweden	G. Bothnia	65 51 N.	24 16 E.	
R. Tortoſa	Eu.	Spain	Medit. Sea	40 47 N.	1 03 E.	
I. Tortola	Am.	Antl. Iſle	Atl. Ocean	18 24 N.	65 00 W.	
I. Tory	Eu.	Ireland	Weſt. Ocean	55 09 N.	8 30 W.	5 30
Toulon	Eu.	France	Medit. Sea	43 07 N.	6 02 E.	
C. Trefalga	Eu.	Spain	Atl. Ocean	36 08 N.	5 58 W.	
I. Tremiti	Eu.	Italy	Medit. Sea	42 09 N.	15 40 E.	
C. de Tres forcas	Africa	Barbary	Medit. Sea	35 30 N.	2 11 W.	
I. Trailles	Aſia	India	Indian Ocean	19 30 S.	101 25 E.	
I. Trinity	Am.	Braſil	Atl. Ocean	20 25 S.	23 35 W.	
I. Trinidada, E. pt.	Am.	Terra Firma	Atl. Ocean	10 38 N.	60 27 W.	
Trinity Bay, Ent.	Am.	Newfoundl.	Atl. Ocean	48 30 N.	52 35 W.	
Trieſt	Eu.	Carniola	Adriat. Sea	45 51 N.	14 03 E.	
Trinquemali	Aſia	I. Ceylon	Indian Ocean	8 50 N.	83 24 E.	
Tripoli	Aſia	Syria	Levant	34 53 N.	36 07 E.	
Tripoly	Africa	Barbary	Medit. Sea	32 54 N.	13 10 E.	
G. Triſte	Am.	Terra Firma	Atl. Ocean	10 19 N.	67 41 W.	
I. Triſtian d'Acunha	Africa	Caſfers	S. Atl. Ocean	37 12 S.	13 23 W.	
Iſ. Tromſound	Eu.	Lapland	North Ocean	70 20 N.	19 00 E.	
Truxilla	Am.	Peru	Pacif. Ocean	8 00 S.	78 35 W.	
Tunder	Eu.	Denmark	Weſt. Ocean	55 00 N.	9 35 E.	
Tunis	Africa	Barbary	Medit. Sea	36 47 N.	10 16 E.	
Turin	Eu.	Italy	R. Po	45 05 N.	7 45 E.	
I. Turks	Am.	Bahama	Atl. Ocean	21 18 N.	71 05 W.	
Turtle Iſland	Aſia	——	Pacif. Ocean	19 49 S.	177 52 W.	
V						
Valencia	Eu.	Spain	Medit. Sea	39 30 N.	0 40 W.	
St. Valery	Eu.	France	Eng. Channel	50 11 N.	1 42 E.	10 30
Valona	Eu.	Turkey	Medit. Sea	40 55 N.	21 15 E.	
Valpariſo	Am.	China	Pacif. Ocean	33 03 S.	72 14 W.	
Van Diemen's land	Aſia	N. Holland	Indian Ocean	43 38 S.	146 27 E.	
Vannes	Eu.	France	B. Biſcay	47 39 N.	2 41 W.	3 45
C. Vela	Am.	Terra Firma	Atl. Ocean	12 15 N.	71 20 W.	
P. Venus	Aſia	Otaheite	Pacif. Ocean	17 29 S.	149 31 W.	10 38
Venice	Eu.	Italy	Medit. Sea	45 27 N.	12 9 E.	
Vera Cruz	Am.	New Spain	G. Mexico	19 12 N.	97 25 W.	
C. Verd	Africa	Negroland	Atl. Ocean	14 45 N.	17 28 W.	
Uhma	Eu.	Sweden	G. Bothnia	63 45 N.	21 10 E.	
Vicegapatam	Aſia	India	B. Bengal	17 30 N.	84 02 E.	
C. Victory	Am.	Patagonia	Pacif. Ocean	52 15 S.	74 28 W.	
Vienna	Eu.	Germany	R. Danube	48 11 N.	16 28 E.	
Vigo	Eu.	Spain	Atl. Ocean	42 14 N.	8 23 W.	
B. St. Vincent	Am.	Paraguay	Atl. Ocean	23 55 S.	45 11 W.	
C. St. Vincent	Eu.	Portugal	Atl. Ocean	37 01 N.	8 58 W.	
I. St. Vincent	Africa	C. Verd	Atl. Ocean	17 47 N.	24 44 W.	
I. St. Vincent	Am.	Carribbee	Atl. Ocean	13 05 N.	61 05 W.	
R. St. Vincent	Africa	Guinea	Eth. Ocean	4 50 N.	7 41 W.	
C. Virgins	Am.	Patagonia	Atl. Ocean	52 23 S.	67 50 W.	
I. Virgins	Am.	Antil. Iſle	Atl. Ocean	18 18 N.	64 14 W.	
Virgin Rocks	Am.	Newfoundl.	Atl. Ocean	46 30 N.	51 30 W.	
Umba	Eu.	Ruſſia	Inland	66 40 N.	34 15 E.	
C. Volo	Eu.	Turkey	Archipelago	39 07 N.	23 23 E.	
R. Voltas	Africa	Guinea	Atl. Ocean	5 52 N.	1 10 E.	
C. Voltas	Africa	Caſfers	Atl. Ocean	28 04 S.	16 18 E.	
Upſal	Eu.	Sweden	R. Sala	59 52 N.	17 47 E.	
Uraniberg	Eu.	Denmark	Baltic Sea	55 54 N.	12 57 E.	
I. Uſhant	Eu.	France	Eng. Channel	48 30 N.	5 [illegible]0 W.	4 30

I. Uſtica

Names of Places.	Cont.	Countries.	Coast.	Latitude.	Longitude.	H. Water.
				° ′	° ′	
I. Ustica	Eu.	Italy	Medit. Sea	38 43 N.	13 33 E.	
I. Vulcano	Eu.	Italy	Medit. Sea	38 29 N.	15 33 E.	
W						
Prin. Wales's Isles	Asia	New Guinea	Endeavour St.	10 26 S.	141 00 E.	
R. Wager	Am.	New Wales	Hudson's Bay	65 28 N.	87 25 W.	6h. 00m.
Wallis's Isle	Asia	———	Pacif. Ocean	13 18 S.	176 20 W.	
C. Walsingham	Am.	New Britain	Hudson's Str.	62 39 N.	77 48 W.	12 00
Wardhus	Eu.	Lapland	North Ocean	70 23 N.	51 12 E.	
Warsaw	Eu.	Poland	R. Vistula	52 14 N.	21 5 E.	
Waterford	Eu.	Ireland	St. Geo. Ch.	52 07 N.	7 42 W.	6 30
Watling Isle	Am.	Bahama	Atl. Ocean	23 42 N.	74 22 W.	
Wells	Eu.	England	Germ. Ocean	53 07 N.	1 00 E.	6 00
Western Isles	Asia	Diemen's la.	Pacif. Ocean	43 36 S.	147 00 E.	
Western Isles { S. point	Eu.	Scotland	West. Ocean	56 46 N.	7 40 W.	
Western Isles { N. point				58 35 N.	6 37 W.	
If. Westmania	Eu.	Iceland	West. Ocean	63 55 N.	17 30 W.	
If. Westrol	Eu.	Lapland	North Ocean	69 15 N.	24 00 E.	
Wexford	Eu.	Ireland	St. Geo. Ch.	52 13 N.	6 56 W.	
Weymouth	Eu.	England	Eng. Channel	52 40 N.	2 34 W.	7 20
Whale's Back	Eu.	Iceland	West. Ocean	63 44 N	17 05 W.	
Whale's Head	Eu.	Greenland	North Ocean	77 18 N.	21 30 E.	
Whale Rock	Eu.	Azores	Atl. Ocean	38 50 N.	24 41 W.	
Whitby	Eu.	England	Germ. Ocean	54 30 N.	0 50 W.	3 00
Whitehaven	Eu.	England	Irish Sea	54 25 N.	3 15 W.	
Whitsuntide I.	Asia	N. Hebrides	Pacif. Ocean	16 44 S.	168 25 E.	
Wicklow	Eu.	Ireland	St. Geo. Cha.	52 50 N.	6 30 W.	
Willis's Isles	Am.	S. Georgia	Atl. Ocean	54 00 S.	38 25 W.	
Windaw	Eu.	Courland	Baltic Sea	57 08 N.	22 20 E.	
I. Wight { N. end	Eu.	England	Eng. Channel	50 47 N.	1 11 W.	
I. Wight { S. end				50 34 N.	1 10 W.	
I. Wight { E. end				50 41 N.	1 00 W.	0 00
I. Wight { W. end				50 41 N.	1 23 W.	
If. Prince William	Asia	———	Pacif. Ocean	16 45 S.	177 55 E.	
William Henry I.	Asia	Society Isles	Pacif. Ocean	19 00 S.	141 6 E.	
Winchelsea	Eu.	England	Eng. Channel	50 58 N.	0 50 E.	0 45
Wintertoness	Eu.	England	Germ. Ocean	53 02 N.	1 22 E.	9 00
Wisbuy in I. Gotland	Eu.	Sweden	Baltic Sea	57 40 N.	19 50 E.	
C. Wrath	Eu.	Scotland	West. Ocean	58 40 N.	4 50 E.	
Wybourg	Eu.	Finland	G. Finland	60 55 N.	30 20 E.	
Y						
Yambo	Asia	Arabia	Red Sea	24 25 N.	38 54 E.	
Yarmouth	Eu.	England	Germ. Ocean	52 55 N.	1 40 E.	9 45
Yas de Amber	Africa	Zanguebar	Indian Ocean	0 00	47 15 E.	
Yellow River	Asia	China	Pacif. Ocean	34 06 N.	120 10 E.	
Ylo	Am.	Peru	Pacif. Ocean	17 36 S.	71 08 W.	
Cape York	Asia	N. Holland	Endeavour St.	10 41 S.	141 39 E.	
York Fort	Am.	New Wales	Hudson's Bay	57 02 N.	92 47 W.	9 10
York, New	Am.	N. England	Atl. Ocean	40 43 N.	74 04 W.	3 0
Youghall	Eu.	Ireland	St. Geo. Ch.	51 46 N.	8 06 W.	4 30
Z						
Zacatula	Am.	Mexico	Pacif. Ocean	17 1[illegible] N.	105 00 W.	
Zacheo	Am.	Antilles	Atl. Ocean	18 24 N.	67 52 W.	
I. Zant	Eu.	Italy	Adriatic Sea	37 5[illegible] N.	21 30 E.	
I. Zanzibar	Africa	Zanguebar	Indian Ocean	6 55 S.	40 10 E.	
Zara	Eu.	Dalmatia	Medit. Sea	44 15 N.	16 65 E.	
N. Zealand { N.W. point	Asia.	———	Pacif. Ocean	34 28 S.	172 44 E.	
N. Zealand { S. point				47 20 S.	167 50 E.	
Zenan [illegible]	Asia	Arabia	Inland	16 20 N.	47 44 E.	
Zuider Sea	Eu.	D. Neth.	Germ. Ocean			3 00

Besides the times of high-water in the preceding table, the following times serve for coasts of considerable extent, and will serve nearly for the places on those coasts.

Finmark, or NNW. coast of Lapland, 1 h. 30m. Jutland Isles 0 h. 0 m.
Friesland coast 7 h. 30m. Zealand coast 1 h. 30m.
Flanders coast 0h. 0m. Picardy and Normandy coasts 10h. 30m.
Biscay, Gallician, and Portugal coasts 3h. 00m.
Irish W. coast 3h. 00m. Irish S. coast 5h. 15m.
Africa W. coast 3h. 0m. America W. coast 3h. 0m.
America E. coast 4h. 30m.

END OF BOOK VI. AND OF VOL. I.